S0-CDK-666

Rehabilitative Audiology

Rehabilitative Audiology

Edited by

Raymond H. Hull, Ph.D.

Director of Audiology
Department of Communication Disorders
University of Northern Colorado
Greeley, Colorado

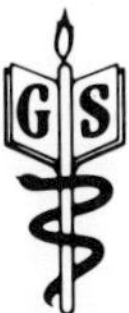

Grune & Stratton
A Subsidiary of Harcourt Brace Jovanovich, Publishers
New York London
Paris San Diego San Francisco São Paulo
Sydney Tokyo Toronto

Library of Congress Cataloging in Publication Data
Main entry under title:

Rehabilitative audiology.

Bibliography
Includes index.
1. Deaf—Rehabilitation. 2. Aged, Deaf—Rehabilitation. 3. Audiology. I. Hull, Raymond H. [DNLM: 1. Hearing disorders—Rehabilitation. WV 270 R345]
RF297.R43 362.4′28 81-7224
ISBN 0-8089-1434-0 AACR2

Grune & Stratton, Inc.
111 Fifth Avenue
New York, New York 10003

Distributed in the United Kingdom by
Academic Press Inc. (London) Ltd.
24/28 Oval Road, London NW 1

Library of Congress Catalog Number 81-7224
International Standard Book Number 0-8089-1434-0
Printed in the United States of America

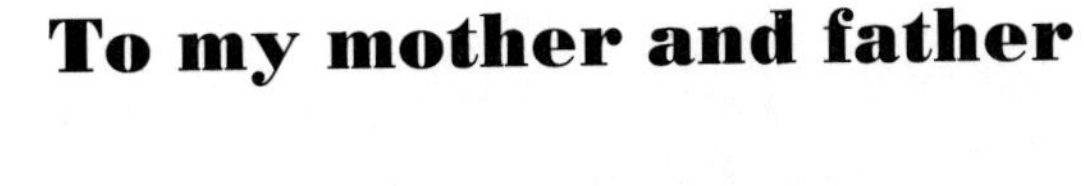

To my mother and father

Contents

B. Counseling the Hearing Impaired Adult

C. Other Aspects of the Process of Aural Rehabilitation for Adults

D. The Vocational Impact and Vocational Rehabilitation Counseling for Hearing Impaired Adults

PART II THE ELDERLY CLIENT

SECTION 1 INTRODUCTION TO AURAL REHABILITATION FOR ELDERLY ADULT CLIENTS

A. Implications and Supportive Procedures for the Confined and/or Multiply Handicapped Hearing Impaired Elderly

Appendixes Materials and Scales for Assessment of Communicative Abilities among Hearing Impaired Adults and Elderly Clients

Preface

The purpose of this book is to provide comprehensive information on the management of hearing impaired people. The book has been divided into two parts in order to examine adequately the problems and procedures for intervention on behalf of two complex populations of hearing impaired persons. Part I concentrates on the adult population, including the younger adult, and Part II discusses the special problems of elderly clients and procedures for serving them. The areas covered include the psychosocial and vocational impact of hearing impairment on both populations, the hearing impaired client's response to the effects, and the processes involved in their aural rehabilitation.

The majority of contributors to this book are audiologists. It is important, however, that a comprehensive treatise on management of the hearing impaired involve professionals from other fields as well. The complex nature of hearing impaired adults and elderly persons, and the services provided them, necessitates an eclectic approach. For example, in Part I vocational-rehabilitation counselors who work with hearing impaired adults prepared the chapters on the vocational implications of hearing impairment from the counselor's point of view and approaches to vocational rehabilitation counseling and placement. It is critical for students and professionals in audiology to be aware of the role of the vocational-rehabilitation counselor as a team member in the aural rehabilitation of hearing impaired adults.

In Part II a number of other professionals were also involved. For example, a well-known psychologist, whose profession is counseling elderly persons, was asked to write the chapter entitled, "Who Are These Aging Persons?" His insights into aging and their effects are marvelous. A sociologist-gerontologist who is knowledgeable of the impact of hearing impairment was invited to author the chapter on techniques for motivational counseling with elderly clients, and it has been a very enlightening treatise.

It is important that our students and professionals also be aware of how the nurse can facilitate efforts on behalf of the hearing impaired elderly client. Therefore, a knowledgeable geriatric nurse practitioner was invited to write a chapter on that topic.

No information is currently available in our texts on the special problems and needs of the multiply handicapped hearing and visually impaired elderly person. A specialist in the area of the deaf and blind elderly was asked to author that chapter. It was a difficult chapter to write, with few available references, but the author presents valuable information on this topic.

The 23 authors who have contributed to this comprehensive treatise on rehabilitative audiology bring with them a wealth of experience and knowledge. They were asked to contribute information on concise, restricted topics so that each topic would receive equal attention. In this way, the comprehensive nature of the book would be achieved within a reasonable number of pages. The combination of the contributors' knowledge and this editor's efforts to meld the topics has, we hope, been fruitful in obtaining this goal.

Various assessment procedures and scales of communication handicap are referred to within this text. They are not, however, restricted to one chapter. It was felt important for them to be discussed within various service contexts because of their variety of uses. Therefore, they are found in Chapter 7, in the discussion on counseling procedures for the adult; in Chapter 19, as part of the discussion on the feasibility of rehabilitating the hearing impaired elderly; in Chapter 23, on modification of hearing aid evaluation and fitting procedures for elderly clients; and in Chapter 27, on evaluation of successes in aural rehabilitation of elderly clients. This manner of presentation will allow the student and professional to view the uses of handicap scales from various vantage points. In Appendixes A through J, various scales of communication are presented with the thoughtful consent of the authors.

The topics selected for coverage in this book were by no means arbitrary. Professionals in audiology, students-in-training, and postgraduates were consulted relative to those topics they felt were critical for preparation to work with hearing impaired people. Although few persons suggested the same topics, a general consensus was reached. Thus, this book is entitled *Rehabilitative Audiology*.

We have attempted to cover a great number of topics in the aural rehabilitation of two complex populations of hearing impaired persons. Therefore, a diverse range of vocabulary and sophistication is acknowledged in regard to the contents of the chapters and the intended readership. We have aimed the text to a broad range of readers, but primarily to junior- or senior-level undergraduate and graduate students and the professional audiologist, speech pathologist, and deaf educator. Other interested readers will include physicians, nurses, psychologists, sociologists, gerontologists, and rehabilitation counselors who have specialized interest in the hearing impaired adult and elderly person.

Lastly, completion of an endeavor of this magnitude is only possible through the unselfish efforts of many people who too often go unsung. I would like to especially thank my secretaries, Betty Chandler and Bonnie Foos, who have tremendously helped me through the trials and tribulations felt during the work of putting this book together. Marybeth Johnson provided typing assistance that was above and beyond the call of duty. I would also like to thank the Director of the School of Special Education, Dr. Bob Sloat, my Audiology faculty, and my students for their understanding when I was so frequently buried beneath the task of completing the work involved in this book.

Raymond H. Hull

Contributors

JEROME G. ALPINER, Ph.D.
Director, Speech and Hearing Department
Porter Memorial Hospital
Denver, Colorado

DANIEL L. BODE, Ph.D.
Associate Professor
Audiology Program
Department of Special Education
California State University of Los Angeles and
Research Associate
Speech Communications Research Laboratory
Los Angeles, California

RICK L. BOLLINGER, Ph.D.
Director, Lauderdale Language and Speech Center
Fort Lauderdale, Florida

SONDRA LV. GERHARDT, M.S.
Group Vice President
Americana Healthcare Corporation
Monticello, Illinois

STEVEN D. GIBBS, M.S.
Audiologist, Birmingham Veterans Administration Medical Center
Clinical Associate, Department of Biocommunication

Schools of Medicine and Dentistry
University of Alabama
Birmingham, Alabama

JACQUELINE M. HEPPLER, R.N., M.S.
Former Assistant Professor
School of Nursing
Geriatric–Nurse Practitioner Program
Continuing Education Division
University of Colorado Health Sciences Center
Denver, Colorado

RAYMOND H. HULL, Ph.D.
Director of Audiology
Department of Communication Disorders
University of Northern Colorado
Greeley, Colorado

PAMELA L. JACKSON, Ph.D.
Associate Professor of Audiology
Department of Communicative Disorders
Northern Illinois University
DeKalb, Illinois

HARRIET F. KAPLAN, Ph.D.
Assistant Professor
Department of Audiology
Gallaudet College
Washington, D.C.

ROGER N. KASTEN, Ph.D.
Professor of Audiology
Department of Communicative Disorders and Sciences
Wichita State University
Wichita, Kansas

JACK KATZ, Ph.D.
Professor, Department of Communicative Disorders and Sciences
State University of New York at Buffalo
Buffalo, New York

LENNART L. KOPRA, Ph.D.
Professor of Speech Communication
Department of Speech Communication
The University of Texas at Austin
Austin, Texas

KEVIN G. MARSHALL, Ed.D.
Clinical Counselor and Rehabilitation Consultant
Cascade Professional Associates
Salem, Oregon

JAMES F. MAURER, Ph.D.
Professor, Speech and Hearing Sciences
Portland State University and
Clinical Audiologist
The Audiology Clinic
Providence Medical Center
Portland, Oregon

ROBERT M. McLAUCHLIN, Ph.D.
Professor and Director
Communication Disorders
Central Michigan University
Mount Pleasant, Michigan

WILLIAM E. MILLER, Ph.D.
Professor of Audiology
Department of Communicative Disorders and Sciences
Wichita State University
Wichita, Kansas

MILLEDGE MURPHEY, Ph.D.
Gerontological Consultant
Fort Myers, Florida

JANE E. MYERS, Ph.D.
Associate Professor and Coordinator
Rehabilitation Counseling Program
University of Ohio
Athens, Ohio

ALLAN W. ORLOFSKY, M.A.
Residential Director
Weld County Community Center
Evans, Colorado

JUDAH L. RONCH, Ph.D.
Psychologist in Private Practice
Poughkeepsie, New York

PERRY THOMPSON, Ph.D.
Professor of Gerontology and Sociology
Gerontology Studies Program
University of Arkansas at Little Rock
Little Rock, Arkansas

ROBERT M. TRAYNOR, Ed.D.
Associate Professor of Audiology
Department of Communication Disorders
University of Northern Colorado
Greeley, Colorado

DAVID TWEEDIE, Ed.D.
Dean, School of Communication
Department of Education
Gallaudet College
Washington, D.C.

GWENYTH R. VAUGHN, Ph.D.
Chief, Audiology and Speech Pathology Service
Birmingham Veterans Administration Medical Center
Professor, Department of Biocommunication
Schools of Medicine and Dentistry
University of Alabama
Birmingham, Alabama

THOMAS P. WHITE, M.A.
Assistant Professor of Audiology
Department of Communicative Disorders and Sciences
State University of New York at Buffalo and
Chief of Audiology
Buffalo Otological Group
Buffalo, New York

PART I

The Adult

Section 1: The Basis of Aural Rehabilitation for the Adult

Raymond H. Hull

Chapter 1: What Is Aural Rehabilitation?

> *Deafness is worse than blindness, so they say—it is the loneliness, the sense of isolation that makes it so, and the lack of understanding in the minds of ordinary people. The problem of the child deaf from birth is quite different from that of the man or woman who has become deafened after school-age or in adult life. . . . But for all of them, the handicap is the same, the handicap of the silent world, the difficulty of communicating with the hearing and speaking world.*
>
> Scott Stevenson*

The aim of aural rehabilitative efforts for the hearing impaired, according to Ballantyne (1977), is to overcome the handicap. That, of course, is the goal of all professionals who deal with the hearing impaired. In discovering the existence of a hearing impairment, assessing its type and degree, and referring the person who possesses it for medical treatment, the audiologist makes that referral with the possibility in mind that the physician can identify the cause and correct it. The referral is made on the premise that the hearing impairment, per se, may be overcome.

If the hearing impairment cannot be treated, the audiologist then assumes the role of the expert in remediation of the handicapping effects of the hearing loss: to help the person who possesses it overcome the communicative, social, and perhaps psychological effects. A team of professionals may become involved, including vocational rehabilitation counselors, a psychologist, a sociologist, a speech pathologist, and of course the audiologist, who will probably coordinate the team. The client's family will hopefully also be involved in the aural rehabilitation treatment process. This task, in its totality, holds tremendous responsibility.

Why, then, is this important area in so many instances presented as a single chapter in texts which deal entirely with the subject of hearing impairment? Only recently have entire texts been written and published which concentrate on ''rehabilitative audiology.''

---

*From Ballantyne, J. *Deafness*. New York: Churchill Livingstone, 1977, p. 215.

This is particularly true in relation to the hearing impaired adult. Only within the past decade have books been published which have concentrated entirely on the adult and aging hearing impaired clients. Earlier texts by the Kinzies (1931), Bruhn (1949), Nitchie (1950) and Bunger (1961) present approaches to speechreading which were, in some ways, designed for adults. But texts which dealt with the effects of hearing impairment on the adult and aging person, approaches to counseling, the psychosocial and vocational impact of hearing impairment, and approaches for remediation did not exist to any degree.

The purpose of the two parts of this text is to provide practical information on this complex topic. It is hoped that the information has been presented in such a way that it is meaningful for both students and professionals. It is also hoped that the readers will provide input back to the editor and authors so that they may learn whether that goal has been reached.

AURAL REHABILITATION—A HISTORICAL LOOK

Aural rehabilitation was not, for a number of years, a popular aspect of the field of audiology. It was sad to see a helping profession develop into one in which the professionals within it, for the most part, isolated themselves from clients who needed professional support and remediation by remaining behind the walls of steel, sound-treated diagnostic rooms. Since the field of audiology had its origin as an aural rehabilitation service during World War II, it has been interesting to note its progress, forward and backward, in that regard.

The military aural rehabilitation programs provided the birthplace for the field of audiology. Veterans Administration hospitals expanded the role of the audiologist and the standards for professionals and equipment. The first training program for audiologists was developed at Northwestern University in the 1940s, and programs expanded rapidly through the 1950s and 1960s. As a young profession, its growing pains were quite evident. As instrumentation became much more elaborate during the 1950s and particularly during the 1960s, and the field became more sophisticated in the area of research, a shift of emphasis toward pure and applied research, in diagnosis of site of lesion of auditory disorders and other medically related areas, became evident. It was apparent that the emphasis among the majority of professionals and training programs was turning toward diagnosis, instrumentation, and research, and away from aural rehabilitation. Results from an automated piece of equipment or from a pure research project were much more tangible than the more vague signs of improvement in social communication observed in an adult hearing impaired client.

The course of working with hearing impaired clients on the improvement of communication skills can be a difficult one. Interaction with hearing impaired adults or aging clients, helping them deal with the emotional impact of hearing impairment and their frustrations and fears, requires that the audiologist become involved on a close professional basis with clients. Unfortunately, insects and humans, even professional humans, often elect to take the path of least resistance. Thus, research and diagnostics became popular, and interest in aural habilitation/rehabilitation of the hearing impaired declined. Courses within training programs in the areas of differential diagnosis of auditory problems, speech and hearing sciences, instrumentation, and experimental audiology expanded rapidly, and new faculty were hired to teach them. Amid the vast array of those glittering courses and the blinking lights of expensive equipment, training programs generally offered a course or two entitled Aural Rehabilitation. When it came to finding a faculty member to teach them, often the lowest ranking faculty member or a doctoral assistant would submit to the task. Students generally reflected the same negative feelings, not only in regard to the course or courses, but also to aural rehabilitation practicum experiences with hearing impaired adults. Some students were known to accept those experiences with the same mental attitude as facing the dentist's drill. But that attitude in most respects does not prevail today. A more humanistic desire to work with *people* is becoming predominant among professionals of audiology training programs and, thus, their students. Prospective students are searching for graduate programs in audiology that permit them to concentrate on learning to provide aural (re)habilitation services. So our field appears to be achieving a healthy balance.

Probably one of the most positive steps taken during the past two decades toward strengthening the professional stature of aural rehabilitation, the professionals who provide those services, and students in training who desire to provide them after graduation, was the origin of the Academy of Rehabilitative Audiology in 1966. The Academy has done much to bring about a renewed awareness of the importance of professional training in aural rehabilitation and those services on behalf of the hearing impaired child, adult, and elderly client. As procedures for providing aural rehabilitative services for the hearing impaired adult and aging become more sophisticated, along with increased emphasis on the need for professional involvement in the fitting and dispensing of hearing aids, the professional prominence of the rehabilitative aspects of audiology continue to grow and expand. But as a primary health care service, both the diagnostic and habilitative/rehabilitative aspects of audiology must carry an equal share of the responsibility in caring for hearing impaired clients. This is also true in the conduct of research to discover new and more effective ways of providing those services.

WHAT IS AURAL REHABILITATION?

What is aural rehabilitation? Aural rehabilitation has for so many years been discussed from within the framework of speechreading, lipreading, visual communication, auditory training, and other subcategories that we have occasionally strayed from the totality of the process. Thus, to discover a definition of "aural rehabilitation" per se is difficult.

The first sentence of this chapter contained a statement by Ballantyne which, as paraphrased, was, "the aim of aural rehabilitative efforts for the hearing impaired . . . is to overcome the handicap." What is the handicap? Elements of the result of hearing impairment may impact greatly on one person but may not be a handicap to another. One person may remain engrossed in despondency over his or her partial loss of hearing, but another may rebound and work with vigor to overcome the difficulties in communication noted as the result of the hearing impairment. One person may demonstrate great social handicap as the result of a relatively mild high frequency hearing impairment, while another person, who possesses a more severe hearing loss, may reveal only a mild handicap occupationally or socially.

If the catalyst for a psychosocial, educational, and/or occupational handicap resulting from either acquired or congenital hearing impairment could be pinpointed, it would probably revolve around the term *communication,* and the interference either receptively, expressively, or both caused by a hearing impairment. A child who possesses a severe congenital hearing loss, whether remediation is begun early or late, will possess a language deficit to some degree which will retard educational and occupational potential; and language delay is the basis for that communication deficit. An adult who acquires a hearing impairment that is of sufficient degree to interfere with the reception of the speech of others may become despondent over his or her difficulties in maintaining a current occupation or functioning on a social basis. Again, the problem centers around interference with communication as the result of the auditory deficit.

So aural rehabilitation and the strategies utilized in the process of aural rehabilitation center around the impact of a loss of hearing on communication and the individual's response to that deficit. In dealing with hearing adults and elderly persons, the majority will have probably possessed normal hearing at some time in their lives and will probably possess normal or near normal language function. In that regard, the impact of the hearing impairment on communicative function reveals itself from innumerable dimensions and avenues.

Each adult and elderly person responds in different ways to an acquired hearing impairment. Each has different demands, either self-imposed or externally imposed, placed upon him or herself. Some will have families who are also impacted upon by the hearing deficit, and others will not. For some individuals, their occupation may require precise and in-depth communication with other professionals or clients, while other persons' occupations require little communication. Some persons may have been greatly involved on a social basis, while others' social lives may have revolved around home and family. A Harvard School of Business graduate whose spouse and parents have always had great expectations of him or her for success in the business world may feel a greater impact as the result of acquired severe hearing impairment than one who desires to be a good rancher, and who is not required to communicate a great deal on his or her ranch in northern Montana.

AURAL REHABILITATION DEFINED

So, what, then, is aural rehabilitation and the provision of aural rehabilitation services on the behalf of those hearing impaired persons? Defined, aural rehabilitation is an attempt at reducing the barriers to communication resulting from hearing impairment, and facilitating adjustment relative to the possible psychosocial, occupational, and educational impact of that auditory deficit. If viewed from the realm of the provision of aural rehabilitation services, it encompasses many facets. These include the following:

Assessment

Assessment of the individual's threshold levels for hearing per se, and determination of his or her ability to hear and understand speech, are the first important steps in the aural rehabilitation process. In the past, in all too many instances, this step was the first and last, except for possible referral on for a hearing aid if one appeared warranted. Few other avenues for remediation of the effects of the auditory deficit were taken. According to Rosen (Note 1),

> As he [the client] takes leave of the audiologist he knows that he has a hearing problem. . . . It is true that the audiologist may have mentioned lipreading, auditory training, or

> training in the use of a hearing aid, but probably did not offer those services himself. Furthermore, the advice was likely to be offered half-heartedly, as if the audiologist was really not aware of or convinced of its value. (p. 42)

Hopefully, this attitude is not as widespread as it appeared to be during the early sixties, but it does still exist to some degree. If the attitude of the audiologist who conducted the audiologic evaluation is such that he or she is not convinced of the value of aural rehabilitative services, the individual who possesses the auditory deficit either may not be referred for them, or may become so discouraged from that audiologist's apparent attitude that even though a referral is made, the client may not keep the appointment. It is discouraging to find audiologists who apparently entered the field of audiology because it is a helping profession, but find themselves feeling uncomfortable when they must relate with hearing impaired people on a face-to-face basis.

Nevertheless, the accurate assessment of the extent of the hearing deficit per se is the first step in the process of aural rehabilitation. With that information at hand, the assessment of the handicapping effects of the hearing loss, the initiation of a hearing aid evaluation, if deemed necessary, and the other steps involved in the total aural rehabilitation program can begin.

Assessment of the Benefits of Amplification

If warranted, assessment of the benefits of amplification for individual clients should be the second step in the aural rehabilitation treatment program, and, if indicated, the fitting and dispensing of the instruments. Correspondingly, with the hearing aid evaluation, however, assessment of the handicapping effects of the hearing loss should be made. In that regard, steps one, two, and three in this sequence must go hand in hand.

It must be stressed that not all persons who possess a hearing deficit can utilize amplification well. But, in the hands of a skilled audiologist who can not only sift through the audiometric data, including those of speech discrimination and the client's dynamic range, but also assess the emotional, social, and occupational consequences of each client's hearing loss and those persons' communicative needs, an accurate determination as to their candidacy for a hearing aid can be made. The hearing aid evaluation is only one part of the total aural rehabilitation program, but it is a critical part. According to Hays and Jerger (1978), the hearing aid evaluation is an (one) important clinical procedure toward the goal of aural rehabilitation of the hearing impaired client, and as such it must be deployed with great skill.

As important as the hearing aid evaluation and fitting, however, are the orientation process and follow-up aural rehabilitation program, which must be designed for each individual. According to Garstecki (1974), many persons who have been fitted with a hearing aid do not return to the audiologist for continuation of the aural rehabilitation program. In most respects, the failure to return lies with the audiologist who may not have emphasized the necessity for those important services, nor were the ongoing hearing aid orientation and aural rehabilitation treatment programs presented as being expected of the client. Hearing aid evaluation and orientation procedures for the adult and elderly client are presented in Chapters 4 and 5, in Part I, and Chapters 22, 23, and 24, in Part II. They are critically important and ongoing components of aural rehabilitation treatment programs.

Assessment of the Impact of the Hearing Deficit

In whatever fashion that is deemed appropriate for individual clients, assessment of the impact of the hearing deficit on individual clients, is, again, critical for formulating a viable aural rehabilitation program which is based upon individual clients' needs. The assessment may include attempts at determining the impact of the hearing loss on the individual emotionally, socially, occupationally, and educationally. In most instances, when dealing with hearing impaired adults and elderly persons, the potential impact of the hearing deficit on the educational aspects of life may not be the most important. Of course, for young adults of school age it becomes extremely important, as it does for those adults or elderly clients who desire to be involved in continuing education programs for occupational advancement or simply for the enjoyment of learning.

There are, at present, a number of procedures that have been outlined for the assessment of the handicap of hearing impairment on the adult or elderly client. In light of the probability of possession of normal to near-normal communicative function prior to the onset of the hearing loss, the impact of the hearing loss on their personal lives, and their occupational or educational goals is, in many ways, a personal thing. Everyone is affected differently.

The results of the audiometric evaluation provide the audiologist with information regarding expected communicative deficits resulting from the hearing loss, particularly when observing the shape of the audiogram notations, the degree of hearing loss, and the client's ability to hear and understand speech. The client's response to that hearing loss is another matter that must be evaluated and taken into consideration as his or her aural rehabilitation treatment program is being developed. The insightful audiologist will be able to observe the more obvious behaviors and respond appropriately to them from the first contact with clients.

Scales of communication and the impact of hearing impairment on the adult and the elderly person that appear to have potential have been developed and are currently available. Those include the Hearing Handicap Scale by High, Fairbanks and Glorig (1964), a paper-and-pencil rating scale that has as its purpose the evaluation of clients' ability to function communicatively in quiet and noisy settings. Others include the Hearing Measurement Scale by Nobel and Atherley (1970). This scale investigates clients' feelings about their hearing impairment, and other parameters including their ability to function in various communication environments. The scale is conducted by personal interview rather than paper-and-pencil format.

Sanders (1975) recommends use of a scale of communication based upon environmental profiles including those of home, social, and work. He stresses the use of profiles which delve into communicative environments which are most important to individual clients.

Another scale of communicative function is the Denver Scale (Alpiner, Chevrett, Glascoe, Metz, and Olsen, 1978). This scale is a paper-and-pencil questionnaire that is individually administered to clients prior to treatment and when treatment is being terminated. The client is permitted to rate him or herself on each question through a seven point semantic differential. Hull (1978) stresses the use of a client self-evaluation questionnaire in which clients rate their ability to function within various communicative environments. Clients then arrange those environments in order from most important to least important. Individual aural rehabilitation treatment programs are designed around those prioritized environments and are also used for evaluation of progress or lack of it.

Clients also confront themselves via videotape prior to treatment and when treatment is terminated. Client self-confrontation regarding their feelings about their ability to communicate with others and their feelings about themselves at that time is used as a part of the process of evaluating improvement or lack of it in treatment. The Hearing Performance Inventory by Giolas, Owens, Lamb and Schubert (1979) examines six categories of a person's response in communication and communicative environments.

Other methods for evaluating communicative function and improvements through aural rehabilitation treatment are discussed in Chapter 9 in Part I and Chapter 27 in Part II.

Evaluation of the impact of the hearing impairment on adult or elderly clients is an important part of the ongoing aural rehabilitation program. It is, however, a difficult task and one that is probably never finished since as clients face new situations, their responses to them may also be different. As physical, occupational, and personal environments change, so do hearing impaired persons' responses to them. Evaluation, therefore, is ongoing, and clients must also be taught to evaluate themselves and their reactions to new communicative environments. Perhaps the most important component of the evaluation process prior to services and upon the decision to terminate them is the client's opinions of his or her ability to function communicatively in their communicating world.

The Treatment Program

A formal aural rehabilitation treatment program is, of course, not separated in any way from the procedures discussed above, but is an extension of them. It involves extensive counseling to facilitate adjustment to the hearing loss (Chapter 7, in Part I, entitled "Facilitating Adjustment," delves into this subject at length), facilitating increased efficiency in communication, including establishment of client priorities in communication and a treatment program centering around them. The procedures used may involve efforts toward greater efficiency of the use of the client's residual hearing, greater awareness and use of visual clues in communication, manipulation of the client's communicative environments, and other specific tasks. Chapters 6, 7, and 8 in Part I and Chapters 26 and 28 in Part II present in-depth discussions of treatment procedures for adult and elderly clients, respectively.

The formal treatment program is certainly not the most important aspect of the aural rehabilitation effort. But for those many clients who can benefit from treatment strategies which may enhance communication in their most difficult environments, it is surely an important aspect of the total process. The most successful aural rehabilitation treatment programs, however, are those in which counseling and hearing aid orientation are carried over as an integral part.

Involvement of Other Professionals

Involvement of other professionals, including the vocational rehabilitation counselor, the social worker, educational personnel, the speech/language specialist, and the psychologist, is important to the ongoing aural rehabilitation program for individual clients who require their services. For elderly clients who reside in the health care facility, involvement of personnel of that facility is necessary. Included may be the activity director, occupational therapist, social worker, nurses, nurses' aides, and others as are necessary for a successful treatment program.

It is incumbent upon the audiologist to call upon other professionals to facilitate the rehabilitation process. It is also important to know when the problems an adult or elderly person is facing are beyond the scope of the audiologists' knowledge and skill, and to be aware of proper referral source. As a team leader in the aural rehabilitation process, the audiologist can function as the catalyst in the development of a truly comprehensive rehabilitation program for those clients who require those additional services. Chapter 12 and 13, in Part I, and Chapters 29, 30, and 32, in Part II, discuss the role of other professionals in the aural rehabilitation program.

Involvement of the Family

A positive involvement of the family and/or a significant other in the client's life can be one of the most strengthening aspects of the aural rehabilitation program both for the adult and elderly client. The words *positive involvement* are stressed because involvement by a nonunderstanding family member, or a friend who in the end decides that he or she does not "have the time" or who otherwise does not desire to become involved, can be damaging. If a spouse, another family member, or another significant other is to be a part of the client's aural rehabilitation program, it is important that he or she be involved from the time of the initial hearing evaluation, and particularly during the period of assessment of the handicapping effects of the hearing loss on the client. As the significant other becomes aware of the impact of the hearing deficit, that person can become an important strengthening component in facilitating adjustment and enhancing communication abilities of the client. The role of the family and significant others in the aural rehabilitation process is discussed further in Chapters 5, 6, 10 and 11 in Part I and extensively throughout Part II.

CONCLUSION

What is aural rehabilitation? According to Costello et al. (1974), in a paper developed by them as members of the Committee on Rehabilitative Audiology of the American Speech-Language-Hearing Association, "audiologic habilitation is designed to assist individuals with auditory disabilities to realize their optimal potential in communication regardless of age, or the age of the person at the onset of the disability" (p. 68). It is a complex process which has as its goal the reduction of the barriers to communication which have resulted from hearing loss. Within its process, a number of professionals and the family may be involved, with the audiologist functioning as the coordinator, or facilitator, of the team. The process is as complex as the client and the handicapping effects of his or her hearing impairment, and unquestionably, it carries great responsibility. Only those audiologists who are willing to accept that responsibility should provide those services. That means emerging from the enclosed sound treated room and coming face to face with people—people who require a close professional relationship and a service which will enhance their ability to function communicatively in a complex and changing world.

REFERENCES

Alpiner, J. G., Chevrett, W., Glascoe, G., Metz, M., & Olsen, B. The Denver scale of communication function, in J. G. Alpiner (Ed.), *Adult rehabilitative audiology*. Baltimore: Williams and Wilkins, 1978, p. 32–34.

Ballantyne, J. *Deafness*. New York: Churchill Livingstone, 1977, p. 215.

Bruhn, M. D. *The Mueller-Walle method of lipreading*. Washington, D.C.: Volta Bureau, 1949.

Bunger, A. M. *Speech reading—Jena method*. Danville, Il.: The Interstate Printers, 1961.

Costello, M. R., Freeland, E. E., Hill, M. J., Jeffers, J., Matkin, N. D., Stream, R. W., & Tobin, H. The audiologist: Responsibilities in the habilitation of the auditorily handicapped. *Journal of the American Speech and Hearing Association,* 1974, *16*, 68–70.

Garstecki, D. C. A behavioral approach toward adult hearing aid orientation. *Journal of the Academy of Rehabilitative Audiology,* 1974, *7*, 9–18.

Giolas, T. G., Owens, E., Lamb, S. H., & Schubert, E. E. Hearing performance inventory. *Journal of Speech and Hearing Disorders,* 1979, *44*, 169–195.

Hays, D., & Jerger, J. A new method of hearing aid evaluation. *Journal of the Academy of Rehabilitative Audiology,* 1978, *11*, 57–65.

High, W. S., Fairbanks, G., & Glorig, A. Scale for self-assessment of hearing handicap. *Journal of Speech and Hearing Disorders,* 1964, *29*, 215–230.

Hull, R. H. Aural rehabilitation of aging persons: Problems and strategies for their solution, in L. Bradford (Ed.), *Audiology—An audio journal for continuing education*. New York: Grune and Stratton, 1978.

Kinzie, C. E., & Kinzie, R. *Lip-reading for the deafened adult*. Philadelphia: John C. Winston, 1931.

Nitchie, E. H. *New Lessons in Lipreading*. Philadelphia: J. B. Lippincott, 1950.

Nobel, W. G., & Atherley, G. R. C. The hearing measurement scale: A questionnaire for the assessment of auditory disability. *Journal of Audiological Research, 1970, 10,* 229–250.

Sanders, D. A. Profile questionnaire for rating communicative performance, in Hearing aid orientation and counseling, in M. C. Pollack (Ed.), *Amplification for the hearing impaired*. New York: Grune and Stratton, 1975.

REFERENCE NOTE

1. Rosen J. *The role of the audiologist in aural rehabilitation*. Unpublished manuscript, University of Denver, 1967.

Jack Katz
Thomas P. White

Chapter 2: Introduction to the Handicap of Hearing Impairment in the Adult: Auditory Impairment versus Hearing Handicap

In order to understand the rehabilitative needs of a client, a battery of audiometric procedures and careful interview should be obtained. Some features of communicative needs can be gleaned directly or indirectly from the auditory tests and intertest relationships. A more complete picture is gained when the communicative difficulties the client faces in his or her communicative world are understood. The audiologic assessment side of the picture tells us how the person responded under certain controlled circumstances within a test environment. It neither tells us whether this is typical behavior nor whether the client routinely faces these types of communicative situations.

In order to make specific recommendations regarding the aural rehabilitative needs of a particular patient, we need to know more about him or her. The same audiometric results may, for example, lead to different recommendations for an infant, a school-age child, a factory worker, a terminally ill patient, and an elderly person. In addition, the individual's own life-style and activities will temper the considerations. It is important that audiologists be aware of what audiometric data can and cannot reveal. The purpose of this chapter is to discuss some of these factors.

At this point, it is well that we consider our terminology. We sometimes confuse cause and effect and measurement with function. We should be free to discuss these matters individually.

DEFINITIONS

In certain conversations, people are likely to use the terms hearing loss, hearing level, hearing impairment and hearing handicap interchangeably. In this chapter, we will delineate them.

Hearing Level versus Hearing Loss

Hearing level (HL) is a measurement made on an audiometer and reported in decibels (dB). Hearing level compares the client's performance to the responses of others in a standard or normal population. It is in essence the dial reading at which the individual responds in a specified manner. *Hearing loss* will be used to indicate a disorder or that hearing ability has been lost (Davis & Silverman, 1970). We would prefer to label a person's 40 dB threshold as a 40 dB HL unless we know what his hearing thresholds were prior to the onset of the problem. If his initial level was −5 dB HL and now it is 40 dB HL, we could specify that he had a 45 dB hearing loss as a result of the disorder. However, with a 10 dB HL prior to the auditory disorder, a person with a 40 dB HL would show only a 30 dB loss.

Hearing Impairment versus Hearing Handicap

The term *hearing impairment* is closely associated with hearing level and is sometimes used interchangeably. It can also relate to measures that are not in dB, such as discrimination scores for speech. Hearing impairment implies that performance is poorer than normal. It is often categorized as mild, moderate, or severe. The term *hearing handicap* refers to the interference that the hearing loss produces. Thus, the influence of the hearing impairment is the hearing handicap.

Relationships of Terminology

The terms described above can best be understood as they relate to individual cases. Two case presentations should clarify their use.

A 42-year-old woman was seen following the onset of tinnitus and hearing loss. The audiometric results revealed a flat *sensorineural loss*. The pure-tone speech frequency average was 45 dB *hearing level* in each ear. These were in good agreement with the speech reception thresholds (40 dB). According to a pre-employment audiogram from three years before, the patient had essentially normal hearing with an average of 8 dB HL in each ear. Thus, there was a 37 dB *hearing loss* associated with the incident. Her *hearing impairment* is classified as mild. The actual *hearing handicap* is greater than this since the patient is employed as a librarian where people tend to speak more softly.

The second case history is that of a 72-year-old man. His hearing problem has been diagnosed as a "presbycusic" loss. His hearing is normal for his age up to 1000 Hz; however, it falls off sharply for the higher frequencies. The *hearing level* at 2000 Hz is 20 dB poorer than at 1000 Hz. Although there is a mild *hearing impairment* for the speech frequencies, the patient reports little difficulty in everyday situations. His wife speaks a little louder to him and he hears well on the telephone or when listening to television played slightly louder than usual.

CONGENITAL VERSUS ACQUIRED HEARING LOSS

One factor which influences the effect of a hearing loss is when it occurs. Severe congenital or prelingual hearing losses (losses prior to the development of language) have a great impact on language, voice, and articulation because the individual does not develop communication in a natural way. This person does not have the constant stimulation of language and accurate feedback of his or her own speech production. Therefore, as an adult he or she may continue to have limitations in language as well as voice and articulation. Prelingual disorders also have a more deleterious effect on social, educational, and vocational aspects of the person's life.

The same type of loss at an older age, especially a catastrophic loss, will be likely to have a profound influence on the individual, but of a much different type. There will be no diminution of the person's language ability and relatively little change in his voice quality. He or she may compensate for a lack of monitoring by increasing volume. Over a period of time, articulatory movements will tend to become less precise, typically affecting the high frequency sibilant sounds first.

The catastrophic loss is usually more devastating in two ways. First, the psychological impact of isolation is much greater than for the person who has known only this condition. Second, word discrimination ability is not as keen as in the adult who has gradually lost his or her hearing over a long period of time. Many clients with progressive hereditary hearing loss have surprisingly good discrimination ability. Over the years they have been able to alter their concepts in a gradual manner. The person with a sudden loss may not know how to listen for the clues to distinguish the singular form of a word from the plural.

Obviously the complex interactions of people, their needs and environments, and the various test indicators provide infinite possibilities. Audiometric results will give us some guidance and general knowledge about the patient, but they fail to reveal things that the patient or his family can tell us. The next section will discuss the contribution of audiometric test results, and the final section will discuss the role of nonaudiometric information.

WHAT AUDIOMETRIC DATA REVEAL

In their simplest form, we can view hearing disorders as reductions of sensitivity, frequency range, and fidelity. Sensitivity can be likened to the decibel variations produced by an attenuator. A reduced frequency range is similar to the effects of an acoustic filter which selectively impedes the passage of certain frequencies and permits others to pass. A lack of fidelity refers to the distortion caused by the nonlinear transmission of a sound due to the breakdown of either peripheral or central structures.

We will first describe the influences of sensitivity (degree of loss) and frequency range (configuration) since they represent the most reliable audiometric information. The disorders of fidelity (clarity), while vitally important, are not as quantifiable. Fidelity and other factors that are less precise reduce our ability to predict handicap from the pure tone information. The audiologist will be most astute by using all of the available information.

DEGREE OF LOSS

One thing that audiometric data reveal is the degree of loss. This information is important because it provides a relative indicator of the handicap the individual may experience. One way of putting the obtained hearing level into perspective is to relate it to a predesigned table which categorizes and classifies various degrees of hearing levels and their predicted handicaps. (See Table 2-1.) By doing this, we may be able to make general statements about the person's hearing function. However, one cannot state with great accuracy the specific effect of the loss. Individuals do not always behave alike and consequently a person may not be consistent with the formulated tables. Thus a table should be used only as a guideline, not as an absolute.

Table 2-1
Relationship of Three Frequency Speech Averages to Typical Hearing Difficulties and Needs*

ANSI (1969) Levels in Decibels	Classification	Approximate† Discrimination	Typical Speech Understanding	Typical Hearing Aid Needs
0–24	Normal	92%	No significant limitations	None except the possible use of special fittings (e.g., CROS, BICROS)
25–39	Mild	82%	Difficulty with faint speech, especially from another room	Occasional use if any
40–54	Moderate	70%	Frequent difficulty with normal speech	Frequent use
55–69	Moderately severe	60%	Frequent difficulty even with loud speech	Group with greatest satisfaction from hearing aid
70–89	Severe	36%	Loud or amplified speech might be understood depending on factors such as type of impairment	Generally good benefit, but depends on discrimination ability and other factors
90 +	Profound	20%	Understanding of speech severely limited even with amplification	Use of hearing aid assists in monitoring the environment

*This information is based in part on that published by Goetzinger (1978). It should be pointed out that this table refers to limitations and needs related to cochlear hearing losses. Conductive, retrocochlear, and central disorders may follow a different pattern of handicap and needs.
†W-22 scores at PB-Max for cochlear cases from Thompson and Hoel (1962), Mongelli (1978), and Katz (Note 1).

Many methods of categorization have been proposed, including those of Davis and Silverman (1970), Green (1978), Goetzinger (1978), and Hodgson (1978). The emphasis of each table varies according to its purpose. These include medical-legal definitions, handicapping effects, rehabilitative needs, and the impact on children versus adults.

The overall effect of the degree of loss is obvious. The greater the hearing level the greater the handicap. However, the actual handicap of a certain degree of loss will vary considerably. Some individuals may have only a slight loss yet have a noticeable handicap. Others may have what would be termed a very significant loss and yet demonstrate relatively little handicap. What makes these paradoxical cases occur is not known for certain, except that individual differences are most certainly a dominating factor. These might include personality, intelligence, motivation, philosophy of life, occupation, and degree of socialization. Individuals who rely heavily on communicative function for their work, such as salespersons, attorneys, and teachers, may notice less significant losses than those who do not (e.g., truck drivers, plant workers). Individuals who tend to socialize more (those who go to parties, plays, and group gatherings) will notice slighter hearing losses sooner than people who tend to stay at home and read, watch television, and relate only to close family members.

CONFIGURATION OF HEARING LOSS

The shape of the audiogram helps to determine the frequency characteristics of the auditory information the individual receives. When we know both the audiometric configuration of the client's hearing and the energy distribution of the incoming auditory signals, we can better understand the frequency information he or she is receiving. One often looks at the best binaural hearing to determine the sounds the client will hear. This is done by noting the better threshold at each frequency for the two ears. Although this approach is a valid one, it is limited in a number of ways. While it does consider HL, it does not consider the locus of lesion, the unilateral/bilateral nature of the loss, and the clarity of the incoming information.

In this section we shall consider the configuration of the hearing loss as if it were produced by an acoustic filter. Despite the limitations of the acoustic filter approach, we can obtain an important source of information that we can use in understanding a client's communicative abilities and deficits. Other variables which influence performance will be considered later.

Flat Configuration

A flat configuration refers to a pure tone audiogram in which there is a relatively small difference in threshold across the frequencies. This does not imply the same dB hearing level throughout. In fact, slightly sloping and jagged patterns are frequently considered flat because they are not extreme enough to be classified as high or low frequency curves.

We can assume that a flat loss will limit the input evenly across the frequencies. The major energy component of speech is in the low frequencies (250 to 500 Hz). Despite their power, they contain relatively little information for identifying monosyllabic words. There is little speech energy in the high frequencies. In the normal listener, essentially complete intelligibility comes from the frequencies 300 to 3000 Hz. The frequencies of speech which contribute most to intelligibility are between 1000 and 3000 Hz. This information can help us to better understand hearing loss as a filter effect.

Because of the distribution of speech energy, a flat loss is likely to affect the high frequency information most severely and the low frequency information least of all. The degree to which the middle frequencies are reduced will determine how much of the speech signal remains for purposes of identification.

High Frequency Configuration

The effect of a high frequency loss is similar to a flat loss for speech because the high frequency sounds are more severely attenuated, or eliminated. It creates, however, an abnormal relationship between the lower and higher frequencies of speech. With this configuration of loss, the presence of normal hearing in the low frequencies is of little benefit for purposes of amplification. It limits the amount of amplification that the patient can benefit from unless the low frequencies are attenuated within the hearing aid or by earmold modifications. The person with a high frequency loss is very much aware of environmental and speech sounds, which contain low frequency information. The individual is not handicapped in his ability to hear the life-saving sounds of a car horn or verbal warning. On the other hand, they experience limited ability to locate the source of sounds and difficulty in blocking out background sounds, or understanding speech from another room.

It is important to observe where the drop of hearing occurs, especially if it occurs within the speech frequencies. Someone who hears only the lower portion of the speech range is often ridiculed for hearing just what he or she wants to hear. This person may respond to his or her name and familiar phrases but is limited when the language is complex or when listening in a poor acoustic environment. The presence of normal hearing levels in the high frequencies appears to be critical when listening in noisy conditions. Many people with high frequency losses will not complain of hearing difficulty except in environments with significant ambient noise. The effect of a high frequency loss may also be reflected in the patient's own speech production of high frequency consonant sounds.

Low Frequency Configuration

A low frequency configuration is the least common, especially among sensorineural cases, and has the fewest disadvantages. Low frequency information is the most powerful and most expendable portion of the speech signal. Thus, from a simple filter effect, the patient retains the most important portion of the frequency range, has good discrimination for speech, and should have an excellent response to amplification. The client's voice quality may be influenced somewhat, but articulation will remain normal depending on which audiometric frequencies are affected.

Saucer Configuration

The saucer curve is occasionally encountered. In this pure-tone pattern, there are better thresholds for the high and low frequencies than those in the mid-range. Thus, the sounds that are most important for speech intelligibility are diminished the most. While this configuration of loss would appear to be extremely handicapping, we often find good performance on speech reception threshold measures and very good discrimination scores. Saucer-shaped losses are frequently congenital. The individual is therefore likely to have refined his or her ability to derive phonemic cues from the higher and lower frequency sounds.

MONAURAL VERSUS BINAURAL HEARING LOSS

Some problems of hearing loss are either minimized or amplified by whether one or both ears are involved. The restrictions placed on individuals as a result of unilateral hearing problems are not, in most cases, primarily those of hearing. While the hearing levels are lowered in the affected ear, the normally functioning ear will dominate and enable the individual to hear in most situations. It is common for persons with a unilateral hearing loss to indicate that they are not generally handicapped in their hearing. An important factor in the person's awareness of a unilateral hearing loss is its degree. The more severe the loss, the greater the likelihood that the individual will be aware of it.

There are some problems that unilateral losses will impose. The most common difficulty is, of course, one whereby the individual has trouble when someone is speaking on the impaired side. The other restriction imposed by a unilateral hearing loss is one of localization. Often, a person with normal hearing on one side and affected hearing on the other will report difficulty in determining the source of sounds in the environment. Another factor which calls attention to the effects of a unilateral difficulty is in the presence of background noise or poor acoustical conditions (e.g., gymnasiums, groups of people talking). In such instances, the person may report considerable difficulty in hearing what is being said. Similarly, a person with a bilateral hearing loss who wears a monaural hearing aid tends to lose the benefits of a binaural system.

TYPE OF LOSS VERSUS THE ASSESSMENT BATTERY

There may be several objectives in evaluating the auditory system, but it is important to obtain as much information as possible as it relates to the handicap being experienced by the client. For example, *conductive losses* are associated with good discrimination ability for speech. Clients with these problems have a greater need for increased volume than they do for improved clarity. Although the communicative effects of conductive loss in the adult are not as severe as an equivalent sensorineural loss, it can produce significant rehabilitative complications. In some cases ear drainage will contraindicate the use of an ear mold, and a conductive overlay on top of a sensorineural problem can limit the use and types of amplification.

Most *cochlear (sensory) losses* reveal some diminished word discrimination ability. There is usually a direct relationship between hearing level and discrimination ability (Thompson and Hoel, 1962). The more depressed the hearing level, the poorer the discrimination score. Disorders of the cochlea produce a variety of audiometric patterns which provide clues as to the etiology. Most cochlear hearing losses are greater in the high frequences than in the low frequencies. This is because presbycusis and noise-induced hearing loss, the most common causes of sensorineural disorder, affect the higher frequencies. Some cochlear losses are greater in the low frequencies than in the high frequencies as observed in cases with Meniere's disease. Others may be flat, as in ototoxic-related hearing loss. Again, these patterns are not mutually exclusive and may have considerable overlap.

Another characteristic of sensory losses is an intolerance for loud sounds. Consequently, this factor must be considered in the use of amplification. In cases with extremely small dynamic ranges, the use of amplification may be contraindicated.

Cochlear losses may also affect the speech and voice of the individual. Because the inner ear functioning is decreased, the internal feedback loop is reduced to the extent that the clients are unable to monitor their own speech and voice patterns normally. This can lead to some articulation disorders as well as reduced vocal inflection and quality. The effect is related to the extent and duration of the hearing loss.

The effects of a *neural hearing loss* are generally more a problem of clarity than of sensitivity. Consequently, audiometric findings will usually show severely depressed word discrimination scores. Some cases may even have essentially normal hearing levels but very poor discrimination ability. The clients may indicate that they hear but do not understand what is being said. The implications of this finding are that people with neural problems are generally poorer candidates for amplification.

Other characteristics of a neural loss as revealed by audiometric findings are fatigue of the auditory system and an unusual tolerance for loud sounds. If considerable tone decay is present, some individuals may have difficulty with amplification because as they receive auditory stimulation their auditory systems slowly and continuously lose sensitivity (Goldberg, 1964). This may require constant adjustments of the volume control on the hearing aid. In some cases, individuals have had difficulty talking on the telephone because the voices get softer and softer.

Intolerance for loud sounds is characteristic of individuals with cochlear hearing losses. Conversely, neural cases do not report this intolerance. They may report no particular discomfort even at the maximum limits of the audiometer. Therefore, if a neural loss is present and a hearing aid is under consideration, the maximum power output of a hearing aid should not contraindicate its use. Unfortunately, many people with neural problems have greater reduction in clarity at high levels of amplification (Jerger & Jerger, 1971).

Central Auditory Dysfunction

In recent years audiologists have become increasingly aware of the influence of *central auditory disorders,* particularly when considering the auditory problems of the elderly. Disorders of the brain and brain stem can have an adverse effect on hearing test responses and central auditory processing.

Karp, Belmont, and Birch (1969) demonstrated significant sensorineural hearing losses in hemiplegic patients. The losses were noted in the ear on the side of the paralysis (in the ear contralateral to the brain lesion). Probably the most common auditory complaint of clients with central auditory dysfunction is the inability to block out background noise. Difficulty in locating the source of a sound is also found in some cases. These symptoms, however, are no different than the symptoms of many patients with purely peripheral dysfunction. Despite the lack of abnormality on peripheral hearing tests, these individuals show slight or, in some cases, significant communicative problems. Often, these individuals reveal depressed performance on central auditory tests. Clients may be particularly handicapped when they have both peripheral hearing loss and central auditory dysfunction, as in cases of presbycusis.

Lesions in certain parts of the brain have been found to produce depressed scores on standard word discrimination tests. Katz and Pack (1975) reported a significant difference in W-22 discrimination scores in patients with lesions involving Heschl's gyrus. In these cases the discrimination was depressed in both ears or in the ear contralateral to the lesion.

Individuals with brain stem lesions may also have auditory difficulties. In some cases the external redundancy of the standard discrimination tests is sufficient to permit them to obtain good scores. However, under complex listening conditions, performance can be expected to go down (Katz, 1970; Jerger & Jerger, 1974).

Performance on central auditory tests can play a vital role in understanding the patient's problem and in arriving at appropriate recommendations. For example, a CROS (Contralateral Routing of Signal) hearing aid which is most beneficial in cases with unilateral hearing losses can be extremely inappropriate for individuals with reduced central auditory function. It is suggested that individuals who have difficulty on the SSI (Synthetic Sentence Identification) with an ipsilateral competing message (Jerger & Jerger, 1974) might well have difficulty utilizing a CROS hearing aid. Other loci of lesion, such as frontal lobe disorders, can disrupt certain auditory functions, but should not contraindicate the use of amplification. With disturbance in Heschl's gyrus or in the brain stem, the likelihood of success is more guarded.

The array of central tests now available provide considerable information for understanding hearing handicap. It would appear that extent and type of central auditory dysfunction will play an important role in determining the appropriate rehabilitative approach.

Tests for Speech Reception and Discrimination

The rehabilitative use of speech tests is invaluable. These results tell us how the individual performs in a test situation and enable us to predict with relative accuracy how the client will get along in his or her environment. Their value lies in the fact that testing is the only controlled way that we can obtain information about the individual's capability for hearing and understanding spoken communication. Numerous speech tests are available. These include tests such as threshold, discrimination, most comfortable loudness (MCL) and uncomfortable loudness (UCL). Results of speech tests also help us predict how well the individual will perform with amplification. If the scores are high, good success with a hearing aid can generally be expected. If the scores are low, the chances of success are reduced.

The interesting yet perplexing finding of the results of speech testing is that they do not tell us for certain how the individual will function in his or her environment. Some persons with reduced word discrimination scores (WDS) communicate with remarkable success. Conversely, there are those who reveal good results in discriminating words but demonstrate poor daily performance and lack of success with amplification. Typically the speech reception thresholds (SRT) and WDS are used in diagnostic evaluations. Much information is obtained; however, by the use of materials which more closely parallel normal conversation. In this regard, there is increasing use of sentences such as the CID Everyday Speech lists, the PAL question-answer type of materials, and the Synthetic Sentence Identification (Jerger, Speaks, and Trammell, 1968). Continuous discourse and speech with competing background noise have also been used to give clues for rehabilitation management. One such battery that has been found to be useful is that by Kalikow, Stevens, and Elliot (1977) called SPIN—Speech Intelligibility in Noise. Another testing approach utilizes time compression of speech. Such tests are becoming useful in identifying individuals who require a greater amount of time to process speech information or who cannot tolerate reduced redundancy. Kasten (1979) and Hull (1979), investigated the use of time-compressed speech to better understand the phonemic and linguistic redundancy requirements in speech perception in hearing impaired older adults.

Other Tests

Other special tests give us clues for purposes of aural rehabilitation. For example, individuals who demonstrate recruitment or acoustic reflexes at reduced sensation levels frequently show intolerance for loud sounds. Some of the diagnostic tests that yield strong cochlear results also suggest that the patient has a reduced dynamic range. This creates a major challenge when amplification is being considered for a client.

Noncochlear results suggest problems that will potentially disrupt communication and hearing aid benefits. For example, Costello and McGee (1967), have discussed the linear relationship between increased tone decay and reduced speech discrimination. Wide traces on the Bekesy audiogram and abnormally large difference limens suggest that the person lacks fine discrimination skills necessary for the analysis of speech. This might reflect itself on the standard discrimination test, and typically is reflected on the more challenging tests. These procedures include some of the central tests like the Rush Hughes difference test (Goetzinger & Rousey, 1959), the Staggered Spondaic Word Test (Katz, 1962), and time altered speech (Quiros, 1961). Reduced performance on these tests have been found to be reflected in life situations, such as in difficult listening environments. Lower performance is also seen among those who have difficulty understanding rapid conversations or foreign accent.

Difficulty in localizing the source of a sound (sound localization/lateralization) also affects speech understanding (Norlund & Fritzell, 1963). One might consider the value of binaural amplification or CROS aids for these people.

The audiometric battery provides information which give clues for contraindicating factors that may have an impact on clients' communication skills. By noting these signs we can counsel the individual more realistically and consider various solutions to their communicative problems.

LIMITATIONS OF AUDIOMETRIC RESULTS

Given a pure-tone pattern, which is described by both frequency and intensity, we can predict with accuracy the individual's sensitivity for speech (SRT) and clarity (WDS) under earphones. However, in attempting to correlate the information derived from a monaural pure-tone audiometric test with the complexities of a noisy, three-dimensional world, for example, the amount of relevant data we can confidently extrapolate becomes greatly reduced. It should be recognized that no amount of audiometric study and quantification can permit us to actually comprehend what a person is hearing or how he or she relates to a given communicative environment. Audiometric data do not allow for individual social or psychological differences. Therefore, in order for the audiometric results to be meaningful, they have to be considered with the particular individual in mind.

There are numerous influences that are important in evaluating the individual's communicative environment. In some ways the client's auditory abilities have already narrowed down the variety of situations in which he or she is accustomed to communicate. Other influences include vocational training, personality features, and socioeconomic status.

CLIENT INTERVIEW

No audiometric battery is so complete as to make a sample of actual communication unnecessary. The audiologist must be highly sensitive to the patient interview and behavioral observations. The interview should contain general and specific information about the person's ability to communicate.

More comprehensive information will be obtained if a family member or friend is present at the interview. By use of the interview technique we are better able to understand the client's ability to function in everyday life situations. The audiologist may also be aided by use of one of the available questionnaires that assess communicative needs.

There are a number of client interview procedures that delve into individual responses to the handicap of hearing impairment. Such scales include those by Alpiner, Chevrette, Glascoe, Metz, and Olsen (The Denver Scale of Communication Function, 1978); High, Fairbanks, and Glorig (Scale of Hearing Handicap, 1964); Nobel and Atherley (The Hearing Measurement Scale, 1970); Sanders (Profile Questionnaires for Rating Communicative Performance in Home, Work and Social Environments, 1975); and others. Scales of communicative function provide important information relative to the impact of hearing impairment on individual clients, and can be utilized as a supplement to standard audiometric data. These scales will be discussed in their various forms and within differing settings later in this text.

In addition to the person's own report, the audiologist will observe the client's ability to handle communication on a firsthand basis. This will take into account factors such as visual and contextual cues, which are not obtained from audiometric tests. Frequently, one of the most important observations is related to the individual's motivation for communication and his interest in obtaining aural rehabilitation services.

EDUCATIONAL, VOCATIONAL, SOCIAL, PSYCHOLOGICAL, AND SOCIOECONOMIC INFLUENCES

It is obvious from the foregoing information that a hearing impairment can have an important effect on communication. Strict audiologic data do not reveal the totality of the handicapping effects of hearing impairment. The relationship is by no means an exact one and depends on many factors related to the individual's hearing and other skills. The following illustrate other potential factors that influence the hearing impaired person's response to an auditory deficit.

Educational

The hard-of-hearing teenager or adult will be extremely challenged in an educational setting. Unlike many situations, the course and the instructor dictate the manner and material to be presented. A minor hearing loss, perhaps even a monaural loss, with some discrimination limitations and poor classroom acoustics could create a significant problem for the student above and beyond the academic challenge. Difficulty in understanding speech as noted earlier in this chapter is related to hearing level, discrimination ability, and room acoustics. Many approaches and devices are being used to manage this educational problem. Sometimes the most successful approach the audiologist can follow is to work with the classroom teacher and possibly recommend room modifications that will be significant in helping the hearing impaired listener.

Vocational and Social

The broad effects of a hearing impairment can be especially realized when considering the vocational aspects of a person's life. Certain vocations result in a greater challenge to the hearing impaired individual. Obviously those that require less oral communication are less handicapping. Other occupations are much more challenging for the hearing impaired person, such as those that require extensive use of the telephone or many group meetings. The audiologist may find him or herself in the position of being able to counsel the client to establish better strategies in handling these difficult situations. The same approach can be used in aiding the client to cope with social situations such as parties and church activities. While the individual may be strongly motivated to overcome his or her vocational handicap, it is not uncommon for clients to avoid social frustrations. Therefore, the audiologist must be sensitive to both potential problem areas. These areas are discussed in depth later in this text.

Psychological

We frequently encounter the client who has relatively good auditory skills but is greatly affected in his or her communicative abilities. Among the important factors that produce this situation may be personality and psychological influences. Individuals who are extremely nervous or shy may not utilize their auditory skills to their fullest. This should show up in the discrepancy between the audiometric results and the client's reported or observed difficulties. While the audiologist is not professionally trained to solve emotional problems, he or she is in an excellent position to encourage, counsel, and direct the individual to sources that can aid the client in these important areas.

Socioeconomic

An individual's socioeconomic status generally enhances or impedes his or her educational and vocational training. It also limits or expands the specific resources at the client's disposal. Fortunately, in recent years more opportunities have been available for the hearing impaired population in general.

In most professional areas the need for accurate communication is demanded. The financial and legal implications of faulty communication can be limiting. The attorney, engineer, physician, teacher, and others are called upon to handle complex communications with great accuracy. Therefore, even minor auditory abnormalities can influence the individual's ongoing activities and threaten his or her livelihood.

In terms of the availability of resources for the hearing impaired, the individual with a higher socioeconomic status is more likely to seek and demand services that will provide help in dealing with his or her environment. The individual with the greater financial resources can more readily avail him or herself of appropriate amplification, as well as aural rehabilitation services and vocational or psychological counseling.

SUMMARY

This chapter concerned itself with the implications of audiometric findings upon rehabilitative needs. Much information can be obtained from basic audiometric procedures that can shed light upon what the auditory capabilities of the hearing impaired are and offer information to aid in developing recommendations regarding the person's needs. Although audiometric data are valuable, the audiologist must be particularly aware of test limitations. There is considerable information that must be obtained through other means. The competent audiologist is one whose evaluations and management recommendations are based upon all areas of input.

REFERENCES

Alpiner, J. G., Chevrette, W., Glascoe, G., Metz, M., & Olsen, B. The Denver scale of communication function, in J. G. Alpiner (Ed.), *Adult rehabilitative audiology.* Baltimore: Williams and Wilkins, 1978, pp. 53–56.

Costello, M. R., & McGee, T. M. Language impairment associated with bilateral abnormal auditory adaptation, in A. B. Grahm (Ed.), *Sensorineural hearing processes and disorders.* Boston: Little, Brown, 1967.

Davis, H., & Silverman, S. R. *Hearing and deafness.* New York: Holt, Rinehart and Winston, 1970.

Goetzinger, C. P. Word discrimination testing, in J. Katz (Ed.)., *Handbook of clinical audiology.* Baltimore: Williams and Wilkins, 1978, pp. 149–158.

Goetzinger, C. P., & Rousey, C. L. Hearing problems in later life. *Medical Times,* 1959, *87,* 771–780.

Goldberg, H. What to do about auditory fatigue. *Hearing Dealer,* 1964, *14,* 12–13.

Green, D. Pure tone air conduction testing, in J. Katz (Ed.), *Handbook of clinical audiology,* Baltimore: Williams and Wilkins, 1978, pp. 98–109.

High, W. S., Fairbanks, G., & Glorig, A. Scale for self-assessment of hearing handicap. *Journal of Speech and Hearing Disorders,* 1964, *29,* 215–230.

Hodgson, W. R. Disorders of hearing, in P. Skinner and R. Shelton (Eds.), *Speech, language and hearing.* Reading, Mass.: Addison-Wesley, 1978.

Hull, R. H. *Aural rehabilitation procedures for the elderly.* Paper presented at the Aspen Symposium on Communication Problems of the Aging, Aspen, Colorado, April 1979.

Jerger, J., & Jerger, S. Auditory findings in brain stem disorders. *Archives of Otolaryngology,* 1974, *99,* 342–349.

Jerger, J., & Jerger, S. Diagnostic significance of PB word functions. *Archives of Otolaryngology,* 1971, *99,* 573–580.

Jerger, J., Speaks, C., & Trammell, J. L. A new approach to speech audiometry. *Journal of Speech and Hearing Disorders,* 1968, *33,* 318–328.

Kalikow, D. N., Stevens, K. N., & Elliot, L. L. Development of a test of speech intelligibility in noise using sentence materials with controlled word predictability. *Journal of the Acoustical Society of America,* 1977, *61,* 1337–1351.

Karp, E., Belmont, I., & Birch, J. Unilateral hearing loss in hemiplegic patients. *Journal of Nervous and Mental Disorders,* 1969, *148,* 83–86.

Kasten, R. N. *Hearing aids and the elderly.* Paper presented at the Aspen Symposium on Communication Problems of the Aging, Aspen, Colorado, April 1979.

Katz, J. The use of staggered spondaic words for assessing the integrity of the central nervous system. *Journal of Audiological Research,* 1962, *2,* 327–337.

Katz, J. Audiologic diagnosis: Cochlea to cortex. *Menorah Medical Journal,* 1970, *1,* 25–37.

Katz, J., & Pack, G. New developments in differential diagnosis using the SSW test, in M. Sullivan (Ed.), *Central auditory processing disorders.* Omaha: University of Nebraska Press, 1975.

Mongelli, C. Central auditory involvement in two geriatric populations measured with the staggered spondaic word test. Unpublished manuscript, University of California, Santa Barbara, 1978.

Nobel, W. G., & Atherley, G. R. C. The hearing measurement scale: A questionnaire for the assessment of auditory disability. *Journal of Auditory Research,* 1970, *10,* 229–250.

Nordlund, B., & Fritzell, B. The influence of azimuth on speech signals. *Acta Oto-Laryngologica* (Stockholm), 1963, *56,* 632–642.

Quiros, J. Accelerated speech audiometry: An examination of test results. Translations of the Belton Institute for Hearing Research (Translated from Interpretation de los resultados obtenidos con loboaudiometria accelerado). *Revista Fonoaudiologica,* 1961, *17,* 128–164.

Reger, S. Pure tone audiometry, in A. Glorig (Ed.), *Audiometry: Principles and practices.* Baltimore: Williams and Wilkins, 1965.

Sanders, D. A. Profile questionnaire for rating communicative performance in a home, work or social environment, in M. C. Pollack (Ed.), *Amplification for the hearing impaired.* New York: Grune and Stratton, 1975.

Thompson, G., & Hoel, R. Flat sensorineural hearing loss and PB scores. *Journal of Speech and Hearing Disorders,* 1962, *27,* 284–287.

REFERENCE NOTES

1. Katz, J. Relationship between pure tone thresholds and W-22 discrimination scores in sensory-neural cases. Unpublished study, State University of New York, Buffalo, 1976.

Pamela L. Jackson

Chapter 3: A Psychosocial and Economic Profile of the Hearing Impaired Adult

Loss of hearing is the most common of all physical impairments. Yet until recently it has received little attention in terms of the psychosocial and economic handicaps that it imposes on the life of the individual. In 1974, Schein and Delk published the results of the National Census of the Deaf Population in a comprehensive book entitled *The Deaf Population of the United States*. This work presents numerous data that describe the extent and the characteristics of the hearing impaired population.

Table 3-1 summarizes prevalence and prevalence rates for hearing losses occurring at various ages. The figure 13,362,842 for the prevalence of all hearing impairments emphasizes the extent of the overall problem. The increase in incidence figures is also apparent if the data are compared to past figures. For example, since the early 1930s, the prevalence rate for deafness has been reported as approximately 1 per 1000. The 1971 rate, however, reported by Schein and Delk indicates a rate for prevocational (prior to 19 years of age) deafness of 2 per 1000, or more exactly, 203 deaf individuals per 100,000. This doubling of the rate in 40 years is attributed to three factors: possible inaccuracies in past counts; differences in definitions which alter the population sampled; or an actual increase in the occurrence of deafness. While all of these do play a part, it is important to add that survival rates of high risk infants have also increased in recent years and will contribute to an overall increase in the number of deaf adults who in the past might not have survived beyond early childhood.

The prevalence and prevalence rates for significant bilateral hearing impairment as they relate to age and sex are shown in Table 3-2. Schein and Delk define significant bilateral hearing impairment as one in which the loss is present in both ears and the better ear has some problem hearing and understanding speech. This category includes deafness which Schein and Delk define as ''the inability to hear or understand speech'' (p. 133).

Inspection of the data in Table 3-2 indicates the expected prevalence of hearing impairment in the 65-and-over age range. The decline in hearing sensitivity with age is well known. The rates in the 24-and-under age ranges are the ones that must be concentrated on, however, especially when future program needs are being considered. Vocational, social, and geriatric programs can then be made aware of their long range responsibilities.

Table 3-1
Prevalence and Prevalence Rates for Hearing Impairments in the Civilian Noninstitutionalized Population by Degree and Age of Onset: United States, 1971

Degree	Age of Onset	Number	Rate per 100,000
All hearing impairments	All ages	13,362,842	6,603
Significant bilateral	All ages	6,548,842	3,236
Deafness	All ages	1,767,046	873
	Prevocational*	410,522	203
	Prelingual†	210,626	100

Reprinted with permission from Schein, J. D. & Delk, M. T., Jr. *The deaf population of the United States*. Silver Spring, Maryland: National Association of the Deaf, 1974, p. 16.
*Prior to 19 years of age.
†Prior to 3 years of age.

Table 3-2
Prevalence and Prevalence Rates for Significant Bilateral Impairment by Age and Sex: United States, 1971

Sex/Age	Number	Rate per 100,000
Both sexes	6,549,643	3,237
Under 6	56,038	262
6 to 16	384,557	852
17 to 24	235,121	862
25 to 44	642,988	1,356
45 to 64	1,870,356	4,478
65 and over	3,360,583	17,368
Females	2,706,124	2,583
Under 6	23,771	227
6 to 16	155,738	701
17 to 24	81,923	568
25 to 44	243,403	990
45 to 64	610,741	2,783
65 and over	1,590,818	14,257
Males	3,843,519	3,938
Under 6	32,267	295
6 to 16	228,819	997
17 to 24	153,198	1,191
25 to 44	399,585	1,749
45 to 64	1,259,885	6,535
65 and over	1,769,765	21,606

Reprinted with permission from Schein, J. D. & Delk, M. T. Jr. *The deaf population of the United States*. Silver Spring, Maryland: National Association of the Deaf, 1974, p. 29.

Table 3-3
Need for Mental Health Services among Deaf People where the 1 Percent, 2 Percent, and 10 Percent Classes Represent Decreasing Degrees of Severity of the Psychiatric Problem

Degree of Hearing Loss	Total Number	Number Needing Services		
		1%	2%	10%
Hearing impaired	13,975,000	139,750	279,500	1,397,500
Significant bilateral loss	6,850,000	68,500	137,000	685,000
Deaf	1,850,000	18,500	37,000	185,000
Prevocationally deaf	430,000	4,300	8,600	43,000

Reprinted with permission from Goulder, T. J. Federal and state mental health programs for the deaf in hospitals and clinics. *Mental Health in Deafness,* 1977, *1*, 14.

PSYCHOLOGICAL PROFILE

The presence of a hearing impairment affects the entire life of the individual, not just his or her ability to perceive auditory cues. The extent of this influence can be illustrated by examining Table 3-3. Even if only the most severe cases are considered, 18,500 deaf individuals are in need of psychological services. Compare that figure with Goulder's estimate that only 727 persons are being served by mental health programs for the deaf and the problem becomes evident (Goulder, 1977). The psychological needs of the hearing impaired population cannot be ignored.

Studies that have attempted to describe psychological and personality traits of deaf persons have been hampered by the communication problem imposed by the hearing loss. Enough information has been gathered, however, to permit several summary statements concerning the psychological profile of the more severely hearing impaired adult. This information is compiled from Schlesinger and Meadow (1972), Levine (1976), Bolton (1976), Schein (1977), and Schein (1978):

1. They tend to be immature
2. They tend to withdraw, especially from communication situations
3. They tend to be less flexible than a normal hearing adult
4. They tend to adhere rigidly to a set routine
5. They tend to demonstrate a negative self-image; this is due in part to a general lack of information concerning the nature of hearing impairment
6. They tend to have a narrow range of interests
7. They tend to show a lack of social judgment
8. They tend to exhibit a lack of regard for the feelings of others
9. They tend to be more naïve than the hearing adult
10. They tend to be more dependent than the hearing adult
11. They tend to be irresponsible
12. They tend to be impulsive
13. They tend to be passive and overaccepting, especially if the loss occurred early
14. They tend to be depressed, but generally in cases where the hearing impairment occurred later in life

It must be stressed, however, that a description of the typical psychological profile of a hearing impaired adult is impossible. The above characteristics are offered only as possibilities, and no one will fit the mold exactly. These traits are frequently observed, but their emergence in any one case will depend on several factors, primarily age of onset and degree of hearing loss. The psychological characteristics of a hearing impaired population are as varied as they are in a normal hearing group. This point is stressed by Bolton when he concludes that the personality characteristics of a hearing impaired population are not due to the hearing loss, but rather they are due to the environment into which the loss places the individual.

SOCIAL PROFILE

The social characteristics of the hearing impaired population can be described in part by examining geographic distribution. Table 3-4 contains a breakdown of the location of this population by region. The highest prevalence rate occurs in the North Central area for the deaf and for the prevocationally deaf groups. The West, however, has the highest prevalence for all hearing impaired. The lowest rates occur in the Northeast for all three groups, and these rates appear to be significantly lower than the other regions. These figures allow at least rough predictions to be made concerning the location of deaf communities which will be in need of rehabilitation services.

Table 3-4
Distribution of Hearing Impaired Population by Regions:
United States, 1971

Regions*	Hearing Impaired	Deaf	Prevocationally Deaf
United States	13,362,842	1,767,046	410,522
Northeast	2,891,380	337,022	83,909
North Central	3,683,226	541,465	135,653
South	4,280,177	562,756	123,260
West	2,508,059	325,803	67,700
	Rates per 100,000 population		
United States	6,603	873	203
Northeast	5,977	697	173
North Central	6,563	965	242
South	6,807	895	196
West	7,170	931	194

Reprinted with permission from Schein, J. D. & Delk, M. T. Jr. *The deaf population of the United States.* Silver Spring, Maryland: National Association of the Deaf, 1974, p. 25.

**Northeast:* Connecticut, Maine, Massachusetts, New Hampshire, New Jersey, New York, Pennsylvania, Rhode Island, Vermont.

North Central: Illinois, Indiana, Iowa, Kansas, Michigan, Minnesota, Missouri, Nebraska, North Dakota, Ohio, South Dakota, Wisconsin.

South: Alabama, Arkansas, Delaware, District of Columbia, Florida, Georgia, Kentucky, Louisiana, Maryland, Mississippi, North Carolina, Oklahoma, South Carolina, Tennessee, Texas, Virginia, West Virginia.

West: Alaska, Arizona, California, Colorado, Hawaii, Idaho, Montana, Nevada, New Mexico, Oregon, Utah, Washington, Wyoming.

Social characteristics of the adult hearing impaired have received more emphasis in recent years. According to Schein and Delk the following summary statements can be made:

The majority of deaf adults have hearing parents. The National Census of the Deaf Population figures show that 91.7 percent of deaf adults fall into this category. Schein and Delk stress the importance of this finding by emphasizing that the majority of parents of these individuals probably had little or no contact with or understanding of hearing impairment prior to its occurrence in their child. This lack of understanding of the problem can affect the social development and adjustment of the individual.

When compared to the general population, deaf individuals marry less often and, when they do, they tend to marry at a later age. This is especially true for men. These data are summarized in Table 3-5. It is interesting to note that the divorce rate in the two populations is very similar. Data from the census also indicated that deaf persons frequently marry other deaf persons, as opposed to hard of hearing or normal hearing individuals, 79.5 percent of the time.

Table 3-5
Percentage Distribution of Marital Status of Deaf Population
Compared to General Population* by Age and Sex: United States, 1972

Respondents' Sex and Age	Marital Status: Single		Married†		Widowed		Divorced	
	Deaf	General	Deaf	General	Deaf	General	Deaf	General
Total	34.1	18.5	60.0	74.3	2.1	3.5	3.8	3.6
16 to 24‡	83.9	57.6	15.4	40.9	0.2	0.2	0.5	1.3
25 to 34	28.3	13.6	77.6	82.0	0.3	0.4	3.8	3.9
35 to 44	17.9	6.3	76.4	87.6	—	1.5	5.7	4.6
45 to 54	13.6	5.9	77.1	84.5	4.1	4.9	5.2	4.7
55 to 64	18.3	6.1	70.1	77.3	7.1	12.8	4.4	3.8
Male	40.3	21.8	55.7	74.3	1.0	1.0	3.0	2.9
16 to 24‡	88.4	67.3	10.6	31.9	0.4	—	0.4	0.7
25 to 34	38.3	17.6	58.5	79.2	—	0.1	3.2	3.0
35 to 44	22.8	7.5	72.0	88.5	—	0.5	5.2	3.5
45 to 54	16.3	7.3	77.5	87.2	1.1	1.5	5.1	4.0
55 to 64	20.8	5.8	73.7	87.4	4.2	3.5	1.4	3.3
Female	27.5	15.4	64.5	74.3	3.3	5.9	4.7	4.3
16 to 24‡	78.1	48.8	21.3	49.2	—	0.3	0.6	1.8
25 to 34	24.6	9.7	71.5	84.7	0.3	0.9	3.6	4.8
35 to 44	12.0	5.2	81.7	86.7	—	2.5	6.3	5.6
45 to 54	11.1	4.5	76.7	82.0	6.9	8.0	5.3	5.4
55 to 64	16.0	6.4	66.7	68.2	10.0	21.2	7.3	4.1

Reprinted with permission from Schein, J. D. & Delk, M. T., Jr. *The deaf population of the United States*. Silver Spring, Maryland: National Association of the Deaf, 1974, p. 39.
*Source: Statistical Abstract of the United States: 1972.
†Includes persons who are separated.
‡General population rates do not include persons 16 and 17 years old.

There are fewer children born to deaf women than to normal hearing women. Also, children born into families in which at least one parent is prevocationally deaf have normal hearing 88 percent of the time.

Additional data on the social characteristics of the deaf are being compiled by Emerton at the National Technical Institute for the Deaf and are described by Johnson (1978). The information is being gathered through a battery of tests that is being designed to obtain a social profile of a deaf individual within five areas. Although it is stressed that the data are still preliminary, the following statements by Johnson are made based on profile results from 295 of the entering students at NTID:

1. In terms of social knowledge, about 13 percent performed at a level expected for college students, 32 percent performed at a high school level, and 55 percent performed at an unsatisfactory level for employment.
2. In terms of social decision making, 95 percent needed improvement, while 84 percent needed improvement in social reasoning.
3. In terms of various levels of interaction, interpersonal was significantly better than group interaction, but it was still relatively low.
4. In terms of social behavior, about 66 percent were considered to be performing at a college level, while 34 percent needed improvement.
5. In terms of career development, 78 percent were below college level. This included performance on tests that measured work-related skills and attitudes.

Again, as with psychological factors, it is important to stress that these characteristics must be considered only as general trends. Rehabilitative programs must still be tailored to individual needs and not to a sterotyped group.

ECONOMIC PROFILE

The economic problems of the severely hearing impaired adult population appear to involve both unemployment and underdevelopment. A large part of the problem may be attributed to the myths concerning deafness and ignorance on the part of many employers as to the capabilities of the hearing impaired. In a survey of Baltimore manufacturing firms, 32 percent of the employers indicated that deafness was the handicap that would most likely prevent them from hiring an applicant. Total deafness ranked fourth after total blindness, mental retardation, and epilepsy (Fellendorf, Atelsek, and Mackin, 1971).

The unemployment data compiled by Schein and Delk indicated that the problem was less severe for deaf men than for the general population. Deaf men showed 2.9 percent unemployment, as compared to 4.9 percent for men in general. Deaf women on the other hand, showed 10.2 percent unemployment as compared to a general female unemployment figure of 6.6 percent. The greatest unemployment for the deaf was seen in the 16-to-24-year age group for both men and women.

If the principal occupations of the severely hearing impaired population are compared to the principal occupations of the general population, part of the unemployment problem is revealed. This comparison is made in Table 3-6. The majority of deaf workers are in the craftsman and operatives areas and have traditionally been in positions that allow little upward mobility. The occupations requiring a great deal of communication, on the other hand, are seldom held by a deaf individual.

Table 3-6
Percentage Distribution of Employed Deaf versus General Population, Adults (16 to 64 Years of Age), by Principal Occupation: United States, 1972

	Percentage of Population	
Principal Occupation	Deaf	General
All occupations	100.0	100.0
Professional and technical	8.8	14.2
Managers and administrators (nonfarm)	1.4	11.0
Sales	0.5	6.4
Clerical	15.0	16.9
Craftsman	21.3	12.7
Operatives, nontransit and transit	35.9	16.2
Laborers (nonfarm)	6.2	5.0
Farmers, farm managers, and farm laborers	1.6	4.0
Service workers	9.2	13.5
Private household workers	0.2	—

From *Hearing and Deafness,* 4th ed., by Hallowell Davis and S. Richard Silverman. Copyright 1947, (©) 1960, 1970 by Holt, Rinehart and Winston, Inc. Copyright (©) 1978 by Holt, Rinehart and Winston. Reproduced by permission of Holt, Rinehart and Winston.

A primary indicator of the economic status of the hearing impaired population is individual income level. Schein and Delk report a median personal income level for deaf individuals of $5915, as compared with a median level of $8188 for the general population. Those in the professional and technical occupation category earn the most, as might be expected. The authors also note that yearly earnings were the least for the congenitally impaired population, while income was the highest for those whose hearing loss occurred after the age of six.

SUMMARY

The information presented in this chapter offers an emerging profile of the psychosocial and economic characteristics of the adult deaf population. It must be stressed that this is also a changing profile. In light of new educational opportunities, improved training programs for professionals who deal with deafness, and the emergence of advocates for the rights of the handicapped, the profile will be altered. Hopefully, in time, the differences created by a loss of hearing will be minimized.

REFERENCES

Bolton, B. Introduction and overview, in B. Bolton (Ed.), *Psychology of deafness for rehabilitation counselors*. Baltimore: University Park Press, 1976, pp. 1–18.

Fellendorf, G., Atelsek, F., & Mackin, E. *Diversifying job opportunities for the adult deaf*. Washington, D.C.: Alexander Graham Bell Association for the Deaf, 1971.

Goulder, T. J. Federal and state mental health programs for the deaf in hospitals and clinics. *Mental Health in Deafness*, 1977, *1*, 13–17.

Johnson, D. D. The adult deaf client and rehabilitation, in J.G. Alpiner (Ed.), *Handbook of adult rehabilitative audiology*. Baltimore: Williams and Wilkins, 1978, pp. 172–221.

Levine, E. S. Psycho-cultural determinants in personality development. *Volta Review,* 1976, *78,* 258–267.

Schein, J. D. Psychology of the hearing impaired consumer. *Audiology and Hearing Education,* 1977, *3,* 12–14, 44.

Schein, J. D. The deaf community, in H. Davis and S.R. Silverman (Eds.), *Hearing and deafness* (4th Ed.). New York: Holt, Rinehart and Winston, 1978, pp. 511–524.

Schein, J. D., & Delk, M. T. Jr. *The deaf population of the United States.* Silver Spring, Maryland: National Association of the Deaf, 1974.

Schlesinger, H. S., & Meadow, K. P. *Sound and sign: Childhood deafness and mental health.* Berkeley: University of California Press, 1972.

Section 2: The Aural Rehabilitation Process
A. Amplification

Roger N. Kasten

Chapter 4: Determination of the Need for Amplification

Advances in the technology of hearing aids over the past 20 years have been tremendous. Indeed, at the present time there are hearing aids available with gain values between 10 and 20 dB and with saturation sound pressure level (SPL) values in the 80–90 dB range. There also are instruments with gain in excess of 80 dB and saturation sound pressure levels approaching 150 dB. At the same time, aids can be built or modified to provide an extended low frequency response, a broad flat frequency response, or a very peaked high frequency response. Aids have been designed that can be worn on the body, at the location of the ear, or in the ear. Magnitude of hearing loss or shape of audiometric configuration no longer appears to be a deterrent to successful hearing aid use.

Although such advances have enhanced success rates among those who require amplification, the task of adequate and accurate fitting of amplification is still far from simple. All too frequently we come in contact with the individual who has owned two, three, four or more hearing aids and who indicates that he or she will never again purchase another hearing aid because none of them are any good. While it is true that many of these individuals have come in contact with inappropriate amplification, it is also true that many appropriate amplification systems have come in contact with inappropriate individuals. The purpose of this chapter will be to discuss many of the factors important for the determination of need for amplification.

PSYCHOLOGICAL ACCEPTANCE

Carhart (Note 1) discussed the minimum criteria for a hearing aid being considered for recommendation for use. He pointed out that a hearing aid should not cause any special problems for the user. He also strongly stated that the potential hearing aid user should be psychologically ready for the hearing aid, and more importantly, the hearing aid should be psychologically acceptable to the individual. These are factors that must be kept continuously in mind during an initial evaluation for potential hearing aid use.

Consider, for example, the individual who indicates he or she will only consider a hearing aid built into eyeglasses. This is a logical statement for a potential hearing aid user to make until we observe that the individual uses eyeglasses only sporadically and frequently employs them as an extension of the hand in the process of emphatic gesturing. Such individuals may be either consciously or subconsciously making the point that they are not yet psychologically ready for hearing aid use. Consider also the trial lawyer who indicates that he genuinely needs help in the courtroom situation but refuses the use of amplification because he feels that a hearing aid will make him look incompetent and unreliable. In these instances, we are dealing with individuals who see the hearing aid as psychologically unacceptable.

Most likely, all audiologists or hearing aid dealers could come up with examples of these apparently cantankerous and unreasonable adults. Indeed, what we are usually viewing are individuals whose fear of this unknown and foreign device has overridden their need for help. It is essential, however, that we not forget the psychological problems that can develop concurrently with the assessment for hearing aid use.

ATTITUDES

Attitudes of the Client

It would appear that many clients do not voice their sentiments regarding hearing aid use until they reach what they see as a point of no return. At that time, they suddenly apply unreasonable conditions to potential hearing aid use and offer unfavorable attitudes or opinions regarding amplification in general. All too often we attribute this condition to poor motivation. Rather than motivation, however, what we may be viewing is a psychological rejection. The audiologist would be in a far better position if a genuinely favorable and optimistic outlook regarding hearing aid use had been developed prior to the consumer's negative reactions. The psychological rejection of amplification usually appears on a purely emotional level. If these rejections are brought forth prior to any consideration of the real values and benefits to be derived from hearing aid use, the audiologist or hearing aid dealer is placed on the defensive and is put in a position of having to defend his or her recommendation for hearing aid use. On the other hand, if a favorable, optimistic attitude toward hearing aid use is generated at the very beginning of the total evaluative process, a negative reaction on a purely emotional level becomes far more difficult for the individual to defend, particularly to him or herself.

Attitudes of the Family

Another primary determinant of need and potential success is the attitude of the user's family toward amplification. In most instances, it is not enough to work with a potential adult hearing aid user, but rather it is necessary to work with a family that will have in it an adult hearing aid user. Negative family reactions can frequently undo the most diligent counseling and fitting procedures developed by the audiologist. Most individuals view hearing aid use with fairly definite preconceived ideas. These ideas are generated from persons they have known in the past or from stories they have heard about hearing aids or hearing aid users. When the ideas have a negative cast, the purveyors of gloom will always be able to find situations to demonstrate that their concepts are correct.

Family members should be brought into the counseling scheme at the earliest possible time. Husbands, wives, or children should be made to understand fully the magnitude of the problem. This can be most easily accomplished by having one or more family members seated in the test room with the potential hearing aid user so that they can actually experience the intensity levels needed to overcome the hearing loss. Frequently, family members are aware that the potential hearing aid user has had difficulty hearing and understanding speech, but they are shocked when they experience the intensity level that must be used for a minimal understanding of speech and the pattern of discrimination errors that occur with material that they themselves find readily understandable. This process can do much to make family members champions of the cause. They often become highly supportive and are willing recipients of information regarding hearing aid use and communication in general.

We find family members frequently are critical factors in determining not only need for amplification but potential success with amplification. An adult may have a truly demonstrated need for amplification in a variety of settings. If these settings represent difficult listening situations, the potential for success can be unlimited. With knowledgable and understanding family members, the difficult listening situation can be structured or at least understood so that the lack of complete communicative improvement will not be self-defeating.

Motivation

A major psychological factor to be recognized within the adult population is individual motivation. The adult may demonstrate a genuine need for amplification but if motivation is lacking, the likelihood for successful hearing aid use is sharply restricted. Stated differently, a lack of motivation does not affect a person's need for amplification but does have a genuine influence upon his or her potential use.

Improper motivation can be the result of many divergent factors. Individuals may completely fail to realize the extent of the problem that they are experiencing. They may, in fact, be relatively well satisfied with the amount of auditory input they are receiving and be unwilling to make a change that will force an alteration of their accepted life style. They may have had experiences with others who have attempted hearing aid use and have found it to be unacceptable and truly unsuccessful. They may react to the cost of a hearing aid and rationalize that something so small cannot be worth that much money. Whatever the reason, as long as they can justify not trusting the device, they can justify not wanting it. Proper motivation is not something that can be readily taught. Indeed, it is a concept that must often be learned as a result of self-discovery.

Potential hearing aid users can be shown the amount of help that they can obtain. We can demonstrate their change in performance in conversational listening settings. We can allow family members to become enthused and excited over the change in performance that can be observed. We can demonstrate that hearing aids can be worn successfully and can provide improvement in many situations. What we cannot do is force someone to change his or her attitude. The poorly motivated adult is much like the horse that can only be led to water. The ultimate decision, transcending observable need, is a decision that will have to be made by each and every potential hearing aid user. The poorly motivated adult, already accustomed to making his or her own decisions, if forced into hearing aid use can find many excuses to demonstrate that his or her original distrust of the instrument was well founded. When this situation occurs, we simply become party to the individual's internalized belief that he or she has no need or can achieve no success. In short, while motivation, as a factor, does not affect the real need for amplification, it can have an overwhelming effect on the individual's self-assessment of his or her need for amplification. The audiologist must, of necessity, be very cautious in dealing with the poorly motivated potential hearing aid user since an overly aggressive approach to the acquisition of amplification can reinforce the already abundant negative viewpoint.

THE DEGREE AND CONFIGURATION OF THE HEARING LOSS

It should be clear at the very beginning that the degree and configuration of a hearing loss are not actually determinants of an individual's need for amplification. The person's need and desire for help are the primary determinants. The degree and the configuration of the hearing loss will not determine the need, but will determine, at least in part, the degree of success that the user may experience.

Over the years, a rule of thumb seems to have emerged which indicates that people with less than 40 dB loss (re: American National Standards Institute [ANSI], 1969) in their better ear do not need amplification. In fact, Silverman and Pascoe (1978) state, "Generally, if the hearing level for speech in the better ear is worse than 40 dB, a hearing aid is needed." Some audiologists have objected to such rulings and have placed hearing aids on individuals with a hearing loss less than 40 dB, based primarily upon the individual's stated need. These pioneers of hearing aid fitting were actually following a concept learned many years ago by traditional hearing aid dealers. Need for amplification is not based upon a numerical value pulled from an audiogram, but rather upon the stated needs expressed by the potential hearing aid user.

In fact, viewed objectively, it seems rather presumptuous to state a numerical lower limit beyond which a hearing aid is not needed. Rather, it seems far more logical to free ourselves from the enslavement of the numerical values obtained from an audiogram and utilize instead the life-style and the expressed needs of the affected individual. Indeed, if one considers the communicative environment of the trial attorney, the librarian, the loan officer in a bank, or the mother concerned about hearing the faint cries of a new baby, it is difficult to rationalize any decibel value as representing a cutoff intensity for the determination of need for amplification.

Mild Hearing Losses

Mild hearing losses simply call for mild amplification systems. As a general rule, the individual with a very mild hearing loss has a specific need for audiotory help and can become a very successful part-time hearing aid user. Stated differently, hearing aid use should be tailored to the unique needs of the individual. Obviously, not all individuals with very mild hearing losses will demonstrate a need for amplification. Where needs become apparent, however, we should all be responsive to the desires of the individuals and should not glibly inform them that their hearing is "still too good."

Table 4-1
General Guide to the Relationship between Hearing Loss and Need for Amplification, Based on Pure Tone Average of Speech Reception Threshold in the Better Ear

Hearing Loss in dB re: 1969 ANSI* Norms	Need for Amplification
0–25	No need
25–40	Part time need for special occasions
40–55	Frequent need
55–80	Area of greatest satisfaction
80+	Great need—partial help

*American National Standards Institute.
Reprinted with permission from Hodgson, W.R., & Skinner, P. *Hearing aid assessment and use in audiologic habilitation.* Baltimore: Williams and Wilkins, 1977, p. 129.

Hearing Losses of Greater Degree

As we consider the broad continuum of potential hearing losses, it should be clear that the need for amplification will increase as the magnitude of the hearing loss increases. When the unaided speech reception threshold exceeds 40 dB, we should realize that the individual is now experiencing major difficulties with the reception and understanding of average conversational speech. If we make the logical assumption that successful reception and understanding of speech is a primary determinant in the need for amplification, then need for amplification will increase markedly as the hearing loss exceeds the level of average conversational speech.

Additional increases in the magnitude of the hearing loss bring forth additional needs on the part of the hearing impaired person. The individual is not only cut off from speech communication, but is progressively excluded from environmental sounds and even primitive contact with the world around him or her. As a guideline, once the hearing loss exceeds a level of 60 dB in the better ear, the individual is deprived of most environmental contact with events of low to moderate intensity. Commonplace events like the ringing of the telephone, the opening or closing of doors, the running of automobile engines, or the ringing of doorbells become lost. The need for amplification when the hearing loss reaches these levels is concerned not only with the proper delivery of usable speech but with maintaining contact with environmental activities. Hodgson and Skinner (1977) have presented the general guide relating to need for amplification which is shown in Table 4-1.

Note that Hodgson and Skinner label the hearing loss range from 55 to 80 dB as being the "area of greatest satisfaction." This is not necessarily meant to indicate that adults whose thresholds fall in that range will receive more satisfaction from amplification than any other, but simply to indicate that adults whose thresholds fall in that range are so dependent on amplified sound that they express the greatest degree of satisfaction from it. Individuals in this hearing loss category are sufficiently isolated from speech and environmental sound that social or vocational pursuits are markedly restricted unless amplification is utilized on a routine basis.

Not surprisingly, as the magnitude of the hearing loss increases, the degree of acoustic isolation increases and the need for continuous amplification increases. Beyond the 80 dB hearing level, need for amplification is at its greatest, but the potential for successful hearing aid use is restricted. Stated differently, every hearing aid user will reject amplification that reaches or exceeds his or her thresholds of discomfort or pain. This means that as the magnitude of the hearing loss increases, the dynamic range of sound available through a hearing aid is progressively reduced. Thus, the adult with a severe to profound hearing loss may be able to achieve only a markedly restricted dynamic range due to the close proximity of his or her threshold of hearing and pain. This can readily explain why many adults with severe to profound hearing losses indicate that they use their hearing aids to retain a degree of contact with their environment but actually find the hearing aids have only marginal value for the process of speech communication. Even with this complaint, however, the severely to profoundly hearing impaired adult, with appropriate auditory training and hearing aid use, can still maintain close contact with the acoustic environment and can prevent the syndrome of isolation and withdrawal that is frequently associated with the nonamplified individual.

The Adult Deaf

We must recognize that many people classified as ''adult deaf'' have not and will not use hearing aids. Some of these individuals indicate that they have never used a hearing aid and do not believe that amplification would be of any benefit to them in their present life-style. Others indicate that they have tried to use hearing aids in the past but have been unsuccessful with them. It is this writer's opinion that both of these explanations are accurate and are a reflection of the marginal auditory care that has been available to the deaf in the past. Recently, however, Gauger and McPherson (1978) reported on a program being carried out at the National Technical Institute for the Deaf which is designed to introduce college-age deaf individuals to successful hearing aid use. They utilized NTID students who had not previously used amplification or who had been unable to use amplification successfully and reported an encouraging degree of success. Their program has recently been made available from the National Technical Institute for the Deaf and should be utilized by audiologists who find themselves working with an adult deaf population.

Configuration of Hearing Loss

If we turn our attention to configuration of hearing loss as a determinant of need for amplification, we again find an optimistic picture. While it is true that some hearing loss configurations are far easier to fit than others, we have reached a point in technology where configuration of loss, as a single factor, should not be a primary determinant to successful hearing aid fitting or use.

Hearing aids are presently available with extended low frequency emphasis, with a broad, relatively flat frequency response, and also with a sharply increased high frequency response. Figure 4-1 gives an indication of the extent of low frequency emphasis that is now available. Figure 4-2 shows the extent to which a relatively flat frequency response configuration can be achieved. Figure 4-3 portrays the degree of high frequency emphasis that can be achieved with present-day technology. As a matter of fact, hearing aid frequency response can be modified, either through hearing aid circuitry or through earmold modification, to provide virtually any type of frequency response characteristic needed for complex fitting schemes. While it has been relatively common in the past to

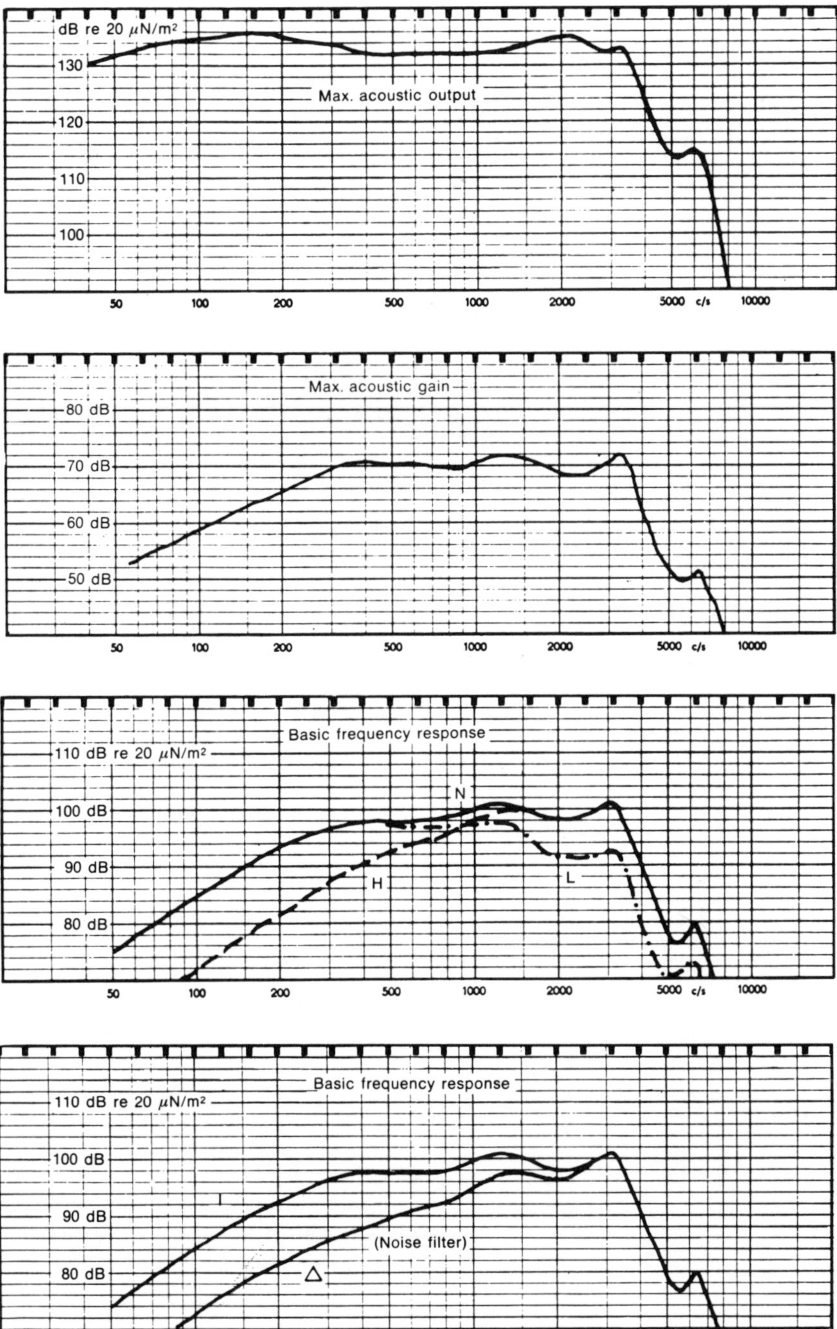

Fig. 4-1. Frequency response characteristics of Danavox Model 727 PPE. (Reprinted with permission from Danavox Inc., Eden Prairie, Minnesota.)

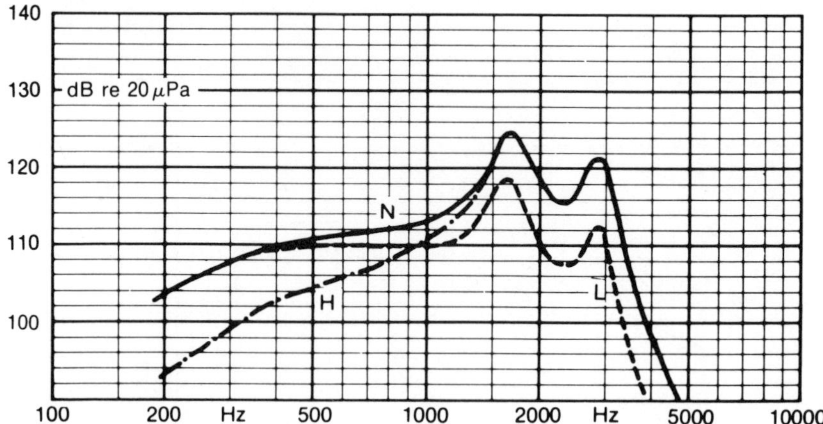

Fig. 4-2. Frequency response curve and effect of tone control—characteristics of Oticon Model P11P. (Reprinted with permission from Oticon Corp., Somerset, New Jersey.)

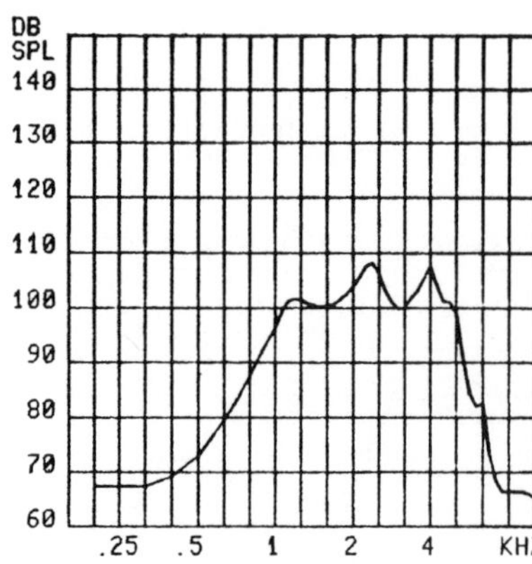

Fig. 4-3. Frequency response run at 60 dB input—characteristics of Siemens Model #66 H. (Reprinted with permission from Siemens Hearing Instruments, Inc., Union, New Jersey.)

depend on a broad and flat frequency response characteristic for the most successful fittings, both high or low frequency response modifications are now obtainable. Indeed, a great deal of effort has been put forth within the hearing aid industry to design hearing aids with limited low frequency amplification and a relatively spiked high frequency response characteristic. A careful examination of the manufacturer's specification sheets for currently available hearing aids will reveal the preponderance of models providing predominantly high frequency amplification.

The Difficult-to-Fit Client

The one category of individuals still creating significant problems in terms of appropriate hearing aid fitting are individuals with a relatively narrow high frequency loss who complain of reduced speech discrimination ability or deteriorating quality of sound input. Often, the narrow range of hearing deficit will be centered around 4000 or 6000 Hz. For the most part, these individuals are describing a very real problem in terms of their perceived auditory deficit. Attempts to provide these individuals with a very narrow spike of amplification appropriate for their specific needs have met with only limited degrees of success. These individuals, in the clinical setting, tend to complain of overamplification or tend to indicate that the hearing aid system does not improve their perceived deficit to the degree that they anticipated. They may, in fact, describe sound as having a relatively hollow quality. They also describe amplified sound as being relatively strident.

These individuals may very well be the one category with whom present technology is yet unable to deal successfully. Although present hearing aids can be tailored to provide a variety of unique frequency response characteristics, the sharply accentuated or spiked frequency response, particularly in the higher frequency region, is not easily achievable.

LEVELS OF SOPHISTICATION

The Audiologist

As we deal with the needs of the hearing impaired population, the audiologist or hearing aid dispenser must be fully conversant with all of the developments within the hearing aid and earmold industries. In many respects this also means that to meet the needs of each specific hearing impaired adult, it is frequently necessary to be conversant with the full armamentarium of systems provided by a variety of hearing aid manufacturers or earmold manufacturers. The individual involved in the fitting or dispensing of hearing aids can no longer be content with a cursory knowledge of products available from a single manufacturer or supplier. As sophistication in product design has increased, sophistication in the fitting of the product must also increase.

The Client

When we speak of sophistication, we must also consider sophistication on the part of the hearing aid user. We have, in recent years, seen the advent of hearing aid systems with multiple control settings. In addition to single units with variable controls, we have also seen an increase in the recommendation and fitting of the contralateral routing of signals (CROS) or front routing of signals (FROS) family of instruments. As all of these instruments have increased in complexity, the level of expertise required of the hearing aid user has increased proportionally. With the CROS family of aids, for example, most evaluators or fitters of hearing aids have dealt with adults who attempt to cope with the instrument but reject it after a brief period of use. The reasons they give are frequently rather nondescript, since they do not wish to admit that the device simply is too complex for them to master.

When we deal with the individual whose unique requirements demand the utilization of one of the CROS family of aids, it is imperative that time be spent in teaching the individual to become the master of the instrument. Unless the hearing impaired person can reach this stage of sophistication, it really makes little difference how much he or she is in need of amplification. If the adult cannot learn successfully to use the device, the practicality of the situation will override the need for the hearing aid and the instrument will be rejected. The audiologist is forced into making a choice when dealing with this type of individual and when attempting to meet the unique needs of the hearing impaired adult in terms of amplification. If the individual's specific requirements demand an instrument of some complexity, then a great deal of additional time must be spent with the person or with the family in teaching them a mastery of the instrument. If complete mastery of the instrument cannot be achieved, then it is absolutely necessary to move to a less complex, and perhaps even less suitable, hearing aid. At any rate, when we consider the need of the individual for amplification, we must pay careful attention not only to the strict auditory manifestations, but also to the ability of the individual to control his or her own amplification system.

TOLERANCE

Tolerance problems with hearing aids have been a matter of controversy for many years. In the true American tradition, individuals fitting hearing aids have attempted to provide the maximum possible amplification to each hearing impaired person. In accomplishing this task, we have attempted to provide a hearing aid with enough amplification that it can, at least in part, overcome the effects of the threshold hearing loss. At the same time, we strive to provide an instrument that will retain, as much as possible, the natural clarity of speech. In addition, we have attempted to provide each hearing impaired person with as much amplification as possible without having the amplified sound cause discomfort or pain.

The absolute degree of success in achieving these three goals has been a matter of real concern. We are aware that many hearing impaired individuals have purchased hearing aids and yet refuse to use them. We are also aware that many hearing impaired individuals have purchased several hearing aids and are unsatisified with all of them. Unfortunately, there are no stable figures which will allow us to determine what percentage of the total population of hearing aid owners turn out to be hearing aid rejectors. Also, we really have no definitive data which will allow us to speak accurately to the situation that causes hearing aid owners to reject their instruments. Briskey (Note 2) estimated that 70 percent of the hearing aid owners who reject their instruments do so because the saturation sound pressure level is too great. Stated differently, he is indicating that these people experience tolerance problems with loud sound and ultimately terminate hearing aid use rather than live with this new problem. Clinical experience, and discussions with others involved with the fitting of hearing aids, would suggest that Briskey's estimate is probably quite accurate.

Comfort versus Discomfort

A number of methods have been used over the years to determine an individual's threshold of discomfort or threshold of pain. Measurements have been made using pure tones, narrow band noise, single speech words, cold running speech and acoustic reflexes. All of these methods have real value, but the ultimate accuracy of each method is only as great as the individual conducting the measurement. One of the major problems we have had to deal with in accurate fitting of hearing aids to adults is the establishment of a saturation sound pressure level that will not violate the hearing impaired individual's loudness reaction. Fitters of hearing aids have rigorously attempted to provide the hearing impaired person with as high a saturation sound pressure level as possible, since that will give to the hearing impaired individual a maximum of acoustic dynamic range. If this attempt is successful, the hearing impaired individual receives as much sound as his or her auditory system is capable of receiving. The intent of this effort is laudable.

Unfortunately, it appears that many hearing aid fittings violate the hearing impaired individual's demand for comfort. The reasons for this violation may be many. A great number of evaluations of hearing aid performance are conducted in very quiet settings. The individual appears to be able to handle loud sound in the quiet setting but finds everyday environmental sound to be more than he or she is capable of utilizing. The actual process of determining a threshold of discomfort or threshold of pain may be the real culprit. In many instances, hearing impaired individuals are instructed to indicate when sound has become uncomfortable or painful. They are told that they should pick the point where they would no longer wish to receive any more sound or to identify that intensity which just borders on either discomfort or pain. In this type of situation, many hearing impaired adults listen to the instructions, view the procedure as some type of test, and resolutely attempt to provide the best possible performance for the examiner. In so doing, they wait until the last possible moment and finally identify their tolerance level at some intensity greater than their real tolerance level. If the evaluator or fitter of hearing aids accepts these responses without question, the ultimate usage of the instrument by the hearing impaired individual is in jeopardy.

Since tolerance ceilings for loud sound can vary markedly among hearing impaired persons, it is critical that the measurement of this type of threshold value be accomplished carefully and accurately. There is no reason at the present time for an individual with a tolerance ceiling of 96 dB SPL to be less successful in hearing aid use than an individual with a tolerance ceiling of 130 dB SPL, except in special cases. As the tolerance ceiling is reduced, the hearing impaired individual must learn to exist with a reduced dynamic range, which is often realistically accomplished by utilizing a reduced gain. This can be accomplished with peak clipping instruments through an actual reduction in the amount of gain available from the instrument, or can more easily be accomplished through the use of one of a variety of compression systems. With the compression or automatic gain control systems, the gain of the hearing aid is automatically manipulated in the presence of loud environmental sounds so that the aid is not driven into saturation. If only a peak clipping aid is appropriate for the specific individual, the available gain from the aid must be kept sufficiently low in order to prevent having the instrument driven repeatedly into saturation. The peak clipping aid can prevent sound from becoming uncomfortably loud, but in the process may generate excessive amounts of harmonic distortion if the instrument is repeatedly driven into saturation. With this in mind, it is frequently advisable to turn to automatic gain control circuitry whenever possible, in order to provide comfortable sound without high levels of signal distortion.

No rigid rules exist that dictate potential users' satisfaction as a function of aided tolerance levels. It is vitally important, however, that the individual's aided tolerance levels be measured with any instrument considered for fitting. For example, if a person can comfortably tolerate environmental sound in the range from 80–90 dB SPL with the aid at its use setting, he or she will probably be able to function with that particular instrument without any adverse tolerance reactions. If, in the aided setting, the hearing impaired person can only tolerate levels in the 70–80 dB SPL range, the hearing aid may well be inappropriate, or the individual will need extensive counseling and orientation in order to achieve successful hearing aid use. On the other hand, with the hearing aid at the use setting, if the individual can only tolerate environmental sounds of less than 70 dB SPL, it is highly unlikely that the instrument is performing appropriately for that person's specific needs. It is also unlikely that the person will be able to achieve successful hearing aid use with that particular fitting. Obviously, intensity values of the type just described are nothing more than guidelines, but these guidelines do tend to delineate rather clearly the potential for success with specific hearing aid systems.

Overamplification

One question that is frequently asked is, "Can a hearing aid do any damage to the hearing that I have left?" For adults, the answer to this question must be made indirectly. Harford and Markle (1955), Macrae (1968), Kasten and Braunlin (1970), and Jerger and Lewis (1975) have all indicated the damaging effect that relatively high-powered hearing aids can have upon the residual hearing of children. Indeed, the Food and Drug Administration (1977) feels that the evidence is sufficiently strong that their regulations require certain high-powered instruments to carry the warning, "Caution: This hearing aid has a maximum sound pressure level capability greater than 132 decibels (dB). Special care should be exercised in selecting and fitting hearing aids of this type as there may be risk of impairing the remaining hearing of the hearing aid user." The FDA regulation clearly does not differentiate between the potential effect of high intensity amplification on children or adults.

It seems reasonable to assume, however, that relatively high output hearing aids which have a deleterious effect upon the residual hearing of children can have the same type of effect on the hearing of adults. Unfortunately, almost all audiologic investigations in this area have tended to center upon children because children make up a more captive population. The one investigation that utilized adult subjects was conducted by Naunton (1957) and does not seem appropriate for this discussion. Naunton chose to use in his subject population a large number of individuals with otosclerosis who effectively possessed a built-in pad between the hearing aid receiver and their cochleas. Thus, although the adults in Naunton's investigation failed to show threshold shifts, the subject population that he selected was such that a lack of threshold shift was almost guaranteed.

Since clear documentation exists that changes in threshold level can result from hearing aid use with some children, it seems reasonable to require very close monitoring of threshold levels in adults who utilize high-output hearing aids. It is rarely adequate to rely upon the hearing aid user exclusively to report the existence of threshold change, but rather the audiologist or the hearing aid fitter must carefully monitor the progress of adults utilizing high-powered instruments.

PSYCHOSOCIAL AND VOCATIONAL FACTORS

There is a relatively simplistic point of view that states that any adult with a hearing loss is a potential candidate for a hearing aid. Unfortunately, many factors intervene which can effectively negate the need for amplification. The audiologist or hearing aid fitter must be very sensitive to the overall life-style of the hearing impaired adult before making a firm hearing aid recommendation based upon the existence of a hearing loss alone.

The Life-Style of the Client

Controversies have existed for years over whether a hearing loss is the same as a hearing impairment. Frequently, we come in contact with adults who display a real hearing loss but whose life-style genuinely reveals no hearing impairment. The adults who fall into this category are those who are not denying the existence of a problem, who are not psychologically rejecting potential hearing aid use, who are not poorly motivated, and who are not attempting to be objectionable. Rather, they are individuals for whom the hearing loss does not pose a real problem. They frequently come to the attention of the audiologist because one individual in their total environment has suggested the possibility of a hearing loss.

For the most part, these are adults who live in a family environment that already generates enough intensity to overcome effectively the loss of sensitivity. Their spouses or children already are compensating for the potential problem, and they really do not see the individual with a hearing loss as one who possesses a significant problem. Often, these individuals engage in social activities that are designed in such a way that a hearing loss does not represent a hearing impairment.

If we consider the large groups of adults whose hobbies include such activities as trap or skeet shooting, square dancing or water skiing, it is genuinely difficult to justify the recommendation of a hearing aid to improve social contacts. On the other hand, if we consider the large number of social activities or hobbies that call for solitary participation, it is equally difficult to justify a hearing aid recommendation based upon improved social awareness alone.

A careful examination of individual life-style will readily reveal the existence or lack of a true hearing impairment. In those instances where the hearing loss does not result in a real hearing impairment, we accomplish little by trying to convince the adult with a hearing loss, or the family of that adult, that he or she truly does have a problem. Indeed, the problem in these situations tends to lie with the audiologist or the hearing aid fitter for overzealously trying to supply help where help is neither needed or wanted.

The audiologist or the hearing aid fitter must carefully consider the life-style described by the adult with the hearing loss in order to determine accurately whether a problem is being denied or whether a problem truly does not exist. This is particularly important when the individual with the hearing loss is the only person providing information relating to his or her life-style. The existence of a real hearing impairment quickly determines the course of events to be followed in the remediation process. As stated earlier, most individuals who describe an auditory problem can be helped by means of amplification and remediation. An attempt to proceed with the evaluation and fitting of amplification for the individual who does not perceive the existence of the impairment, or who does not have an impairment, can only result in confusion, suspicion, and distrust.

Vocational Considerations

Determining the need for amplification on the basis of vocational problems tends to be far more manageable. The individual who experiences auditory problems in a conventional vocational communicative setting can very often receive a great deal of assistance from amplification. Unfortunately, many hearing impaired adults experience significant communicative problems in a highly noisy and chaotic work environment and genuinely hope for relief from this situation through the use of a hearing aid. Unaided difficult listening in that environment will frequently only become more difficult listening in a more chaotic environment when a hearing aid is worn. In our clinical program we have dealt with a number of individuals whose prime complaint centers around problems generated in a noisy work environment. Not one adult with this type of complaint has demonstrated successful hearing aid use on the job. The difficult unaided listening situation simply becomes a more difficult aided listening situation and the aid is rejected as a poor investment.

Again, the audiologist or the hearing aid fitter needs to explain carefully the potential for success to the hearing impaired adult. It would, indeed, be unfortunate if a hearing impaired adult who was experiencing great difficulties with his or her hearing aid in noisy work conditions totally rejected hearing aid use for all occasions because of lack of success in that one environment. Careful counseling and sensitive orientation can direct the adult toward successful hearing aid use in situations away from the more unsuccessful ones.

SUMMARY

The primary determinant for successful hearing aid use among the adult hearing impaired is the adult him or herself. A properly motivated, psychologically accepting, and knowledgeable adult can become a successful hearing aid user under most conditions. We genuinely need to place greater reliance upon the distinct needs and strengths of the hearing impaired individual and spend less time pontificating over the numerical values derived from the audiogram. This is not to imply that the audiogram is not important. Indeed, the audiogram is critical for successful hearing aid fitting, but is not the only factor for consideration. A comprehensive understanding of the unique characteristics of the hearing impaired adult's life style, coupled with a knowledge of the individual's communicative strengths and weaknesses and his or her specific biases and beliefs, can do much to enhance success in determining the real need for amplification and the potential for success in the use of amplification.

REFERENCES

Carhart, R. C. Personal communication, 1962.

Gauger, J. S., & McPherson, D. L. A support system for hearing aid evaluations. *Journal of the Academy of Rehabilitative Audiology,* 1978, *11*, 66–90.

Harford, E., & Markle, D. M. The atypical effect of the hearing aid on one patient with congenital deafness. *Laryngoscope,* 1955, *65*, 970–972.

Hodgson, W. R. & Skinner, P. *Hearing aid assessment and use in audiologic habilitation.* Baltimore: Williams and Wilkins, 1977.

Jerger, J. F., & Lewis, N. Binaural hearing aids; are they dangerous for children? *Archives of Otolaryngology.* 1975 *101*, 480–483.

Kasten, R. N., & Braunlin, R. J. Traumatic hearing aid usage: A case study. Paper presented before the National Convention of the American Speech and Hearing Association, New York, 1970.

Macrae, J. H. Deterioration of the residual hearing of children with sensory-neural deafness. *Acta Otolaryngologica,* 1968, *66*, 33–39.

Naunton, R. F. The Effect of hearing aid use upon the user's residual hearing. *Laryngoscope,* 1957, *67*, 569–576.

Silverman, S. R., & Pascoe, D. P. Counseling about hearing aids, in H. Davis and S. R. Silverman (Eds.) *Hearing and deafness.* New York: Holt, Rinehart and Winston, 1978.

U.S. Food and Drug Administration. Rules and regulations regarding hearing aid devices; Professional and patient labeling and conditions for sale. *Federal Register,* 1977, 9286–9296.

REFERENCE NOTES

1. Carhart, R. C. Personal communication, 1962.
2. Briskey, R. Saturation sound pressure level and the utilization of hearing aids. Presentation at Wichita State University, Wichita, Kansas, 1975.

Robert M. McLauchlin

Chapter 5: Hearing Aid Orientation for the Adult

Hearing aid orientation should be an essential service associated with all hearing aid selection and hearing aid reevaluation procedures conducted with adults. This chapter explores the need for hearing aid orientation services and emphasizes the importance of individualized planning. Additionally, it suggests involving family members and friends in the orientation process and employing user evaluation scales to assess attitudes, experiences, knowledge, and user performance. This chapter then reviews a variety of hearing aid orientation services, with emphasis on those services that should be common to all hearing aid orientation programs, and discusses the implication of audiologists' dispensing hearing aids. Finally, it speculates on prospects for improved hearing aid orientation services.

NEED FOR HEARING AID ORIENTATION

Members of the audiology profession frequently have expressed the need for hearing aid orientation services for the persons they serve, and many have stated that they offer these rehabilitative services. Problems, however, have occurred with hearing aid users availing themselves of these services or with specialists providing services in an effective and efficient manner. Panel V of an American Speech-Language-Hearing Association (ASHA) Conference on Hearing Aid Evaluation Procedures (Castle, 1967) made the following statement: "All hard-of-hearing patients who receive hearing aids, whether the first hearing aid or a change of aid, should receive hearing aid orientation" (p. 53). ASHA guidelines on the responsibilities of audiologists in the rehabilitation of the auditorily handicapped (1974) emphasized that hearing aid users and their families should be provided information about the use of amplification. The guidelines also mentioned the need for periodic reassessment of the amplification device and the person's adjustment to it. According to these guidelines, professional skills are considered essential in helping hearing impaired persons to improve attitudes and behavior. Many audiology facilities offer hearing aid orientation services, according to survey data. Based on a survey of 214 audiology service programs related to type of service offered, Burney (1972) found that about 87 percent of the programs reported offering "hearing aid orientation."

Many hearing aid users are in need of hearing aid orientation or at least more comprehensive and realistic orientation services, as indicated by the following surveys.

1. A U.S. Public Health Service Survey (1964) revealed that 36.6 percent of persons obtaining hearing aids were unsatisfied and not wearing their aids.
2. Market Facts, Incorporated, conducted a household survey in 1971 commissioned by the National Hearing Aid Society and Hearing Aid Industry Conference (Walker, 1974). Of the hearing impaired respondents not wearing hearing aids, 15 percent indicated they had tried amplification but received no benefit. Of the respondents wearing hearing aids, 58 percent complained about their aids or about related services.
3. According to Rassi and Harford (1968), 38 percent of the respondents on a questionnaire sent to persons who obtained hearing aid selections at Northwestern University reported some problems in adjusting to their hearing aids. Problems included listening in the presence of background noise, hearing amplified speech clearly, and regulating the telephone and gain control. Many of the persons experiencing problems expressed no interest in participating in any additional hearing aid orientation program. Only 25 percent of the respondents indicated any interest in this type of program. Moreover, only about 25 percent of the respondents returned for a recommended hearing aid recheck following a procurement of wearable amplification.
4. In a review of clinical data from the Callier Center for Communication Disorders (Roeser, Campbell, & Brown, 1976), 41 percent of the persons for whom hearing aids were selected did not return to the center for a hearing aid check and follow-up services.
5. A survey conducted for the National Hearing Aid Society by Payne and Payne Consultants (1974) revealed that 37.8 percent of 184 hearing aid purchasers experienced initial negative reactions such as "too loud" or "tinny or raspy." Thirty-seven percent reported having "trouble" with their earmold. When asked if "you are now having trouble with your hearing aid," 18 percent indicated "Yes" and 16.8 percent were "not sure."

Some of the dissatisfaction with wearable amplification can be attributed to unnecessary and inappropriate fittings. This dissatisfaction may result from a distribution system in which the financial needs of sales people with limited knowledge about hearing impairment and amplification are pitted against the rehabilitative needs of hearing impaired citizens. An Intradepartmental Task Force on Hearing Aids of the U.S. Department of Health, Education and Welfare (1975) made the following statement after reviewing studies conducted by consumer interest groups:

> The New York City and Baltimore surveys noted that in over 40 percent of the cases studied, dealers recommended the purchase of a hearing aid when hearing health professionals had determined that the patient could not benefit from the use of such a device. (p. 23)

Similar results were found by consumer interest groups in Michigan and Minnesota, according to this Task Force. Therefore, some of the dissatisfaction with and nonuse of hearing aids by consumers reported in these surveys probably are due to the fitting of unnecessary or inappropriate aids by sales people who have limited knowledge about hearing and wearable amplification.

However, some of the problems encountered by prospective hearing aid users are to be expected and frequently are predictable even when wearable amplification is necessary and appropriately selected. In a survey of hearing aid users whose aids were selected at hearing and speech centers (Blood & Danhauer, 1976), 9.4 percent were dissatisfied with the services. Reasons for the dissatisfaction included "aid is only usable in quiet," "little discussion of practical problems of using hearing," and "can't hear too well." Eleven percent responded that they were not "counseled" about their hearing aid.

These data from surveys thus suggest an appreciable need for hearing aid orientation services and a need to improve the quality of orientation services presently being offered.

INDIVIDUALIZED HEARING AID ORIENTATION PLANNING

As is the case with all rehabilitative procedures, hearing aid orientation cannot be packaged for uniform use with all hearing handicapped persons. Individualized planning is essential for achieving success with any hearing aid orientation program. Panel IV participants in an American Speech-Language-Hearing Association Conference on Hearing Aid Evaluation Procedures (Castle, 1967) recognized that a single hearing aid orientation program is not adaptable for all persons. A brief explanation of the use and maintenance of hearing aids may suffice for previously successful users, whereas an extensive orientation program may be necessary for other persons, according to this panel. The range and extent of hearing aid orientation services should vary with persons depending on individual factors, including:

1. Age of onset and progression of hearing impairment
2. Severity of impairment
3. Present age
4. Previous experience with and understanding of hearing aids
5. Attitude of hearing aid wearer about the use of amplification
6. Attitudes of family members and associates concerning the hearing aid wearer and hearing aid use
7. Personal interests
8. Intelligence and language abilities
9. Complexity of the hearing aid system being used
10. Intended use of the hearing aid
11. The amount and success of previously received rehabilitation
12. The presence of any concomitant impairments such as blindness, mental retardation, psychiatric disorders, or arthritis in the hands

An excellent model of individualized planning for handicapped persons is found in a federal regulation for implementing the education of all handicapped children (US Office of Education, 1977). Even though the model is entitled "Individualized Education Program (IEP)" and is specifically intended for children, the major aspects of this model are applicable for planning hearing aid orientation and other rehabilitative services for adults according to individual needs. There is a written statement indicating what services are needed and appropriate. The statement also includes information on present levels of performance; long range goals and short term objectives; projected dates for initiation and duration of services; services to be provided; and appropriate objective criteria and assessment procedures as well as time lines for determining whether short term objectives are being achieved. Other important aspects associated with IEPs include frequent review, and if deemed necessary, revision of the written program; family and client participation in writing the program; multidisciplinary planning; and programmatic evaluation. Most of these required provisions of the IEP for handicapped children were also mandated earlier for eligible handicapped adults under the Rehabilitation Act of 1973 (US Congress, 1973) in a section entitled "Individualized Written Rehabilitation Program."

Individualized planning is not a new concept for professionals in communicative disorders. In fact, what is required in an individualized education or rehabilitation program is no more extensive than what has long been considered professionally appropriate practice in audiology and speech-language pathology.

INVOLVEMENT OF FAMILY AND FRIENDS IN HEARING AID ORIENTATION

Why is it important to involve family members and friends of hearing aid users in hearing aid orientation programs? There are several reasons, but perhaps the most pervasive is that communication is a social interaction between persons who interchangeably speak and listen. Thus, as the sophistication of the persons who interact with the hearing aid user increases relative to hearing impairment and amplification, substantial improvements in communication can be anticipated.

For example, the wife who habitually has raised the level of her voice during the past five years when speaking to her husband to accommodate his unaided moderate bilateral hearing loss may require some orientation. Without some advice and possibly direct orientation, the wife may continue to speak to her husband in her habitual loud voice and will be perceived by him as speaking too loudly when he is wearing his hearing aid. This situation obviously could contribute to a deterioration in social interaction and satisfactory hearing aid use. An inappropriate solution is for the husband to turn the gain of the hearing aid down when listening to his wife. Unfortunately, the situation may be resolved in this manner without appropriate hearing aid orientation. Resolving the situation in this way might lead to frequent adjustments of the gain control when conversing with his wife and others or with his wife while listening to a radio or television adjusted for his aided comfortable listening level. It also could perpetuate any irritation the family members and friends might have been experiencing in listening to the wife's loud voice. Therefore, both the husband and wife must be advised, and preferably shown during orientation sessions, how to share in the responsibility of helping each other adjust to hearing aid use and achieve improved social interaction.

For another example, satisfactory adjustment to hearing aid use can be jeopardized by family members and friends who have unrealistic expectations about wearable amplification. This can happen even when the hearing aid user clearly understands the limitations of amplification for his or her type of hearing impairment and attempts to explain those limitations to family members and friends. These limitations often have to be explained and demonstrated to family members and friends before understanding occurs. More importantly, the persons who communicate frequently with the hearing aid user should understand how they can help to compensate for residual communicative problems which exist even with the use of amplification by the hearing impaired person.

The user's aided speech discrimination ability, the presence of varying types and intensities of background noise, the direction from which the noise and speech are coming, the speaker's articulation and vocal pitch, the familiarity of the user with the topic of conversation, the distance between the speaker and hearing aid user, the speech reading ability and visual environment, and other factors can all improve or hinder a hearing aid user's ability to perceive a spoken message. For purposes of illustration, assume that a wife has a moderate bilateral loss in hearing sensitivity and a moderate and severe impairment in speech discrimination ability for the left and right ears respectively, and is wearing an aid in the left ear. The husband can appreciably improve his social interation with her by knowing that he may have to (1) initially gain her visual as well as auditory attention; (2) move closer to her; (3) speak to her on her left side; (4) initially identify the topic of conversation; (5) reduce the background noise or improve the speech-to-noise ratio; (6) increase the environmental light or move away from the window with the sun at his back; and (7) remove the pipe from his mouth, before she will perceive a spoken message correctly.

Other reasons for participation of family members and close associates in hearing aid orientation programs may include less confusion about information provided in hearing aid orientation sessions because of the presence of additional listeners who have normal hearing and thus have less chance of perceiving spoken information incorrectly; participation in planning and understanding orientation activities to be performed outside of a clinical setting; and enthusiasm because of being included in the planning and orientation process.

Even a working group of the National Academy of Sciences (1972) recommended that financial support might be provided for a trial period to provide pertinent information to relatives, friends, and occupational associates of hearing impaired adults.

The ultimate hearing aid orientation occurs in the daily communicative activities of the hearing aid user. Therefore, a successful rehabilitation program involves orientation directly or indirectly of all participants in the user's communicative activities. While it is possible in many instances to assist hearing aid users in how to help family members and friends adjust to the person's use of amplification, direct participation of these people in a professionally provided hearing aid orientation may substantially enhance the chances of a successful adjustment to hearing aid use in social, educational, and vocational settings.

USER EVALUATION SCALES

Routine employment of a user evaluation scale is strongly encouraged in assessing hearing aid orientation success. If designed appropriately, a rating scale may serve as a daily or weekly schedule for the hearing aid user to follow and complete during the first few weeks or months of hearing aid use. For example, the user can be asked to take five minutes during each day to check the appropriate responses to several questions and record any new comments or questions. Such a scale is useful in determining the appropriateness of the hearing aid selection and success in hearing aid orientation. Moreover, the scaled data and comments provide information which is helpful in modifying future hearing aid orientation programs and hearing aid selection procedures to better serve hearing impaired adults.

Rating scales developed for assessing communication handicap (High, Fairbanks, & Glorig, 1964; Noble & Atherley, 1970; Alpiner, Chevrette, Glascoe, Metz, & Olsen, 1971; Sanders, 1975; and Giolas, Owens, Lamb, & Schubert, 1979) are useful in helping to determine the settings in which prospective or current hearing aid users are encountering difficulty listening as well as to determine the users' and their associates' attitudes toward their hearing impairments. Rupp, Higgins, & Maurer (1977) have developed a scale to predict the feasibility of hearing aid use for aging persons, thus making it more directly applicable to hearing aid orientation. These scales are discussed in detail in other sections of this text. Finally, Gauger (1978) has developed a series of rating scales and other materials for orienting deaf college students to hearing aid use. These materials are easily adapted for use with other adult hearing aid users.

Working Group 65 of the Committee on Hearing, Bioacoustics, and Biomechanics at the National Academy of Sciences (1972) expressed a need for better and more routine use of user evaluation scales. According to this group, the scales should include the user's assessment of speech intelligibility while wearing the hearing aid in a variety of settings; factors associated with hearing aid acceptance such as ease and comfort of use and social interactions; and the degree of "perceptual" or "cognitive" fatigue related to hearing aid use.

Throughout the following discussion of hearing aid orientation services, frequent reference will be made to using rating scales to quantify attitudes, experiences, knowledge, and user performance.

HEARING AID ORIENTATION SERVICES

Hearing aid orientation may involve only a brief explanation of the adjustments on a newly selected hearing aid for a long-time, sophisticated and successful adult hearing aid user. At the other end of the continuum, individual needs may necessitate an extensive program, including the following information and services:

1. Information about the component parts and controls of hearing aids
2. Practice in fitting, adjusting, and maintaining hearing aids
3. Information about the individual limitations as well as benefits to be derived from amplification
4. Information about why a particular aid was selected
5. How to begin using a newly selected hearing aid
6. Situational training
7. How to trouble-shoot hearing aid problems
8. Knowledge about the legal rights of hearing aid users
9. Counseling
10. Auditory training
11. Speechreading
12. Motivational training
13. Speech production training

Hearing aid orientation need not be restricted to a limited time frame following the selection and fitting of hearing aids. Orientation may continue for several weeks or many months until persons achieve their fullest understanding of hearing aid use and maximum potential performance in operating and communicating with particular amplifying devices. Certain aspects of hearing aid orientation, such as explaining about the component parts and adjustments of hearing aids and the anticipated limitations as well as benefits to be derived from amplification, sometimes might be presented prior to performing a hearing aid selection. Thus, this author suggests that hearing aid orientation not be limited to any specific rehabilitative services or time frame. Moreover, hearing aid orientation programs sometimes are developed for particular groups of hearing aid users, such as the military population (Carhart, 1946), the mentally impaired (Moore, Miltenberger, & Barber, 1969), the deaf college student (Gauger & McPherson, 1978), and the aging (Fay & Smith, 1977, and Hardick, 1977).

Hearing Aid Orientation in Retrospect

Hearing aid orientation was an extensive and integral part of aural rehabilitation programs even at the inception of the audiology profession. Carhart (1946) described the hearing aid selection procedures used with military personnel during World War II, which included activities designed to familiarize adults with hearing aid use. These activities, interestingly, were all carried out prior to the final selection of an individual's hearing aid. The major emphasis on hearing aid orientation in this World War II hearing aid selection program is apparent when reviewing the three goals: (1) to obtain a hearing aid having optimal efficiency in everyday situations for each client; (2) to provide the client with an understanding of hearing aids, establish habits of efficient use, and initiate auricular training; and (3) to help the person foster a full psychologic acceptance of hearing aids.

Preliminary to the Carhart hearing aid selection, orientation activities included an explanation about the person's hearing impairment and handicapping conditions, what to expect and what not to expect from wearing a hearing aid, any special problems which might occur, and group instructions about the hearing aid selection procedures to follow.

In an effort to select a manageable number of hearing aids from the total stock of about 200 instruments for further assessment with each individual, the hearing aid selection began with an informal trial of instruments during an interview. Audiometric and case history information also were used in narrowing the selection to 7–10 aids. Certainly, this trial also served to familiarize military personnel with hearing aids.

The second stage involved a 24-hour trial of each preselected aid with a "listening hour" following every trial. Frequently, 25 to 30 persons participated in a single listening hour. Individuals rated 13 different kinds of controlled sounds on a five-point rating scale for each of the preselected hearing aids. The sounds included six musical, three speech, and five environmental selections. A similar rating was done for each person's ability to localize sound, listen over the phone, and experience a 24-hour trial. Finally, a sound discrimination test was administered. Prospective hearing aid users were allowed to adjust their aids for comfort during all of these listening experiences. These ratings, with a weighted score for the discrimination test, were combined and used in eliminating all but three aids for potential selection. The final selection was made from the three remaining aids based on controlled comparisons of these instruments for speech reception threshold, speech discrimination, tolerance, comfort level, and signal-to-noise ratio tests.

Granted, comprehensive hearing aid orientation activities were possible with these prospective hearing aid users because they were a captive audience for an extended period during which their full-time assignment was to be rehabilitated for return to civilian life or active duty. Moreover, the cost of such a program in its entirety for full-time employed civilians might be prohibitive. Despite these limitations for the general adult population, many aspects of this early hearing aid orientation program are being adapted for use today in familiarizing prospective adult hearing aid users to wearable amplification (Garstecki, 1974, and Hardick, 1977).

This lengthy review of the early Carhart hearing aid selection procedure is intended to be a tribute to one of the founders of the audiology profession. Additionally, it is a reminder that hearing aid orientation was an integral part of audiological services from the very outset of the audiology profession and that these early orientation procedures were comprehensive and novel.

Common Hearing Aid Orientation Services for the Adult

Some services should be common to all hearing aid orientations. The user and preferably also family members and associates should receive eight of the previously mentioned 13 services, including

1. Understanding the function of the component parts and adjustments of hearing aids
2. Practice in fitting, adjusting, and maintaining amplification
3. Understanding the limitations as well as benefits to be derived from amplification by the particular user
4. Knowledge of why the particular aid was selected
5. How to begin using a newly selected hearing aid
6. Situational training
7. How to trouble-shoot hearing aid problems
8. How to exercise a hearing aid user's legal rights

Understanding the Component Parts and Controls of Hearing Aids

It is disheartening to evaluate an apparently intelligent adult who purchased a hearing aid a year earlier but is unable to tell the audiologist the location of the hearing aid microphone or the purpose of this component. Adult hearing aid users should be able to name, locate, and describe the functions of the major hearing aid components, including the microphone, amplifier, battery, receiver, cord, (if a body aid), tubing, (if a glasses or behind-the-ear aid), hook (if a behind-the-ear aid), and earmold. Similarly, they should be able to locate and effectively explain the function of the controls on their aids such as the gain control and on-off, tone, and telephone switches.

This author suggests employing a user performance checklist or rating scale to record whether users can satisfactorily name, locate, and describe the functions of the component parts and controls on their hearing aids. An effective hearing aid orientation must go beyond providing information. It must insure that objectives are accomplished by assessing user understanding and performance. Objectives, as always, will have to be tailored to individual needs and capabilities. For example, the level of understanding and performance may need to be set very high for an electronical engineer or the audiologist runs the risk of embarrassing him or herself and insulting the user. This author has explained the ANSI standards for evaluating the electroacoustic characteristics of hearing aids in substantial detail to an engineer for whom a hearing aid was selected. Conversely, understanding and performance levels may need to be set very low, timelines extended for achieving success, and family members or guardians extensively involved when orientating a mentally impaired adult to amplification.

Practice in Fitting, Adjusting, and Maintaining Amplification

A hearing aid user, particularly a new user, needs more than a description and demonstration of how to fit, operate, and maintain his or her newly selected hearing aid. An assessment of the user's ability to perform these tasks is essential to insure that orientation has been successful. Preferably, this assessment should be done at the time the aid is fitted and again at some follow-up appointment within a month. Again, a simple user-performance checklist or rating scale can be employed to record the user's ability to perform the many fitting, adjustment, and maintenance functions associated with the user's hearing aid. Audiologists should rate a hearing aid user's ability, for example, to connect and disconnect tubing and earmolds to a glasses or behind-the-ear hearing aid, insert and remove the earmold from the ear, operate the hearing aid controls, and change a battery. This performance-based assessment should be used for all hearing aid users. Do not assume that a person is adequately oriented to hearing aid use just because he or she has previously worn a hearing aid.

The hearing aid user should be given a list of maintenance suggestions and preferably be provided an opportunity to demonstrate basic maintenance skills. The following suggestions are only examples of what might be included on a maintenance list:

1. Protect the aid against exposure to excessive heat from sources like hairdryers, radiators, heaters, and closed cars on a hot, sunny day.
2. Avoid exposing the aid to excessive humidity as can occur in rain, saunas, steam baths, or when an aid has been placed in a pocket of pants sent to the laundry.
3. Hearing aid users who perspire heavily should place their aid in a container with silica gel at night to remove the moisture.
4. Prevent hairsprays, insecticides, and other sprays from being directed at the aid.
5. Clean the earmold and tubing with mild soap and water or commercially available cleaining solution periodically or when they are blocked; pipe cleaners work well for clearing foreign debris and water from the inside of the tubing and the earmold channel.
6. Keep the hearing aid away from dogs and small children when not wearing it.
7. Routinely remove the aid from the ear and handle it over a soft surface so that if the aid is dropped, the possibility of damaging it is appreciably reduced.

The list containing these maintenance suggestions can be incorporated with other suggestions on how to trouble-shoot hearing aid problems. Hearing aid manufacturers provide some maintenance suggestions in brochures accompanying new hearing aids.

Limitations and Benefits of Amplification

Prospective hearing aid users, as well as their family members and friends, frequently have unrealistic perceptions about the benefits to be derived from wearable amplification. These perceptions range from total lack of benefit to expectation of ''normal'' hearing. Thus, these perceptions must be explored if audiologists hope to achieve success in acquainting hearing aid users and the persons with whom they communicate to amplification. A very positive, though realistic, approach may be required with the person or family member who is extremely skeptical about the benefits of amplification.

Conversely, a skeptical approach may be needed for an individual who expects a hearing aid to resolve all of his or her hearing problems, especially if speech discrimination ability is significantly reduced.

A person's successful performance with amplification depends on an interaction between the person's hearing impairment and the amplifying device. Thus, hearing aid orientation must include the user's thorough understanding of his or her impairment, as well as of the amplifying device, in order to be successful. To select a hearing aid for someone having substantially reduced speech discrimination ability at any intensity level without informing him or her of the limitations of amplification, is to invite a dissatisfied hearing aid user. Other limitations will need to be explained, including sound localization, quality of amplified sound, and the masking and distracting effects of various background noises on hearing aid use. Information may need to be provided about the probability of amplification not helping impairments in auditory memory span, attention, closure, sequencing, or rate of auditory perception. A fluctuating sensorineural impairment of sensitivity and speech discrimination such as may occur in Meniere's syndrome presents an even more complicated set of limitations to be explained to a candidate for hearing aid use. Thorough understanding of these limitations may necessitate demonstrating as well as explaining them to hearing aid users and persons with whom they frequently communicate.

It is helpful to ask a prospective hearing aid user initially to rate how good a candidate he or she is for hearing aid use. A scale can be used which includes the categories excellent, good, fair, poor, and very poor. After completing a comprehensive history, hearing assessment, and hearing aid evaluation, the scale can be used by the clinician either to corroborate the person's prediction or to advise the prospective user that the clinician disagrees with the prediction and why.

Because some limitations are common among hearing aid users, the US Food and Drug Administration (1977) has required that certain disclosures be made to prospective hearing aid users. These disclosures are statements that, first, a hearing aid will not restore normal hearing or prevent or improve a hearing impairment caused by organic conditions, and second, hearing aid use is only one aspect of hearing rehabilitation and may need to be supplemented by auditory training and lipreading instruction.

Why Was a Particular Hearing Aid Selected?

Hearing aid users, if capable of understanding, should be told

1. Why a particular type of hearing aid, such as a postauricular instrument, was selected
2. Why the aid was a particular make
3. Why a monaural aid for the right or left ear or a binaural instrument was chosen
4. Why the particular external controls were chosen and where they should be set
5. Why the type of earmold was selected
6. Why any special features were selected

The inability of a new hearing aid user to tell a close friend why he or she is using the aid in the right ear can result in feelings of insecurity and inadequacy. Conversely, telling the friend that he or she has insufficient hearing or that the clarity of speech is too poor in the left ear to warrant amplification may impart the user's understanding of the impairment and a feeling of adequacy. Moreover, if the new hearing aid user then enlists the friend's help by asking him or her to walk and sit on the user's right side, this demonstrates the user's willingness to discuss and cope with the handicapping condition with friends. A thorough knowledge about one's impairment and hearing aid and an open approach to using the aid for the first time can contribute appreciably to successful hearing aid use.

Using a Newly Selected Hearing Aid

The length of time necessary for satisfactory adjustment to a newly selected hearing aid will vary substantially from person to person, depending on the amount and type of impairment; whether amplification has been used previously; the presence and extent of concomitant handicapping conditions such as mental impairment, spasticity, or visual impairment; the age of onset and progression of hearing impairment; and the person's daily activities. An intelligent long-time successful hearing aid user who has just procured a new replacement instrument might immediately begin wearing the new aid during all of his or her waking hours without needing any formalized hearing aid orientation beyond an explanation of any new or different hearing aid controls. Conversely, a mentally impaired adult who has a long-standing hearing impairment and has never tried amplification may require many months of hearing aid orientation. Typically, a satisfactory hearing aid orientation can be completed for most hearing impaired adults within 2–6 weeks and include the services essential for achieving successful hearing aid usage.

New hearing aid users generally are encouraged to begin using their aids in easy listening situations and progress to more difficult listening experiences. An easy listening situation would involve listening

1. To a single familiar speaker
2. In a quiet environment
3. To a familiar and easy topic
4. While watching the speaker
5. With good lighting on the speaker's face
6. With few visual or auditory distractions

After new users adjust to easy listening situations, the preceding six conditions and others may be varied to increase the difficulty of listening situations. Hearing aid orientation is not complete until clients have adjusted to using their new aids in a wide variety of daily listening activities, and particularly in those situations where they want and need to listen or communicate for social, vocational, or educational purposes.

New hearing aid users can be told to wear their aids as long as they do not experience fatigue, become irritated, or feel soreness of the ear. If they are unable to increase the length of time for wearing their new aids, an audiologist or hearing aid dispenser should be contacted. Additionally, new hearing aid users should be informed of some possible negative experiences, such as difficulty in "tuning-out" background noises which they are unaccustomed to hearing; speech sounding unnatural, including their own; their own speech sounding loud; whistling sound when outside in a wind if wearing an ear-level aid; clothing noise if wearing a body aid; and listening to speech in the presence of background noise.

New hearing aid users should be asked to accomplish specific tasks in adjusting to their new instrument, depending on individual needs and abilities. Persons can also be asked to chart their success in achieving task objectives and to chart satisfaction or dissatisfaction that can be reviewed with the clinician during a follow-up visit. During follow-up visits, user performance scales can be employed to rate the users' abilities to locate, discuss accurately, and operate the hearing aid components and controls; to trouble-shoot hearing aids; and to maintain aids appropriately.

The increased opportunities for hearing aid trials, or return of most of a hearing aid purchaser's money if dissatisfied with the instrument, are substantially changing the approach to hearing aid orientation. Because most of these arrangements are based on about 30 days, including a proposed US Federal Trade Commission rule (1975), hearing aid orientations designed to explore the feasibility of wearable amplification for questionable candidates or to verify the appropriateness of hearing aid selections are being completed within this time limit. Moreover, these increased opportunities may act as a catalyst for audiologists to design compressed comprehensive hearing aid orientation programs for prospective hearing aid users. If the proposed FTC Buyer's Right to Cancel Rule is adopted, these programs probably will become readily available for purchasers and renters of new hearing aids.

Situational Training

An adult hearing aid user, particularly a new one, needs to adjust to using amplification in a variety of specific situations, depending on such factors as type of hearing aid, type and extent of hearing impairment, and social and vocational needs. The hearing aid user should be encouraged to provide the audiologist with a list of situations in which he or she encounters particular difficulty listening. Situations also should be identified which are avoided and where the person experiences frequent frustration. Some situations might be listed by the audiologist for the person to check or rate according to degree of difficulty encountered. These could include the telephone, television, radio, speech of particular persons, theatre, church, group conversations, lectures, work, playing cards, the presence of background noise, and situations when the speaker's face cannot be seen. This information then can serve as a basis for situational training. As mentioned earlier in this chapter under the topic of user evaluation scales, several of these measuring instruments have been published.

Regardless of a new hearing aid user's answers to this type of inquiry, orientation to hearing aid use in some situations should be provided routinely. The user should be shown how to use a telephone effectively if there is sufficient residual hearing, and how to listen to speech and other auditory stimuli in the presence of a variety of background noises originating from different directions. Concerning telephone use, if the new hearing aid user does not understand the functions and location of the hearing aid microphone, it should be obvious that the new hearing aid user is not going to be able to use a telephone appropriately without instruction, particularly if a body-aid has been selected. If a telephone switch was needed and selected, instruction in its use should be provided. Moreover, the user should be informed that the telephone switch will not work on other than some Bell System phones which include those without a grommet or with a blue grommet on the wire leading from the hand-held portion of the phone. Telephone switches cannot be used with phones having a dark grey grommet.

How to Trouble-Shoot Hearing Aid Problems

If hearing aid users sufficiently understand the functions of the component parts and controls of hearing aids, they may intuitively be able to solve many of their own hearing aid problems. This is not intended to suggest that trouble-shooting ability should be left to chance. Quite the contrary, hearing aid users should be told about possible problems that can occur, how to locate the problems, and how to seek a resolution to the problems. A set of used hearing aids exhibiting a variety of problems is very helpful in demonstrating trouble-shooting techniques. Moreover, a chart that lists problems, possible causes, and remedies should be provided to hearing aid users. The clinician can ask the users to study their charts and be prepared to answer questions about them. Preferably, the clients should demonstrate their understanding of the material by locating problems and remedying them with a stock of used aids when they return for another appointment. Hearing aid users should be encouraged to keep this chart with important papers for immediate reference if hearing aid problems arise.

The chart might contain the following problems:

1. Squealing (whistling)
2. No amplification
3. Reduced amplification
4. Intermittent amplification or scratchy, frying, crashing sound
5. Sharp sound (as though in a barrel)
6. "Tinny" or "thin" sound
7. Sound too noisy
8. Reduced clarity of speech
9. Ear canal hurts
10. Problem not describable but a change noticed

Additionally, the chart should list the possible causes, how to locate the problems, and remedies. The chart should indicate clearly which causes can be remedied by the user and which ones should be remedied by an audiologist or hearing aid dispenser. The hearing aid user should be encouraged to call the specialist who selected the hearing instrument if problems arise which the user is unable to resolve. The specialist's address and phone number should be placed prominently on the chart where it can be easily seen.

These charts are available commercially through a variety of sources. Hearing aid manufacturers frequently include these charts in the User Instructional Brochure that is required by the FDA (1977). Two other sources include a booklet by Dodds and Harford (1970) and one of several booklets on hearing aid orientation by Gauger (1978).

Consumer Rights of Hearing Aid Users

Individuals should be informed of their legal rights and options as owners or users of wearable amplification. The cost of hearing aids and most expenses associated with hearing impairment, for example, are allowed as medical expenses in computing federal income tax. Many prospective purchasers of hearing aids may qualify for public or private funds to cover the cost of hearing aids, such as monies available through Medicaid, Rehabilitation Services Administration, Veterans Administration, or employee health benefits. They also should be informed of their legal rights and restrictions under the Labeling and Conditions for Sale Regulation promulgated by the FDA. Certain information must be provided to prospective hearing aid users in the form of a "User Instructional Brochure," as mandated by the FDA. Although many hearing aid manufacturers provided brochures with their instruments prior to this regulation, the extent and uniformity of information varied substantially. This was particularly true concerning electroacoustic characteristics of hearing aids.

As of August 15, 1977, the effective date of the FDA regulation, all hearing aids are to be accompanied by a User Instructional Brochure that contains the following categories of information:

1. Illustration of the hearing aid showing controls, adjustments, and battery compartment
2. Printed material on the operation of all controls designed for user adjustment
3. Description of possible accompanying accessories
4. Instructions on how to use, maintain, and care for as well as replace or recharge batteries
5. How to and where to procure repair services
6. Conditions to be avoided in preventing damage to hearing aids, such as dropping or exposing to excessive heat or humidity
7. Warning to seek medical advice when encountering any side effects, such as skin irritation or increased accumulation of cerumen
8. Statement that a hearing aid will not restore normal hearing nor prevent or improve a hearing impairment caused by organic conditions
9. Statement that with most persons, infrequent use of wearable amplification will not allow them to attain full benefit from hearing aid use
10. Statement that hearing aid use is only one aspect of hearing rehabilitation and may need to be augmented by auditory training and lipreading instruction
11. Warning statement to hearing aid dispensers to advise prospective hearing aid users to see a licensed physician before dispensing aids if any of eight medical conditions exist (see any User Instructional Brochure for these conditions)
12. Notice to prospective hearing aid users indicating, among other things, that hearing aids cannot be sold to individuals until they have obtained a medical evaluation from a licensed physician (preferably one who specializes in diseases of the ear); a fully informed adult may waive the medical evaluation, though such action is strongly discouraged by FDA
13. Selected electroacoustical data obtained in accordance with the Acoustical Society of America (1976) Standard for Specification of Hearing Aid Characteristics (this information may be included on separate labeling that accompanies the hearing aid)

Other information may be included in the User Instructional Brochure if it is not false, misleading, or prohibited by this regulation or by FTC regulations. Audiologists, hearing aid sales personnel, and physicians specializing in diseases of the ear should have a reference copy of this important FDA regulation.

Hearing aid orientation should at a minimum assess the knowledge about or performance with amplification in the eight areas of orientation mentioned above. Remediation can then be provided in those areas of deficiency. Although the other five types of rehabilitative services mentioned may be required as part of some hearing aid orientations, they are not essential for all clients. Moreover, these services will be discussed in more detail in other chapters of this book. Those services, you will recall, are

1. Counseling
2. Auditory training
3. Speechreading
4. Motivational training
5. Speech production training

This author is using the term counseling in a restricted sense to mean providing advice to persons who are having substantive emotional problems in coping with hearing impairment and hearing aid use. Moreover, motivational training might be considered as a subcategory of counseling. Certainly, the 13 components of hearing aid orientation do not represent an exhaustive list of services or the specific categories that other clinicians might choose to use. However, hopefully they constitute a framework upon which comprehensive and quality hearing aid orientation services can be provided based on individualized planning.

AUDIOLOGISTS DISPENSING HEARING AIDS—IMPLICATIONS FOR HEARING AID ORIENTATION

For a long time, audiologists have recognized the implications for unsatisfactory hearing aid adjustment when they are not involved directly with dispensing the device they recommend. Panel VI of an ASHA Conference on Hearing Aid Evaluation Procedures (Castle, 1967) reported that the typical dissatisfied hearing aid user returns to the hearing aid dealer from whom the aid was purchased rather than to the audiologist who selected and recommended the new hearing aid, even though the difficulty may relate to the original recommendation. Audiology members of the American Speech-Language-Hearing Association have been able to purchase hearing aids from manufacturers or suppliers and sell them to consumers on a not-for-profit basis since about 1969 without being in violation of this association's Code of Ethics. Principles Governing the Dispensing of Products to Persons with Communicative Disorders, adopted in September 1974 (ASHA, 1974), and subsequent ASHA interpretations of those principles (ASHA, 1976a, 1976b) provided guidance to ASHA members who chose to dispense hearing aids or other professional related products in accordance with the Association's Code of Ethics.

Principle A stipulated that "products associated with the member's professional practice must be dispensed to the person served as a part of a program of comprehensive habilitative care." The ASHA Ethical Practice Board (ASHA, 1976a) interpreted this principle to mean that "members dispensing hearing aids must be able to provide as a minimum (1) audiologic assessment, (2) hearing aid selection, (3) hearing aid orientation, and (4) counseling. In addition, members dispensing hearing aids also must offer or provide a sound referral plan for other comprehensive rehabilitation services when deemed necessary for the person served." Clearly, ASHA views hearing aid orientation as an essential component of hearing aid selection and dispensing. Even though ASHA (1978) has modified the Principles of Governing the Dispensing of Products to Persons with Communicative Disorders and its Code of Ethics to permit the dispensing of professionally related products for profit, Principle A remains intact as Standard I under Principle of Ethics IV. This author believes hearing aid orientation services can be enhanced substantially if audiologists are more directly involved in dispensing the hearing aids they select.

PROSPECTS FOR IMPROVED HEARING AID ORIENTATION

The future prospects for improved hearing aid orientation services are excellent because of many reasons. Some of these reasons include:

The need for improvement has been identified and is extensive.

The public awareness and understanding of hearing impairment and amplification is improving.

The increasing supply of audiologists and interest of these specialists in rehabilitation is encouraging.
The direct involvement of audiologists in dispensing hearing aids will increase their professional responsibility for ensuring a satisfactory adjustment to amplification.
A body of clinical and research literature is rapidly developing on the topic of hearing aid orientation.
Public and private health, rehabilitation, and education dollars may become available for hearing aid orientation services in the near future.
Federal regulations are mandating the disclosure of selected information to prospective hearing aid users.
Hearing aid user satisfaction and performance scales are being developed and used in ever increasing numbers.
Hearing aid orientation materials packaged in the form of pamphlets, synchronized audio–film strip presentations, and video cassettes are becoming readily available.
The increased national emphasis on individualized planning for the handicapped and family participation in that planning process is becoming a reality,
The capability of computerizing rehabilitation data is increasing.
The potential technological improvements in hearing aids are phenomenal.
The application of implanted hearing aids is increasing.
The selection of hearing aids for increased numbers of the mentally impaired, profoundly and mildly hearing impaired, and the aging is encouraging.

All of these reasons contribute to this author's enthusiasm about the prospects for improved hearing aid orientation services and user satisfaction. However, these prospects can be materialized only through creativity, an expanding base of knowledge, and a dedicated commitment by such individuals as audiologists, rehabilitation counselors, physicians, engineers, speech-language pathologists, hearing aid dispensers, hearing scientists, and teachers of the hearing impaired.

SUMMARY

In view of the available survey data on adult hearing aid user satisfaction, all specialists serving the hearing impaired can make significant clinical and research contributions to improving hearing aid orientation services. This chapter suggests that major contributions can be made by planning according to individual needs; involving persons in the orientation process with whom the hearing aid user frequently communicates; and employing user evaluation scales to assess attitudes, experiences, knowledge, and user performance. Additional contributions can be made if audiologists become more directly involved in dispensing as well as selecting hearing aids. This chapter briefly reviews many of the possible hearing aid orientation services and emphasizes those that should be an integral part of each user's orientation program. The user should understand the functions of the component parts and controls of the hearing aid; know how to fit, adjust, and maintain the instrument; understand the limitations and benefits of wearable amplification; know why a particular hearing aid system was selected; comprehend how to begin using a newly selected device; understand how to use the aid in different and unique listening situations; know how to trouble-shoot hearing aid problems; and recognize the legal rights of hearing aid users. Counseling, auditory training, speechreading, motivational training, speech production training, and other services may be included in hearing aid orientation depending on individual needs.

Hopefully, this chapter will challenge hearing specialists to improve hearing aid orientation services. The prospects for improvement are great given the current technological knowledge and innovations. Only a commitment and expenditure of effort is needed to fulfill the challenge.

REFERENCES

Acoustical Society of America. Specification of hearing aid characteristics. ASA-STD, 1976.

Alpiner, J. G., Chevrette, W., Glascoe, G., Metz, M., & Olsen, B. The Denver scale of communication function. Unpublished Research, University of Denver, Denver, Colorado, 1971.

American Speech and Hearing Association. The audiologist: Responsibilities in the habilitation of the auditorily handicapped. *Journal of the American Speech and Hearing Association,* 1974, *16,* 68–70.

American Speech and Hearing Association. Ethical Practice Board interpretations of principles governing the dispensing of products to persons with communicative disorders. *Journal of the American Speech and Hearing Association,* 1976(a), *18,* 237–240.

American Speech and Hearing Association. Issues in ethics—An open letter to audiologists: Hearing aids and dispensing service charges. *Journal of the American Speech and Hearing Association,* 1976(b), *18,* 854–855.

American Speech and Hearing Association. L.C. 53–78. Adopted by Legislative Council, San Francisco, November 1978.

Blood, I., & Danhauer, J. L. Are we meeting the needs of our hearing aid users? *Journal of the American Speech and Hearing Association,* 1976, *18,* 343–347.

Burney, P. A survey of hearing aid evaluation procedures. *Journal of American Speech and Hearing Association,* 1972, 14, 439–444.

Carhart, R. Selection of hearing aids. *Archives of Otolaryngology,* 1946, *44,* 1–18.

Castle, W. E. (Ed.). A conference on hearing aid evaluation procedures. *ASHA Reports*-2, 1967.

Dodds, E., & Harford, E. *Helpful hearing aid hints.* Washington, D.C. Alexander Graham Bell Association for the Deaf, Inc., 1970.

Garstecki, D. C. A behavioral approach toward adult hearing aid orientation. *Journal of the Academy of Rehabilitative Audiology,* 1974, *7,* 9–18.

Gauger, J. S. *Orientation to hearing aids.* Rochester, New York. National Technical Institute for the deaf, 1978.

Gauger, J. S., & McPherson, D. L. A support system for hearing aid evaluations. *Journal of the Academy of Rehabilitative Audiology,* 1978, *11,* 66–90.

Fay, T. H., & Smith, C. R. A program of auditory rehabilitation for aged persons in a chronic disease hospital. *Journal of the American Speech and Hearing Association,* 1976, *19,* 417–420.

Giolas, T. G., Owens, E., Lamb, L. H. & Schubert, E. D. Hearing performance inventory. *Journal of Speech and Hearing Disorders,* 1979, *44,* 169–195.

Hardick, E. J. Aural rehabilitational programs for the aged can be successful. *Journal of the Academy of Rehabilitative Audiology,* 1977, *10,* 51–67.

High, W. S., Fairbanks, G., & Glorig, A. Scale for self-assessment of hearing handicap. *Journal of Speech and Hearing Disorders,* 1964, *29,* 215–230.

Moore, E. J., Miltenberger, G. E., & Barber, P. S. Hearing aid orientation in a state school for the mentally retarded. *Journal of Speech and Hearing Disorders,* 1969, *34,* 142–145.

National Academy of Sciences—National Research Council. Directions for research to improve hearing aids and services for the hearing impaired. Committee on Hearing, Bioacoustics, and Biomechanics, February, 1972.

Noble, W. G., & Atherly, G. R. C. The hearing measurement scale: A questionnaire for the assessment of auditory disability. *Journal of Audiological Research,* 1970, *10,* 229–250.

Payne & Payne Consultants. A national survey of the hearing aid delivery system in the United States. Austin, Texas, 1974.

Rassi, J., & Harford, E. An analysis of patient attitudes and reactions to a clinical hearing aid selection program. *Journal of the American Speech and Hearing Association,* 1968, *10,* 283–290.

Roeser, R. J., Campbell, A., & Brown, B. The hearing health team . . . A one way street? *Audiology and Hearing Education,* 1976, *2,* 8–11.

Rupp, R. R., Higgins, J., & Maurer, J. F. A feasibility scale for predicting hearing aid use (FSPHAU) with older individuals. *Journal of the*

Academy of Rehabilitative Audiology, 1977, *10,* 81–104.

Sanders, D. A. Hearing aid orientation and counseling, in M. G. Pollack (Ed.), *Amplification for the hearing impaired.* Grune and Stratton, New York, 1975, pp. 363–372.

Topic of the month: Hearing health care in Scandinavia. *Hearing Aid Journal,* 1976, *11,* 13–30.

US Congress. The Rehabilitation Act of 1973, Public Law 93-112. *US Statutes at Large,* 1973, *87:*855–394.

US Department of Health, Education and Welfare. Final report to the secretary on hearing aid health care. The Intradepartmental Task Force on Hearing Aids, 1975.

US Federal Trade Commission. Proposed trade regulation rule for the hearing aid industry. *Federal Register,* 1975, *40,* 26646–26653.

US Food and Drug Administration. Hearing aid devices, professional and patient labeling and conditions for sale. *Federal Register,* 1977, *42,* 9286–9296.

US Office of Education, Bureau of Education for Handicapped Children. Implementation of part B of the education of the handicapped act. *Federal Register,* 1977, 42, 42474–42518.

US Public Health Service. Characteristics of persons with impaired hearing—United States, July 1962–June 1963. National Center for Health Statistics, Series 10, No 35, 1964.

Walker, M. W. Comments on the hearing aid industry's 1971 survey of the hard of hearing. *Journal of the American Speech and Hearing Association,* 1974, *16,* 685–688.

B. Counseling the Hearing Impaired Adult

Harriet F. Kaplan

Chapter 6: The Impact of Hearing Impairment and the Need to Facilitate Adjustment

The sense of hearing is integrally related to communication and interaction with one's fellow beings. To a very great extent, we relate to others through verbal language. When the sense of hearing is impaired, the ability to relate may be impaired as well. Messages may not be interpreted properly because crucial words are missed or because the hearing impaired person does not catch the nuances of meaning conveyed by a rising inflection, a pause, or an emphasis in a particular part of an utterance. Faulty hearing often leads to misunderstanding and inappropriate behavior. It is not difficult to understand why psychological problems arise when significant hearing loss occurs. Helping the individual deal with these problems must be considered an integral part of the total process of aural rehabilitation.

The type of psychological problem and the degree to which it exists varies with the individual, depending on his or her life-style and personality, and the characteristics of the hearing loss. Although there are inevitably individual differences among hearing impaired persons, common adjustment problems are generally observed to one degree or another.

Hearing impaired persons often feel shut off from the world, not only because they can no longer communicate easily with others, but also because some or all of the subliminal auditory clues which permit one to maintain contact with his or her "world" are no longer available. They may react to this depression by withdrawing from social situations and from contact with other human beings. They may even modify vocational aspirations. The outgoing community leader may begin to shun former acquaintances and avoid activities involving communication. The executive may avoid social obligations necessary to maintain his or her position. An extreme example of this type of behavior is the case of the man who as a result of a gradually worsening hearing loss requested a transfer to a position requiring minimal communication despite the fact that the job change would result in significant loss of income and status. The hearing impaired person may not understand that the cause of such avoidances and depression may be directly related to the hearing impairment per se. This lack of understanding may lead to further depression.

EMOTIONAL REACTIONS TO HEARING LOSS

Feelings of Inadequacy

Depression is frequently complicated by feelings of inadequacy. The hearing impaired person often feels that he or she should be able to cope with the hearing loss more effectively and that difficulties in coping indicate weakness. In addition, there may be feelings of shame not only because of a perceived inability to cope and overcome the handicap but also because he or she may have rationalized that the inability to hear normally is associated with other types of abnormality, such as disability in thinking, learning, remembering, or decision-making. This author is acquainted with a hearing impaired lady who constantly apologizes for her hearing loss. Her repeated use of the phrase ''It's my fault'' to explain misperceptions reveals much about her perception of herself as a less than adequate person.

Another example of the shame that is often associated with hearing loss is typified by the gentleman who returned from a trip to another part of the country where the dialect was unfamiliar to him. When asked to tell his aural rehabilitation group about his trip he commented that people spoke very differently than at home and that he had felt terribly ashamed that his hearing loss would not allow him to understand them. Although he acknowledged that differences in speech created difficulty, he still perceived his communication difficulties as ''his fault''

Defense Mechanisms

In most cases, the threat to self-esteem is handled by one or more defense mechanisms. A common defense mechanism is denial. A person may simply not acknowledge the existence of hearing loss because acceptance of the fact that he or she is not completely normal is difficult. That same individual would probably have no difficulty accepting the reality of a visual problem because a visual problem may be viewed with greater objectivity and not be associated with the general adequacy of a person. Denial increases the problem because it makes it more difficult for the hearing impaired person to seek help or accept the need for a hearing aid, which would then cause the hearing impairment to become visible to others. Undoubtedly, we all know hearing impaired people who insist that their communication difficulties would disappear if only people would speak plainly the way they did when that person was younger.

Hostility and Suspicion

Other defense mechanisms are hostility and suspicion. Hearing impaired persons may blame others for their difficulties, accusing them of mumbling or of deliberately cutting them out of the conversation. They may become suspicious, accusing others of saying unpleasant things about them or planning unpleasant situations for them. Laughter may be misinterpreted as ridicule. Carried to extremes, suspicion may resemble paranoia in many ways. Hearing impaired persons may consider themselves persecuted by others, including friends and family. Suspicion or hostility is frequently turned against those who are closest to these individuals (spouses, children, friends), further complicating adjustment. Often hearing impaired persons may react negatively to helping personnel; the doctor, the audiologist, the hearing aid dealer. It is very important for the helping person to realize the true source of this unpleasant behavior and remain objective about it.

The following discussion of the psychological levels of hearing will provide insights for the reader relative to the source of these behaviors.

PSYCHOLOGICAL LEVELS OF HEARING

Ramsdell (1978) has described three psychological levels of hearing for the normal hearing person and the problems which exist correspondingly with loss of hearing at each level.

Primitive Level

At the primitive level, sound functions as auditory coupling to the world. We react to the changing background sounds of the world around us without being aware of it. As Ramsdell states:

> At this level, we react to such sounds as the tick of a clock, the distant roar of traffic, vague echoes of people moving in other rooms of the house, without being aware that we do hear them. These incidental noises maintain our feeling of being part of a living world and contribute to our own sense of being alive (p. 501).

When this primitive function is lost, acute depression may occur. Since the primitive level of hearing is not on a conscious level, the hearing impaired person may not be aware of the cause of the depression. Frequently, the depression is attributed to his or her own inadequacy in coping with the hearing impairment.

The severity of the depression will be greatest among persons who experience a sudden hearing loss, whether it is through trauma, surgery (e.g., acoustic tumor removal), or other causes. Fortunately, hearing loss of sudden onset most frequently occurs in one ear only, although bilateral losses do occur.

Depression due to the loss of the primitive level will occur in the individual with slowly deteriorating hearing as well. It is more insidious, occurring more slowly, but the resulting depression may be equally great. In some instances the depression may be even greater because the person may not be aware that his or her hearing is deteriorating. Informing the client of the true cause of the depression will help alleviate some of the problem, although this knowledge will not eliminate it entirely.

The loss of the primitive level is a problem in severe to profound bilateral losses. According to Goodman's system of classification, this would include hearing losses of 70 db HL or greater (Goodman, 1965). If low-frequency sensitivity is only mildly impaired, the primitive level is likely to be maintained, since many low-level background sounds contain low-frequency sound energy.

Warning or Signal Level of Hearing

At the warning level, sounds function to convey information about objects or events. The doorbell indicates that we have a visitor. Footsteps indicate that someone is coming up the stairs. A siren indicates that an emergency vehicle is approaching. A fire alarm indicates danger. Since warning sounds are frequently intense, loss of the warning level is generally found among persons who possess severe to profound losses. However, some warning sounds are of low intensity, and may be missed by persons with less severe hearing losses. These are mainly distant sounds, such as the horn of an automobile or the whistle of an approaching train.

Insecurity

When an inability to hear warning sounds exists, it is understandable that feelings of insecurity may result. Recently a number of hearing impaired adults of this author's acquaintance expressed concern about not being able to hear smoke alarms in the event of a fire. Complaints of hearing impaired parents who could not hear their babies resulted in the development of electronic visual signals which respond to a baby's cry. Still another example of insecurity resulting from warning level difficulties is the lady who refused to sit with her back to a door for fear that she might not be able to hear and protect herself from an intruder. That same lady installed multiple dead-bolt locks on her apartment door to increase her feeling of security. This problem was partially alleviated by a device which caused lights to flash when her door was manipulated in any way.

Annoyance

Feelings of insecurity are closely related to feelings of annoyance due to disruption of normal patterns of life by loss of hearing at the warning level. The hearing impaired person who can no longer hear his or alarm clock may oversleep in the morning and suffer penalties at work as a result. When the ring of the telephone can no longer be heard, social activities may be curtailed or business opportunities lost. These are very real problems to the hearing impaired adult.

Localization Problems

Localization problems may be considered a special type of ''warning level'' difficulty. As Ramsdell points out, with some noises the nature of the noise itself provides information about the probable direction. The sound of an airplane will always come from overhead. However, with many noises the nature of the noise alone is not sufficient to predict direction. Since in order to predict direction we need approximately equal sensitivity in both ears, the inability to localize sound is a special problem for persons who possess unilateral losses. What we do not always realize, further, is that localization problems also exist for the individual with a bilateral hearing loss who is aided monaurally.

The insecurity and annoyance from warning level difficulties can best be dealt with by training the hearing impaired person to be more visually aware of the environment and by providing ''devices'' that will allow him or her to hear warning signals. This will be discussed in greater detail in Chapters 7 and 9.

Loss of Aesthetic Experiences

For some individuals sound provides aesthetic experience. The musician who can no longer attend concerts or the opera because the music that was once pleasurable is now hopelessly distorted may be experiencing deterioration in the quality and pleasure of his life. Unfortunately, the use of amplification cannot always provide a remedy for this particular problem. Depression and/or frustration may result. For some people the inability to hear the sounds of nature may represent the loss of their most pleasant aesthetic experience. I am reminded of the young man who possessed a severe hearing loss whose first reaction to his new aid was ''I can hear the wind rustling the leaves.'' An important dimension of his life was thus restored.

Symbolic Level of Hearing

At the symbolic level we are dealing with sound as language, and as a major method of communication. Nearly all hearing impaired people have difficulty in this area to one degree or another. Although the hard-of-hearing or deafened adult does not suffer the delayed language development characteristic of the congenitally deaf child, he or she does face the problem of communicating under conditions of reduced verbal redundancy imposed by impaired auditory reception. For the normal hearing individual, spoken language contains many clues to meaning which occur simultaneously. For example, when a sentence is spoken, the listener acoustically and visually perceives the individual words. The listener, further, makes use of linguistic clues inherent in the sentence, situational clues, prosodic features of the sentence such as stress and inflection, and nonverbal clues such as facial expressions in the interpretation of meaning. The hearing impaired person, however, depending on the degree, type, and configuration of loss, does not have all of these clues available to him or her. The fewer auditory clues available, the more likely this person is to misinterpret what is heard, with consequent embarrassment, frustration, and social penalty. This situation is worsened if the communication environment contains background noise, competing speech, or other auditory or visual distractions.

At Home

The home can be a source of tension because of communication difficulties. More often than not, a hearing impaired person will complain of difficulty understanding his or her spouse. There are a number of reasons for accentuation of communication problems in the home. First, there is more opportunity for interpersonal communication and consequently more opportunity for difficulty. Second, the hearing impaired person expects his or her family to be more understanding of the special problems resulting from hearing loss than nonrelatives, but then experiences disappointment when he or she finds that is not the case. Third, households tend to be noisy places. About a year ago this author measured the sound pressure level in her kitchen with the water running, the refrigerator going, and the radio turned on. The noise level on the C scale of the sound level meter was *100 dB SPL*.

Typical of the problems in the home is the problem of a client who complained that he could use his hearing aid comfortably everywhere but at home because his family had no consideration for his needs. His children, for example, slammed doors when they entered the house and played rock music at high intensity levels. At the dinner table everyone talked at once, making it impossible for him to sort out one conversation from another. Kitchen appliances were in use from time to time during dinner, creating unbearable noise. And worst of all, his wife insisted on communicating with him from another room, raising the level of her voice when asked to repeat, but not coming into his line of vision. His solution to these problems was, first, to not use his hearing aid at home, and second, to minimize communication with his family. Several conferences with the entire family, which included discussions of hearing loss and the resulting limitations imposed upon listening, improved the situation for our client. Unfortunately, not all families are equally adaptable. When conflicts already exist within a family, the presence of a hearing loss can accentuate them. The hearing impairment can be used as a weapon by either the hard-of-hearing person or other family members.

At Work

Work-related problems are common. The extent and nature of the difficulty will depend on the nature of the hearing loss itself and the type of job the person holds. The greater the amount of communication required and the greater the need for precision of understanding, the more difficulty the client is likely to experience. The executive who must attend and conduct meetings is likely to be penalized if he or she misinterprets what is to be heard. The receptionist who has difficulty understanding speech on the telephone may be in danger of losing his or her job. This is particularly true if one of the receptionist's primary responsibilities is to correctly perceive names, addresses, and phone numbers. The physician who finds it increasingly difficult to monitor a patient's heartbeat with a stethoscope may find it more and more difficult to function professionally. All of these work-related problems create anxiety and frustration. If not dealt with, the anxiety and frustration complicate the already existing communication problems. The vocational impact of hearing impairment and the role of the vocational counselor will be discussed further in chapters 12 and 13.

At School

The adult or adolescent in school often has special problems. Classrooms are rarely quiet places. Ross (1972) reported that signal-to-noise ratios were found to vary between +1 and +5 dB. It is often difficult for a normally hearing individual to interpret correctly exactly what a teacher is saying under these conditions, particularly when lecture material is new and complex. This task is immeasurably more difficult for a hearing impaired student, since he or she must attempt to function efficiently in spite of an auditory system that will distort the incoming speech signal even under favorable conditions.

Not only are many classrooms noisy, but they tend to be reverberant to one degree or another. Classrooms which contain large areas of rigid, smooth surface and few absorbent materials such as drapes or carpets tend to be highly reverberant. Such room conditions further distort speech and add to the burden of the hearing impaired student. These conditions, moreover, retard the efficient use of a hearing aid. Teachers are not always aware of the special needs of the hearing impaired individual, and do not always project themselves or their voices adequately. Teachers will occasionally speak with their backs to the class while writing at the blackboard, thus reducing the intensity of their voices at the level of the ears of the students. That position, further, makes speechreading impossible. Another barrier to speechreading faced by the student who possesses a hearing loss is the need to take notes. One cannot concentrate on interpreting visual clues and write at the same time. All of these problems tend to limit educational opportunities for hard-of-hearing adults, with consequent vocational imitations.

Some individuals may seek out special classes for the deaf where special arrangements are made to meet the needs imposed by hearing loss. However, educational opportunities for hearing impaired adults are generally limited. Furthermore, most hard-of-hearing individuals who have known normal hearing for most of their lives identify more readily with the normal hearing population than with the prelingually deaf and find that classes for deaf adults do not meet their needs. These problems often cause frustration, depression, and the development of unhealthy defense mechanisms. The adult with acquired hearing impairment often finds that opportunities for education or retraining are few.

Social Activities

For many adults, sudden or increasing hearing loss results in a restriction of social activities. The impaired speech intelligibility that develops exposes the hearing impaired individual to the danger and embarrassment of misinterpretation of what is said. As a result he or she may react inappropriately and be exposed to ridicule. It is a rare person who possesses enough ego strength to continually ask people to repeat what has been said, explaining that he or she has a hearing loss. Even well-meaning friends do not always succeed in making the hard-of-hearing person feel comfortable. Normally hearing people feel uncomfortable themselves when they know a listener is not understanding what they are saying. Often they are at a loss as to how to make the hard-of-hearing listener understand better, particularly when the hearing impaired person attempts to "bluff" and does it badly. Both partners in the conversation may attempt to deny the existence of the hearing loss, but communication is disrupted and speaker and listener are embarrassed.

When the hearing loss is severe or has been present for a long time, speech may deteriorate. In that case, the hearing impaired person may not be clearly understood when he or she is the speaker in the conversation. This adds to the possible social penalties imposed by the hearing impairment.

Conversational difficulties increase exponentially in difficult listening situations. Following a conversation which is alternating between members of a group can be an extremely difficult experience, particularly when background noise is present. A dinner party can be extremely anxiety-provoking. A client, the wife of an executive, told of the strategies she developed to cope with these situations. She always made it a point to sit next to someone with a loud voice and then managed to manipulate the conversation so that she could do most of the talking. In this way, she could also minimize conversation with other guests. It was a great relief to her when her husband accepted a new position that did not require her to attend dinner parties.

Social activities are further limited when a hearing impaired individual can no longer enjoy the theater or lectures. Just as in face-to-face conversations, the person must cope with speakers or actors who may not project adequately, speech which shifts rapidly from one person to another, poor room acoustics, or the loss of loudness sensitivity imposed by his or her hearing loss.

More and more, as social activities become restricted, the hearing impaired person experiences isolation and loneliness. Resignation to this state may ultimately be accepted, or it may be met with aggression. The individual may deny the reality of his or her problem and attribute a shrinking social life to the maliciousness of others. Regardless of whether the problem is met with resignation or aggression, the hearing impaired person suffers deterioration in the quality of his or her life-style.

Other Problems at the Symbolic Level

There are other practical problems associated with loss of hearing at the symbolic level. Every hearing impaired person has at one time or another encountered the rude person who doesn't understand hearing problems. A former college teacher with a severe bilateral hearing loss entered a post office with the intention of mailing a package. When the clerk asked her whether she wanted insurance, she politely asked him to repeat the question. He responded with "What's the matter? Are you deaf or just plain dumb?"

A closely related problem involves the difficulty encountered by many hearing impaired persons in obtaining certain public or health services. Hearing impaired persons are, for example, at a definite disadvantage when dealing with the law. In recognition of this fact, a legal center for the deaf has been established a Gallaudet College. Further, most hospitals do not make special provisions for communicating with hearing impaired patients, nor are personnel aware of their communication problems. A lady friend told with wry amusement of her difficulties communicating with the nurses in the recovery room following surgery. None of the hospital personnel knew of her hearing loss or that she used a hearing aid. She could not inform them of her problem because a tracheotomy tube prevented speech. Although she was able to smile at the experience in retrospect, at the time she felt helpless, frightened, and angry, not amused.

A special problem at the symbolic level is loss of ability to use the telephone. The telephone message has become an integral and necessary part of our lives. Not only does it facilitate socialization, but it is also a vehicle for transmitting warnings. The mother who cannot use a telephone to call the doctor when her child is ill is at a great disadvantage. In addition, the telephone is essential for business. Although many business or professional people express a desire to hide from their telephones, they would find the lack of the pesky device a great hinderance to the management of business.

The hearing impaired person who cannot understand speech conveyed by telephone or who cannot hear the telephone ring is affected in every aspect of his or her life. Social contacts are reduced because friends and family cannot be easily contacted. Vocational opportunities are limited to the minority of jobs not requiring use of the telephone. Finally, the inability to use the telephone to summon help is threatening indeed, particularly for the individual who lives alone.

The problems resulting from loss of hearing at the symbolic level all involve deterioration of easy communication. To one degree or another, all hearing impaired persons suffer from these problems and their consequent emotional reactions. Both the problems and the reactions to them need to be dealt with by the helping professional.

INDIVIDUAL DIFFERENCES

Thus far we have been talking in generalities. Obviously, the specific problems a hearing impaired person will face and corresponding reactions to them will depend on his or her personal life-style. A very pertinent description of some of the personality characteristics of the hearing impaired adult is presented by Goetzinger (1978). The personality traits listed by him include introversion, despondency, hopelessness, sense of inferiority, fear, super sensitivity, bitterness, brooding, persecution complex, suspicion, apathy, and listlessness. Goetzinger adds that such descripters as cruelty, egocentrism, selfishness, and lack of sympathy are also "generously" used to describe the adult hearing impaired. He states that possible reasons for behaviors that may prompt such descripters for the hearing impaired by hearing persons "include the extra effort which must be exerted to meet the demands of the environment, head noises, the absence of sound itself, the threat of limited employment opportunities and second class citizenship" (p. 461).

The impact of hearing loss on family interactions will depend to a large extent upon the dynamics of that person's family situation. In families with existing conflicts, the hearing loss may add additional strain. For example, one gentleman confided that he cannot use his hearing aid at home because his wife deliberately makes noise to make its use difficult. When the family is supportive of the hearing impaired individual, problems related to the hearing loss may be resolved more easily through family education.

The occupation of the client determines what kind of work-related problems the hearing loss creates. If the individual does not need to attend meetings or use the telephone, difficulty hearing in these situations will not exact vocational penalties. On the other hand, if precise communication is required in these or other difficult situations, the hearing loss may be a much greater problem to the individual. A salesman will not experience the same difficulties as a bookkeeper; a musician may suffer from loss of hearing far more than a writer; a mother of young children will have different problems than the woman with grown children.

The personality characteristics of a hearing impaired individual and the type of social life to which he or she has been accustomed determine the degree of psychological adjustment needed in the social sphere. The person who is sustained by pursuits not involving others, and who prefers to spend his leisure time reading or painting, will not experience the same problems as the person who is deeply involved in civic activities. The person with a keen need for musical experience will feel a far greater loss if he can no longer appreciate a concert than the person who has never enjoyed music.

Since each hearing impaired person is first and foremost an individual with a unique personality and life-style, the first step in facilitating adjustment to the hearing loss is to identify the specific problems experienced by that individual. Chapters 7 and 27 will discuss various scales of hearing handicap which are designed to do precisely that, particularly as they relate to facilitating adjustment to a hearing loss.

CHARACTERISTICS OF THE HEARING LOSS

The nature of the hearing loss itself helps determine the types and severity of adjustment problems that may exist. Although a more severe loss has greater effect on all three psychological levels of hearing, adjustment to a milder sensitivity problem may be equally difficult. A mild loss will not cause problems at the primitive level and possibly not at the warning level. However, the problems at the symbolic level may be as great as, although different from, those encountered with a more severe deficit. A person with a severe loss may be able to use amplification more effectively than a person with a mild impairment, particularly if large air-bone gaps exist in ears that are found not to be medically treatable. As a result, the former individual may find him or herself communicating far better than the latter. The person with a mild loss is at a particular disadvantage when his or her hearing is characterized by good low-frequency sensitivity and a severe loss in the high frequencies. Such an individual has minimal difficulty recognizing that another person is speaking, but far greater difficulty in interpreting what is heard. The problem is not one of insufficient loudness, but rather one of too much distortion. Hearing aids tend to handle acuity problems far better than problems of speech distortion, although with new innovations present in modern hearing aids, including earmold modifications, many people who possess high-frequency hearing loss can be successfully fitted. But there are still those who cannot use hearing aids effectively because of normal or near-normal hearing for the low frequencies.

Audiometric Configuration

With a sloping configuration into the high frequencies, problems imposed by background noise tend to be more acute than with a flat configuration because ambient noise is largely a low-frequency phenomenon and tends to mask the high-frequency components of speech that are so important for intelligibility. The person with the high frequency loss complains "I hear but I don't understand." Further complicating the problems encountered is the fact that the person may not realize that the communication difficulties result from the nature of the hearing loss. He or she may attribute those problems to failing mental processes, as may others in the environment. A person who cannot successfully adjust to amplification, may blame him or herself for not trying hard enough and may consider the lack of success an indication of inadequacy. It is very important that such individuals have complete understanding of the limitations imposed by their specific hearing losses.

The person with the unilateral hearing loss has special kinds of communication problems. Impairment at either the primitive or warning levels may not be noted, and no difficulty in hearing or understanding speech may be experienced so long as it is delivered to the good ear. However, if speech occurs on the side of the poor ear, by the time it reaches the good ear it is considerably attenuated. Tillman, Kasten, and Horner (1975) have described this phenomenon, which they call the "head shadow" effect. The listener will experience difficulty interpreting what he or she hears because the intensity of the signal is inadequate and because some distortion has occurred. The hearing impaired adult with this problem must turn so that the good ear faces the source of sound. Most importantly, the client must understand the nature of the problem in order best to cope with it.

Another problem unique to the person who possesses a unilateral hearing loss is determining the direction of an oncoming sound. The inability to localize accurately can create problems at the warning level, where determining direction of a signal can be very important. Fortunately we have available amplification devices to remedy this situation.

A third and perhaps the most common complaint of individuals with unilateral loss is difficulty discriminating speech in the presence of competing noise. In order to differentiate the two signals perceptually, binaural hearing is necessary. In the more common situation, involving speech coming from the front and the noise surrounding the listener, all signals converge on the one good ear. The person with the unilateral loss does not have two ears with which to sort out the competing signals.

Onset of Loss

The hard-of-hearing adult generally has experienced normal hearing throughout childhood and adolescence, has developed normal language, and has been educated in regular schools. He or she does not reveal the speech and language deficits so common to the prelingually deaf. However, possible psychological problems, although different, may be equal or more severe. The child who has never known normal hearing does not perceive him or herself as a person who has experienced a loss. This child has always identified him or herself as a hearing impaired person and cannot mourn for what has never been known. Although hearing on the primitive level may not be experienced, the child does not experience the depression so typical of this loss among the deafened adults, because auditory coupling with the environment has never been known. In contrast, the person who has experienced an auditory deficit later in life must adjust to a change in his or her mode of dealing with the world. Niemeyer (1971) states this quite well:

> The person afflicted by late hearing impairment has taken the experience of hearing for granted: to him the loss of adequate hearing means a drastic change of life: he compares his present handicap with his earlier condition as a normally hearing person and begins to look at himself and his companions from a different angle (p. 1).

In the elderly, the sense of isolation and loneliness due to deteriorating hearing is perhaps most acute, since social opportunities tend to become restricted with age even when hearing is relatively normal.

When an adult incurs a sudden total loss of hearing, severe emotional upset can be expected. The individual has been transformed from a normal hearing person to one completely cut off from normal interaction with his or her fellow human beings overnight. He or she has not had time to acclimate gradually to this new condition or to make necessary adjustment. This person may experience a period of mourning or self-pity. This period of time can be quite unbearable for family and friends. Yet most important during this period is the family's emotional support and their adjustment to the loss.

Sudden hearing loss is often unexplained. The afflicted person may fear losing some other sense without warning or, if the hearing loss involved one ear only, may fear the loss of the other ear in the same manner. This author recalls a female client who acquired a total unexplained sudden hearing loss in one ear, who had also suffered a mild digestive upset the previous day. She attributed both problems to food poisoning, which she thought was incurred at a restaurant where she had eaten. For a year following the loss of hearing, she shunned all restaurants and was reluctant to accept dinner invitations even at homes of friends.

ADJUSTMENT TO AMPLIFICATION

When a person feels a loss of self-esteem because of an inability to hear normally, he or she has a tendency to conceal the hearing loss. The fear is often related to the possibility that people will view him or her as mentally abnormal. To such an individual, a hearing aid is a visible indication that he or she is an inferior person. Even though it may be recognized logically that there is no truth to those fears, emotionally that person may not be able to accept the use of the aid. Even when the hearing aid can be completely hidden from view, the problem of acceptance is not solved for some people. For the person who denies the auditorily based problem, the fact that a hearing aid must be worn represents tangible evidence of his or her inferiority. It matters not if anyone else is aware of that "badge of shame." This author has found these feelings especially prevalent among adolescents, where peer identification and acceptance are overriding concerns. Related to the perceived stigma of the hearing aid is the concern of some persons about masculinity or feminity. Many adolescents and adults fear that hearing loss and its visible badge, the hearing aid, will make them less attractive to the opposite sex.

If a hearing impaired individual does succeed in working through the emotional objections to amplification, the usual expectation is that the decision to use an aid will result in restoration of good hearing. In many cases of sensorineural hearing loss, as stated earlier, the hearing aid cannot restore the good hearing that the individual once knew, particularly under conditions of competing noise. As long as a conversation is carried on with one person in a quiet room, the person may be satisfied with the performance of the instrument. In most cases, however, group conversation and listening against a background of noise will be difficult with the hearing aid as well as without. If the hearing impaired person is not properly prepared for the limitations of amplification and the adjustment necessary to use it well, he or she will be disappointed during attempts to use the aid. Many hearing aids are "worn" in the dresser drawer for this reason. Once the aid is discarded, the hearing impaired person may feel even more isolated from normal communication, and perhaps even more depressed, since all hopes of solving those problems through the mechanical prosthesis have not been fulfilled.

Not all hearing impaired people can use hearing aids successfully. There are those who make an honest effort to adjust to amplification but find for various reasons that communication is not improved. It is very important that such individuals understand that their lack of success with amplification is a function of the characteristics of their hearing problems and not due to lack of character or motivation.

CONCLUSIONS

In meeting the needs of the hearing impaired adult it is essential to go beyond accurate diagnosis and selection of amplification. At every stage of the rehabilitation program, understanding and acceptance of the problems imposed by hearing loss are necessary. Only then can the client handle his or her communication problems in a positive way. In order to come to terms with a hearing loss, the hearing impaired person needs the support of not only the audiologist but also of his or her family and friends.

In this chapter, the various problems imposed by hearing loss and typical reactions to these problems have been discussed. It has been stressed that each hearing impaired person is an individual and must be understood in terms of his or her own unique set of problems. Only by clearly defining the mechanics underlying a client's behavior can therapist and client together work to facilitate adjustment to the problems imposed by the hearing loss.

REFERENCES

Goetzinger, C. P. The psychology of hearing impairment, in J. Katz (Ed.), *Handbook of Clinical Audiology,* (2nd ed). Baltimore: Williams and Wilkins, 1978, pp. 447–468.

Goodman, A. C. Reference zero levels for pure-tone audiometers. *Journal of the American Speech and Hearing Association,* 1965, *7,* 262–263.

Niemeyer, W. Psychological aspects of hearing-aid fitting, parts 1 and 2. *Maico Audiological Library Series,* Vol. 9, Report 10, 1971.

Ramsdell, D. A. The psychology of the hard-of-hearing and the deafened adult, in H. Davis and S. R. Silverman (Eds.), *Hearing and Deafness.* New York: Holt, Rinehart and Winston, 1978, p. 501.

Ross, M. Classroom acoustics and speech intelligibility, in J. Katz (Ed.), *Handbook of Clinical Audiology,* (1st ed.). Baltimore: Williams and Wilkins, 1972, pp. 756–771.

Tillman, T., Kasten, R., & Horner, J. The effect of the head shadow on the reception of speech, in M. D. Pollack (Ed.), *Amplification for the Hearing-Impaired.* New York: Grune and Stratton, 1975, p. 254.

Harriet F. Kaplan

Chapter 7: Facilitating Adjustment

The adjustment problems of the hearing impaired adult can be attributed to at least two major factors among many: loss of self esteem due to altered sensory capabilities and reactions to resultant feelings of inadequacy; and the penalties imposed by society. The task of the professional is thus twofold. Through educational and personal-adjustment counseling (Sanders, 1975), the client must be helped to accept him or herself as a hearing impaired person and to understand the limitations imposed by the hearing problem. Once this is achieved the client can be helped to manipulate his or her environment in such a way that the penalties imposed by that environment are minimized. Environmental manipualtion may involve use of listening aids, modification of communication situations, and education of family, friends, and associates.

The first step in the rehabilitation process is the definition of problems specific to the client. In the first part of this chapter, various behavioral scales available to delineate these problems and how this information can best be used in the treatment process will be discussed. That section is followed by a discussion of what is involved in the counseling environment. The counseling process may be divided into two aspects: facilitation of attitudinal change and provision of information. In the vast majority of cases, these aspects interact and result in behavioral change. This part of the chapter discusses what the person needs to know about hearing loss in general, his or her hearing loss in particular, hearing aids, and how best to cope with difficult listening situations. In addition, information is presented on what is involved in the establishment of an atmosphere in which the clients can modify negative feelings that they may have developed about themselves. It is important for the therapist to realize that only the client can modify his or her attitudes and resultant behavior, that the therapist's role is that of facilitator; the one who creates a situation in which change can occur.

Modification of the environment is as important as modification of the behavior of the hearing impaired individual. In this section of the chapter, education of family and others important to the client is discussed, as is use of listening aids. One of the most effective ways to reduce anxiety and frustration is to modify situations to maximize ease of communication.

The final section of the chapter contains a description of the management of one hearing impaired adult to illustrate how the various techniques discussed can be used together to facilitate adjustment.

DEFINITION OF THE PROBLEM

In order to provide meaningful assistance to the hearing impaired client, it is necessary to obtain information on the specific communicative difficulties encountered in his or her daily activities. Not only is it important to identify specific difficult listening situations, but also to assess feelings and attitudes of the client toward communication and toward him or herself as a hearing impaired person.

There are several behavioral scales available to evaluate communication functioning. All are designed to be administered prior to initiation of therapy.

CASE HISTORIES

To one degree or another the traditional case history explores areas of communicative difficulty. In the typical case history procedure, the audiologist probes difficulties with group conversation, listening in noise, use of the telephone, work-oriented situations, listening in church, and others. The interviewer also attempts to obtain some estimate of the individual's motivation to cope with his or her difficulties by environmental modification and by use of amplification. Hardick (1977) discusses the use of the interview procedure in some depth. However, the case history interview provides only a general overview of the client's communicative difficulties. It does not provide quantitative information about degree of difficulty in various situations, nor generally does it sufficiently and systematically probe the specific social, vocational, and interpersonal situations creating problems. The case history can be thought of as a screening tool, but a more precise communication evaluation is necessary in order to plan a program of rehabilitation that meets the client's specific needs and allows the audiologist to observe progress as it occurs.

HEARING HANDICAP SCALE

Perhaps the first scale designed to explore the effect of hearing loss on the activities of daily living was the Hearing Handicap Scale (High, Fairbanks, & Glorig, 1964). This is a self-report, pencil-and-paper type of scale designed to evaluate the client's experiences involving speech communication in quiet and noise, and to a lesser extent audition of background noises and warning signals. There are two forms, each containing 20 items, which have been found to correlate highly (High, et al., 1964). A typical test item is as follows: "Can you carry on a conversation with one other person when you are on a noisy street corner?"

The client must answer each item by responding to a one-to-five scale representing a response continuum based on frequency. The following verbal landmarks have been assigned to the numbers:

1. Practically always
2. Frequently
3. As often as not
4. Occasionally
5. Almost never

The advantages of this scale include:

It has been carefully standardized on a young middle aged adult population and thus the overall percentage score can be used to indicate degree of handicap.

The scale includes items probing many problem areas dealt with in rehabilitation.

Since there are two highly correlated forms, the scale can be used to measure progress.

The disadvantages of the scale include:

The scale items are homogeneous in nature and depend to a large extent on hearing sensitivity (Giolas, 1970).

The scale does not include items designed to probe vocational difficulties or feelings of the individual about his or her hearing loss, or about him or herself as a hearing impaired person.

Although there is high consistency between forms, there has been no attempt to measure test-retest reliability, either group or individual. Unless the audiologist is confident of the reliability of the client's responses on a scale, he or she cannot use that scale to measure progress over time as a function of rehabilitation.

The standardization procedures were used on a test sample with mixed, but predominantly conductive hearing losses. It is uncertain whether results would be similar with adults having pure sensorineural losses of presbycusis.

There is some question as to the appropriateness of a pencil-and-paper questionnaire with disabled people, particularly the elderly (Noble, 1972, Noble & Atherley, 1970). Although interviewer bias is not present with a questionnaire test, there is some question whether complete information or correct information is always obtained. In an interview situation where rapport between interviewer and client is present, there is greater likelihood of obtaining correct information because of greater client cooperation and understanding of the questions. It is this author's personal experience that an interview procedure is essential with the geriatric or poorly educated client.

DENVER SCALE

The Denver Scale of Communication Function (Alpiner, Chevrette, Glascoe, Metz, & Olsen, 1978) is also a pencil-and-paper questionnaire designed to assess subjectively the communication function of hearing impaired adults with acquired hearing loss. It is administered by giving to each client, prior to initiation of therapy, a questionnaire which allows the client to judge him or herself on communication function using a seven point "semantic differential" continuum. The 25 items are divided into four categories—family, self, social-vocational, and communication—in order to assess difficulties in each area so that therapy procedures can be developed to meet specific needs. The same scale is to be administered after completion of therapy to allow assessment of progress. The judgments of the client on both the pre- and postherapy scales are plotted on a graph which has an ordinate ranging from "agree" on the bottom to "disagree" on the top. Should improvement occur, the scores on the later test will be closer to the top of the graph. A sample item of the Denver Scale follows:

I now take less of an interest in many things as compared to when I did not have a hearing problem.

Agree _____ _____ _____ _____ _____ _____ _____ Disagree

Comments:

A complete discussion of the Denver Scale as well as the test items and profile form can be found in Chapter V of *Amplification for the Hearing Impaired,* edited by Michael C. Pollack (Alpiner, 1975), and in Chapter 3 of *Handbook of Adult Rehabilitative Audiology,* edited by Jerome G. Alpiner (Alpiner, 1968). This scale and others are found in the Appendix to this Text.

The major advantage of this scale over the Hearing Handicap Scale of High, Fairbanks, and Glorig is that it probes not only difficult listening situations but also feelings and attitudes of the hearing impaired person. This scale can also be given to normal hearing friends and relatives to measure their attitudes toward the hearing impaired adult.

The Denver Scale is still in pilot form; standardization information needs to be obtained. McNeill and Alpiner (Note 1) in 1975 performed a test-retest reliability study and found that overall reliability when individual scores were pooled was both statistically and clinically acceptable (above 0.7). Individual categories (family, self, social-vocational, communication) were equally reliable. However, when subjects were looked at on an individual basis, 63 percent were unreliable from test to retest. Since the scale is designed to be used to compare individuals to themselves over time, this variability in individual reliability is a serious problem. Kaplan, Brown, and Feeley (1978) modified the Denver Scale, converting it into an interview form for use with a geriatric population, and performed a test-retest reliability study. Their results were similar to those of McNeill and Alpiner. Group reliability was good, but individual test-retest reliability was unacceptable for a significant number of subjects.

The problems inherent in a self-report format discussed in connection with the Hearing Handicap Scale apply to the Denver Scale as well. There is also some question whether all clients are able to grasp the concept of the semantic differential used in the Denver Scale. Kaplan et al. found that in an interview procedure, geriatric clients had difficulty with the semantic differential. Some experienced problems remembering what the scale points meant and most had difficulty deciding between degrees of agreement or disagreement. Responses tended to fall at the extremes of the continuum.

HEARING MEASUREMENT SCALE FOR DISABILITY

The Hearing Measurement Scale was developed by Noble and Atherley in 1970 for the measurement of auditory disability in those who possess a cochlear sensorineural disorder. The scale consists of 42 items grouped into seven sections. Four of the sections are concerned with description of specific disabilities in auditory capacity (e.g., difficult listening situations). The other three sections are concerned with hearing handicap, or the emotional reactions to difficult listening situations plus the opinion of the individual about his hearing. Each item is weighted in the scoring procedure to reflect its relative importance with regard to everyday hearing handicap. Test-retest reliability has been evaluated using male subjects suffering from noise-induced hearing loss and has been found high. However, individual test-retest reliability measures have not been reported.

Noble and Atherley chose to use an interview technique rather than a paper-and-pencil format because they felt that the interview situation would provide more complete and truthful responses. They felt that they could control for interviewer bias; that is, the tendency for different interviewers to score verbal responses differently on a semantic differential scale, by using the same interviewer in a test-retest situation. McCartney, Maurer and Sorenson (1977), in their comparison of the Hearing Handicap Scale and the Hearing Measurement Scale, discuss the differential effects of the interview and self-report procedures.

Although the Hearing Measurement Scale was not developed specifically as a comparative pre- and posttherapy measure, it can be used in that way much in the same manner as the Denver Scale. With both tools, however, the problem of individual test-retest reliability must be resolved.

PROFILE QUESTIONNAIRE FOR RATING COMMUNICATIVE PERFORMANCE

Sanders (1975) recommends a somewhat different approach to defining specific areas of difficulty. He suggests using profile questionnaires for specific environments, such as home, school, occupational, and social environments. The profiles used should depend upon the individual needs of the client being evaluated. Each individual profile would contain a number of statements, each of which would be given a rating by the client ranging from +2 (little or no difficulty understanding) to −2 (great difficulty understanding). In addition, the client would be instructed to rate the frequency with which the situation is encountered on a 1–3 scale. By multiplying the value of the rating of the statement by the frequency of occurrence, one would obtain a weighted value, indicating the importance of that situation to the individual. The same profile can be used for assessment of posttherapy performance. To this date, statistical analysis of this technique has not been reported.

The most recent scale developed is the Hearing Performance Inventory of Giolas, Owens, Lamb, and Schubert (1979). It is a scale of 158 items. A sample item is, "At the beginning of a conversation, do you let a stranger know that you have a hearing problem?" The client has a choice of responses ranging from "almost never" to "practically always." This is a paper-and-pencil-type activity and covers a wide range of communication situations. The authors feel the scale can be used to develop a profile of communication difficulty to aid in planning therapy or to compare a client's assessment of his or her difficulty with the family's assessment of the problem. The Hearing Performance Inventory appears to be a promising tool, but it would be more useful if it were less time consuming. In addition, it was developed for use with a hard-of-hearing young- and middle-aged adult population. Its use with a prelingually deaf population is questionable.

ASSESSING THE CLIENT'S NEED FOR AMPLIFICATION

In asessing a client's need for amplification, audiologists customarily examine the degree of hearing loss, the pure-tone configuration, speech discrimination in quiet and in noise, and the presence of tolerance difficulties. All of these factors are extremely important, but there is another factor that is equally important and must be considered when deciding whether or not to recommend a hearing aid. That factor is: *Does the client really want a hearing aid?*

The audiologist may then objectively discuss the positive and negative aspects of amplification for that particular client, leaving the decision to him or her. Even if the client should decide not to try a hearing aid, an aural rehabilitation program should be recommended. Frequently, after a period of aural rehabilitation, the hearing impaired individual begins to feel more positively about the advantages of hearing aid use. For further discussion of this issue, see Sanders, (1975) and Rupp, Higgins, and Maurer (1977).

After the specific communicative and attitudinal problems of the client have been defined, a specific aural rehabilitation program can be developed to meet his or her needs. In addition to speechreading and auditory training exercises, personal adjustment and educational counseling must be included in the program as needed.

PERSONAL ADJUSTMENT COUNSELING

Although in the actual rehabilitation environment facilitation of attitudinal change and provision of information are intertwined, the author is artificially separating them here for purposes of discussion. As was discussed in the second page of this chapter, the personal adjustment counselor functions as a facilitator to help the client modify attitudes about him or herself as a hearing impaired person. Kodman (1967) discusses three facilitative conditions that must be present if the therapist is to be successful.

The first condition is referred to as *accurate empathy*. This refers to the understanding by the therapist of the true feelings that underlie statements the client might make. The therapist then responds in such a way that the client's feelings are reflected back to him or her, so that his or her difficulties can be viewed objectively. For example, a client might say, "Most people don't speak plainly these days. I'd rather read a book than talk to people." The empathetic clinician might reply, "It must be terribly frustrating not to understand people. Let's talk about some of your experiences." As the client begins to relate his or her difficult listening experiences, the therapist can continue reflecting back upon his or her feelings and perhaps in the process lead the client to suggest ways of coping with these situations. This is a nondirective approach. The clients makes decisions based upon an increased perception of his or her situation; decisions are not imposed upon the client. The condition of accurate empathy is as important in a group situation as in an individual session. In the group situation the therapist must reflect the feelings of each member as they are expressed. After a group becomes a cohesive unit, the members of the group may begin to practice accurate empathy toward each other, providing strong positive reinforcement for attitudinal change.

Luterman (1976) describes three levels of questions or statements that he has encountered in his counseling sessions. The first type or level is the *content* question, which actually represents an attempt to seek information. Luterman feels that this type of question is relatively rare in the initial phases of rehabilitation, although audiologists tend to react to most questions as though they were on the content level.

The second kind is the *confirmation* question. Here the client may appear to be seeking information but actually has a strong underlying opinion about his or her question and is seeking a confirming answer. As Luterman states, "Confirmation questions are very tricky and when treated as straight content questions, they invariably result in the phenomenon known as 'putting your foot in your mouth' " (p. 64). For example, a client might ask, 'If I wear a hearing aid, will shouting hurt my ears?' If this question was asked by a hearing aid user whose family generally created a noisy household environment, a positive answer to this question could provoke or intensify conflict. A safe response to such a question might be 'Maybe, what do you think?' In this manner, the client's feelings about this issue might be revealed and a source of conflict brought to the surface where it could be dealt with.

The third kind of question is the *faint knocking* question. This, according to Luterman, "contains an affect the questioner might not be aware of or is not feeling secure enough to reveal." As example of such a question might be, "If I don't wear a hearing aid will my hearing get worse?" A response based on affect might be "Some people feel so self-conscious about wearing hearing aids that they would prefer not using them regardless of the effect on communication. Is that how you feel?"

Most questions or statements can be interpreted on content, confirmation, or affect levels. It is important for the effective counselor to distinguish among the various types of questions and respond appropriately. If the audiologist is not certain that he or she is providing accurate feedback to the client, he or she can respond in the following manner: "I think what you are saying is———. Is that right?"

The second condition is referred to as *unconditional positive regard.* This involves acceptance of the client as he or she is, regardless of any hostility, belligerence, or apparent lack of cooperation. It is sometimes difficult for the novice clinician to accept expressions of negativism from a client and not to consider this behavior personal attack. However, it is important to realize that unpleasant actions or expressions are simply manifestations of the client's problems. A lady in one of this author's aural rehabilitation groups typifies this type of behavior. She originally joined the group with the stipulation that under no conditions would she allow herself to receive a hearing test. Her terms were accepted despite the fact that hearing testing was an integral part of the program. After a semester of group therapy, she apologized for her attitudes, explaining that she had been convinced that we were simply trying to sell hearing aids. She became one of the most hard-working and motivated members of the group, despite other expressions of hostility every now and then. If at the beginning of therapy we had insisted on hearing testing, we would have completely lost her as a client.

A third facilitative condition is *genuineness.* This condition implies a relaxed, friendly attitude toward the client, respect for the client's suggestions, ability to accept criticism, and communication with the client in a manner he or she can easily understand. A genuine clinician does not retreat into professional jargon or assume a pose of superiority because of his or her professional stature. An example of a low level of genuineness is the following:

Client: "I don't think this hearing aid will do me a bit of good."
Clinician: "You're not correct. The tests show a definite improvement with the hearing aid."

A more genuine type of response might be: "Maybe you're right. Why don't you try the aid at home for a few weeks and if it doesn't help, you can return it and get your money back. Let's talk again in a week."

The qualities of accurate empathy, unconditional positive regard, and genuineness can be developed or enhanced through experience. Taping sessions—with the permission of the client, of course—and reviewing the client–clinician interchange later is an excellent way for the novice clinician to improve his or her skills.

Rapport between client and clinician is established during the interview. Not only is this a time to collect pertinent information, but also to convey to the client interest in his or her problems and a genuine desire to help. All questions asked during the interview should be pertinent. This author likes to start interviews in the following fashion: "Before

I test your hearing, I need to get some information about your hearing problem. Why don't you tell me what brings you here today?" Subsequent questions relate directly to the information provided by the client in this early interchange. The interview form is merely a *guide* to make sure that important areas have been covered.

One of the most important goals of personal adjustment counseling is to help the client accept the reality of his or her hearing loss and the need for help. One must not assume that because the client has come to the clinic for evaluation, acceptance of amplification or therapy is inevitable. He or she may simply be appeasing family or friends or perhaps be taking the first tenuous steps toward seeking help while remaining very ambivalent about accepting him or herself as a hearing impaired person. As was discussed earlier in this chapter, it is important for the therapist to assess, through the interview or by the use of an attitude scale, what the client's feelings are and what experiences cause difficulty. There is no point in recommending amplification if the client is not ready to accept it. It is far better to pursuade the individual to enroll in an aural rehabilitation program which includes discussion-counseling in order to help him or her accept the reality of the hearing problem. If necessary, the group discussions can be supplemented with individual counseling. It must be made clear that participation in aural rehabilitation treatment is not contingent on hearing aid use. It must be emphasized that the audiologist is ready to assist with selection of a hearing aid if and when the client becomes ready. It has been this author's experience that many hearing impaired individuals seek amplification and use it well only after a period of aural rehabilitation.

EDUCATIONAL COUNSELING

Educational counseling refers to the provision of information about the following matters:

1. The nature of the hearing loss
2. The problems it creates
3. Difficult listening situations and suggested ways to cope
4. Types of hearing aids
5. Use and care of hearing aids
6. What can be realistically achieved with a hearing aid
7. Problems imposed by the community on hearing impaired persons

Although this type of counseling can be accomplished either in an individual or a group situation, this author feels that the group situation is more effective because experiences can be shared and peer reinforcement can occur. However, participation in a group requires that the individual identify him or herself as a person with a hearing problem. If a client is not ready for this degree of acceptance of the problem, individual therapy is preferable with the goal of ultimate participation in a group.

The Nature of Hearing Loss

Early topics to be discussed include the nature of hearing loss and the communicative problems it creates. The nature of hearing loss should be discussed as it relates to the specific individual. For example, a client may present a high-frequency hearing loss with discrimination difficulty. The client can be told that he or she hears low-pitched sounds fairly well, but has a great deal of difficulty hearing high-pitched sounds. The sound of the voice requires good hearing in the low pitches but the ability to correctly hear sounds like /s/ or /f/ or /th/ requires good hearing in the high pitches. When people have difficulty hearing /f/ and /s/ and /th/ and similar sounds, words tend to get confused with other words. Therefore, the hearing loss allows him or her to know that people are talking but not always to understand what they are saying.

Mechanism of the Ear

Discuss the mechanism of the ear, problems that can occur in different parts of the ear, types and degrees of hearing loss, and communicative problems associated with each type. In a group situation this can be followed by explanations of the audiograms and associated communication problems of various members of the group who agree to public discussion of their hearing problems. Keep the explanations simple and avoid the use of technical terms. These early discussions should reinforce and supplement the information that was given to each client following the hearing evaluation. The goal of these early sessions is to develop understanding by each individual of the nature of his or her hearing problem.

The following is an example of the type of presentation discussed above:

> The audiologist displays an enlarged picture of the pure tone audiogram of one of the clients in the group and says:
>
> "This is Mary Jones's audiogram. If you remember from when we talked about your audiograms, the numbers across the top represent the different pitches you all heard during your hearing tests, and the numbers down the side represent loudness levels. The Xs and Os represent the left and right ears and tell us how loud we had to make each pitch before Mary could just barely hear it. People with normal hearing can hear all pitches between the top of the chart and the '20' line on the graph. Now look at Mary's hearing. Mary can't hear any of the pitches until they reach the '50' line. Remember I said that the loudness level corresponding to the '50' line is the level at which I am talking now. What this means is that without her hearing aid Mary is just barely able to hear what I am saying now. But with her hearing aid on, she can hear the most important pitches around the '20' line, like some people with normal hearing. It makes quite a difference."

This type of discussion leads to many questions about individual hearing problems and development of new insights.

Coping with Difficult Listening Situations

Another important area to be dealt with is difficult listening situations and how to cope. In these presentations, those problem situations identified during the evaluations of the clients should be discussed. Suggestions for handling these situations should be elicited from the group, or the individual if the therapy format is an individual session. Assertiveness training can be easily incorporated into these sessions. It is important for the hearing impaired person to develop the attitude that he or she has the right to understand others and it is acceptable to ask people speaking to him or her to modify their conversation so that they can be understood. Many hearing impaired people do not realize that friends do not know how to help them understand and welcome suggestions.

It is helpful for the clients to learn to distinguish between the following kinds of behavior possible in any situation: aggressive, which involves violation of other people's rights; passive, which involves allowing others to violate your rights; and assertive, in which you protect your rights without violating those of other people. The audiologist might pose the following problem: ''Suppose you meet two friends on a noisy street who are having a conversation. They greet you and try to include you in their conversation but you are unable to follow what they are saying. What might you do?'' The therapist would then try to elicit some of the following examples of assertive behavior:

1. Ask the people to move away from the source of the noise so that you can understand better.
2. Ask one of the two people to briefly summarize what they had been talking about before you entered the conversation.
3. Admit you did not understand and ask for repetition or rephrasing of the idea.
4. Ask the people to speak louder.

The clients would then be asked to give examples of aggressive behavior, such as verbal or physical abuse of the speakers, and of passive behavior, such as saying nothing about the lack of understanding.

Role playing can be incorporated into assertiveness training sessions very effectively to help clients define appropriate behaviors for difficult listening situations. Homework assignments involving the use of these behaviors in actual life situations can follow the role playing sessions and be followed up by discussions at subsequent classes.

A very useful listening strategy for clarifyinng a partially understood message is to ask for repetition of only that part of the message not understood. For example, if the speaker said ''I saw Mrs. Smith in Lord and Taylor yesterday'' and the listener did not understand ''Mrs. Smith'' or ''Lord and Taylor,'' the listener might say, ''Whom did you see yesterday?'' After the speaker responds, the listener might then ask, ''Where did you see Mrs. Smith?'' Providing feedback as to what was and was not understood seems to be more acceptable than simply asking for repetition of the entire message. Appendix A at the end of this chapter provides a list of other suggestions for coping with difficult listening situations.

It is important to realize that it is difficult for many hearing impaired people to be assertive, particularly since they are too often rebuffed. Coping with difficult listening situations in the manner suggested takes practice and development of a thick skin. Be sure that you make your clients understand that you are aware of the difficulties involved in implementing these suggestions.

Combatting Depression

The hearing impaired person needs to understand the psychological changes that can accompany the loss of hearing, particularly the depression that can occur when there is loss of the primitive level. This topic is an extremely important part of educational counseling. Often an important step in relieving this depression is an understanding of the reason for it. Similarly, realization that feelings of insecurity can be traced to loss of the warning level can help the person accept these feelings as logical and allow him or her to learn to cope with them.

There are ways to combat problems at the primitive and warning levels. One of the best ways to restore hearing at the primitive level is to use a hearing aid, even though it may not transmit intelligible speech. In order to cope with loss of hearing at the warning level, the client needs to develop increased visual awareness of the environment. For example, while driving, he or she must pay careful attention to other drivers to become aware of the presence of an ambulance or an accident in his or her path. Visual warning signals in the form of flashing lights can be installed at home to alert him or her to the sound of the telephone, doorbell, or baby crying. All of these possible courses of action should be discussed during group or individual therapy sessions.

Hearing Aids

Much educational counseling regarding hearing aids is needed. It is vital that prospective hearing aid users understand what a hearing aid will and will not do. The limitations of amplification in a noisy situation must be clearly explained, so that disappointment will be minimized when the individual becomes a hearing aid user. The new hearing aid user must also understand, first, that no hearing aid will restore normal hearing, second, that speech may not sound completely natural, and third, that perfect understanding in all situations may not be possible. The prognosis for successful hearing aid use will vary with the individual depending on the type, degree, and configuration of the hearing loss and discrimination problem, and the needs and attitudes of the individual. The person whose hearing difficulties exist primarily in situations where competing noise is a factor will generally be less satisfied with a hearing aid than the person who experiences primarily a problem of insufficient loudness. The demanding person who expects to understand perfectly with amplification in all situations will be less satisfied than his or her more adaptable counterpart who better accepts the limitations of amplification. Therefore, in addition to discussing limitations of amplification in general, the prognosis of the individual seeking a hearing aid should be explained based on his or her specific problems and needs.

Other aspects of hearing aid use need to be discussed. These include:

1. Who needs a hearing aid
2. Description of the hearing aid evaluation procedure
3. Roles of the doctor, audiologist, hearing aid dealer
4. How to most effectively use and take care of the hearing aid

These areas are more completely discussed in Chapter 5.

Consumerism

Discussion of consumerism should be a part of all aural rehabilitation programs. The problems of the hearing impaired in obtaining service from the community are very real. Examples of inadequate services include telephones that cannot be used with hearing aids and the lack of visual warning signals in some smoke detectors. Hearing impaired people need to be able to vent their frustrations regarding these difficulties, and to be made aware of community organizations representing their interests, e.g., the Alexander Graham Bell Association, the Gray Panthers, Consumer Organization for the Hearing Impaired (COHI), and Self Help for the Hard of Hearing (SHHH). They should be made aware of existing and proposed legislation affecting the hearing impaired and should be encouraged to become activists in promoting their own interests. Not only is activism a special form of assertiveness for hearing impaired people but it also requires complete acceptance of themselves as hearing impaired persons.

Speechreading and Auditory Training

Speechreading and auditory training are integral parts of all aural rehabilitation programs. Since this subject is discussed in depth in other portions of this text, only a few words will be included here. In the preparation of speechreading/auditory training lessons, materials relevant to the situations causing communicative difficulty should be used. As the hearing impaired person becomes more familiar with the language and the distractions appropriate to these communicative situations, his or her ability to cope with them increases. In this way, adjustment is facilitated.

EDUCATING THE FAMILY AND ASSOCIATES

Family and Friends

Since communication involves not only the hearing impaired person but also family members, employers, friends, and others, educational counseling of these people is extremely important to the adjustment of the hearing impaired person. Family members or associates must understand the nature of the client's hearing problem and the specific ways communication is affected. It is highly desirable to include spouses, children, parents, or friends in the initial explanation of the client's hearing loss after testing is completed. If these people have accompanied the client to the initial evaluation, they should be present at the counseling session following testing. Other family members or friends should be involved in the client's rehabilitation at a time judged most expeditious by the client and the audiologist. In some cases, it may be wise for the audiologist to initially see family members separately from the hearing impaired individual. This should be considered if strong conflicts exist within the family constellation. These judgments must be made on an individual basis.

The limitations imposed by some types of hearing loss are baffling to the lay person who finds it difficult to understand why some things can be heard easily and other conversational situations are handled poorly. The effect of the high-frequency hearing loss on speech perception, the practical effects of a discrimination problem, and the devastating effects of competing noise or competing speech on the understanding of the hearing impaired person must be carefully explained. For complete understanding, several explanations at different times may be necessary, as is often the case with the hearing impaired person as well. For that reason, normal hearing family members or friends should be encouraged to enter a rehabilitation group with the client. Hardick (1977) feels so strongly about this that he refuses to allow a client to enter his rehabilitation group unless that client is accompanied by such a person.

There is an excellent recording produced by Zenith Radio Corporation and edited by Dr. Aram Glorig (Glorig, 1971) that illustrates, by using filtered speech, how difficult it is to hear when certain speech frequencies are not heard; demonstrates difficult listening situations; demonstrates what speech sounds like through hearing aids adjusted in different ways; and explains a few simple rules for making understanding easier for the hearing impaired person. This author has found this recording very useful for family counseling.

It is important for the family members to understand the limitations of amplification, particularly the fact that a hearing aid may not improve communication at all in noisy situations, or possibly only to a limited extent. It is in the difficult listening situation that the spouse or friend can be particularly helpful. He or she can speak naturally and clearly, make sure to face the light when speaking, rephrase rather than repeat a sentence when it is not understood, and provide clues to meaning in a group conversation. Noisy situations can be minimized. If the family is going out to dinner, a quiet restaurant can be chosen. Social activities can be modified to favor small rather than large group activities.

It is valuable to identify specific situations in the home that create special difficulty by using the case history or behavioral scale information. Then family and client together can discuss ways to minimize these difficulties without disrupting the life of the household. For example, this type of family counseling session worked well for the man who refused to use his hearing aid at home because of the noise level in the house. After all members of the family voiced their points of view and frustrations (for instance, the children claimed they were forced to shout because their father did not pay attention, even when using his hearing aid), they were able to make constructive suggestions to help alleviate the problem. Some of the suggestions for alleviating the situation were:

The father would wear his hearing aid at home.
He would keep away from the kitchen during meal preparation and clean-up because of the high levels of noise.
The children would not shout, slam doors, or play music at excessive volume.
Everyone would try to communicate with the father in a face-to-face situation and avoid shouting from one room to another.
The father would make a conscious effort to use his speechreading skills.

The family of the hearing impaired client must understand that the adjustment to amplification takes time for many people. The family can provide a great deal of aid and support during this difficult period. Most important, optimal aided communication must not be expected of the new hearing aid user too soon. It is acceptable for the new hearing aid user initially to wear his aid only in quiet situations or only for part of the day.

The person who has had a sudden loss of hearing has a particularly difficult adjustment to make. He or she often experiences a period of mourning or self-pity that can be quite unbearable for all concerned. Most important during this period of mourning is the family's emotional support and their adjustment to the loss. The hearing impaired person must know that his or her feelings are understood and that he or she is not being a burden to the family. Honest discussion of feelings by all family members involved plus specific suggestions to ease communication are very helpful.

There are times when *not* bringing family members into the rehabilitative situation creates additional problems. A parent, child, or spouse may feel resentful that he or she was not included. The case of an 18-year-old girl comes to mind. Without informing her parents, she initiated contact with an audiological facility for help with her discrimination problem. When her father learned of this contact he was furious at not being informed of the problem prior to her evaluation. Several sessions of family counseling were necessary before all members of the family were able to function as a cooperative unit to help the girl with her problem.

Employers

In addition to intervention with the family, it is often necessary to educate employers and fellow employees in ways to optimize communication with the hearing impaired person. Areas of difficulty should be identified by using the case history or behavioral scale and the desirability of intervention should be carefully discussed with the client. If the client feels that intervention on the job would be detrimental, his or her judgment should be respected. If he or she and the employer are receptive, however, the same types of suggestions useful with family and friends are applicable. In addition, modifications to maximize communication can be made in the job environment, such as a telephone amplifier installed on the client's office phone. See Appendix B at the end of this chapter for additional suggestions that can be given to normal hearing individuals important to the hearing impaired client.

Educating School Personnel

The young adult in school may have special problems related to that environment. Not only does he or she need counseling on ways of coping in the classroom, but his or her teachers also need and appreciate suggestions that maximize the probability of success of the hearing impaired student in a class with normal hearing peers. Although we usually think of classroom problems as restricted to children, there are many hearing impaired college students and adults in vocationally oriented programs who need special help with the classroom situation. Interestingly enough, many modifications in teaching techniques designed to help the hearing impaired student will also help the normal hearing students in the classroom. See Appendix C at the end of this chapter for suggestions concerning students with hearing impairment.

It may sometimes be necessary to involve teachers and school administrators in modifying the learning environment for hearing impaired students. Large lecture halls present much difficulty for the person with a hearing problem, regardless of whether he or she uses amplification. Rooms with poor acoustics and teachers who do not articulate clearly also create problems for hearing impaired students. It would be ideal to enroll such teachers in public speaking courses, but this is usually not practical. Often the best way to alleviate such problems is to schedule the student for classes held in small rooms with good acoustics, taught by teachers who speak clearly. Obviously these modifications are not always possible, but their feasibility should be explored.

The Utah State University has developed a program of supportive services for hearing impaired college students involving tutoring, speech and hearing remediation, and classroom and instructional adjustments. This program is discussed in Berg (1972).

AN EXAMPLE OF PATIENT MANAGEMENT

Mrs. Kensington is a 53-year-old woman who had possessed a mild bilateral hearing loss since age 30. She is bilingual, with Spanish as her native language. She had adjusted well to amplification and was able to function as an English teacher in a local high school until two years ago, when her hearing sensitivity dropped dramatically bilaterally. The drop in hearing was accompanied by dizziness and persisted after the dizziness had subsided. Over a period of one month, hearing sensitivity improved to the level of moderate impairment but dropped again as a result of exposure to a fire siren. Antihistamines and vasodilators were administered by her physician in an attempt to improve the hearing but were unsuccessful.

Audiological evaluation revealed a severe bilateral sensorineural hearing loss with poor speech discrimination and a severe tolerance problem. The site of lesion was cochlear. Although binaural hearing aids were fitted, sufficient gain for her degree of loss could not be used for fear of triggering another episode. Therefore, the hearing aids were not completely satisfactory in transmitting intelligible speech. Since her speech understanding was no longer sufficient to allow her to continue teaching, and since she could no longer tolerate the normal noise levels of a school, she was forced to retire from her teaching position.

Mrs. Kensington's first visit occurred after the second sudden drop in auditory sensitivity. She was undergoing otoneurological tests to try to determine the source of the problem and had been referred for an audiological evaluation as part of the diagnostic workup. She appeared depressed and anxious, but hopeful that some medical remedy for her problem would be found. The case history interview and Denver Scale questionnaire revealed:

1. Communication difficulties in almost all situations
2. A feeling of worthlessness because she could no longer work
3. Extreme sensitivity to what she perceived as callousness by anyone with whom she could not communicate
4. Resentment toward her husband because she felt he was unsympathetic toward her problems
5. Fear that another attack of dizziness and further deterioration of hearing could occur at any time

She was eager to try any type of amplification that would improve her communication.

At the conclusion of the audiological evaluation her hearing loss was explained briefly. Detail was avoided because it was the judgment of the audiologist that she could not absorb a lengthy explanation of her hearing status at that time. It was agreed that we would experiment with different types of amplification and start her in a speechreading-counseling program concurrent with the otolaryngologist's attempts to treat the situation medically. Since she was not receptive to enrollment in a group, individual therapy was arranged on a twice-weekly schedule. It was suggested that she ask her husband to attend sessions with her, but she felt that that would not be appropriate.

Each therapy session consisted of speechreading training, educational counseling, and discussion of her problems. Various modifications of her binaural hearing aids were tried during these sessions to find an optimal arrangement for her. Some time was spent during each therapy session in hearing aid orientation activities. Auditory training, aside from hearing aid orientation, was not attempted because removal of visual clues proved too frustrating, and competing speech or noise could not be used for fear of triggering dizziness. Goals of therapy were:

1. To improve communication by improving speechreading skills
2. To teach ways of better handling difficult listening situations
3. To help her view communication partners, particularly her husband, in a more realistic and less threatening manner
4. To help her identify warning signs of an impending attack of dizziness so that she could either leave the situation or take one of the pills her doctor had given her for control (her doctors had been able to find a medication that would prevent or minimize attacks)
5. To find a hearing aid that would provide maximal speech intelligibility
6. To help her seek another source of employment or volunteer work that would restore a sense of self-worth

During the first semester of therapy her speechreading skills improved rapidly. That, in combination with tactics designed to help with difficult listening situations, improved her handling of communication sufficiently to allow some improved self-confidence. She also learned to recognize impending symptoms of an attack of dizziness earlier and thus became more willing to enter situations where noise might be present.

At the end of the first semester she felt that she was ready to enter group therapy. At first she was fearful that she would not be accepted by the group because her hearing would be far worse than anyone else's. However, it quickly became apparent that others in the group suffered equally great or more severe hearing losses and were managing to cope with them. She found the group a source of support in her attempts to adjust to her own problems and also found that she in turn could be of help to other group members. Her ability to assist others served to enhance her feeling of worth. Initially she did not ask her husband to participate in the group, but after seeing that other spouses were present she agreed to invite him. The information that he received from these sessions has brought them closer together and has eased the strains at home.

She is still a member of the group. Her speechreading skills are still improving, as is her ability to handle difficult communication situations. These skills partially compensate for the less than optimal speech intelligibility provided by her hearing aids. She has joined a local self-help group whose purpose is to improve services for the hearing impaired, and is well on her way to becoming an activist. She has had one attack of dizziness, triggered by noise exposure, but has experienced no further deterioration of hearing. Her reaction to this attack, however, was markedly different than previously. She simply attributed it to the fact that she had delayed the taking of a pill and considered it a warning that she must be more vigilant to minimal symptoms in the future. Perhaps most important, she is currently negotiating a position as an English language tutor to Spanish-speaking hearing impaired adolescents.

REFERENCES

Alpiner, J. G. Hearing aid selection for adults, in M. C. Pollack (Ed.), *Amplification for the hearing impaired*. New York: Grune and Stratton, 1975, pp. 145–205.

Alpiner, J. G., Chevrette, W., Glascoe, G., Metz, M., & Olsen, B. The Denver scale of communication function, in J. G. Alpiner (Ed.), *Handbook of Adult rehabilitative audiology*. Baltimore: Williams and Wilkins, 1978, pp. 53–56.

Berg, F. S. A model for a facilitative program for hearing impaired college students. *Volta Review*, 1972, *74*, 370.

Giolas, T. G. The measurement of hearing handicap, *Maico Audiological library series*. Maico Hearing Instruments, Minneapolis, Vol. 8, report 6, 1970.

Giolas, T. G., Lamb, S., Owens, E., & Schubert, E. Hearing performance inventory. *Journal of Speech and Hearing Disorders*, 1979, *44*, 169–195.

Glorig, A. (Ed.). *Getting through: A guide to better understanding of the hard of hearing*. Chicago: Zenith Radio Corporation, 1971.

Hardick, E. J. Aural rehabilitation programs for the aged can be successful. *Journal of the Academy of Rehabilitative Audiology*, 1977, *10*, 51–66.

High, W. S., Fairbanks, G., & Glorig, A. Scale of self assessment of hearing handicap. *Journal of Speech and Hearing Disorders*, 1964, *29*, 215–230.

Kaplan, H., Brown, J., & Feeley, J. A modified Denver scale: Test-retest reliability. *Journal of The Academy of Rehabilitative Audiology*, 1978, *11*, 15–32.

Kodman, F. Techniques for counseling the hearing aid client, *Maico Audiological Library Series*. Maico Hearing Instruments, Minneapolis, Vol. 8, reports 23–25, 1967.

Luterman, D. The counseling experience. *Journal of the Academy of Rehabilitative Audiology*, 1976, *9*, 62–66.

McCartney, J. H., Maurer, J. H., & Sorenson, F. D. A comparison of the hearing handicap scale and the hearing measurement scale with standard audiometric measures on a geriatric population. *Hearing Aid Journal,* Oct. 1977, p. 10.

Noble, W. G. The measurement of hearing handicap: A further viewpoint, *Maico audiological library series*. Maico Hearing Instruments, Minneapolis, Vol. 10, Report 5, 1972.

Noble, W. G., Atherley, G. R. C. The hearing measurement scale: A questionnaire for the assessment of auditory disability. *Journal of Auditory Research,* 1970, *10,* 193–214.

Rupp, R. R., Higgins, J., & Maurer, J. F. A feasibility scale for predicting hearing aid use (FSPHAU) with older individuals. *Journal of the Academy of Rehabilitative Audiology,* 1977, *10,* 81.

Sanders, D. A. Hearing aid orientation and counseling, in M. C. Pollack (Ed.), *Amplification for the hearing impaired.* New York: Grune and Stratton, 1975, pp. 323–372.

REFERENCE NOTE

1. McNeill, M. R., & Alpiner, J. G. A study of the reliability of the Denver scale of communicative function. Unpublished data, University of Denver, 1975.

APPENDIX A: HOW TO COPE WITH DIFFICULT LISTENING SITUATIONS

- Ask speakers to speak in a good light and while facing the listener so that speechreading skills can be used.
- Ask the speaker to speak clearly and naturally but not to shout or exaggerate articulatory movements.
- If you do not understand what a speaker is saying, ask the speaker to repeat or rephrase the statement.
- If entering a group in the middle of a conversation, ask one person to sum up the gist of the conversation.
- If someone is speaking at a distance, that person should be asked to stand closer.
- If the speaker turns his head away, ask him or her to face you to permit optimal speechreading and listening.
- If you are attempting to understand speech in the presence of noise, try to move yourself and the speaker away from the source of the noise.
- When in a communication situation requiring exact information, such as asking directions or obtaining schedules for a trip, request that the speaker write the crucial information.
- If the speaker is talking while eating, smoking, or chewing, request that he or she not do so because of the difficulty speechreading.
- A person who has a unilateral loss should be sure to keep his or her good ear facing the speaker at all times.
- If possible, avoid rooms with poor acoustics. If meetings are held in such rooms, request that they be transferred to other rooms with less reveberation.
- If a speaker at a meeting cannot be heard, request that he use a microphone.
- Come early to meetings so that you can sit close to the speaker. Avoid taking a seat near a wall to minimize the possibility of reverberation. This is particularly important for those who use hearing aids.
- If you are going to a movie or to the theater, read the reviews in advance to familiarize yourself with the plot.
- In an extremely noisy situation, limit conversation to before the noise has started or after the noise has subsided. Normal hearing people do this all the time. For example, if a plane goes by and a conversation is going on, most people will halt their conversation and wait until the plane has gone by.

APPENDIX B: DO'S AND DON'TS WHEN TALKING WITH A HEARING IMPAIRED PERSON*

- Don't assume the hearing impaired person is intellectually impaired.
- Do give the hearing impaired person a chance to be involved in the communication process.
- Do position yourself so that maximal light shines upon your face—not on the hearing impaired person.

---

*This list was developed in conjunction with a group of hearing impaired adults enrolled in an aural rehabilitation group.

- Do not shout unless there is an acute emergency. Speak in a normal audible voice directed toward the hearing impaired person. This helps to eliminate distortion. Your loud voice calls others' attention to a difficult speaking situation.
- Do use clear, distinct articulation.
  —Don't clip word endings or mumble.
  —Don't overarticulate.
  —Speak to the hearing impaired person as you would want someone to speak to you!
  —Maintain good posture when you speak. This improves articulation and projection of the voice, making it easier for the hearing impaired person to understand.
- Don't speak with your back to the hearing impaired person.
- Don't use facial contortions and exaggerations of normal facial gestures. Use natural facial expressions. Unnecessary use of eyes, eyebrows, smile, or body movements is distracting.
- Don't use excessive body movements. Avoid talking while moving around. Use natural gestures.
- Don't talk with your mouth full, while chewing gum, or while smoking.
- Don't speak with objects such as hands, paper, or a microphone in front of your mouth. This is distracting.
- Don't stand too close to a hearing impaired person while speaking. Breath odors or mouth moisture may cause the listener to instinctively withdraw and this withdrawal may be interpreted as unfriendliness. In addition, it is difficult to speechread when the speaker is too close.
- Do give the hearing impaired person the topic of conversation. Don't force him to guess. (e.g., "We are talking about ———".)
- Do restate what you've said when you detect the hearing impaired person has misunderstood. Look for clues of misunderstanding (e.g. facial expressions, inappropriate responses). However, don't assume the listener will misunderstand and repeat everything. You'll be a bore and you'll insult his or her intelligence. As a last resort, write to the hearing impaired person.
- Don't show annoyance with the hearing impaired person's questions. He or she is trying hard to understand.
- Do speak to, not about, the hearing impaired person.
- Do help the hearing impaired person manipulate the environment, to allow communication in as noise-free an atmosphere as possible.
- Do encourage the hearing impaired person to rest. Listening and looking continually are fatiguing tasks.
- Do not startle a hearing impaired person. Attract his or her attention before speaking (e.g., lightly stomp on the floor or switch the light). A good way to get the attention of a hearing impaired person is to gently tap his or her shoulder with your forefinger two or three times. Wait for a reaction and then speak. When the hearing impaired person is at a distance, wave your hand and smile. Find out how he or she likes to be aroused from sleeping. A good way is to tap him or her on the shoulder or knee gently and speak in his or her better ear.
- Do respond to the hearing impaired person's questions or statements with more than one word. (For example, the question "What do you want to eat?" can be logically answered with the words "meat, beet, bean, meal", all of which look alike. How-

ever, if you use a sentence such as "I'd like some rare meat", the word "meat" is not likely to be confused with the other words.

- Do use stress on key words, inflections for questions, and pauses between lengthy statements. Be careful, however, to use adult language—you're not addressing a child. If necessary, repeat the key word and spell it.
- Do go to the hearing impaired person. Don't require him or her to listen and lipread over excessive distances—but don't get too close.
- Do attempt to be on the same level as the hearing impaired person so he or she doesn't have to lipread a person whose face is too high or too low.
- Do listen to the hearing impaired person.

APPENDIX C: HELPING THE HEARING IMPAIRED STUDENT

- Preferential seating is important to anyone with a hearing problem. The hearing impaired adult will usually know what position in a classroom is best for him or her. However, since the focus of attention may change during a lecture, the student should be assured that any change of seat will not be considered disruptive.
- The teacher should be careful to speak only when the hearing impaired student can see his or her lips. The following situations should be avoided if possible:
  —Talking with one's back to the class, as when writing on the blackboard.
  —Standing in front of a window or a bright light. The light should be shining in the speaker's face, not the student's eyes.
  —Teaching from the back of the room where the student cannot see.
  —Walking around the classroom while talking.
- The teacher should:
  —Speak in a careful yet natural manner. Avoid exaggerated lip movements.
  —Restate or rephrase statements when the student fails to understand.
  —Not cover his or her face with a hand or a book while reading.
  —Not stand too close to a student who must lipread. He might have to tilt his head back to see the speaker's face, causing unnecessary strain and fatigue.
- A hearing impaired student relies heavily on written material to obtain information. It is helpful to inform him or her in advance what material will be covered on a particular day so that pertinent material can be read in advance.
- It is not possible for the hearing impaired student to use visual cues in class and take notes simultaneously. The teacher can either prepare special lecture notes or request that a fellow student share notes with the hearing impaired student.
- The teacher should use the blackboard or the overhead projector as much as possible. If the written material must be copied by the students, lecturing should not occur at the same time.
- Oral tests should never be given to a hearing impaired student.
- The teacher should be available for extra tutoring. The hearing impaired student should be encouraged to meet with the teacher after class for explanation of material not understood.

C. Other Aspects of the Process of Aural Rehabilitation for Adults

Daniel L. Bode
David Tweedie
Raymond H. Hull

Chapter 8: Improving Communication through Aural Rehabilitation

One of the basic premises that is apparent is that some form of rehabilitative activity should accompany the discovery of a hearing loss. An examination of traditional literature dealing with aural rehabilitation procedures, however, leaves one less than satisfied. Research in various areas of aural rehabilitation are marginally applicable to the process of therapy.

Investigators have explored various aspects of speechreading and auditory training, but these processes appear to be global and thus difficult to quantify. Attempting to use these data in the determination of a treatment focus for particular clients becomes difficult. Further, in spite of subjective evaluation that certain strategies of aural rehabilitation are more effective than others, definitive validation of treatment techniques is still missing. The complexities of auditory impairment in its varying degrees of severity along with the variability of persons affected result in challenges that are both fascinating and frustrating.

The most successful approaches would appear to be those that address and incorporate specific therapy procedures as well as other needs of clients as they relate to the impairment of hearing and their communicative needs. It has been known for some time, for example, that the use of vision alone is not as efficient as a combination of the use of vision, the client's residual hearing, and environmental cues which enhance the totality of human communication. The latter philosophy will be stressed throughout this chapter.

This chapter will address a number of avenues and approaches to aural rehabilitation. It must be remembered, however, that the complexities observed within hearing impaired adults require a client-oriented approach to aural rehabilitation. Using a ''method'' without considering the specific needs of given clients may result in inadequate treatment.

TECHNIQUES FOR IMPROVING COMMUNICATION AMONG HEARING IMPAIRED ADULTS: PAST AND PRESENT

Before addressing current issues involved in the process of aural rehabilitation for adults, a review of factors involved in the use of vision and audition in communication is appropriate.

Lipreading

The visibility of the phonemes of speech has not been found to be sufficient for total reliance in communication for most persons. It has been difficult, however, to extinguish the term "lipreading" and its connotations of vision-alone.

Early definitions of lipreading, for example Bruhn (1949), stressed the eye as literally taking the place of the ear. She felt that the eye could be trained to distinguish the visible characteristics of the movements of the speech mechanism. Such descriptions of lipreading have been passed on through the years, and the term still tends to denote such strict concentration on the visualization of speech.

Other early methods of lipreading stressing the primary use of vision were those of the Kinzies (1931), Bunger (1961)—the Jena Method—and Nitchie (1950). In the early to middle part of this century, however, it was undoubtedly more necessary to emphasize the visual mode in communication when providing therapy for hearing impaired adults. As stated by McCarthy and Alpiner (1978), the visual-only methods stressed in early attempts at aural rehabilitation were emphasized due to lack of efficient amplification systems.

A review of those early methods is appropriate since it is from these that our more current procedures have evolved or deviated.

The Mueller-Walle Method

Martha Bruhn introduced the Mueller-Walle method in 1902. This method was strictly analytic in its approach. It stressed development of lipreading skills through kinesthetic awareness of the movements in speech production. It involved rapid, rhythmic syllable drills since it was felt that the syllable is the basic unit of words, that in turn, comprise sentences, and should be subconsciously recognized. Bruhn viewed lipreading as training the eye as well as the mind, and felt that it involved visual, auditory, and motor memory. Her plans for lipreading lessons were divided into four parts:

1. Definition of the movement(s) of the new sound to be studied, contrasting the movements of the new sound with the ones previously studied
2. Written work
3. A story or talk that incorporated the new sound
4. Group practice or a period of questions

Jena Method

Anna Bunger and Bessie Whitaker introduced the Jena method of lipreading. The method was developed by Karl Brauckmann of Germany. Bunger (1944 and 1961) outlined Brauckmann's method, which emphasizes the audible, visible, movement, mimetic, and gesture forms of communication, including syllable and rhythm. The movement form was thought of as being complete for all persons no matter what the level of hearing, since not all movements of the muscular system for speech are completely visible. The mimetic form was viewed as incomplete but an important component of communication. Brauckmann also believed that the gesture form was not complete, but that it complements all others above.

Bunger (1961) states that the first aim of persons who desire to learn lipreading is to develop awareness of the movements of speech and to learn how they feel. This was called kinesthetic awareness, and it was then to become a substitute for audition.

The method included an explanation of the formation and composition of syllables. The consonants were presented and classified under the categories of production, including lips, tongue, and tongue–soft palate. The consonants were combined with words for practice. The consonants were said aloud, and then the client said them. Clients were asked to concentrate on the manner of articulation for their production, and to categorize them in accordance with the three areas above.

The rhythmic component of this method included a basic rhythmic pattern that was established to accompany the syllable drills such as hand clapping, tapping, or ball bouncing. The aim of this aspect was to alert the client to the feeling of speech movements as he or she talks and to imitate visible speech movements as another person is speaking.

The materials used included the above syllable exercises, grammatical forms, and stories and conversations.

The Nitchie Approach

In 1903, Edward Nitchie introduced an approach that was intended to break away from the more analytic approaches. His method advocated a "whole thought" approach to lipreading by emphasizing a working relationship between mind and eye. This mode of thinking paved the way toward a more psychological-synthetic basis for lipreading. Stress was placed on grasping the whole of the message when not all auditory information was available. This was in contrast to the philosophies of Bruhn and Bunger, which stressed working with the analytic components of words. Elizabeth Nitchie (1950), Edward's wife, revised his materials and added additional ones. The integrity of Edward's wholistic approach was retained. Ordman and Ralli (1957) utilized Nitchie's approach and, with the aid of Elizabeth, developed lifelike materials for use in lipreading lessons.

The Kinzie Approach

The Kinzie sisters, Cora and Rose, designed a lipreading approach and materials that evolved from a philosophy that incorporated portions of those by Mueller-Walle and Nitchie, and is considered a synthetic approach. Their method involved a graded sequence of lipreading lessons based upon varying levels of lipreading ability for both children and adults. The grading of the lessons was completed so that individuals could progress from one level of skill to the next at their own rate.

In the development of their materials, several rules were established. They were as follows:

1. Sentences that were definite should be used.
2. Sentences should be natural in their structure.
3. Word selection should also be natural.
4. Sentences should be interesting, pleasing, and rhythmic.
5. All sentences must be dignified.

Within their story sections, they chose those that were short and humorous. They felt that these held the greatest value for beginners and intermediates. They also chose stories about famous people for these two levels. They felt that higher level literary selections were most appropriate for advanced clients.

Within their lessons, explanations of articulatory movements for sound production were made, including sample words that contained those sounds and contrasting words. Vocabulary lists preceded sentence work. More advanced lessons included stories and accompanying questions. Mirror work in relation to sound production was advocated during lipreading practice. They also stressed the use of voice during lessons to aid clients in the use of their residual hearing. Their materials for adults included 36 lessons on movements of sounds, 36 lessons on stories, and 18 lessons utilizing homophenous words.

The methods reviewed above were generally administered to clients in strict, unalterable ways. When clients had progressed through the lessons to the point of completing them, or had advanced in their lipreading skills to their apparent maximum, they were dismissed. The actual success rate is still unknown, although many clients apparently felt that they had benefited. And some probably did. In one way or another, they were perhaps better able to understand the speech of others in spite of the fact that they did not have the advantage of amplification devices.

According to Hull (1979), however, strict methods of lipreading which are presented as a structured sequence of lessons are now generally felt to be unsatisfactory for two basic reasons:

1. After the sequence has been completed, clients generally emerge unchanged in their ability to communicate with others. Even though individual clients may thank the audiologist who provided the lipreading sessions by saying such polite things as, "I surely learned a lot," or "Thank you, your lessons were *very* interesting," they may have concluded that they did not improve.
2. Those approaches do not lend themselves to a basic need in the process of aural rehabilitation. That is addressing specific communicative difficulties that clients face on a daily basis, and aiding them to function more efficiently in spite of their auditory deficit.

The strict approaches described above, and others like them, are based on the assumption that if the lessons are adhered to and learned, they will aid hearing impaired people to identify the visual clues of speech. In that regard, then, it was felt that they should likewise be able to communicate better within their everyday worlds. Although the assumption appeared rational to those who advocated the use of those strict and relatively unalterable approaches, it is generally not a valid one (Hull, 1979).

The Efficiency of Vision in Communication

Research on the benefit of the visual-only mode in communication has likewise revealed a much less than optimistic picture. A number of investigators have studied the efficiency of vision in speech reception. The purpose of the majority of those investigations was to study the reciprocal benefits of vision and audition. For example, studies by Heider and Heider (1940), Utley (1946), DiCarlo and Kataja (1951), O'Neill (1954), Hutton (1959), Woodward and Barber (1960), Brannon (1961), Erber (1969), Binnie and Barrager (Note 1), Hull and Alpiner (1976), and Erber (1979) have concluded that vision alone contributes only approximately 50 percent to speech intelligibility when no auditory information is available. Erber (1969), for example, confirmed that for essentially inaudible speech, intelligibility scores in vision-alone conditions remain at about 50 percent. Hull and Alpiner (1976) reported that among young adults who possessed normal language function, approximately 50 percent of linguistically and phonemically balanced words within sentences could be identified in conditions of vision alone. They also found that only about 30 percent of sentences could be identified relative to their content when subjects were forced to depend upon vision as the only sensory modality.

The Complement of Audition to Vision

Erber (1979) again demonstrated that vision alone under optimal conditions permits only about 50 percent intelligibility. For children who possessed a severe sensorineural hearing loss, vision alone was attributed approximately 35–41 percent intelligibility. However, this study, like others, demonstrated the considerable complement of vision to audition and audition to vision. For example, in utilizing a systematic mechanism for manipulating the amount of visual clarity available to subjects (plexiglas placed at various distances to simulate visual acuity of from 20/20—normal—to 20/400—severe visual deficit), Erber (1979) found a 44 percent advantage when clear visual clues were available and combined with audition at a comfortable level. This advantage was maintained in spite of a simulated severe high frequency hearing loss (450 Hz low-pass filter with a 35 dB rolloff per octave). Even with the existence of the simulated high frequency hearing loss, scores increased from 54 percent intelligibility for single words in the vision-alone mode at 20/20 vision, to 98 percent when the distorted auditory mode was also introduced, demonstrating the complement of vision to low frequency hearing.

Erber (1979) also utilized the same procedure for the visual mode with severely hearing impaired children. The results from identifying content words within sentences indicated that the benefit of their dominant sensory modality (vision) is great under optimal conditions (20/20 vision) but still only allows for approximately 33 percent intelligibility. When their amplified residual hearing was combined with clear vision, their intelligibility scores increased to 68 percent. For profoundly hearing impaired children who were studied, the contribution of the auditory modality was found to be only 6 percent. However, the combined auditory and visual score was 47 percent. When vision was reduced to replicate a severe loss of vision, scores dropped to 4 percent. Again, the complement of audition is evident, but proportionate to the degree of auditory impairment. In working with adventitiously hearing impaired adults, however, the majority are found within the mild and moderate to more severe categories, where the complement of audition to vision and vice versa is very evident.

According to Hull (1979), the reasons for the lack of definitiveness in the visual-only reception of speech are probably that some phonemes look alike; some phonemes are difficult to identify because they are not visible by observing the lips (only about one third of the phonemes of American English are readily recognizable by observing the face of the speaker); and there is a general lack of redundancy of the visemes of speech relative to the comprehension of verbal messages. Audition, even at minimal levels, adds greatly to the synthesis and closure required to comprehend speech.

Other studies that confirm the complement of audition to vision include those by O'Neill (1954), Sumby and Pollack (1954), Miller and Nicely (1955), Prall (1957), Hutton, Curry and Armstrong (1959), Van Uden (1960), Erber (1971), Binnie, Montgomery and Jackson (1974), and Hull and Alpiner (1976).

Although it is important for clients to recognize the benefits of vision in communication, particularly in adverse listening environments, the efficient use of their residual hearing should be brought to a high level of awareness during aural rehabilitation. They should be made aware not only of the limitations imposed by their impaired hearing, but also of the amount of residual hearing available for use. Both should also be discussed in light of the efficient and complementary uses of audition and vision in communication.

IMPROVING COMMUNICATION SKILLS

Up to this time, the discussion in this chapter has centered on some early traditional methods used in attempts at improving hearing impaired persons' ability to communicate in their worlds and the benefits and limitations of the sensory modalities used in verbal communication and in most forms of aural rehabilitation.

As noted earlier, the approaches to aural rehabilitation for adults that appear to be most effective are those that are wholistic. That is to say, there is more to resolving the communication deficit resulting from an adventitious hearing loss than learning to use residual hearing and complementary visual clues. That is not to say, however, that these aspects are not extremely important in the process.

The most critical aspect of the process of aural rehabilitation is the client. This is where some of the earlier approaches may have lost their validity. Current philosophies which stress wholistic approaches to aural rehabilitation services for the adult include those by Fleming, Birkle, Kolman, Miltenberger, and Israel (1973), Binnie (1976), Colton (1977), Tannahill and Smoski (1978), Alpiner (1978), Hull (1979), and many others. Fleming et al, for example, state that although approaches to aural rehabilitation treatment may vary from therapist to therapist, this type of variation is good *only* if it still meets the specific needs of clients. Tannahill and Smoski stress that regardless of the age of the client or the degree of loss, each individual must be considered in light of his or her background, current needs, and life-style, and the anticipated demands on his or her communication skills.

Binnie (1976) presents a wholistic view when he states that,

> A philosophy that undergirds relevant aural rehabilitation is that every hearing impaired adult has the right to receive all of the services he or she needs to effect maximum communication efficiently . . . Aural rehabilitation involves a team approach, including participation by otology, audiology, psychology, vocational rehabilitation, and education. (p. 217)

Alpiner (1978) further stresses the need for taking the whole client into consideration when assessment and treatment are being planned. According to Hull (1979),

> Although the majority of the problems hearing impaired adults encounter revolve around a decreased ability to communicate with others especially in adverse listening environments, each client faces uniquely individual problems as a result of his or her auditory deficit. In order for aural rehabilitation treatment to be appropriate and meaningful for clients, the approach must relate to their specific problems and communicative needs. (in press)

In other words, it appears that audiologists are currently adhering to philosophies that address aural rehabilitation as a many-faceted process, that goes beyond speechreading and auditory training. Again, however, the latter aspects are usually part of the process.

Table 8-1
Training Exercises for the Use of Vision in Communication*

Visual Perception
Perceptual field
Peripheral field
Synthetic ability
Figure ground recognition
Attention Span
Tachistoscopic training (speed of reception)
Visual closure (training in the ability to exclude the irrelevant and to organize materials on the basis of observed similarities)
Predictabilities
Sentence completion practice
Word guessing

*Data from O'Neill and Oyer (1961).

Approaches to Aural Rehabilitation Treatment

More traditional, but contemporary, approaches include those of O'Neill and Oyer (1961). In their discussion of visual training, they refer to a number of avenues to train the hearing impaired individual to use vision more fully as a means of communication (Table 8-1).

O'Neill and Oyer suggest that the visual form training accomplishes two purposes for the lipreading client. Those are, first, the development of visual concentration, and second, the development of synthetic ability.

O'Neill and Oyer also present a suggested approach to training clients in the combined use of visual and auditory clues. They state,

> The initial stages of aural rehabilitation give training without voice so that the hard of hearing person can focus his attention upon the visual aspects of speech. If such an approach is not employed from the beginning, the auditory channel will be used exclusively and the subject will not try to make use of the visual cues. Only because of this initial 'sensory' isolation will the individual be alerted to the use of lipreading alone. (pp. 74–75)

Even though their rationale for the visual-only training has merit in some instances for some clients, many audiologists today are avoiding unisensory approaches, particularly with adult clients.

The O'Neill and Oyer approach to the combined use of vision and audition includes beginning with combined practice in environmental noise conditions—in other words, not in an ideal communication environment. They recommend beginning at a 0 dB signal-to-noise ratio. They continue with:

1. Progress from words utilizing lip sounds to words with open articulation (vowel) sounds
2. Auditory discrimination of isolated sounds
3. Amplified sound, introduced first at threshold, and then gradually increased to make a smooth transfer from vision to combined vision with audition
4. Association of gestures and facial expression with quality and rate of speech

5. Use of phrases, sentences, and stories
6. Story retention (thought level rather than words or sentences), assessed by multiple-choice tests

A summary of the first four weeks of lessons, as described by O'Neill and Oyer, is as follows:

First day: Explanation of purpose of program. Discussion of the value of combined practice. Demonstration of contributions of vision alone, audition alone, and vision and audition together.

Second day: Fifteen minutes of practice on "speech without auditory cues," followed by fifteen minutes of practice on "speech without visual cues."

Third day: Initial listening in noise practice.

Fourth and fifth days: Thirty minutes of practice understanding individual words against interfering noises. Individual monosyllabic words in contrasting pairs are used in the practice.

Sixth and seventh days: Practice in listening without auditory cues. Paired words differing only in vowel composition. Fifteen minutes of practice with vowel discrimination against a noise background (recordings of various environmental noises).

Eighth and ninth days: Review of practice with selected consonants and vowels as incorporated in monosyllabic words.

Tenth day: Discussion of hearing aids and how they assist in lipreading. Discussion of benefits of hearing aids and effects of auditory "sets," and discussion of critical listening and viewing.

Eleventh day: Practice in speech discrimination. Sentences and phrases. Viewing alone, auditory alone, and combined. Listening against noise backgrounds using phrases.

Twelfth and thirteenth days: Intelligibility practice with sentences, without voice, with voice, in noise and in quiet.

Fourteenth and fifteenth days: Practice in rapid response to sentences.

Sixteenth day: Demonstration of "whole" approach with magazine covers. Stressed recall of thoughts. Presented description of pictures with no voice, low voice, and conversational voice.

Seventeenth day: Work on developing tolerance for noise. Discuss fact that noise has semantic as well as acoustic aspects.

Eighteenth day: Practice on colloquial forms using following subject areas: newspapers, automobiles, magazines, and cigarettes. Use of intermittent noise backgrounds with combined approach.

Nineteenth day: Situation practice. Discussion of people and objects in the clinic. Go over daily newspaper items, short stories from Reader's Digest and Saturday Evening Post. Use of white noise as background.

Twentieth day: Start incorporating tachistoscopic practice with five- and six-digit numbers presented at 1/50 of a second.

Another approach includes that presented by Sanders (1971) who states, "As one might expect, formal lipreading lessons are highly structured. . . . The lesson is divided into separate units, each of which concentrates upon a particular aspect of visual communication" (p. 311). Even though Sanders advocates approaches to aural rehabilitation that utilize audition, vision, and the special communicative needs of the client, he cites the following more traditional approach in sequence, based on the approach suggested by Nitchie:

Stage one: Increasing awareness of articulatory movements
Stage two: Recognition of articulatory movements
Stage three: Practice words related to articulatory movements studied in stage two
Stage four: Sentences utilizing the practice words from stage three. Alternatives to sentences include 20 cards, on each of which is written an answer to questions. The instructor presents the questions, and the client selects the card that contains the appropriate answer, or vice versa for variety's sake. True-or-false questions on various topics and connected discourse using anecdotes, dialogue, or stories on various interesting topics are also advocated.

Sanders stresses that even though formal approaches to lipreading can be utilized for both adults and children, they "should not detract the teacher from grasping every opportunity to meet the (special) needs . . . both of individual students and of the group" (p. 318).

Costello (1974) also presents an approach that is traditional in nature, but involves more than a formal approach to the use of visual and auditory clues in communication. It emphasizes current methodologies in aural rehabilitation, and involves the following components:

1. Evaluation of peripheral and central auditory disorders
2. Development or remediation of communication skills through specific training methods
3. Use of electronic devices to increase sensory input (auditory, vibratory, and others)
4. Counseling regarding the auditory deficit
5. Periodic reevaluation of auditory function
6. Assessment of the effectiveness of the procedures used in habilitation

Current Approaches

McCarthy and Alpiner (1978) suggest a "progressive approach" to aural rehabilitation treatment that is based on modifying either the clients' behavior and attitudes, the clients' environment or a combination of both. In modifying the clients' behavior and attitudes, the emphasis is on developing the willingness to:

1. Admit the existence of the hearing loss and its handicapping effects
2. Admit the hearing loss to others
3. Take positive action to minimize communication difficulties by asking others to repeat and speak more clearly, and asking for selective seating (p. 98)

According to these authors, the sequence of their approach is as follows:

1. Audiologic and hearing aid evaluation
2. Assessment of communication function
3. Identification of problem areas due to hearing loss
4. Verbal discussion within the group regarding problems
5. Admission of hearing loss to themselves and to others
6. Modification of behavior, attitudes, and environment
7. Willingness to utilize amplification in nonthreatening therapy sessions

8. Reduction of stress in communication situations
9. Willingness to utilize amplification outside of therapy sessions
10. More effective communication with normal hearing persons
11. Termination of therapy (p. 100)

This approach concentrates on the psychological impact of hearing impairment, and the client's response to the deficits experienced in his or her environment. This philosophy seems appropriate for portions of an aural rehabilitation treatment program, and addresses important areas to be covered. It is stressed, however, that not all audiologists are trained as counselors, and those should not venture into areas where problems (emotional or otherwise) require counseling by professionals trained to do so.

Hull (1979) presents a wholistic approach to aural rehabilitation treatment that is presented in its entirety in Chapter 26, in Part II of this text. It involves counseling, hearing aid orientation, designing a program (for increased communicative efficiency that is based on individual client's prioritized needs), specific treatment procedures, and evaluation of successes (or lack of them).

This approach lends itself to both younger and older adult clients. Its premises are that, first, each client has special priority needs that revolve around his or her frequented communicative environments; second, most clients can benefit from specific treatment techniques that are based on language factors that, if brought to a greater level of awareness, aid in communication; and third, the majority of hearing impaired adults complain of difficulty communicating in noisy or otherwise distracting environments. Practice in learning to cope in those environments can be of common benefit to most clients.

Aural Rehabilitation

In the end, however, specific approaches, alone or combined, rarely fit the needs of all hearing impaired clients. It is best, then, for audiologists to develop a philosophy regarding aural rehabilitation and then, taking that philosophy, extract, remold, and design programs that fit individual client's communicative needs.

What, then, is aural rehabilitation? A wholistic philosophy that would serve audiologists well was written by Braceland (Note 2). He states that rehabilitation, in its broadest sense, encompasses a philosophy that a handicapped person has the right to be helped to become a complete person, and not only to be restored as much as possible to usefulness and dignity, but also to be aided in reaching his or her own highest potential. This is a far reaching philosophy that should guide all persons who work in helping professions. In aural rehabilitation, however, such a philosophy should guide the audiologist to serve the needs of individual clients. Thus, not every hearing impaired adult should be placed in aural rehabilitation treatment groups, nor do all require extensive hearing aid orientation, nor do all require special amplification devices.

Such a philosophy suggests that, for some, the process of aural rehabilitation may involve a session or two to resolve a specific problem the client is experiencing within a specific communicative environment, and perhaps several more brief contacts to assess progress. Another may only require a hearing aid orientation program with a few follow-up visits for adjustments of the hearing aid and suggestions for more efficient use of the aid in difficult listening environments. Other visits may be for hearing and hearing aid reevaluation and words of encouragement. Others, however, will require more lengthy and comprehensive aural rehabilitation programs.

In any event, there are guidelines that will aid in the planning and execution of efficient aural rehabilitation programs for adult clients. The following are some principles that seem important both to rehabilitative procedures and to the rehabilitation program. This description is not exhaustive and is not intended to supplant the good judgment of an individual audiologist. In the absence of an extensive body of knowledge surrounding these topics, we are offering considerations which have guided us, and which practicing clinicians have reported or demonstrated to us.

Auditory and visual stimuli should be presented to the client with maximum clarity during initial sessions. The client should experience a maximum degree of success in the initial phase of the therapy process. Not only will this success motivate him or her to continue to attempt speechreading or to make the auditory discriminations necessary to comprehend, but the client will begin to develop a pattern for approaching more difficult listening situations. By this procedure he or she will initiate informal data collection and preparation for the more difficult listening situations to come later in therapy or in day-to-day living.

Auditory and visual stimuli initially should be presented with sufficient redundancy of cues that the client experiences both successful performance and acquisition of knowledge regarding the receptive communication task. In the normal reception of communication, redundancy constantly reinforces our "best guess" regarding the probable message. The positive feedback about our first best guess gives us the courage to make the next guess. Each cue adds data to help us make a decision and reduce our fear of the next dubious situation.

The clinician should serve as a model of a person who functions as an effective communicator. Clear, articulate speech without unnatural overarticulating, which tends to confuse persons attempting speechreading, should be the norm. Appropriate intensity levels of speech for maximum intelligibility in varying listening situations should be sought. Unintentional masking of visible speech by hand or head movements should be noted and avoided.

Therapy and practice material, both auditory and visual, should be selected for general and specific applications, i.e., for those situations common to most communicators and for those circumstances unique to the individual client. The unique communication needs of the client must be addressed in the therapy session. Varying occupations, social, and environmental conditions require the audiologist to prepare his or her client for realistic communication. Practice sessions should be undertaken with the problems of real life situations in mind.

Clients should not only be informed of the clinician's general and specific objectives, but should also formulate their own goals, some of which should be co-managed with the clinician's, while the remainder are the client's responsibility. Since auditory rehabilitation is a learning process, the client must be made aware of his or her part and responsibility. Too often, audiologists have applied the medical model of treating the symptom. In a learning, or more appropriately a *re*learning process, the therapist is only part of the process and the client's degree of active involvement is of paramount importance. Carryover to real life situations cannot and will not be fully accomplished unless the client is totally aware of personal responsibility.

Clinicians should establish an explicit catalog of possible methodologies to achieve specific objectives and then review this information during planning of individual therapy. Varying approaches to therapy should be gleaned from the literature. Novel approaches developed by colleagues or individual clinics should be attempted and evaluated for future use.

Both individual and group therapy programs should be available to clients. Communication is a dynamic process that must be developed with varying speakers and in varying situations. The client–therapist model is only one approach and should not be the only one considered. Group sessions should be structured to permit not only a "dry run" for the objectives of an individualized lesson, but also for practice with different speakers. The group situation also permits the client to discuss with peers the communication problems common to each member.

Clients should be instructed regarding alternative listening strategies appropriate for specific communication situations. The clinician should explain to the client why certain situations are more difficult than others in which to communicate. The client explains that the aid set at the prescribed level helps in a one-to-one situation, but in groups he or she may not understand the conversation clearly.

Here the client should be informed that this is to be expected in certain noise situations and that an alternative listening approach may be to turn down the aid and rely more on speechreading. This approach should be encouraged in a few similar situations to help determine if it is a viable alternative. Other difficult situations should be discussed for the purpose of developing alternative strategies. These will add to the client's confidence in knowing that there are many ways of attempting to overcome difficult communicative environments.

Clients should be instructed regarding alternative response criteria appropriate for specific communication events. Many clients seem to adopt avoidance and/or withdrawal behaviors during situations requiring their participation in the communication act. Responses may include a range of behaviors from total noninvolvement in specific communication situations to the other extreme, attempting to dominate the conversation. Therapy planning might include activities that directly involve principles of effective interpersonal communication.

Systematic practice during and outside of therapy sessions should be given high priority by both the clinician and the client; at the same time, spontaneous practice opportunities should not be ignored by either party. A balance needs to be maintained between systematic and nonsystematic therapy activities. The two extremes are to be avoided, that is, boring and repetitive drills versus completely open-ended and nonstructured sessions. Each clinician needs to calibrate the therapy approaches so that some activities on the continuum between these extremes are included, but with neither end dominating the general or specific aspects of the program.

Since successful communication is exciting and satisfying, therapy activities also should contain sufficient opportunities for similar positive interactions and experiences. Therapy does not have to be static in all aspects. Interesting but still challenging training activities can be planned. Establishing a relaxed and satisfying communication relationship with clients is an ingredient of successful interaction that appears to be discussed infrequently. Developing and maintaining motivation are important potential effects of a relationship wherein humor, active involvement, and dynamic interaction are part of the therapy program and not the exception.

Any opportunities for improving the speech expressiveness of the client's family, friends, and others should be exploited. Too often, it seems, clinicians concentrate exclusively upon the client, with little or no attention given to significant others who are important to the client. Interviews and discussions with family and friends might be of substantial importance to the client. General improvement in the communication expressiveness and effectiveness of these individuals could reduce the client's difficulties as much as, if not more than, therapy activities directed only to the client.

Development of assertive influence on the communication environment by the client should be an essential component of therapy. Assertiveness, without aggression, can be an important therapy objective. The client can learn to stage-manage situations and communication events to maximize the probability of successful communication. Reducing background noise levels, decreasing the distance from a talker, optimizing lighting for speechreading cues, and requesting that the talker use clearer speech and appropriate gestures are examples of areas where the client can become assertive and active in improving the communicative circumstances.

Clients should be encouraged to establish and maintain a balance between dominance and submissiveness during communication events. The client may need counseling directed at emphasizing and demonstrating the give-and-take of many communication situations. Again, a balance between dominating and withdrawing behaviors might be explored during therapy. Acceptance of realistic expectations also could be addressed. Few of us can claim successful communication with even the majority of persons with whom we come in contact. In short, the client may be assuming too much personal responsibility for communication events.

Counseling activity should be considered essential to the effectiveness of other components of the therapy relationship. Counseling skills seem essential to the success of any therapy relationship. Audiologists are becoming more and more aware of this, and some training institutions are including formal courses and practicums in counseling as part of the curriculum. Counseling may be one of the most important activities involved in auditory rehabilitation. If this is true, then major attention and effort will need to be directed toward developing counseling skills in graduate students and in practicing audiologists.

Developing technology should be incorporated into therapy activity on an experimental basis, and resulting judgments of specific equipment for specific purposes should be shared with other practitioners. Technological aids, in addition to hearing aids, should be applied through the aural rehabilitation program. These include, as examples, telephone amplifiers, teletypewriters, prerecorded practice materials for home use, videocassette auditory-visual training systems, and radiotransmission devices for specific social or vocational situations. Such existing technology can be used to enhance communication for clients with special needs. These devices are discussed in depth in Chapter 9.

CONCLUSIONS

There are several questions requiring attention by those who offer or recommend rehabilitative audiology services. These have been asked many times but the answers are elusive:

Is auditory and visual training a form of ''language'' training? If so, how do we relate these procedures to contemporary descriptions of linguistic usage? If not, is such training a prerequisite for successful language usage?

Who should be responsible for auditory and visual training? Teachers? Audiologists? Speech and language pathologists?

How can we enhance interdisciplinary communication among those who participate in the rehabilitation process?

How can we assess effectiveness of auditory and visual training?

What principles can be agreed upon and generalized from the present limited knowledge?

How does one orient beginning students to the nature and scope of rehabilitative audiology?

The need exists for effective interdisciplinary cooperation regarding auditory rehabilitative services, with a continuing effort to revise our philosophies and approaches in dealing with those who have hearing impairment. This can be enhanced through communication with other disciplines about respective professional activities and through implementation of the team approach. Public sharing of what we are doing, how we are doing it, and which approaches seem to be most effective are needed. Problem-oriented studies are necessary to stimulate interdisciplinary communication and to develop professionals who not only appreciate the team approach but also seek its realistic achievement.

In this chapter we have presented varying philosophies and approaches to aural rehabilitative treatment. It behooves the reader to extract those portions that will be of direct benefit to his or her clients. We must continually remain vigilant to the special needs of individual clients. Some may require specific strategies to address particular problems in communication that are peculiar to them. Others may benefit from speechreading/lipreading instruction to complement their residual hearing. Whatever the assessed needs of clients, the audiologist must be flexible and knowledgeable in offering those services.

REFERENCES

Alpiner, J. G. *Handbook of Adult Rehabilitative Audiology*. Baltimore: Williams and Wilkins, 1978, p. 267.

Binnie, C. A. Relevant aural rehabilitation, in J. L. Northern (Ed.), *Hearing Disorders*. Boston: Little, Brown, 1976, pp. 213–227.

Binnie, C. A., Montgomery, A. A., & Jackson, P. L. Auditory and visual contributions to the perception of selected English consonants. *Journal of Speech and Hearing Disorders*, 1974, *17*, 619–630.

Brannon, C. Speechreading of various materials. *Journal of Speech and Hearing Disorders*, 1961, *26*, 348–354.

Bruhn, M. D. *The Mueller-Walle Method of Lipreading*. Washington, D.C.: The Volta Bureau, 1949, p. 114.

Bunger, A. M. *Speech reading—Jena method*. Danville, Illinois: The Interstate Press, 1944.

Bunger, A. M. *Speech reading—Jena method*. Danville, Illinois: The Interstate Printers and Publishers, 1961, p. 109.

Colton, J. Student participation in aural rehabilitation programs. *Journal of the Academy of Rehabilitative Audiology*, 1977, *10*, 31–35.

Costello, M. R. The audiologists: Responsibilities in the habilitation of the auditorily handicapped. *Journal of the American Speech and Hearing Association*, 1974, *16*, 68.

DiCarlo, L. M., & Kataja, R. An analysis of the Utley lipreading test. *Journal of Speech and Hearing Disorders*, 1951, *16*, 226–240.

Erber, N. P. Interaction of audition and vision in the recognition of oral speech stimuli. *Journal of Speech and Hearing Research*, 1969, *12*, 423–425.

Erber, N. P. Auditory and audiovisual reception of words in low frequency noise by children with normal hearing and by children with impaired hearing. *Journal of Speech and Hearing Research*, 1971, *14*, 496–512.

Erber, N. P. Auditory-visual perception of speech with reduced optical clarity. *Journal of Speech and Hearing Research*, *22*, 212–223.

Fleming, M., Birkle, L., Kolman, I., Miltenberger, G., & Israel, R. Development of workable aural rehabilitation programs. *Journal of the Academy of Rehabilitative Audiology*, 1973, *6*, 35–36.

Heider, F. K., & Heider, G. M. A comparison of sentence structure of deaf and hard of hearing children. *Psychological Monographs*, 1940, *52*, 42–103.

Hull, R. H. Aural rehabilitation in adults, in N. J. Lass, L. V. McReynolds, J. L. Northern, & D. E. Yoder (Eds.), *Speech, hearing and language*. Philadelphia: W. B. Saunders (in press).

Hull, R. H., & Alpiner, J. G. The effect of syntactic word variations on the predictability of sentence content in speechreading. *Journal of the Academy of Rehabilitative Audiology,* 1976, *9,* 42–56.

Hutton, C. Combining auditory and visual stimuli in aural rehabilitation. *Volta Review,* 1959, *56,* 316–319.

Hutton, C., Curry, E. T., & Armstrong, M. B. Semi-diagnostic test materials for aural rehabilitation. *Journal of Speech and Hearing Disorders,* 1959, *24,* 318–329.

Kinzie, C. E., & Kinzie, R. *Lipreading for the Deafened Adult.* Philadelphia: John C. Winston, 1931.

McCarthy, P. A., & Alpiner, J. G. The remediation process, in J. G. Alpiner (Ed.), *Handbook of adult rehabilitative audiology.* Baltimore: Williams and Wilkins, 1978, pp. 88–111.

Miller, G. A., & Nicely, P. E. An analysis of perceptual confusions among some English consonants. *Journal of the Acoustic Society of America,* 1955, *27,* 338–352.

Nitchie, E. H. *New lessons in lipreading.* Philadelphia: J. B. Lippincott, 1950, p. 251.

O'Neill, J. J. Contributions of the visual components of oral symbols to speech comprehension. *Journal of Speech and Hearing Disorders,* 1954, *19,* 429–439.

O'Neill, J. J., & Oyer, H. J. *Visual Communication for the Hard of Hearing.* Englewood Cliffs, New Jersey: Prentice-Hall, 1961, p. 163.

Ordman, K. A., & Ralli, M. P. *What people say.* Washington, D.C.: The Volta Bureau, 1957, p. 117.

Prall, J. Lipreading and hearing aids combine for better comprehension. *Volta Review,* 1957, *59,* 64–65.

Sanders, D. A. *Aural Rehabilitation.* Englewood Cliffs, New Jersey: Prentice-Hall, 1971, p. 373.

Sumby, W. H., & Pollack, I. Visual contributions to speech intelligibility in noise. *Journal of the Acoustic Society of America,* 1954, *26,* 212–215.

Tannahill, J. C., & Smoski, W. J. *Introduction to aural rehabilitation,* in J. Katz (Ed.), *Handbook of clinical audiology.* Baltimore: Williams and Wilkins, 1978, pp. 442–446.

Utley, J. Factors involved in the teaching and testing of lipreading through the use of motion pictures. *Volta Review,* 1946, *38,* 657–659.

Van Uden, A. A sound-perceptive method, in A. W. G. Ewing (Ed.), *The modern educational treatment of deafness.* Washington, D.C.: The Volta Bureau, 1960, pp. 3–10.

Woodward, M. F., & Barber, C. G. Phoneme perception in lipreading. *Journal of Speech and Hearing Research,* 1960, *3,* 212–222.

REFERENCE NOTES

1. Binnie, C. A., & Barrager, D. C. Bi-sensory established articulation functions for normal hearing and sensorineural hearing loss patients. Paper presented at the Annual Convention of the American Speech and Hearing Association, Chicago, 1969.

2. Braceland, F. J. The restoration of man. Donald Dabelstein Memorial Lecture, presented at the Annual Conference of the National Rehabilitation Association, Oct. 9, 1963.

Gwenyth R. Vaughn
Steven D. Gibbs

Chapter 9: Alternative and Companion Listening Devices for the Hearing Impaired

While society is concentrating on the mainstreaming of hearing impaired children, vast numbers of hearing impaired adults are being excluded from the work force, community functions, and relationships with families and friends. Given the ecological problems posed by noise and other acoustic inadequacies, traditional aural rehabilitation techniques have, in many instances, not resolved the problems of hearing impaired listeners, nor of their normally speaking or speech impaired associates who wish to communicate with them. Further, hearing aids are not always found to be beneficial. But as part of a total aural rehabilitation program, hearing impaired persons deserve to be made aware of alternatives to hearing aids that may be more efficiently utilized and, in many respects, may be economically more feasible.

LISTENER/TALKER RIGHTS

Listeners and talkers have the right and the need to participate in interpersonal communication. Most modern environments are pervaded by noise and reverberation to such a degree that oral/aural communication can be highly unsatisfactory in personal, social, educational, vocational, cultural, and recreational settings. The resulting frustration of both listeners and talkers may contribute to rejection, isolation, and inactivity.

Although great progress has been made in regard to hearing aids, few hearing aid users find them truly satisfactory in noisy or otherwise distracting environments. Many users state that they cannot understand speech while in an automobile, walking on the street, or on personal business involving those listening/talking environments in which bank tellers, receptionists, drive-in personnel, clinic clerks, and other talkers speak from behind some type of enclosure.

Because of noisy environments, many hearing impaired persons are unable to communicate satisfactorily with their physicians and nurses, their on-the-job supervisors and

Some of the information included in this chapter was presented at the Mini-Conference on Elderly Hearing Impaired People, White House Conference on Aging, Washington, D.C., January 11–13, 1981, and may be found in the report on the conference (in press).

Table 9-1
Listening/Talking Environments—Situation Summary

Number of Listeners/ Talkers	Personal/Social	Educational	Vocational	Cultural/ Recreational
Equipment Related Media One Listener/One Source		Video Radio Record/tape player	Dictation equipment	Television Radio Record/tape player Movies
Telephone One Listener/One Talker	Conversation Business contacts	Conferencing	Conversation Answering machine Intercom	Conversation with family and friends
Interpersonal Communication One Listener One Listener/One Talker or One Source	Clinical diagnosis, treatment, and counseling Religious settings Conversation "Teller" windows Receptionists	Tutoring Lectures	Interview Instruction Supervision Selling	Automobile Table games Restaurant
One Listener/Small Group of Talkers	Group conversation Family groups Party groups Home dining table Backyard parties Alerting spouse or child	Seminar Panel discussion	Group conversation Table conference	Restaurant Home dining table Automobile Table games Walking outside Group conversation Parties
One Listener/ Medium Group of Talkers	Table conversation Parties	No public address system Conference/ classroom Lecture room	Group conversation Table conference	No public address system Group conversation Parties

co-workers, ministers, counselors, teachers, family members, and friends. They find interpersonal communication difficult when attending staff meetings, eating in restaurants, going to parties, playing card games, and talking with grandchildren.

Many hearing impaired persons cannot understand television and radio broadcasts—a problem they try to solve by turning up the volume, much to the dismay and frustration of normally hearing family members.

The telephone is an important communication instrument. The adventitiously severely hard of hearing have had only three options: utilizing the telecoils on their hearing aids, buying telephone amplifiers, or purchasing a teletypewriter.

Some telephones are not compatible with the telecoils; some persons do not benefit from telephone amplifiers presently on the market; and most family members and friends

Number of Listeners/ Talkers	Personal/Social	Educational	Vocational	Cultural/ Recreational
Several Listeners Several Listeners/ One Talker or One Source	Church (with or without public address)	Auditorium Lecture room (with or without public address)	Table staff meeting Small group meeting	Public address: Arena Auditorium Theater Movies
Several Listeners/ Small Group of Talkers	Group conversation Table conversation	Seminar Panel discussion	Group conversation Table conference	Public address or talkers: Arena Auditorium Theater Movies Games Restaurant Parties Group conversation
Several Listeners/ Medium Group of Talkers		Conference/ classroom Lecture room Public address		Public address or talkers: Arena Auditorium Theater Movies Games Restaurant Parties Group conversation

do not have teletypewriters, and, further, may not be able to afford them. The barriers to telephonic listening/talking have been enormous for hearing impaired persons. In this chapter, SPACE IB, C, and D as well as SPACE IIIA, B, C, and D will address amplification of speech reception at the listener's end.

For persons who cannot benefit from any amplification, VisiCom will be discussed as providing an inexpensive, easily available communication device to overcome the problems of listeners and talkers over the telephone. VisiCom utilizes Touchtone® to activate an LED readout on the small, portable VisiCom device that allows the hearing impaired person to receive graphic messages over the telephone.

Table 9-1 reflects some of the listening/talking environments in which hearing impaired persons experience difficulty in understanding speech.

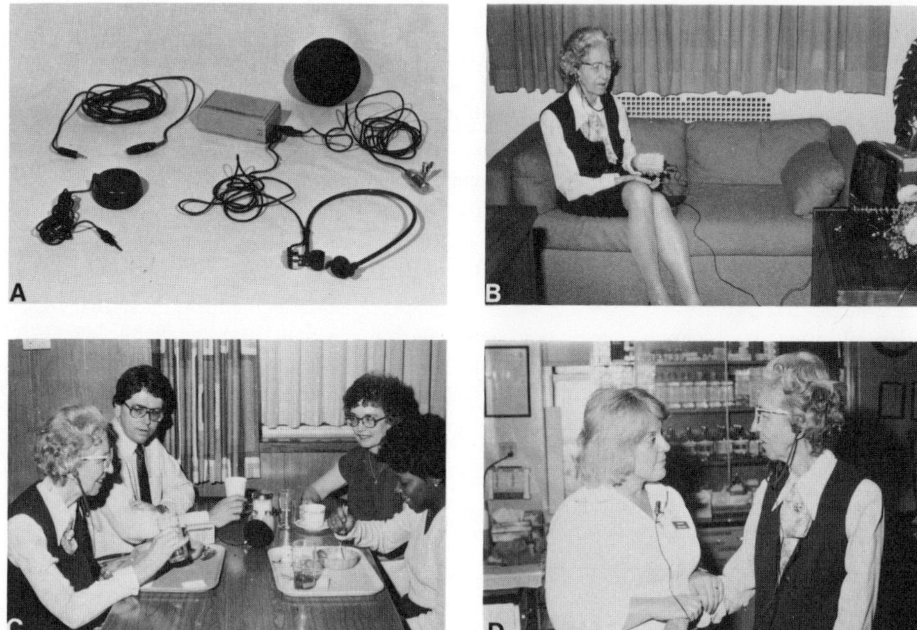

Figure 9-1. SPACE listening devices IA and IB. (A) SPACE I components. *Clockwise, from upper left:* extension cord, amplifier, windscreen, microphone, headphone, and telephone earpiece. (B) SPACE IA used with television. *From left:* headphone, amplifier, and extension cord. (C) SPACE IB in use in a small group. *From left:* headphone, amplifier, and microphone in windscreen. (D) SPACE IB in a clinical setting. *From left:* microphone on speaker's lapel, headphone, and amplifier in listener's pocket. (Photographs courtesy of Audiology-Speech Pathology Service, Birmingham Veterans Administration Medical Center, Exchange of Medical Information Program, EC-H-CO Annual Report, 1980.)

IDENTIFICATION OF ALTERNATIVE AND COMPANION LISTENING DEVICES

In order to address the problem of noisy listening/talking environments, alternative and companion amplification devices have been identified and studied at length in regard to their effectiveness. These devices have been named SPACE (Situational/Personal Acoustic Communication Equipment). Although these systems were originally identified by an Exchange of Medical Information Project of the Veterans Administration as being useful for older adults, their application has equal, if not greater importance, for hearing impaired children and for young and middle-aged adults. The impact of the SPACE devices upon interpersonal communication affirms the right of listeners and talkers to hear and be heard.

The SPACE devices provide advantageous signal-to-noise ratios through delivery of the speech signal directly from the talker to the listener's ear; portability and wearability of amplification systems that require no permanent installation or architectural modifications; amplification at a reasonable cost ($60–$1,000); and commercial availability.

The types of SPACE devices include Hardwire, Infrared, FM-to-Auditory Trainer, and FM-to-Personal Hearing Aid.

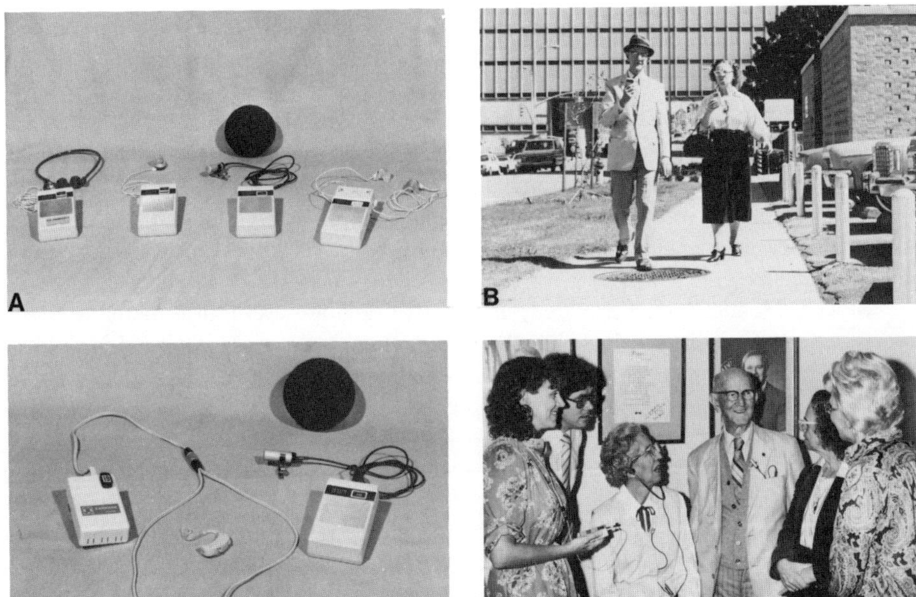

Figure 9-2. SPACE listening devices IB, IIIA and B, and IVD. (A) SPACE IIIA and IIIB. *From left:* earphone and FM transmitter, earmold and FM receiver; windscreen, microphone and FM transmitter; and FM receiver. (B) SPACE IIIA or B used out of doors. *From left:* earmold, FM receiver (in man's hand), FM transmitter (in woman's hand), and microphone (on woman's lapel). (C) SPACE IVD. *Clockwise, from upper right:* windscreen, microphone, FM transmitter, neck loop with hearing aid, and FM receiver. (D) SPACE IVD, IB, IIIA or B, self-wired. *From left:* neck loop, microphone, transmitter (in woman's pocket), and receiver; earphone, microphone, and amplifier (in woman's pocket); earmold, receiver (in man's pocket), microphone, and transmitter (in man's pocket). Two FM transmitters on same frequency can not be used simultaneously. (Photographs courtesy of Audiology-Speech Pathology Service, Birmingham Veterans Administration Medical Center, Exchange of Medical Information Program, EC-H-CO Annual Report, 1980.)

Descriptions of SPACE Listening Devices

The SPACE listening devices are divided into four categories, according to the type of signal transmission utilized.

Hardwire

SPACE IA. SPACE IA utilizes an earphone plugged directly into television, radio, and other similar equipment. The SPACE IA stethoscope earphone has a detachable button receiver that can be used with a standard snap-in earmold. An extension cord allows the listener to move farther from the source (Figure 9-1a).

SPACE IB. SPACE IB uses the earphone described above, with an amplifier and microphone or telephone pickup. The microphone may be placed near a television or radio speaker, near a talker, or in a windscreen in the center of a table for group communication. The telephone pickup allows the unit to amplify telephone conversations (Figures 9-1a through 9-1d, and 9-2d).

SPACE IC. SPACE IC requires a special ear-level hearing aid that may be connected directly to the television, radio, or stereo, with a special input cord. An extension cord may also be used.

SPACE ID. SPACE ID uses a body hearing aid plugged directly into the television, radio, or stereo. An extension cord may also be used.

The advantages of SPACE I devices include large, easily adjusted controls, low cost, usefulness as part-time or occasional amplification, excellent signal-to-noise ratio, and good fidelity.

SPACE IA and B are hardwired, inexpensive, and are useful in listening to radio, television, stereo, and the telephone. When the microphone of IB is placed in a windscreen (Figure 9-1c), it is effective for use in small groups, around a conference or dining table, in an automobile, in interviewing and conducting business, and in clinical settings (Figure 9-1d).

The parts for SPACE IA and B are available at electronic equipment stores or a designated distributor (see the appendix to this chapter). SPACE IA and B are suitable for persons with normal hearing or those with mild to severe impairments who do not object to the cords. SPACE IC and D utilize personal hearing aids with an external input capability and cord to plug into the television, radio, or SPACE IB amplifier.

The user of SPACE IB can place the microphone in a strategic location on his own clothing, such as a tie, lapel, collar, or belt. The SPACE IB microphone will pick up talkers within a small group.

The amplifier fits easily in a pocket, allowing for easy adjustment of the volume control. The SPACE IB wire can be bound together with a plastic bag twist-tie or rubber band and also placed in a pocket.

Insertion of the stethoscope earphone in the listener's ears reduces background noise and provides bilateral hearing (Y-cord). This may improve listening in noisy environments.

Replacing the stethoscope earphone with the user's own snap-in earmold can make the SPACE IA and B less conspicuous. In addition, acoustic modifications of the earmold can be made. Since the stethoscope earphone cuts out some of the background noise, the degree of hearing in the ear without an earmold must be considered before opting for one-ear amplification in noisy listening/talking environments.

When an earmold is substituted for the stethoscope earphone, only one cord to the snap-in earmold is visible. This holds true for SPACE IC and D when they are combined with the amplifier of SPACE IB. With these combined systems, amplification can be controlled both at the ear level and at the amplifier.

Thus, by "self-wiring" of the hearing impaired person for both reception (microphone) and amplification, SPACE IB provides a strong and unobtrusive listening ally (Figure 9-2d).

"Self-wiring" converts SPACE IB into a type of "body hearing aid." Most users report that they hear better with SPACE IB than they do with their own body aid. Microphone placement, level of amplification, and stethoscope earphone, if used, may contribute to this improved listening capability.

The effective use of SPACE IB depends upon listener hearing loss, signal-to-noise ratio, the amplification level needed by the listener, and distance of talkers from microphone.

In certain listener/talker environments when the talker is behind a barrier such as a bank teller's window or when the noise level is extraordinarily high, the listener may need to hold or place the microphone closer to the talker or to a sound source such as a television, radio, or public address speaker. When listening to the latter, the background noise will have to be sufficiently low to provide a satisfactory signal-to-noise ratio.

Voice amplifier. The SPACE IB amplifier and microphone can be utilized as a voice amplifier. Some hearing impaired persons prefer to attach the amplifier to the telephone earpiece by using the magnetic earpiece. This arrangement without the stethoscope earphone serves very well as a telephone amplification device for group listening.

Another combination utilized by hearing impaired persons is to plug the amplifier into the television set or to place the microphone next to the television speaker so that the signal comes through the amplifier rather than the earphone. An extension cord permits the listener to sit at a distance from the sound source. Since this option increases the sound level in the room, normally hearing listeners may find this option unsatisfactory and insist upon use of the earphone by the person with the hearing impairment.

Speech pathologists may wish to recommend the SPACE IB as a voice amplifier for talkers with voice problems or who have been laryngectomized and speak with low volume. It is a very inexpensive amplification device that works well in automobiles and other noisy environments in which a spouse or friend cannot hear the talker. In this case, a choice may be made by the listener to use earphones or just the amplifier unit with the microphone placed close to the talker.

Infrared

SPACE IIA. SPACE IIA includes a transmitter plugged into a broadcast unit and a stethoscope receiver.

SPACE IIB. SPACE IIB utilizes a transmitter plugged into a broadcast unit, a barneckloop receiver, and a personal ear-level hearing aid with telecoil.

SPACE IIC. SPACE IIC includes a transmitter plugged into a broadcast unit, a receiver, and a personal ear-level hearing aid with an external input capability.

SPACE IID. SPACE IID includes a stereo transmitter plugged into a stereo source, and a stereo receiver.

SPACE II devices are moderately priced when used in small rooms, with the cost increasing as the listening area is expanded. Use of infrared requires no permit or license. General usage includes theaters and churches, with small units being appropriate for use with television and radio.

Infrared devices provide good fidelity and signal-to-noise ratio. The receivers are portable and do not restrict the listeners' movements within a room, as long as no object comes between the transmitter and receiver. Infrared signals do not interfere with other listeners outside the room. Eavesdropping is a problem only if the listener places himself outside a window in line with the transmitter.

A number of theaters are utilizing Infrared systems. Receivers are checked out to theater patrons for the performance. The cost of the receiver is charged to the user's credit card. At the end of the performance, the user returns the receiver, and a small fee is charged. Infrared systems can be used effectively in theaters, churches, and with home television. They do not, however, offer the owner-user the broad application available with SPACE III FM devices.

SPACE II requires that the receivers be directed toward the transmitters. Listeners who sit in the front may be below the transmission line. The range of the transmitter is dependent upon its size. The larger the transmitter, the more expensive it is. The range of the SPACE II devices is shorter than that of the SPACE III and IV FM devices.

Infrared devices are not completely portable. Transmitters all require 110 volt AC power and cannot be used in an automobile, outdoors, or in any situation where an AC outlet is not available.

FM-to-Auditory Trainers

SPACE IIIA. SPACE IIIA consists of a microphone and portable FM radio transmitter, radio receiver, and earphone. The microphone may be placed on the talker, near a TV, radio, or public address speaker, or in the center of a conference table (Figure 9-2a, 9-2b, and 9-2d).

SPACE IIIB. SPACE IIIB uses a microphone and portable FM radio transmitter, and a binaural receiver with gain and frequency response controls and greater amplification capability. This unit may be used with severely to profoundly hearing impaired individuals (Figure 9-2a).

SPACE IIIC. SPACE IIIC is the same as IIIA and IIIB. SPACE IIIC uses a mixing transmitter to receive signals from several microphones transmitting on different frequencies and retransmit the signal on one or more channels for a number of listeners. The individual transmitters and receivers consist of the FM units described above.

SPACE III listening systems are the same auditory trainers used in school rooms for hearing impaired children. They offer wide application. Older adults, or anyone with normal hearing or a hearing loss who cannot function well in environments with poor acoustics and/or noise, will find that SPACE III permits more normal communication. The units are wireless and permit great flexibility in interpersonal communication situations. The devices are portable and offer a transmission range of 300 feet in open areas. This makes them ideal for large or small meeting rooms, churches, lecture halls, theaters, small groups at parties, conference or dining tables, interviews and business transactions, clinical situations, automobiles, walking down the street (Figure 9-2b), use with television and radio, and use with the telephone.

SPACE IIIC is a recent development in FM equipment for use with multiple talkers. SPACE IIIC makes it possible to transmit from a number of microphones to a common mixer that then retransmits on one or more frequencies compatible with the frequencies of the listeners' FM receivers.

SPACE III devices may be used in all the situations described for SPACE I. The units do not restrict the user's movements or detract from his or her appearance with wires. These devices may be used with the transmitter located in the center of a conference table, protected by a windscreen, or with the transmitter and receiver both placed on the listener.

The main disadvantages include regulation of the transmitters by the Federal Communications Commission, the possibility of eavesdropping by anyone with a receiver within the transmitter's range, and the relative high cost of the units.

FM-to-Personal Hearing Aid

SPACE IVA. SPACE IVA uses the microphone and FM transmitter to transmit to an FM receiver that is acoustically coupled to the user's hearing aid.

SPACE IVB. SPACE IVB uses the microphone and FM transmitter to transmit to an FM receiver that is electrically connected to a direct input hearing aid.

SPACE IVC. SPACE IVC uses the microphone and FM transmitter to transmit to an FM receiver which magnetically couples to the telecoil of the user's hearing aid through a magnetic Velcro® loop adapter.

SPACE IVD. SPACE IVD uses the microphone and FM transmitter to transmit to an FM receiver that is coupled to the telecoil of the hearing aid through a magnetic neck loop (Figure 9-2c and 9-2d).

SPACE III FM transmission is combined with personal hearing aids in each of the SPACE IV devices. These amplification systems use acoustic, electrical, or magnetic pickup. The quality of the telephone coil in the personal aid affects the quality of the reception in the latter. For the hearing aid user, these units allow the improvement in signal-to-noise inherent to other SPACE systems, while not requiring physical or acoustic adjustment to different earmolds or receivers.

SPACE IV demonstrates the principles of compatibility with the listener's individual aid, yet provides an extension of FM capability that enhances signal-to-noise ratio for both listeners and talkers. SPACE IV devices can also be utilized in the listening/talking environments described for SPACE I and III devices.

These devices are completely portable and cosmetically acceptable, but have the same disadvantages as SPACE III. The units are relatively expensive, are regulated by the FCC, and allow possible eavesdropping by unauthorized listeners.

Table 9-2 suggests which SPACE devices can be effectively utilized in noisy listening/talking environments.

VisiCom: Visual Communication Equipment

The VisiCom is a new device designed by the staff and consultants of the EC-H-CO Project for hearing, speech, and language impaired persons who need assistance in communicating by telephone or face to face. It is lightweight, pocket-sized, rechargeable, and completely portable. The VisiCom displays information transmitted over telephone lines on an LED readout. The information originates from standard Touchtone® telephones or from portable Touchtone® pads acoustically coupled to the mouthpiece of a dial telephone.

The VisiCom is for use by hearing impaired persons who are able to speak sufficiently well to be understood over the telephone, or by speech impaired persons who have good hearing. Two persons who both have hearing and/or speech impairments can communicate with each other if both have VisiComs and some type of Touchtone® capability. VisiComs are commercially available.

The advantage of the VisiCom for most adventitiously hearing impaired persons is that only one VisiCom is required, instead of two units as is necessary with teletypewriting devices. Since the majority of the telephones are now Touchtone®, persons

Table 9-2
SPACE Devices (Situational/Personal Acoustics Communication Equipment)*

Situation	Hardwire (I)	Infrared (II)	FM, FM/Aid (III,IV)
Media			
TV, radio	I ABC&D	II ABC&D	III,IV ABC&D
Individual	I ABC&D	II ABC&D	III,IV ABC&D
Group	I ABC&D	II ABC&D	III,IV ABC&D
Interpersonal			
One-to-one	I BC&D		III,IV ABC&D
Several-to-one	I BC&D†		III,IV ABC&D†
Conference	I BC&D†	II ABC&D	III,IV ABC&D†
Automobile	I BC&D†		III,IV ABC&D†
Restaurant	I BC&D†		III,IV ABC&D†
Telephone	I BC&D		
Groups			
Educational settings	I A,‡ I BC&D†	II ABC&D	III,IV ABC&D
Clinical settings	I A,‡ I BC&D		III,IV ABC&D
Vocational settings	I A,‡ I BC&D	II ABC&D	III,IV ABC&D
Familial settings	I A,‡ I BC&D†	II ABC&D	III,IV ABC&D
Dining	I A,‡ I BC&D†		III,IV ABC&D†
Group	I A,‡ I BC&D†		III,IV ABC&D†
Recreational	I A,‡ I BC&D†		III,IV ABC&D†
Public address			
Church	I ABC&D§	II ABC&D	III,IV ABC&D
Lecture rooms	I ABC&D§	II ABC&D	III,IV ABC&D
Theater		II ABC&D	III,IV ABC&D
Arena (very large)			III,IV ABC&D

*A combination of I and II can be used for multiple listeners, if there is no public address system available. For use in group listening, SPACE IA, C, D, and IIA, B, C, D, must be used with media that has one jack input for individual listening and two jacks for individual and group listening simultaneously. SPACE IC and D must be combined with IB for use in interpersonal communication.
†Enhances reception with windscreen.
‡SPACE IA for one listener in group of several talkers.
§With preferential seating.

wishing to telephone a hearing impaired person need no special equipment. Port-a-Tone pads and Soft Touch™ Dials are easily available, if Touchtone® service is not available. The Soft Touch Dial is very inexpensive.

APPENDIX: SOURCES OF EQUIPMENT DISCUSSED IN THIS CHAPTER

SPACE IA and IB can be purchased at electronic stores or from VisiCom Inc., P.O. Box 43247, Birmingham, AL 35243.

SPACE II equipment is available at IPAS Inc., 1440 Broadway, Suite 2250, New York, NY 10018.

SPACE IIIC has been developed by H.C. Electronics, Camino Alto, Mill Valley, CA 94941. SPACE IC and ID, SPACE IIIA and IIIB, and SPACE IV are available from hearing aid manufacturers and distributors.

Port-a-Tone Terminals may be purchased from Dictation Equipment, 1911 South 27th Avenue, Birmingham, AL 35209.

Soft Touch™ Dials are available at BUSCOM Systems Inc., 4700 Patrick Henry Drive, Santa Clara, CA 95050.

Pamela L. Jackson

Chapter 10: Techniques for Speech Conservation

Speech characteristics and therapy techniques for prelinguistically hearing impaired clients are well documented in the literature. The degree of auditory impairment and the extent of the resulting handicap for this population have drawn the attention of researchers and clinicians alike. Their efforts have resulted in a documented body of literature which is the basis for communication training programs throughout the United States.

There is, however, another subgroup of the hearing impaired population that is often overlooked in these descriptions of speech behaviors. That group is the adventitiously hearing impaired who have losses that occurred after speech and language skills had developed normally. With the onset of the hearing loss, speech monitoring ability may diminish, and in time, changes in speech production may occur. The task facing clinicians who deal with this clientele is one of conservation of already existing skills rather than the development of new ones. Maintenance of intelligibility is the goal.

SPEECH CHARACTERISTICS OF THE HEARING IMPAIRED ADULT POPULATION

A description of the typical speech characteristics of this population is nearly impossible because there is no typical case. Many factors and their interaction are responsible for the amount of deterioration that occurs after the hearing impairment develops. These factors are listed below.

Degree of Hearing Loss

If the hearing loss is of such a degree as to allow at least partial monitoring of speech, the problem will be less severe than if no speech monitoring is possible. In the majority of cases of adventitious hearing loss, the onset is gradual and the degree is mild enough that no change in speech production is noticed.

Configuration of the Hearing Loss

Configuration and degree of hearing loss interact to impose a certain amount of distortion on the incoming auditory signal. For example, a precipitous high-frequency hearing loss will either nullify or distort sibilant or high-frequency voiceless consonant sounds. The configuration will be a prime determiner of speech monitoring ability.

Age of Onset

In general, the more years of normal hearing a client has, the better will be his or her oral speech skills. Even though this statement has been found to be true, the relationship between age of onset and oral speech skills is still a complex one. Binnie, Daniloff and Jackson (Note 1) reported on the case of a child who incurred a profound, bilateral hearing loss as a result of spinal meningitis when he was five years, five months old. Prior to his hospitalization, he reportedly showed no indications of speech or language problems. Approximately six weeks after his illness began, the subject was seen for auditory management, which included periodic tape recording of his spontaneous speech as well as his responses to the screening portion of the Templin-Darley Tests of Articulation (1969). Testing was conducted at two-week intervals for a period of nine months. Phonetic, spectrographic, and perceptual analyses of the tapes were conducted and revealed increases in word duration, increases in duration variability, a rise in fundamental frequency (Fo), less variation in pitch inflection, the syllabification of final consonants, and significantly depressed speech intelligibility scores. Even within a nine-month period, the speech of this five-year-old had markedly changed.

The age factor must be considered a critical determiner of speech deterioration when other, older cases are compared to this five year old. For example, consider the case of a client who incurred a sudden, profound hearing loss at age 21 due to antibiotic treatment for a kidney infection. Even several years following the onset, speech intelligibility remained intact, with only minor sibilant distortion being noted. Prosodic features remained unaffected. Other cases of similar etiology have been reported, however, in which speech deterioration was much more extensive and intelligibility was markedly affected.

The influence of age of onset of hearing loss on speech intelligibility has never been systematically explored. The need for such an investigation is supported by the concluding statements made by Kent (1976) following his survey of acoustic studies of speech development. He concluded that the variability of speech motor control progressively diminishes, beginning by age three years and continuing until the child is eight to twelve years of age. At that point adult stability is achieved. This development of precise motor control occurs, therefore, after the majority of speech sounds have already reached the point where they are phonetically acceptable. This statement implies that eight to twelve years of age may be a critical dividing line for predicting speech deterioration following the onset of a hearing loss.

Hearing Aid History

Ideally, amplification will be employed shortly after the hearing loss is discovered, so that speech monitoring ability is maintained. The time amplification is first initiated and the success that is achieved in restoring discrimination ability will influence how severe speech deterioration will be.

Accompanying Problems

The presence of mental retardation, learning disabilities, neuromuscular problems, and other similar disorders will possibly affect speech skills in adventitiously hearing impaired just as in the congenitally hearing impaired population.

Table 10-1
Phoneme Production Errors

Consonant Errors	Vowel Errors
Failure to distinguish between voiced and voiceless consonants	Vowel substitution
Consonant substitutions	Misarticulation of diphthongs. Two types of errors may occur: (1) the diphthong may be produced as two separate vowels, or (2) one component of the diphthong, usually the second, may be omitted.
Excessive nasality	
Misarticulation of consonant clusters. Two types of errors may occur: (1) one of the sounds may be dropped from the cluster, or (2) the sounds may be produced so slowly that additional syllables are added when /ə/ is inserted between the cluster elements.	Diphthongization of simple vowels
	Neutralization of vowels so that the production approaches /ə/
	Nasalization of vowels
Misarticulation of abutting consonants in different syllables with /ə/ being inserted between the final consonant of one syllable and the initial consonant of the next.	
Omission of initial consonants	
Omission of final consonants	

Need to Use Speech

As with the congenitally hearing impaired, speech skills are largely dependent upon the need for continued oral communication. This continued use may need to be accompanied by reinforcement and monitoring to insure that skills are maintained.

The type of speech problem that occurs with acquired hearing loss will vary widely, and as a result, each case must be evaluated for individual patterns. The error patterns that occur may involve a combination of three different components, including articulation, voice, and rhythm and timing.

Articulation

The phoneme production errors involved in the speech of the deaf have been thoroughly described in the classic study by Hudgins and Numbers (1942) and are summarized in Table 10-1.

Which of these errors appear in the speech of the adventitiously hearing impaired depends on the factors mentioned earlier. Based on the information from Chapter 2, certain predictions can be made as to which speech sounds may deteriorate in the presence of a particular hearing loss. Based on that information and according to Calvert and Silverman (1975), common errors involve omissions and distortions of the sibilants, especially /s/, that were described above. These errors can be explained in part by comparing them with acoustic characteristics of the speech signal. In general, speech sounds that are more difficult to hear are more often in error. Each sound contains energy

Table 10-2
Voice Disorders in the Hearing Impaired

Strength	Resonance	Placement	Inflection
Lacking voice	Hypernasality	High pitch	Lacking variation
Lacking control of volume	Hyponasality	Low pitch	Erratic variation
Weakness		Gutteral voice	
Harshness		Erratic changes	
Breathiness			

at several frequencies which means that a given audiometric configuration may remove only part of the identifying information and result in a distortion. The sound may be detected based on lower frequency cues but may no longer be understood, thus resulting in faulty auditory monitoring and possible distorted output.

Voice

The disorders of voice that can occur in a hearing impaired population have been listed by Magner (1971) in Table 10-2.

The specific characteristics of voice that occur in an individual will also vary greatly. It has been shown, however, that subtle quality and resonance differences occur early in the speech deterioration process of adventitiously hearing impaired adults. These changes may be due, at least in part, to the speaker's attempts to replace the decrease in auditory monitoring ability with an increase in tactual-kinesthetic feedback.

Rhythm and Timing

Hudgins and Numbers (1942) reported three types of rhythm patterns that occur in the speech of the deaf: correct rhythm, abnormal rhythm, and nonrhythm. They also emphasized the importance of speech rhythm on overall intelligibility by indicating that its contribution was equal to that of consonant articulation.

The relationship between rhythm and intelligibility was also supported by Hood and Dixon (1969) in their study of the physical characteristics of speech rhythm of deaf speakers. For the purpose of their investigation, they defined speech rhythm as being composed of intonation changes, loudness changes, and two temporal factors, relative syllable duration in a sentence and rate of utterance of a sentence. They concluded that deaf speakers showed less fundamental frequency and intensity variation and greater duration of both syllables and total utterances than did normal hearing speakers. They also found that ratings of rhythm proficiency were highly correlated with the two duration measures and slightly related to intensity variation. No relationship existed between rhythm proficiency ratings and fundamental frequency variation.

A great deal of research concerning the timing and rhythm patterns of deaf speech was reviewed by Nickerson (1975). He offered the following conclusions:

1. Deaf speakers use a slower speaking rate than normal speakers
2. Deaf speakers do not make a large enough duration difference between stressed and unstressed syllables
3. Deaf speakers' pauses are more numerous, longer, and/or inserted at inappropriate places

Table 10-3
The Initial Receptive Communication Evaluation

Pure tone air and bone conduction testing
Speech audiometry
A sensitivity measure such as a speech reception threshold (SRT) or a speech detection threshold (SDT)
A discrimination measure such as the W-22 word lists
Immittance testing
Site of lesion testing

4. Deaf speakers use inappropriate rhythm or syllable grouping
5. Deaf speakers demonstrate some timing problems related to speech sound production

As with articulation and voice problems, the rhythm characteristics of an adventitiously hearing impaired person will vary considerably depending on the factors summarized earlier. It appears, however, that once speech rhythm patterns are well established, they are maintained more accurately than articulation and voice patterns. In view of their importance in speech intelligibility, however, rhythm and timing must not be overlooked.

DIAGNOSTICS FOR SPEECH CONSERVATION

Receptive Skills

In order to obtain a complete evaluation of the communication problem created by the hearing loss, both receptive and expressive skills must be explored. The initial receptive evaluation would include the items listed in Table 10-3. This information should give the audiologist information to aid in medical diagnosis, to serve as a guide for aural rehabilitation recommendations, and to predict communication difficulty.

Based on the results of the initial testing, aural rehabilitation may be recommended. The receptive portion of the diagnostic evaluation would continue with a hearing aid evaluation and additional communication evaluation to assess skills with the recommended aid. Additional tests or areas of exploration may include:

1. SRT/SDT
2. Discrimination in quiet and in noise using materials with different levels of redundancy. Examples of materials are word tests, such as the W-22, WIPI, and CAT; phoneme tests (i.e., consonant and/or vowel confusion tests); and sentence tests such as the C.I.D. Everyday Speech Sentences.
3. Prosodic feature perception tests such as measures of stress pattern recognition in words and/or in sentences

The key point that must be remembered in performing an evaluation of receptive skills is that the examiner is looking for the starting point for auditory training as well as attempting to obtain a measure of communication difficulty in normal listening situations. These goals may be met, at least in part, through discrimination testing using the standard W-22 word lists in quiet, but in many cases this procedure may be inappropriate.

In some instances, the use of the W-22 word lists may result in scores near 100 percent, and yet the client reports communication difficulty. The listening task must be made more difficult in some way to find the fine dividing line between success and failure. This may mean increasing the difficulty of the listening task by increasing the complexity of the material (i.e., a sentence test such as the CID Everyday Speech Sentences), by reducing the redundancy of the materials (i.e., a phoneme recognition task), or by increasing the level of background noise.

In other cases, the W-22 word lists are too difficult and the errors are so numerous and random that no patterns emerge that can be systematically incorporated into auditory training. In these instances, the task must be made easier and this usually means selecting a closed-response set of materials. In many cases a test such as the Word Intelligibility by Picture Identification Test (WIPI) (Ross and Lerman, 1971) is appropriate even though the standardized norms do not apply, since the task can also be performed by adults with more severe losses. Written multiple-choice response forms can be created to eliminate a picture-pointing response for adults. The point is that in the evaluation of receptive skills for communication purposes, the audiologist must look for a level of task difficulty where some success is achieved and yet systematic errors are made. This will be the starting level for auditory training.

The final area of auditory diagnostics involves an assessment of prosodic feature perception. The importance of this area should be fairly obvious in view of the documented importance of prosodic features in the intelligibility of speech of the deaf (Hudgins and Numbers, 1942). At present, few tests exist that probe this area of prosodic feature perception in the hearing impaired. One is the CID-CAT (Erber and Alencewicz, 1976) or the expanded version of the same concept, the CID-MONSTR. The CAT consists of four words in each of three different stress pattern categories (monosyllable, trochee, and spondee), while the MONSTR consists of ten words in each of the three categories. In either case, the concept is the same. The test is scored in two ways: first by percentage of words recognized correctly and second by percentage of stress pattern recognition. In other words, if a monosyllable is presented and a monosyllable is the response, it is counted as correct in the prosodic feature scoring even if the exact word is incorrect. In many cases of severe to profound hearing loss, the client is unable to receive enough phonetic information through the auditory channel only to recognize the words, and yet he can perform the stress recognition task because he can at least feel the patterns. Auditory training may need to start at a prosodic feature level to prevent speech deterioration in the stress and rhythm areas.

A second test which is available to probe prosodic feature perception is the Stress Pattern Recognition in Sentence test or the SPRIS (Jackson and Kelly-Ballweber, Note 2). This 48-sentence test consists of four repetitions of each of 12 simple sentences. Each sentence consists of four monosyllabic words. For each repetition of a sentence, a different word is stressed, thus giving a slightly different connotative meaning to the utterance. The subject's responses are scored in the same way the CAT is scored, first by percentage of correct sentence identification and second by percentage of correct sentence stress pattern identification. This test has also been shown to be appropriate with an adult hearing impaired population.

When the receptive diagnostic information is pulled together, the aural rehabilitationist has an indication of how much distortion the hearing loss is imposing on the incoming speech signal. This is derived from the audiogram, which is a frequency-by-intensity plot of sensitivity across the frequency range. The speech results are an indication of how well the client is using his or her residual hearing. Those areas of auditory perception that are now more difficult for the adventitiously hearing impaired become the core of auditory training to maintain his or her speech monitoring ability. It is this speech monitoring ability that is the key to speech conservation.

Expressive Skills

Articulation

Evaluation of the expressive speech skills of the adventitiously hearing impaired population follows the same basic principles as any speech evaluation. The client's articulation characteristics are evaluated with various types of materials under various conditions. The clinician is interested in obtaining information concerning usual speech sound production, error contexts and consistency, and stimulability of error sounds.

Evaluation of speech sound production: word level. Several tests are commercially available to probe phoneme production at the word level, but the general thrust of the materials is toward consonant production in a younger population with pictures being used to elicit responses. Any of these materials would serve the purpose with an adult population, if written word lists rather than pictures were used as the stimulus items.

While vowel articulation may not be of primary importance in the typical normally hearing client, it is of major concern in the speech productions of the hearing impaired population. Errors in vowel production are common in the congenitally impaired client, and as mentioned earlier, vowel errors in the form of resonance changes may be among the first to appear in the speech of the adventitiously hearing impaired. For this reason, it is critical that a test of articulation ability be selected that will probe vowel as well as consonant productions.

For the evaluation of the speech skills in a hearing impaired population, Berg (1976) recommends the Templin-Darley Tests of Articulation (Templin and Darley, 1969) or his own shortened version of this test. The Templin-Darley Tests of Articulation were designed as a basic tool of the speech pathologist to assess speech production skills at the word level of children age three to eight years. The stimulus materials consist of 57 cards with two to four pictures per card that are used to elicit responses. There are also printed lists of words and sentences for use with older clients for whom pictures may be inappropriate.

These 141 items comprise the Revised Diagnostic Test. In order to increase the versatility of the test, the items are combined into two specific tests and also into several groupings of sounds to meet specific purposes in testing articulation. Various units in the test are presented in Table 10-4.

Berg's shortened version of the Templin-Darley test consists of 67 items from the 141 original words chosen to sample all vowels and diphthongs; all single consonants in the prevocalic position of words; the voiced stops /b/, /d/, and /g/; the sibilants /s/, /z/, /ʃ/, /ʒ/, /tʃ/, and /dʒ/, and the glides /r/ and /l/ in the postvocalic position; and several blends involving /s/, /r/, and /l/ with other phonemes. His suggested recording form and list of stimulus words are found in Table 10-5.

Each item in this table contains the phoneme to be tested and the stimulus word that is to be used in eliciting the production. Berg also presents pictures that can be used with children to elicit a verbal response. In the case of the hearing impaired young adult,

Table 10-4
Various Units in the Templin-Darley Tests of Articulation

The 50-item Screening Test

A 42-item Grouping of Consonant Singles, composed of 22 initial and 20 final consonants, which probes the client's mastery of consonant production.

The 43-item Iowa Pressure Articulation Test, which explores the adequacy of velopharyngeal closure by assessing the adequacy of oral pressure for speech sound production (Morris, Spriestersbach, and Darley, 1961).

Groupings of Consonant Clusters intended to determine the consistency of the speech sound production in various phonetic contexts.

> A 31-item /r/ and /ɚ/ Cluster Grouping made up of two- and three-phoneme clusters
>
> An 18-item /l/ and /l̩/ Cluster Grouping made up of two- and three-phoneme clusters
>
> A 17-item /s/ Cluster Grouping made up of two- and three-phoneme clusters
>
> A 9-item Miscellaneous Consonant Cluster Grouping

Groupings of Vowels and Diphthongs

An 11-item Vowel Grouping

A 6-item Diphthong Grouping made up of five diphthongs and one consonant-vowel combination

---

a word list to be read by the client may be substituted. The position of the phoneme within the word is specified by the I (initial or prevocalic), M (medial or intervocalic), or F (final or postvocalic) beside the word.

The recording form provides a blank for scoring the acceptability of the production. Any scoring code can be used, but a suggested system would be to mark an omission with "om," a substitution with the phonetic symbol of the error sound, and an addition with the phonetic symbols. If the clinician's ear is trained to pick up fine production differences, a scaling system may be used to differentiate various levels of distortion. An example of one such system might be:

1 = *Correct production.* The sound is produced correctly with no distortion.
2 = *Mild distortion.* The distortion would be noticeable only to the trained listener.
3 = *Distortion.* The distortion would be noticeable to the layman but would not be annoying.
4 = *Marked distortion.* The distortion would distract the average listener from the speech content.
5 = *Severe distortion.* The distortion is so severe that the sound is not recognizable.

The importance of such a system must be stressed. A distortion of an articulation may occur in varying degrees, and the severity of the problem may be determined by the severity of the distortions in addition to the number of phonemes involved. The clinician must be careful to judge an articulation as a distortion even if it only mildly deviates from accepted standards. The productions of the hearing impaired must be judged relative to normal hearing articulation and not judged as acceptable as long as it is intelligible. Intelligible speech may very well be distorted speech.

Additional commercially available tests to probe articulation skills at the word level include the Fisher-Logemann Test of Articulation Competence (1971) and the Goldman-Fristoe Test of Articulation (1969). The Fisher-Logemann Test of Articulation Competence consists of 109 picture stimuli on 35 bound cards intended for use with adults as well as children. Eleven of the cards may be used as a screening test. The test explores the production of all English phonemes, both vowels and consonants, and provides for errors to be analyzed in terms of distinctive features.

The Goldman-Fristoe Test of Articulation was developed for the main purpose of assessing consonant articulation ability. The test materials consist of 35 pictures of objects or activities. The client names the pictures or answers questions to provide a total of 44 responses. Even though vowels are not specifically probed, the Sounds-in-Words Subtest contains all of the vowels and diphthongs except /u/, /ɑ/, and /ɔɪ/ and, therefore, could be used for that purpose.

Evaluation of speech sound production: sentence level. When attention is focused on a particular phoneme in a word articulation test, it may be possible for the client to produce it correctly. Yet when the same sound occurs in conversation, it is omitted, distorted, or erroneously produced in some way. For this reason, it is important to explore the ability of the adventitiously hearing impaired adult to produce speech sounds in sentences or in conversation as well as in isolated words.

Several tests are also available to probe articulation ability at the sentence level. One is the Templin-Darley Tests of Articulation mentioned earlier. The sentence portion of this test consists of 141 items constructed and organized to evaluate the same speech sounds as the word portion. A second test is the sentence form of the Fisher-Logemann Test of Articulation Competence. It consists of 15 sentences printed on a single card and designed to test all English speech sounds. The sounds within the sentences are arranged so that each voiced-voiceless cognate pair of consonants is tested in the same sentence. Consonants having no cognate are grouped into sentences according to manner of production. The last four sentences probe vowel productions with the sounds being arranged in terms of place of articulation. A third test for sentence articulation is the Sounds-in-Sentences Subtest of the Goldman-Fristoe Test of Articulation. This subtest was developed to assess systematically speech sound production in a context similar to conversational speech. The material consists of two stories that are read by the examiner while the client watches sets of four or five pictures. The subject then repeats the story in his or her own words, using the pictures to guide the narrative and thus the words in the speech sample. The result is content-controlled speech that approximates conversational speech.

Evaluation of error contexts and consistency. It is very possible that the misarticulations that occur in a specific phonetic context do not occur in others. This inconsistency of productions creates a need to examine speech sound articulation ability in more than one context. This type of evaluation is possible with the Templin-Darley Tests of Articulation since certain consonants occur in a number of different clusters. The

Table 10-5
Recording Form for Berg's Shortened Version of the Templin-Darley Test of Articulation*

1. p (i)	pipe ____	34. s (f)	mouse ____
2. t (i)	two ____	35. sm-	smoke ____
3. k (i)	cat ____	36. skr-	scratch ____
4. b (i)	bicycle ____	37. -ks	socks ____
5. d (i)	door ____	38. z (m)	scissors ____
6. g (i)	girl ____	39. z (i)	zipper ____
7. m (i)	mittens ____	40. z (f)	ties ____
8. n (i)	nose ____	41. -lz	nails ____
9. ŋ (f)	ring ____	42. ʃ (i)	shoe ____
10. f (i)	fence ____	43. ʃ (m)	dishes ____
11. ɵ (i)	thumb ____	44. ʃ (f)	fish ____
12. v (i)	valentine ____	45. ʃr-	shred ____
13. ð (i)	there ____	46. ʒ (i)	Zhivago ____
14. w (i)	window ____	47. ʒ (m)	television ____
15. tw-	twins ____	48. ʒ (f)	mirage ____
16. b (f)	tub ____	49. tʃ (i)	chair ____
17. d (f)	slide ____	50. tʃ (m)	matches ____
18. g (f)	dog ____	51. tʃ (f)	watch ____
19. i (m)	feet ____	52. dʒ (i)	jump ____
20. I (m)	pin ____	53. dʒ (m)	engine ____
21. ɛ (m)	bed ____	54. dʒ (f)	cage ____
22. æ (m)	bat ____	55. ɚʤ	large ____
23. ʌ (m)	gun ____	56. ɝ	bird ____
24. ɚ	car ____	57. r (i)	red ____
25. ɑ (m)	clock ____	58. r (m)	arrow ____
26. ʊ (m)	book ____	59. pr-	presents ____
27. u (f)	blue ____	60. dr-	drum ____
28. o (m)	cone ____	61. str-	string ____
29. ɑu (m)	house ____	62. -mɚ	hammer ____
30. e (m)	cake ____	63. l (i)	leaf ____
31. ɑI (f)	pie ____	64. l (f)	bell ____
32. ɔI (f)	boy ____	65. gl-	glasses ____
33. s (i)	sun ____	66. -tl	bottle ____
		67. -lt	belt ____

Adapted with permission from Berg, F. S. *Educational audiology: Hearing and speech management*. New York: Grune & Stratton, 1976, p. 168.
*The i, m, and f indicate initial, medial, and final position of the test phoneme within the word.

results may reveal one or more contexts in which the speech sound is correctly produced. This information, in turn, will serve as an aid in the remediation process.

Berg (1976) recommends the Deep Test of Articulation by McDonald (1964) to explore error contexts in the speech of hearing impaired children. This test would also be appropriate for use with an adventitiously hearing impaired adult population. The materials consist of both a picture and a sentence version with the items being designed to test the articulation of the following 13 speech sounds in several phonemic contexts: /s/, /z/, /r/, /l/, /ʃ/, /tʃ/, /dʒ/, /θ/, /ð/, /k/, /g/, /f/, and /v/.

The information obtained from such a probe may reveal one or more contexts in which the speech sound is correctly produced. This in turn allows selection of appropriate materials for training when kinesthetic and visual feedback mechanisms are being used to lead to correct production in all contexts.

Evaluation of stimulability of error sounds. In planning a speech conservation program, it is extremely helpful if information is available concerning the susceptibility of a particular sound to remediation. While Snow and Milisen (1954) indicate that prognostic information can be obtained by comparing productions obtained from pictorial and oral articulation tests, it is not known whether this information would apply to an adventitiously hearing impaired population in which articulation skills are deteriorating rather than developing. It is known, however, that those sounds which are the most susceptible to correction are the easiest to incorporate into a kinesthetic feedback program since the target is already closely approximated.

The suggested procedure for stimulability testing (Milisen, 1954) involves having the client watch and listen carefully while the examiner produces the sound two or three times. Then the client is to imitate the production. This procedure is to be carried out using all sounds that were misarticulated on the previous test and should place the sounds in speech of varying complexity (i.e., in isolation, in nonsense syllables, and in words). The task is repeated twice and the best response is recorded.

Specific materials for probing error stimulability include some of the tests already discussed. The Templin-Darley Tests of Articulation include directions for determining how well the client can produce the error sounds when furnished with optimal auditory-visual stimulation. The directions indicate that each sound is to be presented in isolation, in a syllable, and in a word as well as in a consonant cluster within a word. The Goldman-Fristoe Test of Articulation also includes a Stimulability Subtest where the simplest level of production is the syllable followed by words and simple sentences.

Two tests have been specifically designed to probe stimulability of error sounds. The first is the Carter-Buck Prognostic Articulation Test (1958) which consists of a spontaneous word portion and an imitated nonsense syllable portion. The second is the Van Riper-Erickson Predictive Screening Test of Articulation (1968) which consists of nine imitation tasks, placing sounds in isolation, syllables, words, and sentences. Since both of these instruments were developed to predict which children will master their articulation errors without therapy, it is uncertain whether these materials could be applied to an adventitiously hearing impaired population. However, even though the normative scores will not apply, the concept may still be applicable.

Voice

Evaluation of the voice characteristics of the adventitiously hearing impaired client could be conducted on several levels. One might be by direct observation of the laryngeal mechanism by a physician to investigate any physical change in structure. This should always be done in cases of vocal deviation in order to rule out any underlying pathological cause.

A second level for voice evaluation is at the listening level, where the clinician's ear is used to make a value judgment concerning the acceptability of the voice production. Since intelligibility is seldom affected by voice changes only, the clinician must decide whether a deviant voice is an inappropriate voice based on age, sex, regional, and physical considerations.

The third level of voice evaluation is the acoustic level. This involves direct physical measurement of the various parameters of the voice, such as fundamental frequency, fundamental frequency variation, intensity, and periodicity. Several instruments are available for such measurement as well as for feedback in therapy and are reviewed in the appendix.

The typical voice evaluation involves systematically obtaining a representative sample of the client's communication skills. Ideally, this sample is tape-recorded for future reference. The verbal behavior should include a sample of conversational speech, impromptu speech such as telling a story, oral reading, or singing, and automatic speech such as counting or naming the days of the week. The sample should then be carefully listened to for deviations in laryngeal function (tension, breathiness, harshness), pitch level and variability, intensity, and resonance. This information will describe the client's typical vocal behavior.

A second part of the voice evaluation involves additional probes aimed at further assessing vocal capabilities. Procedures designed to evaluate laryngeal function include the following:

Ask the client to produce an /ɑ/ with a gradual soft onset (i.e., /hɑ/). Listen for a sudden abrupt onset of voicing at both loud and soft intensities.
Listen specifically for how voice is initiated in the various speech samples. That is, listen to whether it occurs with a hard or a soft glottal attack.
Time three sustained productions of /ɑ/ using normal air intake. Listen for efficient use of air. A client with normal breath support should be able to produce the sustained vowel for 12 to 13 seconds.
Observe what happens to vocal quality with changes in intensity.
Stand behind the client and place your finger on the thyroid cartilage. Feel for the presence of laryngeal tension during phonation.
Have the client clear his or her throat and listen for a potential change in clarity.

Procedures aimed at evaluating pitch level and variability include:

Ask the client to produce a clear /ɑ/ at the lowest pitch level possible and then to slide through the scale to the highest level he or she can reach without going into falsetto phonation. This will give an indication of the client's pitch range.
Ask the client to produce a vocalized sigh. This should occur near his or her habitual pitch level.
Compare the client's pitch level during oral reading with that of a sustained vowel.
Compare the client's pitch level at various intensities.
Look for the direction, frequency, and extent of pitch breaks.

Procedures for the evaluation of intensity include the following:

Observe what changes occur in intensity level with changes in pitch.
Have the client vary his or her pitch at a given intensity and observe the control that can be achieved.
Observe the client's intensity at various rates.
Note whether the client is using clavicular or diaphragmatic breathing during phonation.

Finally, procedures for the evaluation of resonance include:

Observe velopharyngeal mobility on vocalization.
Listen for variation of nasality with different vowels.
Listen for changes in nasality with increased loudness.

Following the overall voice evaluation, specific problems in laryngeal function, pitch, intensity, and resonance will be identified in various contexts. As in articulation testing, the next step is to evaluate the stimulability of the various errors. Again, this information will influence decisions for therapy and will be beneficial when tactual-kinesthetic feedback is being stressed for the hearing impaired individual.

Rhythm and Timing

The diagnostic evaluation of the rhythm and timing characteristics of the speech of the adventitiously hearing impaired involves analysis of the same type of speech sample that was collected for the evaluation of voice changes. In this case the clinician judges the utterances for the following rhythm characteristics: overall rate (i.e., too fast, too slow, monotonous), uncontrolled variability, patterned rate, phrasing, variation in syllable duration, and variation in pause duration.

TECHNIQUES FOR SPEECH CONSERVATION

In the 1974 report from the ASHA Committee on Rehabilitative Audiology, Costello (1974) and her associates stated that the single most important component of the aural rehabilitation program was the selection and fitting of the hearing aid. The earlier the use of amplification is initiated and the success that is obtained in restoring usable hearing, the less chance there is that the ability to monitor speech will deteriorate. However, in cases where auditory monitoring is lacking, auditory training and speech-reading training will be integral parts of the speech conservation program. If the auditory skills that are achieved with amplification are insufficient to allow auditory monitoring, kinesthetic monitoring must be substituted and may be reinforced with visual and/or vibrotactile training aids.

Speech conservation training may include several areas of emphasis depending on which expressive skills are being affected by the hearing loss. These areas include articulation, voice, and rhythm training.

General Therapy Procedures and Principles

The comprehensive speech perception and production diagnostic evaluation will uncover specific problems that may potentially develop or that have already started to develop with the decrease in auditory feedback. The goals in the speech conservation program, therefore, are, first, to maintain existing production skills that are in danger of deteriorating, and second, to correct any errors that have already developed as a result of the adventitious hearing loss.

Several methodologies are available for speech production training and each varies somewhat in principle and procedures. In general, however, the majority of techniques involve presentation of a model production by the clinician followed by an imitated response from the client. The role of the clinician in this paradigm is one of orienting the client to the task, stimulating the production, listening carefully to the response and judging its acceptability, offering immediate feedback and reinforcement, and providing continuous evaluation of progress. The procedures are designed to shape the articulation, voice, or rhythm error into a correct production. Changes in behavior across time can be charted using procedures such as precision therapy described by Waters, Bill, and Lowell (1977).

Van Riper (1972) has outlined the stages of articulation therapy in a very comprehensive way that includes numerous suggestions for training. While ear training techniques receive a major emphasis in his program, he stresses that the clinician is free to choose other techniques to stimulate correct production. This production is considered at four specific operational levels and progression from one to the next is suggested but not required. Therapy can be initiated at whatever level seems appropriate. These four successive levels are

1. The isolated sound level
2. The syllable level
3. The word level
4. The sentence level

From this last step, carryover into controlled conversation and finally into everyday speech is initiated.

Within this framework, Van Riper outlines four steps to be used in training the error sounds at each of the four levels. These steps can be described as follows:

Have the client identify the error and the standard of production for the specific sound. This stage normally involves ear training aimed at drawing attention to the specific characteristics of the sound in question so that the client will begin to discriminate it from incorrect productions. Obviously, this task may be difficult for the adventitiously hearing impaired client, so some modification is needed.

With a hearing impaired population, this stage can be considered one in which the client learns the characteristics of the sounds that may potentially or that have already started to deteriorate. This involves auditory training and speechreading training, which will be integral components of the speech conservation program. It also includes vocabulary building of terms such as those listed by Fisher (1975), which will be used in the correction process. This might include terms such as *harsh, hoarse, glottal attack, denasal, voiced,* and others. It must be remembered that this stage involves no production on the part of the client. It involves only structured input and comparison.

Have the client scan and compare his or her own utterance with the standard. This step also involves ear training, but now it is intended that the client carefully listen to his or her own productions rather than to the speech of others. It is assumed at this stage that the client clearly understands the characteristics of the target to which comparisons are made with his or her own approximations.

Again, at this stage, modification is needed for a hearing impaired population. What is really involved at this level is self-monitoring through whatever perceptual channel is needed. Hopefully, residual hearing will play a major role, especially with amplification. Visual, tactual, and kinesthetic feedback information is used to supplement the auditory channel.

Van Riper stresses that this monitoring ability will occur at various times relative to each production as therapy progresses. Initially the error will be recognized after it occurs, next while it is happening, and finally it can be identified and hopefully corrected before the production.

Have the client vary his or her production until the correct sound is achieved. At this stage, the new sound is being taught to the client. Van Riper explains that this must occur at all levels mentioned earlier (isolation, syllable, word, sentence, and conversation) through a process in which the client is taught to vary his utterance. Five methods are outlined for approaching this task: progressive approximation, auditory stimulation, phonetic placement, modification of sounds that are produced correctly, and key words.

The first method, progressive approximation, is Van Riper's method of choice. It involves shaping the response and rewarding productions that are progressively approaching the target.

Auditory stimulation involves ear training followed by imitation of the correct production. With the hearing impaired client the approach should be termed auditory-visual stimulation, stressing the inclusion of speechreading cues which must be emphasized. The success of this method will vary depending on the amount of residual hearing and the success of amplification.

Phonetic placement, the third method, involves the clinician instructing the client in the specific placement and movement of the articulators for the production of each sound. The position is analyzed and changes in positioning are suggested. Application of this approach involves the use of a mirror, diagrams, and models to guide placement.

The fourth method mentioned is modification of correct sounds. This method involves having the client produce a sound which he or she can do correctly and then gradually vary the production to approximate the target for the error sound. For example, the client may be instructed to slide the tongue forward from a /ʃ/ production to approximate the /s/ which is normally in error.

Finally, the key word method requires utilization of words in which the defective sound can be produced correctly and thereby makes use of information obtained from the evaluation of error contexts described earlier. Emphasis is placed on the sound within the contexts where success is achieved and the production is then introduced in isolation and in other words. Kinesthetic and auditory monitoring from one area to the next is stressed.

Another method for obtaining correct sound production is the motokinesthetic method described by Young and Stinchfield-Hawk (1955). This method may have had application with a hearing impaired population since auditory stimulation is supplemented by tactile stimulation. This method is based on the assumption that by manipulation of the client's articulators, the clinician can establish tactile and kinesthetic feedback patterns. The client, therefore, passively produces the sound as the clinician manipulates the articulators until the movement pattern is established.

Have the client stabilize the correct sound production so that it becomes automatic. This stage involves activities at each level of complexity designed to strengthen the new sound production so that it occurs automatically without any conscious effort. To achieve this goal, Van Riper suggests such activities as simultaneous writing and talking, babbling, unison speech, and negative practice. It is important that this stage not be overlooked until the production has stabilized in all contexts and has become a natural part of the client's speech repertoire.

Within the framework just outlined, the clinician is free to deal with the speech production errors that have been identified. Specific techniques within the areas of articulation, voice, and rhythm are needed to accomplish various remediation goals. Several sources are now commercially available that delineate remediation techniques for individual speech sounds and various voice and rhythm disorders. The reader is urged to refer to these sources for specifics. They include books by Calvert and Silverman (1975), Fisher (1975), Haycock (1941), Ling (1976), Magner (1971), and Vorce (1974).

Articulation Training

In articulation training, the ability to imitate a correct sound depends to a large degree on the ability to perceive the model. In cases of adventitious hearing loss, this means using visual and tactile stimulation in addition to auditory. Several of the references, therefore, stress the need for the use of a mirror and somewhat slower speech to emphasize the positioning of the articulator.

Tactile cues are also outlined and described by the various authors to be used to improve feedback during stimulation. As an example, production features can be cued in the following ways:

1. Voicing (vowels and /b, d, g, v, ð, z, ʒ, dʒ, m, n, ŋ, l, r, w, j/) can be cued by feeling the vibration at the side of the throat and then contrasting it with voiceless productions
2. Nasality (/m,n,ŋ/) can be cued by feeling the vibration at the side of the nose
3. Plosives (/p, t, k, b, d, g/) can be cued by the pulse of air that can be demonstrated by holding a strip of paper or the back of a hand in front of the mouth
4. Fricatives (/f, θ, s, ʃ, tʃ, v, ð, z, ʒ, dʒ/) can be cued by the flow of air that can be demonstrated by holding a strip of paper or the back of a hand in front of the mouth

These tactile cues can be used in the initial shaping of the sound but should soon be faded as more emphasis is placed on kinesthetic feedback. They are appropriate in isolation, syllables, or words but may not prove successful at the sentence level.

Voice Training

Remedial treatment of voice disorders involves establishing new habits or preventing bad habits from forming. The same basic therapy outline is used. First the problem must be identified and then analyzed in terms of its specific defect. Next, the voice must be varied in some way, and eventually the new voice must be located through successive approximation. Stabilization of the new voice in communication is then stressed.

The texts mentioned earlier also offer suggestions for the remediation of voice disorders. A few examples are summarized in table 10-6.

Rhythm and Timing Training

With an adventitiously hearing impaired adult population, errors in rhythm and timing can be prevented or corrected (for the most part) by reviewing the importance of stress and rhythm and by reviewing some already established rules. This may be accomplished by employing some form of prosodic notation in the therapy session to stress phrasing, stress, and inflection rules.

Several such notation systems are available, but one that appears fairly straightforward is presented by Calvert and Silverman (1975). They suggest a system that indicates pitch changes with a curving line, loudness by the height of a horizontal line above a syllable, and duration by the length of the line. Slash marks are used to indicate phrasing. They then present the following illustration:

"Yesterday was a beautiful day/but today//it's terrible."

These markings can then be incorporated into activities that draw attention to the importance of stress, rhythm and timing in speech perception and production.

Table 10-6
Suggestions for the Remediation of Voice Disorders

To correct excessive harshness:

Conduct exercises to reduce laryngeal tension such as head rotation and alternate tension and relaxation

Improve speech breathing

Emphasize easy vocalization through the use of aspirated voice onset

To correct excessive breathiness:

Improve speech breathing

Have the client count and increase the number he or she reaches on one inhalation

Increase loudness somewhat

Have the client grip his or her chair or hold a book at shoulder height and count while the increased laryngeal tension is felt

To correct pitch problems:

Work on sustaining vowels at an even, optimum pitch level

Write *high* at the top and *low* at the bottom of a blackboard to give visual feedback as pitch is lowered and raised

Use a resonating object such as a balloon, a cardboard tube, or metal, and have the client feel the high and low vibrations

To correct intensity problems:

Improve speech breathing

Again, use a resonating object to demonstrate intensity changes

To correct resonance disorders:

Lower vocal pitch or increase vocal intensity slightly to reduce general nasality

Alternate productions of /ŋ/ and /ɑ/, first slowly and then more rapidly stressing kinesthetic awareness

Combine alternate /m/ and /n/ productions, again emphasizing the feeling of the nasal resonance

DEVELOPMENT OF COMMUNICATION ASSERTIVENESS

Even though specific programs of receptive training and speech conservation are being conducted, the adventitiously hearing impaired adult is still faced with the problem of maintaining a healthy attitude toward communication. It is all too easy to withdraw socially and admit defeat in difficult listening or speaking situations. If this happens, a vicious circle is formed, for it is only through continuous practice that speech skills can be maintained if the hearing loss is severe. Because of this, the need often arises for assertiveness training and counseling to change attitudes toward the hearing impairment. This assertiveness training can be an integral part of the aural rehabilitation program along with hearing aid orientation, speechreading, auditory training, and speech conservation.

Communication assertiveness involves, first of all, motivation. This motivation is obviously for the client, but it should also involve family members. Their role in the maintenance of speech skills is critical, so it is important that they also understand the consequences of the auditory impairment. Next, specific problem communication areas must be identified and the client must be desensitized so that he or she no longer avoids difficult situations. At this point the client becomes involved in receptive training and speech conservation work, so that the client learns to vary his or her behavior in positive ways and gradually to approximate more correct productions or improved speech monitoring skills. These newly learned skills are then stabilized in general communication situations.

Speech conservation, therefore, involves not only training in specific monitoring and production skills, but also support for communication in general. The clinician must be aware that a hearing loss will affect many phases of the client's life, and all need to be considered in an aural rehabilitation program.

REFERENCES

Berg, F. S. *Educational audiology: Hearing and speech management*. New York: Grune and Stratton, 1976.

Calvert, D. R., & Silverman, S. R. 1975. *Speech and deafness*. Washington, D.C.: Alexander Graham Bell Association for the Deaf, 1975.

Carter, E. T., & Buck, Mc K. Prognostic testing for functional articulation disorders among children in the first grade. *Journal of Speech and Hearing Disorders*, 1958, *23*, 124–133.

Costello, M. R. The audiologist: Responsibilities in the habilitation of the auditorily handicapped. *Journal of the American Speech and Hearing Association*, 1974, *16*, 68–70.

Erber, N. P., & Alencewicz, C. M. Audiologic evaluation of deaf children. *Journal of Speech and Hearing Disorders*, 1976, *41*, 256–267.

Fisher, H. B. *Improving voice and articulation* (2nd ed.). Boston: Houghton Mifflin Company, 1975.

Fisher, H. B., & Logemann, J. A. *The Fisher-Logemann test of articulation competence*. Boston: Houghton Mifflin Company, 1971.

Goldman, R., & Fristoe, M. *Goldman-Fristoe test of articulation*. Circle Pines, Minnesota: American Guidance Service, Inc., 1968.

Haycock, G. S. *The teaching of speech*. Washington, D.C.: Alexander Graham Bell Association for the Deaf, 1941.

Hood, R. B., & Dixon, R. F. Physical characteristics of speech rhythm of deaf and normal-hearing speakers. *Journal of Communication Disorders*, 1969, *2*, 20–28.

Hudgins, C. V., & Numbers, F. C. An investigation of the intelligibility of the speech of the deaf. *Genetic Psychology Monographs*, 1942, *25*, 289–392.

Kent, R. D. Anatomical and neuromuscular maturation of the speech mechanism: Evidence from acoustic studies. *Journal of Speech and Hearing Research*, 1976, *19*, 421–447.

Ling, D. *Speech and the hearing-impaired child: Theory and Practice*. Washington, D.C.: Alexander Graham Bell Association for the Deaf, 1976.

Magner, M. *Speech development*. Northampton, Massachusetts: Clarke School for the Deaf, 1971.

McDonald, E. T. *A deep test of articulation*. Pittsburgh: Stanwix House, Inc., 1964.

Milisen, R. 1954. A rationale for articulation disorders. The disorder of articulation: A systematic clinical and experimental approach. *Journal of Speech and Hearing Disorders,* 1954, *Monograph Suppmenent 4,* 5–17.

Morris, H. L., Spriestersbach, D. C., & Darley, F. L. An articulation test for assessing competency of velopharyngeal closure. *Journal of Speech and Hearing Research,* 1961, *4,* 48–55.

Nickerson, R. S. Characteristics of the speech of deaf persons. *Volta Review,* 1975, *77,* 342–362.

Ross, M., & Lerman, J. *Word intelligibility by picture identification*. Pittsburgh: Stanwix House, Inc., 1971.

Snow, K., & Milisen, R. Spontaneous improvement in articulation as related to differential responses to oral and picture articulation tests. The disorder of articulation: A systematic clinical and experimental approach. *Journal of Speech and Hearing Disorders,* 1954, *Monograph Supplement 4,* 45–49.

Templin, M. C., & Darley, F. L. *The Templin-Darley tests of articulation*. Iowa City, Iowa: University of Iowa, 1969.

Van Riper, C. *Speech correction: Principles and methods* (5th ed.). Englewood Cliffs, New Jersey: Prentice-Hall, Inc., 1972.

Van Riper, C., & Erickson, R. L. *Predictive screening test of articulation*. Kalamazoo, Michigan: Western Michigan University, 1968.

Vorce, E. *Teaching speech to deaf children*. Washington, D.C.: Alexander Graham Bell Association for the Deaf, 1974.

Waters, B. J., Bill, M. D., & Lowell, E. L. Precision therapy—An interpretation. *Language, Speech and Hearing Services in Schools,* 1977, *8,* 234–244.

Young, E. H., & Stinchfield-Hawk, S. *Moto-kinesthetic speech training*. Stanford, California: Stanford University Press, 1955.

REFERENCE NOTES

1. Binnie, C. A., Daniloff, R. G., & Jackson, P. L. Phonetic disintegration following sudden hearing loss. Presented at the American Speech and Hearing Association Convention, Houston, Texas, November 20–23, 1976.
2. Jackson, P. L., and Kelly-Ballweber, D. Auditory stress pattern recognition in sentences. Presented at the American Speech and Hearing Association Convention, Atlanta, Georgia, November 16–19, 1979.

APPENDIX: VISUAL AND VIBROTACTILE SPEECH TRAINING AIDS

One of the central concepts in speech conservation with the adventitiously hearing impaired is the effective use of amplification and auditory training to make maximum use of residual hearing. There are several cases, however, where additional sensory cues are needed to provide monitoring in speech conservation programs. Several devices are commercially available that were designed to provide visual and/or vibrotactile information, and a few are described below in terms of their general purpose, the type of information they provide, and where additional information can be obtained.

Kay Sonograph

This instrument provides visual cues for consonant and vowel articulation, duration, voice, pitch, and nasality. The cues are in the form of a printed spectrogram which is a time-by-frequency-by-intensity representation of the acoustic parameters of speech. This printout becomes a permanent record.

Contact: Kay Elemetrics
12 Maple Avenue
Pinebrook, New Jersey 07058

Series 700 Sound Spectrograph

This instrument provides visual cues for consonant and vowel articulation, duration, voice, and pitch. The cues are in the form of a printed spectrogram which becomes a permanent record.

Contact: Voice Identification, Incorporated
P.O. Box 714
Somerville, New Jersey 08876

Speech Spectrographic Display

This instrument provides visual cues for consonant and vowel articulation, duration, voice, and pitch. The cues are in the form of a video spectrum display with a frequency range of 100–5000 Hz. Two time scales, 0.75 or 1.5 seconds, are available. There is also an option for a two-channel split-screen display for clinician-client comparisons.

Contact: Spectraphonics, Incorporated
1531 St. Paul Street
Rochester, New York 14621

LUCIA Spectrum Indicator

This instrument provides visual cues designed to give feedback in vowel and voiced-voiceless fricative training. The instrument displays frequency by intensity spectral information in light displays. Intensity is represented in ten levels of 3.5 dB each and frequency information covers a range of 180–6800 Hz. There is also a mirror attached to the front of the unit for speechreading cues.

Contact: SI America
255 South 17th Street
Philadelphia, Pennsylvania 19103

Visible Speech Apparatus

This instrument provides visual cues for the training of fricative and plosive consonants, vowels, and pitch. The display is a light indication system which provides spectra of speech sounds. Frequency is displayed with 16 bandpass filters and covers a range of 90–8000 Hz. The intensity of each column is in 10 dB steps. Color coding on the display indicates fundamental frequency and first and second formants.

Contact: Precision Acoustics Corporation
55 West 42 Street
New York, New York 10036

Video Articulator

This instrument provides visual cues for place and manner of articulation, nasality, pitch, and duration. The display is a modified Sony 7-inch television set. Cues are changes in the basic circle pattern which represent changes in vocal fold and vocal tract configurations. Pitch and duration readouts are also available.

Contact: Amera, Incorporated
P.O. Box 627
Logan, Utah 84321

Vocal-2

This instrument provides visual cues for word stress patterns, fundamental frequency, and /s/ phoneme production. The visual display is on a split screen with an example placed on the top and client trials on the bottom. It displays intensity by time patterns, frequency by time patterns, or /s/ information.

Contact: Madsen Electronics
1807 Elmwood Avenue
Buffalo, New York 14207

Speech Therapy System

This instrument provides visual cues intended for use in articulation, phonation, loudness, and stress training. The visual display is a 6½-inch diagonal screen with an amplitude-by-time oscilloscopic output. The screen is split for clinician-client comparison.

Contact: Hearing Evaluation and Acoustic Research, Incorporated
732 N.W. 19th Street
Portland, Oregon 97209

Talk Time

This instrument provides visual cues for training in loudness, duration, vocal attacks, stress and intonation, rate, and voiced-voiceless consonant articulation.

Contact: Voice Identification, Incorporated
P.O. Box 714
Somerville, New Jersey 08876

S-Indicator

This instrument provides visual and tactile information to train /s/ as well as other voiceless fricatives. The visual cues are from a display panel with a meter and a light to indicate the quality of the /s/ production. There is an optional vibrator which also signals a correct /s/.

Contact: SI America
255 South 17th Street
Philadelphia, Pennsylvania 19103

"S" Indicator Model S-1

This instrument provides visual information to train /s/ articulation from isolation to connected speech. The visual cues are in the form of an indicator light.

Contact: Guinta Associates
67 Leuning Street
South Hackensack, New Jersey 07606

"S" Indicator

This instrument provides a visual display for training /s/ articulation. The visual cues are in the form of a meter and a light indicator.

Contact: Matrix Research and Development Corporation
533 Main Street
Acton, Massachusetts 01760

F_o-Indicator

This instrument provides visual cues to train pitch level, intonation, phonation, voiced versus voiceless articulation, and breath control. The visual cues are from a meter and from red and green lights that monitor the limits of the frequency range. A contact microphone is held against the throat, and the rate of vocal fold vibration is measured within a range of 50–550 Hz.

Contact: SI America
255 South 17th Street
Philadelphia, Pennsylvania 19103

"F" Meter

This instrument provides visual cues to train pitch level, intonation, phonation, voiced versus voiceless articulation, and breath control. The visual cues are in the form of a meter and indicator lights.

Contact: Matrix Research and Development Corporation
533 Main Street
Acton, Massachusetts 01760

N-Indicator

This instrument provides visual cues for training nasalization, denasalization, and phonation. A contact microphone is held against the nose, and the intensity of nasal vibration is shown on a meter. The panel also has a green and a red light to signal when the production is below or above a 50 percent deflection point.

Contact: SI America
255 South 17th Street
Philadelphia, Pennsylvania 19103

"N" Indicator

This instrument provides visual cues to be used to train nasalization and denasalization. A contact microphone is held against the nose and nasal vibrations are indicated by a meter and a light.

Contact: Matrix Research and Development Corporation
533 Main Street
Acton, Massachusetts 01760

TONAR II

This instrument provides visual cues to be used in the detection and modification of nasality in continuous speech. It can also provide fundamental frequency and intensity information. The information is presented in the form of calibrated printouts called tonagrams, which display sound from the nose, sound from the mouth, and a nasal-to-oral ratio. The frequency range is 70–5000 Hz.

Contact: Quan-Tech Division KMS Industries, Incorporateed
43 South Jefferson Road
Whippany, New Jersey 07891

Spright

This instrument provides visual information for training phonation, intensity, and duration. The feedback is in the form of a display of ten red lights spanning a 40 dB intensity range. The louder the voice, the more lights come on.

Contact: Electronics Incorporated
502 East LaSalle
South Bend, Indiana 46617

Voice Lite

This instrument provides visual and tactile cues for use in training phonation, loudness, duration, stress and rhythm, voiced versus voiceless articulation, nasality, and breath control. The visual cues are provided by a translucent dome with a light that reacts to sound. Brightness of the light is intensity related. The unit has an optional microphone that indicates nasality, and it also has an optional tactile stimulator.

Contact: Behavioral Controls, Incorporated
P.O. Box 480
Milwaukee, Wisconsin 53201

Sound Lamp

This instrument provides visual information for use in training phonation, duration, loudness, stress and rhythm, voiced versus voiceless articulation, and breath control. The visual cues come from a white glass globe with a light that reacts to sound. Brightness of the light is intensity dependent.

Contact: Hal-Hen Company
36-14 11th Street
Long Island City, New York 11106

COVOX Vibrotactile Aid

This device consists of a hand-held vibrator to be used in providing tactile information for pitch, phonation, duration, stress and rhythm, and voiced-voiceless articulation.

Contact: Av-Alarm Corporation
2734 Industrial Way
P.O. Box 2488
Santa Maria, California 93454

Mono-fonator and Poly-fonator

The mono-fonator is designed for individual use, while the poly-fonator is designed for use by one to four clients. This instrument provides tactile information for use in training stress, duration, phonation, and some phonetic features. The clinician or client speaks into the microphone and the vibrational cues are produced by a vibrator placed on the hand. Earphones are included for auditory information.

Contact: Siemens Corporation
Hearing Instrument Division
685 Liberty Avenue
Union, New Jersey 07083

Daniel L. Bode
David Tweedie

Chapter 11: Considerations for Determining the Quality of Aural Rehabilitation Services

It is not the purpose of this chapter to review past and current attempts at assessing improvements among clients in their ability to communicate and/or cope in various communicative environments. Those are reviewed within varying service contexts in Chapter 7, in Part I of this text, and in Chapters 19 and 27, in Part II. Rather, the focus of this chapter is a description of some of the major principles, as well as problems, involved in determining the quality of audiologic services in aural rehabilitation. The intent is to suggest that practitioners conduct their professional activities with confidence that these efforts are important, although often not presently amenable to scientific measurement. Principles of determining assessment and treatment successes, or lack of them, that may serve to reduce the complexity of the topic will be addressed.

Determining the success of auditory rehabilitative efforts with adult clients implies that their communication behaviors are assessed before, during, and after the remedial activity. Under these ideal circumstances, we also should be able to compare any observed behavioral changes with those expected from other hearing impaired individuals not participating in our intervention efforts, i.e., members of a "control" group. The person receiving professional services should show positive changes, while an individual not receiving these services should show few if any changes. These basic premises become complex and difficult under less than ideal circumstances. Ideal situations rarely exist except under narrowly defined laboratory conditions. Even then, the precision required for laboratory studies often reduces the scope of communication behaviors to such specific experimental dimensions that generalization of results is extremely limited. A partial solution is to use the client as a self-control with before and after measures.

Two circumstances facing the clinician are important to consider. First, many of the potentially important benefits of aural rehabilitation services are not amenable to direct assessment/measurement. Second, the positive results of these rehabilitation services might not be apparent until sometime after the professional relationship ceases.

In the first instance, a client's attitudes may change positively as a result of the services. Such changes may not be detected initially by either the clinician or the client. Experienced clinicians have observed two related extremes. The first is a situation wherein the client feels no change has taken place but the clinician has observed some change. In the opposite situation, the client extols the benefits while the clinician is perplexed because observable changes are not evidenced. If we identify possible outcomes, then, there are four alternative results: client and clinician both observe change; client observes change, clinician does not; client observes no change, clinician does; and the least desirable circumstance, neither party observes positive changes. Professionals are very aware of these possible outcomes and recognize them as expected when working within the behavioral sciences. Student clinicians often expect near 100 percent success rates and that both the client and the clinical supervisor will recognize these changes. Relatively few practicum experiences are needed to illustrate the optimism of these expectations.

The second problem associated with assessment of the benefits of aural rehabilitation services is that observable changes may not result until after direct contact has terminated. Both clinicians and clients may expect almost immediate results. These expectations often are not realistic and can interfere with the rehabilitation process. Attitudes such as these can result in feelings of frustration and discouragement if not recognized and dealt with constructively as part of the professional relationship. Both client and clinician need to be aware of this possible component of therapy and not be distressed by presumed lack of progress. Our main point here is that long-range benefits should not be ignored in assessment. It is important to be aware that lack of observable, positive change does not necessarily imply lack of success.

In summary, positive benefits of aural rehabilitation services may not be directly observable, and long-range benefits from professional contacts may result. Many of these factors are not easily assessed by the clinician responsible for their eventual occurrence.

QUESTIONS REGARDING ASSESSMENT PROCEDURES

Whenever the topics of assessment and evaluation are discussed, questions of reliability and validity should be raised. Too often in the past, these questions have been avoided, particularly in assessment of the success of aural rehabilitation. Since there are no readily available and widely used instruments for pre- and postservice assessment having demonstrated reliability and validity, the evaluation task is immediately increased to difficult proportions. Without reliable and valid assessment tools, how can a clinician determine success or nonsuccess of professional intervention? What guidelines for assessment can be suggested? Who is and is not providing successful service? When does one terminate services, either because they are unsuccessful or because the client has reached a plateau of maximum improvement? How can a clinician continue accepting financial compensation for rehabilitative activities when there are limited procedures for demonstrating the worth of these services? In order to suggest answers to these questions, basic concepts of reliability and validity need to be emphasized.

Reliability

Reliability is essential to assessment. It refers to the consistency of scores obtained by the same individual on different occasions. If a given score is obtained at one time, then a clinician should have reasonable confidence that the same or similar score would result from an immediate reassessment of the individual. Without knowledge of reliability, conclusions about the person's behavior should be made with caution.

Associated with test reliability is *error variance*. This is essentially any contributing condition not relevant to the purpose of the test. In any given assessment situation, there are usually many sources of error variance. Two major objectives of assessment are to maximize *true* variance in test scores while minimizing *error* variance. Even when true variance is maximized, however, error variance may still be too high for practical use of the test.

The reliability of a test needs to be known prior to its widespread use for making important decisions. For example, in diagnostic site-of-lesion testing in clinical audiology, it is generally accepted that any single test is usually not sufficiently reliable for confident interpretation. Thus, the concept of a test battery approach has been used for many years. This approach basically requires the administration of a number of different tests, with interpretation based on the pattern and consistency of results. If the pattern is equivocal, then additional test procedures or repetition of the original tests is indicated.

A similar situation exists in assessment of the effectiveness of aural rehabilitation efforts. It seems appropriate to maintain the following conceptual framework: use many assessment tools, analyze the consistency of results, and reach conclusions accordingly. Until assessment tools demonstrate repeatable results with the same individuals, careful use of these tools is necessary.

Validity

Validity is an additional important concept in assessment. Here the concerns are what the test measures and how well it does so. The least desirable type of validity is so-called face validity, also called "faith" validity. This refers not to what the test necessarily measures, but to what it appears to measure. Essential to other types of validity is the concept of a criterion. A test is judged to be valid only if it accurately predicts a given criterion either within or outside the testing situation.

An example of a difficult assessment circumstance, with regard to validity, is the clinical hearing aid evaluation. Audiologists have attempted for decades to identify test procedures which would validly determine the "best" hearing aid(s) within clinical test rooms (sound-isolated to reduce uncontrolled sources of error variance). These efforts for internal validity have achieved some degree of success. However, the objective of external validity has not been as easily achieved or as thoroughly addressed. Little is known about whether the "best" hearing aid selected within a clinical test situation is also the best hearing aid for the variety of listening conditions in the client's everyday life. Trial periods with a hearing aid and systematic follow-up are advised to achieve some degree of external validity.

The question of validity of assessment tools can become quite complicated. The validity of a test not only must be determined but also the validity of the criterion or criteria used to establish the test's validity. An extreme but realistic example of this exists when a clinician needs a valid test, but to determine its validity, an internal or external criterion must be defined. Measures of the criterion are then needed, using valid tools for measurement. And so, conducting clinical research to define and assess reliably and validly an individual's "communication" abilities remains a major challenge.

PRINCIPLES OF ASSESSMENT OF QUALITY OF SERVICES

Given the limitations of many procedures for assessment of the quality of services, it is necessary for audiologists to establish a general philosophy and approach to the evaluation of clients, their rehabilitation needs, and the success of clinical efforts. The following principles are offered not as definitive or universally accepted practices, but as general guidelines that may be helpful at various times to individual audiologists. Again, it is incumbent upon each clinician to establish his or her own operating principles.

Assessment in auditory rehabilitation should include reliable and valid audiometric testing. There should be little, if any, separation between audiology and aural rehabilitation; that is, between diagnostic activity and responsible audiologic rehabilitation work. Traditionally, some audiologists have seen themselves only as diagnosticians and have left rehabilitation activity to other professions. An audiologist ideally should be responsible for total case management in nonmedical areas. This does not mean that the audiologist should be, or even attempt to be, all things to all people. Rather, he or she should coordinate and assume responsibility for rehabilitative services for a given hearing impaired individual. In a comprehensive approach, the clinical audiologist should assume responsibility for insuring that appropriate follow-up services are available, and then should be an active participant in the actual provision of these services.

Assessment is most effective when the client understands the test procedures and the interpretation of test findings. The client's active participation in assessment can be extremely important. Lack of active participation, insufficient understanding of the task, or confusion regarding what is expected during the assessment can contribute to increases in error variance and a consequent reduction in the reliability and validity of evaluation procedures. Simple, direct instructions and brief explanations of each task can substantially improve both the assessment process and the results obtained. A few moments thus spent should not be viewed as wasted time. Just the opposite is true. Completion of the task may be accomplished more rapidly and with less chance of needed repetitions of the procedures due to misunderstandings and subsequent errors.

Interpersonal relationships between client and clinician are an important component of assessment procedures. There can be considerable benefits if the client and clinician are able to establish a cooperative, comanagement relationship. If the two are not seeking the same or similar assessment goals, clinician and client can effectively cancel each other's efforts. Though not always possible, establishment of common understanding of objectives and procedures should improve the reliability of results and contribute toward maintenance of a strong and positive professional interaction.

Establishment of a counseling relationship should be a major priority. Since it is our assumption that the same person assessing communication abilities will be providing the treatment services, it is important that a counseling relationship be established at the outset of contact with the client. Too often, a person conducting an evaluation, perhaps in an attempt to be objective, treats the client insensitively and with little regard for the client as a person. Objectivity and sensitivity, however, are not mutually exclusive characteristics of an audiologist.

Clients can be treated as unique individuals and still be viewed quite objectively. It is important to realize that this balance is not easily achieved. Rather, it is much easier to become objective at the expense of a human relationship with the client. The opposite also can occur. Either extreme is to be avoided as a typical professional stance.

A case history is essential to the interpretation of test findings. An initial interview with a client should coincide with the assessment stage of a clinician–client relationship. This interview should result in a case history including, at a minimum, the following components: objective dates and events; the client's reaction and interpretation of these facts; and the clinician's interpretation of both the reported events and the client's perceptions of them. Too often, only the objective components result from an interview. The other two perspectives are important in a comprehensive assessment and sometimes can be as useful as formal test results in describing and understanding present functioning of the individual.

Reliability and validity of test results should be viewed on a continuum. There are many domains in which our tools have some reliability and validity but not as much as we would ideally like to have available. The opposite is also true, since some tools provide more information than is needed. It is essential that assessment procedures continue to be used, at the audiologist's discretion, even though many of them fall short of having ideal characteristics. They can still provide some information which, in combination with other tests or other sources of information, is useful in the clinical appraisal process. Often, the sum of components having less than ideal reliability and validity can result in a valid overall assessment.

Testing should be viewed as a dynamic rather than a static process. An audiologist usually has a far greater number of assessment tools available than he or she can realistically use with a given client. It is necessary, then, to have a point of departure in testing, but with flexibility in determining subsequent components in a test battery. Ideally, selection of the second test should be dependent upon the client's responses to the first test, selection of the third test based on responses to the second, and so forth. This flexible and dynamic approach to assessment seems to have advantages over administration of tests that are independent of the client's ongoing performance. Adjusting the testing conditions to the individual, rather than the opposite, is the fundamental principle here.

Audiologists should be ''calibrated'' with as great a concern as given to calibration of test equipment and procedures. Since any test or battery of tests requires interpretation, the individual doing the interpretation must be highly skilled. Here is one of the most difficult tasks facing clinicians and others responsible for clinical training programs. The art of test interpretation in aural rehabilitation is not a skill easily learned or taught. An audiologist often must interpret not only tests he or she has directly administered, but also those administered by other professional specialists. This is a considerable challenge and an important responsibility. An audiologist often finds that he or she must integrate information from physicians, teachers, psychologists and others, and then interpret this data in terms which are appropriate to a hearing impaired individual. The operational acquisition of this difficult-to-learn skill defies easy description or implementation, but its achievement is of considerable importance.

The rights of a client to respect, privacy, and intelligent counseling as part of assessment procedures should be given high priority. The goal here is to include the client in all aspects of decision-making regarding the planning of a rehabilitation program. Granted, there may be circumstances wherein a particular client might not be directly involved in the planning process, but these instances should be relatively few with adults. Treating the client with respect, protecting his or her rights to privacy, and providing counseling about assessment procedures and results, can contribute substantially to successful professional interactions and consequent achievement of auditory rehabilitation goals.

Hearing aids should be considered a necessary but not sufficient end product of aural rehabilitation. For years the hearing aid evaluation and selection procedure has been viewed by many as a terminal activity, i.e., that audiologic responsibility for client welfare ends with a recommendation for a hearing aid. Follow-up services often have not been considered to be the direct responsibility of the audiologist. The issue of who, then, is responsible for these services continues to be a major issue. We believe that the work of audiologists should involve all aspects of client care, including speechreading instruction, auditory training, speech and language therapy, manual communication, and counseling regarding hearing handicap. The hearing aid selection process should be only one component in the total audiologic service to hearing impaired clients.

Assessment tasks should be viewed within a communication assessment framework, ideally including description of receptive language performance. The philosophical position here is that assessment procedures should encompass more than measures of a person's speech receptive ability. For example, monosyllabic speech discrimination scores via auditory, visual, and combined modalities, while providing important information, are not sufficient for judging either the individual's communication ability or his or her potential. As one component of a battery of tests, these scores can be very helpful, but to limit assessment to these tasks seems inappropriate. The use of connected speech (phrases and sentences) is important, in order to validly assess receptive/perceptive performance. A paradox of assessment with hearing impaired listeners is that monosyllables are often used to obtain reliable results, but with questionable validity; whereas if sentences are used, having at least face validity, difficulty is encountered obtaining reliable results. A fundamental problem is that a test cannot be valid if it is not at the same time reliable. Tests of sentence and other connected speech stimuli continue to be needed for thorough clinical appraisals.

Auditory training, speechreading instruction, and assessment should be conducted simultaneously or concurrently. A particularly important aspect of assessment is consideration of combined evaluation and instruction; that is, conducting assessment in such a way that instructional information is also obtained. The theoretical ideal is that both goals be achieved simultaneously, or concurrently. If these dual objectives could be achieved, our knowledge of a listener's communication abilities might increase dramatically. Testing and instruction conducted at the same, or at least adjacent, times could provide considerable information regarding performance.

Some aspects of aural rehabilitation are amenable to this type of diagnostic therapy, for example, speechreading instruction and auditory training. The use of videotape and newly developed computer-controlled testing and training materials, with listener responses recorded for either on-line or later analysis, is a means for giving listener practice and at the same time allowing assessment of performance with auditory, visual, and combined signals.

FUTURE DEVELOPMENTS

It seems that some exciting prospects exist and can be predicted. First, the research literature in aural rehabilitation has begun to increase substantially. Second, audiologists interested in providing rehabilitation services are becoming more visible in their activities. Third, external pressures are demanding a greater involvement by audiologists in the provision of rehabilitation services. Fourth, the growth of private practice opportunities for audiologists and the increasing potential for employment in the schools and in programs for geriatric citizens suggests that audiologic rehabilitative services are going to be both accepted and expected. Fifth, many graduate students and beginning practitioners in audiology seem to be highly motivated to involve themselves in rehabilitative work and to advance the art and science of this aspect of the profession.

The result of all of the above developments, if mutually reinforcing, should be a continuing increase in the quality and effectiveness of services offered to the public. Given the developing emphasis upon accountability within the various health services, these increases may be more and more mandated by federal regulation, professional standards, and consumer demands.

Reliability and Validity

In this chapter, we have considered questions of reliability and validity of assessment procedures. We have suggested that a balance is needed between impossibly high demands for stable and accurate results, thereby failing to use procedures that give some information, and the other extreme—indiscriminate use of procedures having little logical or demonstrated usefulness. We expect that attention in training programs will become more directed than at present toward developing these skills in student clinicians. Achievement of this balance probably cannot be a terminal objective for one- or two-year graduate programs. Time and experience beyond the limitations of formal graduate study seem necessary to develop and refine these clinical skills.

Inclusion of the Client in Decision-Making

The integration of diagnostic and rehabilitative skills by individual clinicians should continue to be an objective. Inclusion of the client in all major aspects of decision-making will be an important new dimension to clinical practice in auditory rehabilitation. The interpersonal relationship between client and clinician will then assume even greater importance than at present. Consequently, questions of counseling effectiveness will demand greater attention by audiologists. Dynamic participation and responsiveness in the rehabilitation process by both client and clinician will be essential. The rights of clients to respect and privacy during this process will need to be given heightened consideration.

The Treatment Program

The coordination and integration of hearing aid selection and orientation, auditory and visual communication training, and related counseling activities will require increased operational skills by the individual clinician. Too often in the past, these services have been fragmented and offered in a noncomprehensive aural rehabilitation environment. Again, the individual audiologist will need to become basically competent in varied aspects of assessment and therapy in order for these services to be integrated in clinical practice. Increased training (coursework and practicum) in counseling seems essential to this process.

True "prescription" of hearing aids may be a viable objective as present research and clinical experiences are collated and distilled to achieve the practical objective of satisfactory and satisfied hearing aid use. For too long, we have not been able to close the gap between what is known about hearing aid use and the selection and adaptation process. It is encouraging to observe instances where this gap is being narrowed, where researchers and clinicians are cooperating and communicating with each other.

Assessment of Communication

As we focus more and more on the person with a hearing impairment, then the need for communication assessment, rather than just audiometric evaluation, becomes obvious. Ideally, the often artificial boundaries between the professions of audiology and speech and language pathology might be eliminated. If the objective is communication therapy for a person with hearing impairment, then the skills, interests and activities of these two professions are not mutually exclusive, but are highly interdependent.

Perhaps in the near future we will improve our ability to assess nonverbal components of a person's behavior, such as response latency, listening strategies, and listener response criteria. So-called ''body language'' cues also probably contribute a significant amount of information to the effectiveness of communication with a hearing impaired individual. Assessment of the importance of these cues remains a challenge to those involved in evaluation of auditory rehabilitation services.

Client Evaluation

Inclusion of provisions for client evaluation of the success of audiologic services is needed. For example, is the acceptance or rejection of a hearing aid due to the aid, to the extent of an audiologist's professional services, or to the client's attitudes toward acknowledging a problem and accepting visible evidence of it?

The client's judgments should be given appropriate consideration, including judgments such as changes in self-acceptance and motivation, in attitudes toward communication, in self-confidence and assertiveness, in situational control during difficult listening conditions, and so forth. These and other psychosocial factors may prove to be important indices of the success of auditory rehabilitation. Judgments of family members, friends, and coworkers also might be important sources of information regarding effectiveness of audiologic services.

The increase in the number and extent of communication disciplines and services during the past several decades suggests that the benefits to individuals with hearing impairment will continue to show positive gains. An increase in effectiveness of our procedures for *assessing* these benefits and for reporting these gains to our colleagues and to the public is needed and should be given high priority in the coming years.

SUGGESTED READINGS

Alpiner, J. G. Evaluation of communication function, in J. G. Alpiner (Ed.), *Handbook of adult rehabilitative audiology*. Baltimore: Williams and Wilkins, 1978.

Hodgson, W. R. and Skinner, P. H. *Hearing aid assessment and use in audiologic habilitation*. Baltimore: Williams and Wilkins, 1981.

Noble, W. G. *Assessment of impaired hearing: A critique and a new method*. New York: Academic Press, 1978.

O'Neill, J. J., & Oyer, H. J. Aural rehabilitation, in J. Jerger (Ed.), *Modern developments in audiology*. New York: Academic Press, 1973.

Oyer, H. J., & Frankmann, J. P. *The aural rehabilitation process: A conceptual framework analysis*. New York: Holt, Rinehart and Winston, 1975.

D. The Vocational Impact and Vocational Rehabilitation Counseling for Hearing Impaired Adults

Kevin G. Marshall

Chapter 12: The Vocational Impact of Hearing Impairment as Viewed by the Vocational Rehabilitation Counselor

In Western society, probably no other single elective variable influences a person as comprehensively as the choice of work. Employment, as the primary determinant of a person's economic situation and subsequent standard of living, is a major social discriminator. It determines the type of activity and environment the person will be immersed in for nearly one third of his or her life, and is a predominant factor in making the majority of daily life decisions, such as when to eat, sleep, take vacations, and the like. Psychologically, the type, level of remuneration, and physical setting of the employment determine which social values are ascribed to different jobs. Subsequently, the job often becomes a yardstick by which many persons measure the worth of themselves and others.

It has been over 40 years since Congress mandated the 40-hour work week, and since that time many gradual but major changes have taken place. Education and training have become pre-eminent, women have entered the job market in larger numbers and in leadership roles, wages and benefits have increased manyfold, new industries and vocations have been created, and other entire labor areas have vanished. Between 1959 and 1965 alone, 6,000 new jobs were listed in the *Dictionary of Occupational Titles,* and 8,000 others became extinct (Williams & Vernon, 1970). A national trend towards white-collar jobs and increasing technical knowledge and mechanization, combined with a shrinking demand for low-level, unskilled labor, presents a discomforting outlook for individuals or segments of our populace who are not keeping pace with our increasingly sophisticated and mobile society. Projections from all sectors of the economy and the business world indicate that increased sophistication and refinement of job skills will continue at an even more accelerated rate for the foreseeable future, and that increased technical expertise and flexibility will be required of members of the labor force just to maintain current job and income levels.

The potential impact of this situation on the hearing impaired population has implications ranging from severe to devastating. These effects, some possible solutions, and the role of the hearing professional in minimizing or alleviating many of these potentially negative occurrences will be the focus of this chapter. It should be noted that the author sees the audiologist as an extremely important link between the hearing and the deaf segments of the population, and perhaps the most widely distributed group of professionals available to act as advocates, proponents, and information disseminators for and to deaf and hearing impaired people.

THE SITUATION

Historically, deaf and severely hearing impaired people have frequently been viewed with suspicion by people with normal hearing and often seen as different or even frightening. They have regularly been the objects of jokes and scorn, and have been forced to contend with general prejudicial attitudes of a society ignorant of the true nature of their disability. Even today, the "deaf and dumb" label prevails in a surprisingly large segment of our society, and numerous myths and erroneous ideas are widely held. The stigma remains, and the result is that this one segment of our population reflects a lower than average socioeconomic level based not on potential, but on circumstance.

The educational and socioeconomic discrepancy between hearing impaired and hearing members of our society is not an innate, unchangeable entity. Rather, it is a socioculturally created situation imposed upon this group, however inadvertently, by a hearing society which constitutes the vast majority and makes the rules by which deaf and hearing impaired persons must live (Marshall, 1978). Despite the evidence, which shows the hearing impaired population to have vocational and intellectual potential equivalent to its hearing peers (Vernon, 1969), severely hearing impaired people most frequently enter the work force in various lower manual skill areas. An extensive survey, conducted in 1959 by Gallaudet College and the National Association of the Deaf, showed a heavy concentration of deaf persons in skilled and semiskilled manual occupations, including three fourths of the men and three fifths of the women. These figures contrast sharply with those for the total population; about two fifths of all men and one fifth of all women hold jobs at these levels. Over one half of the employed deaf were in manufacturing industries, contrasted with one fourth of the total population (Lunde & Bigman, 1959). Although more recent information indicates that some changes have occurred, statistically very little improvement has been actually realized despite the efforts of educators, legislators, rehabilitation counselors, and others. The most widespread impact of severe hearing impairment then, is not unemployment but rather underemployment. Most severely hearing impaired persons can and do find some type of work, but too frequently their true potential or ability is not known or considered by the employer and, thus, never has opportunity for full realization.

Three primary reasons why the aforementioned situation still basically prevails are:

1. Historically, the educational systems developed for severely hearing impaired persons have not been able to adequately prepare them for full, competitive employment in the hearing world. Although current educational and career development programs are greatly improved over their predecessors, many deaf adults are the products of the previous programs.
2. Increasing demands of our technological society are offsetting many of the gains made in existing career development programs and the training and education of severely hearing impaired children.
3. The general public still harbors numerous half-truths, fears, and much misinformation about hearing impaired people. Until the public and employers better understand

and accept deafness and hearing impaired people, attaining a vocational niche based on ability and potential will not occur for this faction of our population.

In all three of these areas, audiologists are seen as having a potentially strong influence in working towards problem resolution and true parity for hearing impaired persons with the hearing population. By acting as facilitators and proponents, new and more accurate information can be infused into existing structures. Input from hearing impaired people and the professionals working directly with them allows others who have only secondhand knowledge about them to observe and interact with these "different" individuals. This direct contact and interaction can only serve to promote less fear, more cooperation, and true understanding. If this process can be initiated and propagated at a grass-roots level by the audiologist, not only will his or her own job become easier, but also he or she can gain some degree of personal satisfaction from helping to resolve one of the greatest discrepancies of our modern society.

THE CLIENT

The audiologist should become aware of the vocational potentials and liabilities of the hearing impaired person with whom he or she is working before attempting to become involved in any vocational advocacy on that person's behalf. Good intentions will seldom suffice in an interview with a potential employer who is concerned with facts, abilities, liabilities, and just possibly a little personal curiosity. Also, a brief warning seems in place at this time. This consists of a caution to not generalize or stereotype actions or behaviors to "the deaf" or to hearing impaired persons. There is no special psychology of deafness. These are individuals leading their lives and basing their beliefs, as we all do, on past experiences and on the information available. Since they do share a similar disability, some common experiences will influence some of them in similar ways. However, they should be regarded as what they are—individuals, more different than alike—who share impaired hearing only secondarily.

Educational Status

Educationally, severely hearing impaired people have fared quite poorly in the United States until very recently. For many years, numerous schools and programs have been educating "deaf" people. The methods, theories, and techniques used have varied widely, and the results have often been less than positive. The most extensive survey of the educational achievement of the severely hearing impaired included 93 percent of deaf students 16 years or older in the United States (Boatner, Stuckless, & Moores, 1964). Only 5 percent achieved a tenth grade level or better, 60 percent were at grade level 5.3 or below, and 30 percent were functionally illiterate. Meanwhile, the average worker today spends 33 percent more years in school than his or her predecessor (Friedman, 1967). The outcome of these divergent educational practices, coupled with all-too-frequent late diagnosis of severe hearing loss and inconsistent application of therapeutic and remedial techniques, is a group of individuals with a true handicap in the area of competitive employment.

When engaging in any career planning or job development, an individual educational assessment should always be obtained for the hearing impaired person if classroom educational skills are going to be needed on a particular job or in the training for the job. A high school diploma or other school record may give some indication of the person's experiences and abilities, but will probably not accurately indicate specific skill and ability levels compared with hearing peers. Care should be taken to select an evaluator who is experienced in testing severely hearing impaired persons and who can communicate in the mode and at the language level of the individual being assessed. Also, the audiologist should become knowledgeable in the basics of the evaluation instruments used and the interpretation and meaning of the results to that individual. Employers and personnel officers too frequently look only at test scores and results without considering the variables which can skew results unfairly (and drastically) for hearing impaired applicants. A thorough understanding of the applicant by the hearing advocate will facilitate his or her ability to intercede with relevant data and input when appropriate.

Social Status

On a social–personal level, severely hearing impaired persons constitute a near-normal cross-section of our society. However, at least partially as a result of the less-than-accepting, often second-class treatment and status they are accorded in a hearing world, deaf persons tend to seek out and associate most frequently with others who are also deaf. This is well documented in the literature and it seems neither surprising nor unhealthy for individuals to want to associate with others who accept them, who have many similar concerns, and who share the unique mode of communication, sign language. This association, over a period of years, has evolved into a distinct subgroup, or subculture, within which most social and religious interactions of deaf persons take place and most marriages occur (Marshall, 1978). In fact, over 90 percent of all deaf men and 95 percent of all deaf women marry other deaf people (Rainer, Altshuler, Kallman, & Deming, 1963).

The major conflict that seems to arise from belonging to this subculture is that nearly all jobs occur outside of its boundaries. When placed on a job surrounded only by normal hearing, oral persons, the non-oral hearing impaired person is effectively isolated. Even if he or she does have some oral skills, many deaf persons are difficult for the inexperienced hearing person to understand. If the co-workers avoid or exclude the deaf person or, even worse, tease or patronize him or her, true communication and understanding are lost or never achieved, and an undesirable situation is created. In point of fact, the primary reason for job loss or change by deaf persons is not lack of skill or ability, but unsatisfactory socialization. Inclusion and peer acceptance is a nearly universal requisite for self-acceptance and satisfaction, and a need not easily denied. Any situation, job-related or otherwise, which does not promote positive self-concept is tenuous at best and will probably be short-lived.

Job Placement and Retention

The five most commonly identified personal variables noted by this author, which are seen as detrimental to successful job search, placement, and retention by severely hearing impaired individuals, are:

1. *Communication problems.* The individual cannot adequately communicate with hearing persons either by voice or written notes.

2. *Educational deficit.* This includes low language comprehension, poor reading and mathematical skills, etc.
3. *Lack of "real world" experiences.* Limited knowledge of how the working world functions, how to ride buses and travel independently, ability to handle personal finances, understanding the importance of reliability and dependability, inability to care for own living needs, and general naiveté.
4. *Actual limitations occurring because of the inability to hear.* Nonuse of telephones, fire alarms, signals, etc.
5. *Feelings of exclusion,* social and otherwise, from other employees and the employer.

These five variables should be kept in mind by the audiologist when working as an advocate for full employment of deaf individuals. Although changing the entire situation and/or personality of the client is neither possible nor desirable, helping him become aware of the most prevalent pitfalls and hazards will facilitate open communication and provide a more clear grasp of the reality of the situation, and should assist in the formulation of a plan of action which can minimize the occurrence of problems.

One final consideration in terms of the vocational impact of hearing impairment is a general lack of knowledge by many congenitally hearing impaired people regarding the expectations about the work situation itself, which often places them in a less-than-competitive position relative to their hearing counterparts. Vicariously acquired "savvy" plays a prominent role in employee attitude, acceptance, satisfaction, and success. Several common examples of this "missed" information are:

There is no perfect job, and there is some dissatisfaction with every job. In all of the vocational training, educational testing, positive "pep talks" and the like, seldom is a deaf student prepared to expect the bad days and imperfections that exist in every job. As a result, when these times inevitably arise, the unprepared person may feel that a major problem has surfaced, and generalize these negative feelings to the total job or to him or herself.

There are subtle rules, traditions, and courtesies which must be followed even though they may not be written or stated outright. When these unwritten rules are broken or not adhered to, supervisors, managers, and/or co-workers can become unpleasant, or worse. Two examples are: deferring to senior employees in certain situations and (not) parking in specially designated areas.

Change is necessary and to be expected. The job market, job skills, and consumer demands are subject to frequent and rapid changes, mandating flexibility and adaptability as necessary components of the personal makeup of individuals in the working pool. The average worker will most likely change his job skill four or five times in his working life. Given these facts and the inevitability of vocational change, a "mental set" towards change should be held in the minds of all workers. In most training facilities and programs for the deaf, emphasis on specific skills or jobs takes precedence over building a general, lifetime career concept.

Any attempt to summarize the true impact of hearing impairment on employment and employability seems a nearly impossible task. Capsulizing the obvious problem areas such as education and communication ability here is not difficult, but actual problem resolution becomes more so. A great deal of the impact comes about as a result of intangibles—attitudes and subtle nuances which are nearly impossible to identify, much less quantify. Despite the potential to function on an equal footing with hearing peers, finding the opportunity to demonstrate this potential without bias often becomes a nearly insurmountable task for the severely hearing impaired individual, without assistance and understanding.

In all likelihood, the audiologist will not have the time or the expertise to effectively evaluate and resolve every facet of a deaf person's vocational plight. However, an understanding and appreciation of the situation and its background predisposes him or her to work toward successful mobilization of other resources and to figure significantly in the resolution of the many seemingly insurmountable problems in the person's vocational milieu.

THE EMPLOYER

To be maximally effective in facilitating the employment situation for severely hearing impaired persons, it is necessary to understand some of the variables involved in the situation. Although it is difficult to generalize certain attributes to all employers and potential employers, a number of given considerations usually exist in the business world, since companies are all presumed to be in business to produce a profit. Altruism on the part of the proponent is a probability, but in and of itself it will most likely not be a swaying consideration to most businessmen. Four basically universal considerations should be kept in mind when dealing with persons from the business sector:

Efficiency is directly related to amount of profit. If employees are careless, slow, or unreliable, the end product of the company (and thus the profit) will diminish in either quality or quantity, or both.

Overhead and other operating costs and expenses are to be kept to a minimum, as they are subtracted directly from income and thus affect the profits. If employees are careless or unskilled with equipment and facilities, repairs and down time cost the company additional money through lowered production.

Training and supervision are essential to maximal production. If employees are difficult to train or supervise, efficiency and overhead may both be negatively affected.

Public relations and positive company/product image with the general public are usually considered necessary for successful merchandising of the product or service provided. Positive image and personnel/employee relations are also seen as necessary to the successful operation of a company. If a specific employee is a negative influence on the internal or external company image or on personnel attitudes he or she will be seen as a liability.

If any employer can be shown that involvement with any person or group of persons such as the severely hearing impaired will enhance any of these four areas, he or she will frequently be interested in at least obtaining more information about the situation. Conversely, if the employer holds negative biases towards a specific group, whether accurate or not, he or she will avoid involvement for the good of the company.

Much potential as educator, facilitator, and myth breaker exists here for the audiologist. A number of concerns, myths, and questions are frequently surfaced by potential employers when faced with hiring their first deaf person. If the audiologist has done his or her homework and can factually address the honest concerns of the employer, citing precedents, laws, insurance rates, competitor involvement, and specific skills of the individual concerned, the chances of positive results will be greatly enhanced. At this point, bringing a rehabilitation counselor or employment counselor into the picture may be desirable. An additional expert in current specifics of the employment picture can be beneficial to all parties involved. Frequently, however, the audiologist will remain the expert on most aspects of deafness unless another specialized professional can be located. The other consideration is that the first contact made with an employer usually sets the stage for future success or failure. The audiologist should be prepared to make these initial contacts and to set the stage in a manner that facilitates further followup contacts by himself or any other professional.

Although finding employment for the severely hearing impaired person is of paramount importance, it should be remembered that the employer also needs accurate, reliable information. If a client is placed in employment based on inaccurate or incomplete information, no positive credibility is being created for the advocate, the deaf population, or the individual involved. Being a proponent in the true sense means being personally sold on the client for what he or she actually is and can be, not just because he or she is a hearing impaired person in need of a job. When all parties involved are aware of the expectations, limitations, and special considerations which may be involved, the highest probability of success is attained.

ROLE OF THE HEARING PROFESSIONAL

When the audiologist embarks upon an endeavor as comprehensive and as important as assisting an individual in selecting, preparing for, and locating his or her chosen vocation, a few suggestions may help to ease the burden. This author, functioning as a rehabilitation counselor specializing in the area of hearing impairment, found the following general guidelines to be of value when dealing directly with clients and employers:

1. Be certain your (hearing impaired) client is making his or her own choices and that you have not accepted the responsibility for making decisions that should be made by the client.
2. There is no substitute for possessing all of the relevant facts regarding the client, the employer, and the general job situation. Be adequately informed and prepared before you make the initial contact with a prospective employer.
3. Do not rely on emotion and altruism on the part of the employer to gain a job for your client. Employment based on facts and on probability of success is most likely to promote positivism and success.
4. When investigating a possible job for your client, find out who actually makes the hiring and firing decisions. Often, it is not the seemingly obvious person, but rather a line foreman, supervisor, or even a "screening" secretary. If your client cannot maneuver through the informal outer office maze before reaching the formal personnel hiring procedure, he or she will be excluded by default before actually having the opportunity to apply for the job and be considered based on his or her merits.
5. The client should be ready for a job physically, psychologically, and socially, and should have the necessary skills or abilities to succeed on the job.
6. Involve your client in his or her own job search. Doing activities for instead of with a person gives him or her little or no personal investment in the success of the outcome.

Although this list is far from comprehensive, the majority of frequently occurring job placement problems were found to be related to one or more of these areas.

As *the* professional in the community, viewed by most hearing people as the expert on deafness and all related considerations, the audiologist has a professional obligation to work as an advocate of the deaf community and to help bridge the gap that separates the hearing impaired and hearing segments of our society. It is likely that he or she does, in fact, possess more information relative to hearing impairment and its physical and psychosocial concomitants than any other individual in most communities. Properly applied, this professional's efforts can effectively diminish the devastating impact upon the educational, socioeconomic, personal, and vocational aspects of the lives of deaf people in that community.

Examples of specific personal and community actions the hearing professional can undertake to reduce the vocational impact of deafness are:

Advocate early screening, identification, and treatment programs. Early identification of a hearing loss means more remediation and a lessening of the factors which differentiate the deaf faction of our society from the hearing.

Educate the community in general about the impact hearing impairment has on an individual and his employment. Explode the myths and decrease irrational fears, if possible. Remember, the people being addressed constitute the population of potential employers in the community. A general lack of accurate knowledge about deafness is surprisingly widespread, and a small, regular freeing-up of time to spread accurate information now can prove invaluable further down the way.

Become knowledgeable about the general employment situation in your area and the resultant implications to deaf and hearing impaired persons. National economic concerns as well as local trends can influence the success or failure of a vocational plan of action.

Become familiar with other resources and potential resources for deaf and hearing impaired persons in your area. Assess the available education, training, and social service opportunities in the vicinity and locate professionals such as physicians, educators, and rehabilitation counselors who have knowledge of deafness and experience with deaf persons. Find out if there are social clubs or organizations of deaf people in the community.

Do the primary job in your hearing specialty area comprehensively, creatively, and thoroughly. Work toward development of new techniques, prostheses, warning devices, etc., which will enable hearing impaired persons to be more competitive and independent. Follow through and follow up on first efforts (i.e., elimination of the hearing aid "dresser drawer syndrome" in hearing impaired adults). Provide any professional reports to the community in understandable, application-oriented language, and contribute to a team approach towards alleviation and remediation of the inequities or problems which exist.

Show personal concern and demonstrate a willingness to become involved with hearing impaired persons in your area. Get to know them, learn sign language, demonstrate to other hearing people that hearing impaired persons are people first and hearing impaired secondarily.

The much overused cliché, "actions speak louder than words," seems an appropriate summation of the above. By personal example, and with a surprisingly small initial investment of time and energy, the audiologist can serve as a catalyst to speed up the gradually improving but still slow and tedious process of reducing the negative impact of hearing impairment, vocationally and otherwise, to these individuals.

SUMMARY AND CONCLUSIONS

An overwhelmingly negative impact on equal vocational opportunity for deaf and hearing impaired persons has been identified and documented in this chapter. Unlike the social and personal variables of a hearing impaired individual's life where he or she may choose to exclude the hearing faction of the world, employment most frequently is found outside the confines of this subculture. Competition with hearing counterparts is necessary, and usually a deaf person has a definite competitive disadvantage. The result has been the systematic relegation of these people to lower socioeconomic positions in our society than their potential and efforts warrant.

Recent encouraging changes have taken place, due primarily to pressure exerted by various professionals and advocacy groups, and by hearing impaired people themselves. Legislation such as Public Law 94-142, which mandates equal educational opportunity regardless of handicap, and Section 504 of the Vocational Rehabilitation Act, which assures equal access to services and employment in any organization, agency, or company that deals with the Federal Government, will do much in the future to accelerate the improving climate for hearing impaired and other handicapped persons. It remains to be seen, however, whether the increases mentioned here can gain enough momentum to catch up to and overcome an economy which is speeding ahead, undaunted by the special needs of a few.

The true key to resolution of this disparity seems to lie not so much in the treatment of the ills, or the end result which has developed from ignorance, prejudice, and neglect, but in interceding at the earliest moment with adequate diagnosis, treatment, and education and in mobilizing and coordinating the efforts of the various professionals, employers, and others involved. Audiologists as professionals have a major role to play in minimizing the devastating impact hearing impairment has had on full vocational actualization of these individuals. Preparation to meet this challenge has already begun and needs to continue at an accelerating pace to accomplish the task.

REFERENCES

Boatner, E. B., Stuckless, E., & Moores, D. F. *Occupational status of the young adult deaf of New England and the need and demand for a regional technical-vocational training center*. West Hartford, Connecticut: American School for the Deaf, 1964.

Friedman, M. The changing profile of the labor force. *AFL-CIO American Federationist*, 1967, *74*, 7–14.

Lunde, A. S., & Bigman, S. G. *Occupational conditions among the deaf*. Washington, D.C.: Gallaudet College Press, 1959.

Marshall, K. G. *A comparison of the self concepts of normally hearing offspring of deaf parents with those of normally hearing offspring of normally hearing parents*. Greeley, Colorado: University of Northern Colorado, 1978.

Rainer, J., Altshuler, L., Kallman, F., & Deming, G. (Eds.). *Family and mental health problems in a deaf population*. New York: Columbia University Press, 1963.

Vernon, M. Sociological and psychological factors associated with hearing loss. *Journal of Speech and Hearing Research*, 1969, *12*, 541–563.

Williams, B. R., & Vernon, M. Vocational guidance for the deaf, in H. Davis & S. R. Silverman (Eds.), *Hearing and deafness*. New York: Holt, Rinehart and Winston, 1970, p. 477.

Allan W. Orlofsky

Chapter 13: The Process of Vocational Rehabilitation Counseling and Placement for the Hearing Impaired Adult

The process of vocational rehabilitation counseling and the role of the rehabilitation counselor is an area in which many professionals in the field of communication disorders are not familiar. It is important that in the rehabilitative process, professionals such as the audiologist, the otologist, the speech pathologist, and the hearing aid specialist become familiar with the vocational rehabilitation services that may be available within the community for their clients. Only through the utilization of many professionals in the rehabilitation process can the total individual be served. To effect the goal of rehabilitation, or habilitation, and to assist the hearing impaired client to participate as a contributing member of society, all professionals dealing with the individual must be aware of the community resources available.

The importance of useful and purposeful work in our society has been well documented. According to Menninger (1964), "One of the ultimate results of the maturing process is the ability to work consistently with satisfaction to himself and to others" (p. xiii). The psychological needs met by meaningful employment are also well documented. These needs apply to individuals with sensory impairments as well as to the unimpaired population.

Vocational rehabilitation services to the severely hearing impaired have been generally unavailable, and where available to the majority of the estimated ten million individuals under the age of 65 who may benefit from those services, such services have been limited. It has been estimated that the annual loss of earning power due to acoustic impairments exceeds $1.5 billion (Porter, 1975).

DEFINITION OF VOCATIONAL REHABILITATION COUNSELING

Thompson and Barret (1959) define vocational rehabilitation counseling as a process in which the counselor thinks and works in a face-to-face relationship with the disabled person in order to help him or her both understand his or her problems and potentialities and carry through a program of adjustment and self-improvement to the end that the person make the best obtainable vocational, personal, and social adjustment. Vocational rehabilitation has also been defined by Lankenau (1969) as a process which has many facets. Primarily it is an attempt to prepare a handicapped person for gainful employment. This process may be complicated by a variety of physical, mental, educational, social, and family problems. Therefore, the process involves not only the rehabilitation counselor, but social workers, psychologists, physicians, educators, and employers as well. This chapter is intended to acquaint those professionals in the communication disorder field with the process of vocational rehabilitation counseling.

HISTORICAL LOOK AT VOCATIONAL REHABILITATION

Vocational rehabilitation serivces, as a federal and state grant-in-aid program, were started during the administration of Woodrow Wilson in 1920. The Legislative Rehabilitation Act was introduced as the Smith-Fess Act. This act was known as the Civilian Vocational Rehabilitation Act and was an outgrowth of the Soldier Rehabilitation Act passed in 1918. The initial Federal act, passed on a temporary basis, provided funding to the states on a one-to-one matching basis with the funds intended to provide vocational guidance, training, occupational adjustment, prothetics, and placement services only. The Rehabilitation Act was supported as temporary legislation until 1935, when it became continuous federal policy.

The Seventy-eighth Congress, in 1943, greatly broadened the scope of rehabilitation by the passage of Public Law 113. The new act offered much more liberal financing and significantly broadened the concept of rehabilitation by providing medical, surgical, and other physical restoration services. The Eighty-ninth Congress, in 1965, amended the Vocational Rehabilitation Act by passing Public Law 333. This amendment created a category known as Extended Evaluation Services, whereby a counselor could evaluate a client for up to 18 months before having to make a determination of rehabilitation eligibility. This procedure greatly increased the ability of vocational rehabilitation services to be extended to more severely handicapped individuals. The act also eliminated economic need as a prerequisite for services and gave the states the ability to determine their own economic need criteria. This allowed some services to be provided regardless of the financial condition of the client.

Public Law 112, passed by the Ninety-third Congress in 1973, placed emphasis on vocational rehabilitation services to those individuals with the most severe handicaps. The legislation defines severe disability as "that physical or mental impairment which seriously limits the functional capacity (mobility, communication, self-care, self-direction, work tolerance, work skills) of a handicapped individual to the extent that a person is unable, to a substantial degree, to cope with the physical or mental demands of gainful employment and whose rehabilitation normally requires multiple services (restorative, compensatory training, selective placement) over an extended period of time" (Department of Health, Education, and Welfare, 1974).

According to the act, deaf people with resulting severe speech deficit are to be considered severely disabled and receive priority service. In this instance, the hearing loss must exceed 70 dB in the better ear in spite of amplification and/or medical treatment.

The Counselor

Most rehabilitation counselors employed by state and federal programs are specifically trained in the area of vocational rehabilitation counseling at the masters degree level. In addition, certification through the Commission on Rehabilitation Counselors Certification, a branch of National Rehabilitation Counseling Association, was instituted in 1975. In order to be granted certification, the counselor must exhibit competencies through written evaluation as well as practical performance assessed while serving an internship under the direction of a certified counselor in the field.

There has been a growing awareness among rehabilitation administrators of the need to have counselors on their staff who have the ability to communicate with deaf and hearing impaired clients. Further, most state vocational rehabilitation programs now have counselors specifically trained in manual communication to work with a hearing impaired caseload. Although specifically trained counselors may not be available throughout entire states, they are often available in urban population centers which contain larger numbers of hearing impaired individuals. They can also be available to serve as consultants to counselors in rural and low-population rehabilitation offices.

A Team Approach

The successful rehabilitation of a hearing impaired adult will involve professionals from many disciplines. The audiologist and speech pathologist, for example, will need to be joined with other professionals, such as psychologists, physicians, special educators, and vocational rehabilitation counselors, to insure adequate and efficient rehabilitation services for hearing impaired individuals. A unified and coordinated effort must be undertaken by all members of the professional team in order to provide consistent and effective services to the disabled individual. This team must operate throughout the rehabilitation process, with emphasis being placed upon the expertise of certain professionals at a particular point in the hearing impaired individual's process of rehabilitation. The combined efforts of the team are necessary to assist the disabled individual achieve his or her maximum potential to the extent that no single discipline represented in the team could otherwise accomplish.

Coordination of effort is a key element in the successful operation of the team approach. Within the rehabilitation team, the vocational rehabilitation counselor is uniquely qualified to serve this coordinating function. To ensure eventual vocational success, the rehabilitation counselor must include the rehabilitation efforts of all other professionals working with the hearing impaired individual. The state agency rehabilitation counselor will have specific training to assist the individual in the selection of meaningful and realistic goals. The counselor will have access to a wide variety of community agencies necessary for the fulfillment of those goals, and will have available monies to help make these goals a reality.

THE VOCATIONAL REHABILITATION PROCESS

The vocational rehabilitation process starts at the point of referral. Approximately ten percent of persons receiving rehabilitation services are self-referred individuals. Therefore, 90 percent of all people served are referred from other sources. Some of the referral sources on which vocational rehabilitation depends for clients include hospitals, rehabilitation centers, health agencies, physicians, welfare and social service agencies, educational institutions, state employment offices, the Social Security Administration, workmen's compensation, private insurance companies, and knowledgeable professionals in fields dealing with handicapped individuals.

The rehabilitation process, again, commences with referral and the initial interview. The counseling interview is the basic method of securing information about the client. The major source of client information, therefore, is the client him or herself. The type of information gathered at this time would include general directory information such as name, address, birth date, social security number, marital status, and number of dependents. Information regarding the individual's educational background, medical history, vocational history, financial status, and general personal-social history would also be obtained at this time. The initial interview is also utilized to introduce the client to the process of rehabilitation and the steps he or she will be taking to arrive at a satisfying vocational objective. At the conclusion of the initial interview, steps are taken to collect further information which may be necessary for the determination of client eligibility. This further data will consist of a medical evaluation to include, at minimum, for each individual a complete physical examination and a referral to an audiologist for auditory testing. In subsequent counseling sessions, a determination will be made by the counselor and the individual regarding need for further specific evaluation. These evaluations may include intelligence testing, aptitude testing, interest inventories, and, if indicated, psychiatric evaluation.

At the conclusion of a complete evaluation, client eligibility for services is determined using the criteria established in the Vocational Rehabilitation Act. Prior to client acceptance, the counselor must show that the client meets the following requirements:

1. The presence of a physical or mental disability
2. The existence of a substantial handicap to employment
3. A reasonable expectation that vocational rehabilitation services may render the individual fit to engage in a gainful occupation

If after the normal evaluation the third criterion cannot be established, a counselor may place the severely hearing impaired individual into a category known as "extended evaluation." While the client is in the extended evaluation category, the counselor may provide extensive evaluation services necessary to make a determination of the individual's expectation of engaging in a gainful occupation.

The vocational implications of a hearing impaired individual from the view of vocational rehabilitation includes the combination of psychological effects of hearing impairment and the problems of performing in a work setting. At the time eligibility is determined, the vocational rehabilitation counselor must understand and successfully deal with the problems the hearing impaired individual has in the vocational, educational and social–emotional–personal areas. The problem areas identified must be assessed by both the counselor and the client prior to the selection of a vocational objective.

A study of vocationally significant problems encountered among hearing impaired students at Gallaudet College found problems which are of great importance to the rehabilitation counselor working with the hearing impaired (Roy, 1965). They are as follows:

Examples of problems in the vocational area:

1. Lack of job information and experience
2. Lack of knowledge of self
3. Unrealistic goals
4. Dependency
5. Passivity
6. Literal-mindedness
7. No generalization

Examples of problems in the educational area:

1. Poor study habits
2. Lack of reading skills
3. Poor preparation for college work
4. Overload
5. No meaningful goal

Examples of problems in a social–emotional–personal area:

1. Difficulty in social interaction
2. Lack of acceptance of self in the environment
3. Unwillingness to face difficulties
4. Lack of motivation
5. Immaturity
6. Dependence

INDIVIDUALIZED WRITTEN REHABILITATION PROGRAMS

After rehabilitation eligibility has been determined, an Individualized Written Rehabilitation Program (IWRP) is developed jointly by the vocational rehabilitation counselor and the client. The Rehabilitation Act of 1973 mandates joint consultation in development throughout the formation of the Individualized Written Rehabilitation Program and the entire rehabilitation process. The IWRP contains an agreed-upon vocational goal, immediate objectives necessary to fulfill that goal, anticipated dates of initiation and completion of services, evaluation procedures, and schedules. The rehabilitation program specified for the hearing impaired individual in most instances is lengthy and involves many specialty areas. The vocational rehabilitation counselor assumes the responsibility for coordination of the various services necessary to assist the client in reaching the chosen vocational goal.

Upon completion of the Individualized Written Rehabilitation Program document, services necessary to complete the intermediate objectives are initiated. These services may consist of, but are not limited to:

1. Necessary medical, audiological, surgical, psychiatric and hospital services
2. Necessary prosthetic devices such as hearing aids
3. Individual counseling and guidance
4. Vocational training in schools, on the job, by correspondence, or by tutor

5. Interpreter services and aural rehabilitation services
6. Maintenance and transportation during rehabilitation, if necessary
7. Necessary tools, equipment, supplies, licenses, and books
8. Placement on a selected job
9. Follow-up counseling to insure adjustment to and success in the vocational placement

Vocational Placement

Successful and continuing vocational placement is the primary goal of the vocational rehabilitation process. Placement opportunities for hearing impaired individuals, at this time, cover a much wider range of occupations than in past years. Previous occupations such as printing, jewelry engraving, and watch repair so frequently associated with hearing impaired individuals have given way to a range of occupations including both technical and professional areas. This has taken place in part because of the development of specific vocational training for the deaf and hearing impaired as well as social enlightenment.

An aid to placement for the hearing impaired which has supported efforts by the vocational rehabilitation counselor has been Section 503 of the Rehabilitation Act Amendment of 1974. Simply stated, Section 503 required nondiscrimination in the hiring of handicapped individuals by employers participating in federal contracts which were in excess of $2,500. This act mandated that handicapped individuals be actively recruited and given appropriate consideration for employment by those employers. The act specified that employers have an obligation to make accommodations necessary for the hiring of handicapped individuals. Those accommodations might have included the installation of equipment such as volume controls on hearing impaired employees' telephones, restructuring of job descriptions which may accommodate the handicapped individual, and physical or structural modifications which would allow access to the job by qualified handicapped individuals.

Hiring a highly skilled or highly educated hearing impaired individual for a menial or unskilled position was not considered to be within compliance according to Section 503. The act also addressed itself to possible discrimination by employers in promotion, training, and transfer of handicapped individuals.

One of the roles of the vocational rehabilitation counselor in the placement process is the education of employers. The rehabilitation counselor works with employers in the community concerning the many misconceptions about the hearing impaired generally held by the public. Employers are informed about simple and inexpensive workplace modifications, such as a volume control on a telephone, which may mean the difference between vocational success or failure for the appropriately trained and qualified hearing impaired individual.

After placement, it is imperative that the vocational rehabilitation counselor maintain follow-up communication with both the hearing impaired client and the employer. The counselor's responsibility and coordination function does not end with the initial job placement. A period of work adjustment for both the client and the employer will be necessary. During this time, the vocational rehabilitation counselor must be available as a resource person, to answer questions, make appropriate referrals, and help deal with any potential problem areas which might arise to cause the client's position to be in jeopardy.

Postemployment services necessary for an individual to maintain employment successfully can be provided without the necessity for a redetermination of eligibility for a period up to one year after successful closure of the rehabilitation case.

SUCCESSFUL VOCATIONAL REHABILITATION PROJECTS

The Arkansas Rehabilitation Service Project

This project, coordinated by Blake (1970), was an experiment to determine the effectiveness and feasibility of providing rehabilitation services to a multiple handicapped adult deaf population in a residential facility. The majority of clients served in this project were of at least average intelligence but were low achievers. The population comprised, for the most part, some of the state rehabilitation counselors' most difficult cases. The rehabilitation center provided intensive job orientation and extended periods of personal, social, and work adjustment, as well as basic adult education prior to any formal vocational evaluation or vocational training. The center also provided specialized personnel who were specifically trained to communicate effectively with deaf clients.

The study showed that many of the clients referred to the facility made gains in personal, social, and vocational areas. Although gains were made, most of them could not be described as significant. Due to the multiple handicaps of the population served, it was determined that additional specialized personnel and services were needed for effective rehabilitation to take place.

Some of the major recommendations made as a result of this study included:

A comprehensive residential rehabilitation center for the deaf should be established as a permanent model facility for low achieving, often multiply handicapped, deaf adults.

Counseling, guidance and interpreting services should be made available on an organized, permanent basis in metropolitan areas containing large deaf populations.

Professional-level training programs in the area of rehabilitation with deaf adults should be established.

Efforts should be taken to locate, develop, produce, and distribute instructional materials for use with low-achieving deaf adults.

Communication between rehabilitation personnel and deaf clients must be of paramount importance through the provision of services by specialized staff (Blake, 1970).

The New England Project

This project sought to provide deaf adults with rehabilitation services not previously available and to provide these services in a setting with hearing clients. One hundred and twenty-six deaf adults were served during the length of this project. The major service provided was rehabilitation counseling. Other services included psychological counseling, personal adjustment training, and a summer enrichment program. The largest single limiting vocational factor identified in this project was the illiteracy of 47 percent of the clients served. At its completion, the project was judged to have positive effects upon the clients. The final report showed that 60 percent of the individuals served were employed or enrolled in academic or vocational training at the project's end. Some of the recommendations of the project included:

There is a need for sufficient qualified staff proficient in manual communication.

Vocational rehabilitation services provided to deaf adults should be longer and more comprehensive than to the non–hearing impaired population.

Rehabilitation and educational services for the deaf should begin as early as possible and be cooperative in nature in order to prevent or lessen some of the recognized problems faced by deaf adults.

Services in the area of mental health, continuing education, manual language education, and counseling should be developed or expanded in metropolitan ares (Lawrence & Vescovi, 1967).

St. Louis Jewish Vocational Service Project

Hurwitz (1971) utilized a workshop setting to demonstrate vocational and social development for severely handicapped deaf clients. Services provided included basic education, behavioral guidance, and skilled training in a prevocational adjustment workshop. Also included in the project were on-the-job training and job placement. A total of 265 clients were served, with the majority being classified as illiterate. Approximately one half were considered to be multiply handicapped because of other physical or psychological conditions.

At the conclusion of the project, one half of the clients were placed in competitive employment, while approximately 20 percent were recommended for advanced training. The project showed that both on-the-job training and residential placement, particularly in foster homes, were highly effective training approaches for the low-literacy clients involved in the program. At the time of follow-up it was determined that 76 percent of the project clients were self-sufficient, as opposed to 86 percent being financially dependent at the time of referral.

The results of these projects and other studies have shown that vocational rehabilitation services can be effectively delivered to the deaf and hearing impaired population. It has been concluded as a result of these studies that certain factors are important for successful rehabilitation, particularly with low-literate deaf individuals. These programs, further, have demonstrated that the ability to communicate in manual sign language is a prerequisite for the successful vocational rehabilitation of deaf clients. Vocational rehabilitation counselors as well as other team members should also be aware that a deaf or hearing impaired client will probably require a longer vocational rehabilitation program in order to achieve the selected vocational goal than will his or her hearing counterparts.

Personal Adjustment Training in Vocational Counseling

A large portion of the rehabilitation program should include personal adjustment training. Personal adjustment training would include such areas as communication skills, basic education, personal hygiene, marriage and family, leisure time, consumer services, citizenship, and independent living skills. Although not directly related to training in a specific vocational skill area, competence in the areas of personal adjustment is necessary to insure successful vocational placement over an extended time. Along with personal adjustment services, an extended period of work adjustment training should take place prior to the acquisition of specific skill training. At the time of placement, employer education and the importance of continued employer contact cannot be stressed enough. Continued on-the-job counseling, often at very short notice, will be necessary in many instances in order to enhance the probability of the hearing impaired individual's vocational success.

Included in the appendix for this chapter is a list of the addresses of all vocational rehabilitation state offices. Specific information on the field office closest to your area and particular state services for the deaf and hearing impaired can be obtained from this source.

REFERENCES

Blake, G. An experiment in serving deaf adults in a comprehensive rehabilitation center. *Final Report, SRS Grant No. RD-1932-S.* Little Rock, Arkansas: Arkansas Rehabilitation Service, 1970.

Hurwitz, S. Habilitation of deaf young adults. *Final Report, SRS Grant No. RD-1804-S.* St. Louis: Jewish Employment on Vocational Service, 1971.

Lankenau, R. O. Deaf leadership training for community interaction. *Final Report, SRS Grant No. 638-T-69.* Salt Lake City, Utah: National Association of the Deaf, 1969.

Lawrence, C. A., & Vescovi, G. M. Deaf adults in New England: An exploratory service program. *Final Report, SRS Grant No. RD-1576.* Boston: Morgan Memorial, 1967.

Menninger, W. C. The meaning of work in Western society, in H. Botow (Ed.), *Man in a world at work.* Cambridge, Massachusetts: Riverside Press, 1964.

Porter, E. B. Guidelines for the diagnosis, evaluation and remediation of problems of persons with severely impaired hearing. *Final Report, SRS Grant No. 44-P-81008/3-03.* Silver Spring, Maryland: National Association for Hearing and Speech Action, 1975.

Roy, H. L. *The guidance of exceptional children.* New York: David McKay Company, 1965.

Thomason, B., & Barrett, A. M. (Eds.), *Casework performance in vocational rehabilitation.* Washington, D.C.: Office of vocational rehabilitation, 1959.

U.S. Department of Health, Education and Welfare. *Social and Rehabilitation Service Instruction RSA-PI-74-16.* Washington, D.C.: U.S. Government Printing Office, 1974.

APPENDIX: DIRECTORY OF STATE VOCATIONAL REHABILITATION OFFICES

Alabama: 2129 East South Boulevard, Montgomery 36111
Alaska: Pouch F, Alaska Office Building, Juneau 99801
Arizona: 55 East Thomas Rd. Suite 101, Phoenix 85012
Arkansas: 211 Broadway Room 227, Little Rock 72201
California: 714 P Street, Sacramento 95814
Colorado: 705 State Services Building, Denver 80203
Connecticut: 600 Asylum Avenue, Hartford 06105
Delaware: P.O. Box 1190, Wilmington 19899
District of Columbia: 1331 H Street, Northwest Washington 20005
Florida: 725 South Bronough Street, Room 254, Tallahassee 32304
Georgia: 629 State Office Building, Atlanta 30334
Hawaii: P.O. Box 339, Honolulu 96809
Idaho: 209 Easton Building, Boise 83702
Illinois: 623 East Adam Street, Springfield 62706
Indiana: 12 West Market Street, Indianapolis 46204
Iowa: 801 Bankers Trust Building, Des Moines 50309
Kansas: 1145 East State Office Building, Topeka 66612
Kentucky: State Office Building, High Street, Frankfort 40601
Louisiana: P.O. Box 44064, Baton Rouge 70804
Maine: 32 Winthrop Street, Augusta 04330
Maryland: 2100 Gilford Avenue, Baltimore 21218
Massachusetts: 296 Boylston Street, Boston 02116
Michigan: P.O. Box 1016, Lansing 48904
Minnesota: 1745 University Avenue, St. Paul 55104
Mississippi: P.O. Box 1698, Jackson 39205
Missouri: 1616 Missouri Boulevard, Jefferson City 65101
Montana: 507 Power Block, Helena 59601
Nebraska: 707 Lincoln Building, Lincoln 68508
Nevada: 308 N. Currey Street, Carson City 89701
New Hampshire: 64 N. Main Street, Concord 03301
New Jersey: Leber Industry Building 10th Floor, Trenton 08625
New Mexico: Old Capital Annex, Room 116, Santa Fe 87501
New York: 162 Washington Avenue, Albany 12210
North Carolina: 305½ West Martin Street, Raleigh 27602
North Dakota: 418 East Rosser Avenue, Bismarck 58501
Ohio: 240 S. Parsons Avenue, Room 125, Columbus 43215
Oklahoma: P.O. Box 25352, Oklahoma City 73105
Oregon: 680 Cottage Street S.E., Salem 97310
Pennsylvania: 7th and Forresters Street, Harrisburg 17121
Puerto Rico: P.O. Box 1118, Hato Rey 00919
Rhode Island: 40 Fountain Street, Providence 02903
South Carolina: 400 Wade Hampton, State Office Building, Columbia 29201
South Dakota: 804 North Euclid, Pierre 57501
Tennessee: Suite 1400, 1808 W. End Building, Nashville 37203
Texas: 221 East 9th Street, Austin 78701

Utah: 136 E. S. Temple Street, Salt Lake City 84111
Vermont: 79 Main Street, Montpelier 05602
Virginia: P.O. Box 11045, Richmond 23230
Virgin Islands: P.O. Box 630, St. Thomas 00801
Washington: P.O. Box 528, Olympia 98501
West Virginia: P & G Building Washington Street, Charleston 25305
Wisconsin: 1 West Wilson Street, Madison 53702
Wyoming: 305 State Office Building, Cheyenne 82001

PART II

The Elderly Client

Section 1: Introduction to Aural Rehabilitation for Elderly Adult Clients

Judah L. Ronch

Chapter 14: Who Are These Aging Persons?

All too often the answers given to the question posed by the title of this chapter are based on either idealizations, personal experiences generalized to all of the aged, a rapidly growing body of statistics, or, worst of all, ignorance of the realities of aging in America. One of the most prominent gerontologists in the United States, Robert N. Butler, the first Director of the National Institute on Aging of the National Institute of Health, has characterized the aged as "the neglected stepchildren of the human life cycle" (p. 1) (Butler, 1975). In his Pulitzer Prize–winning work, he describes old age as a "tragedy," culminating in the more fundamental question of the book's title: "Why Survive? Being Old in America."

The central characters in the new American tragedy have lately become the newest minority to attract a great deal of attention and have become the focus of medical, political, social, economic, and psychological investigations which hope to generate a fruitful answer to the question, "Who are the aged?"

Our attitudes toward the aged, and at the very least, a covert indication of the way we regard them, could be discerned from the terminology used to designate this segment of society. For many years, the old have occupied a position of respect, and throughout history our vocabulary reflected this attitude. Terms such as senator, alderman, guru, presbyter and veteran all have their roots in the words of various languages for "old," and denoted the position of honor and privilege enjoyed by the aged (Comfort, 1977). Of late, we have adopted "golden age," "senior citizen," and the like, but our colloquial terms still reflect a negative, indeed "vindictive" (Comfort, 1977) regard for old people. Butler cites, for example, the social values placed on aging as seen in expressions such as "fading fast," "over the hill," "old crock," "geezer," "old fogey," and "biddy." Part of the problem, says Comfort (1977), is that "what was once traditionally venerable, often too venerable, is now simply obsolete." When we consider that in the Rome of 2,000 years ago the average length of life was 22 years, in America in 1900 49.2 (Wolf, 1963), and is presently 67.5 years (for Caucasian men) and 74.9 years (for Caucasian women) and has not increased since 1960 (Butler & Lewis, 1977), we realize that as the number of aged increased, they became the "newest underprivileged minority" with which society had to contend (Comfort, 1977). Currently, the aged constitute about 11 percent of the total American population. Using the age of 65 as an arbitrary point of inclusion in the "aged" category (a legacy from Bismarck's assignment of pensioner status to those over this age during the 1880's [Butler & Lewis, 1977]), there are now about 23 million persons in the United States, and 190 million in the world, who are elderly or aged. Of these, 10 million are over 73, one million over 85, and 106,000 over 100 years old in the United States (Butler & Lewis). Clearly, then, this fastest-growing minority in America must be understood and become well-known, if only because it is a minority which we shall all, hopefully, join in due time.

In an attempt to answer the question, or more accurately *questions* posed by the title of this chapter, emphasis will be placed on integrating data about aging with examples of the diverse kinds of people who make up the aged group. Through that information, it is hoped that those who work with the aged might begin to understand the aging process in general as well as aged persons as individuals. Throughout this chapter, references are provided wherein interested readers may find more data with which to answer their own questions about issues raised in the present discussion or in works cited.

THE MANY FACES OF THE AGED

As is true of any group, there is no one prototypical older person, no "average" elder who embodies and represents all the positive and negative aspects of being old. Probably the best way to obtain a quick overview of the aged is to try to illustrate the parameters of the lives of old people in various circumstances. The first presentation is the well elderly.

> Mrs. D. lives alone in a retirement community in Florida and says she enjoys every minute of it. Now 73 years old, she has been a widow for 22 years, and though she has had close relationships with male friends, she is determined not to compromise her independence by remarrying. Her income is derived mainly from dividends on sound investments made by her late husband and herself in the 1930s, and from her Social Security pension. She had worked for many years, both full- and part-time, as the manager of a beauty salon in a fashionable New York City department store, and it is obvious that the meticulous attention to detail she evidences in her appearance now is a long-standing trait which made her a professional success. Mrs. D. looks at least 10 to 15 years younger than her actual age (a source of great pride to her) and is the type of person one wishes to look like "at her age." Playing golf three times a week, volunteering in the gift shop of her local hospital, visiting with her younger sister, who lives nearby, and a regular Saturday night bridge game are only a few of the activities which keep her vital and satisfied. When her current male companion is in town (he spends the rest of the year in the North), they attend local cultural and social events or go out to dinner.
>
> Mrs. D. maintains a very optimistic, organized approach to life, and one is left with the definite impression that she has been this way all of her adult life. She is very fortunate to enjoy good health, economic security, and close ties to her sister and three brothers and their wives who live in nearby communities.

> Mr. J. is now 78 years old and lives in a city of 35,000 in New York State. Born in New England, he came to this city while in his mid-teens with his family. Typical of his generation, Mr. J. completed 10 years of formal education and then went to work in a foundry, the first of a number of semiskilled jobs. When the Great Depression occurred, he found

employment as a fireman and stayed at that occupation until he retired on pension and Social Security at age 65. He lives in a single family house with his wife of 37 years, not far from the family home in which Mr. J. was raised. His two sons reside in the same city and see Mr. and Mrs. J. quite frequently.

Since his retirement, Mr. J. follows nearly the same kind of daily routine as when he worked. Because he worked nights, he learned to make use of his free daytime hours, and continues to this day taking odd jobs, such as helping friends and neighbors with home maintenance projects, socializing with community friends of long standing, and frequent visits with former co-workers and friends at the firehouse. He still arises early in the morning, goes out for a walk to get the newspaper, occasionally attends church during the week, stops to chat with friends he meets on the street. This routine seldom varies. He assists in some household tasks, particularly the family laundry (he also insists on doing his children's), and some cooking. He is physically healthy and robust. His membership in community groups is, as always, on the non-active joiner level, but he reads about the doings of these groups with intense interest. He has by consensus been designated a local "expert" on pension and union matters, a skill which has grown primarily out of his need to look after his own interests. Typical of Mr. J., he shares this information as he shared his labor and skills in home maintenance in the past.

Both Mrs. D. and Mr. J. represent the successful retirement life-style typical of many moderate-income elderly. While not wealthy, they are secure and in good health, and have the support provided by close family ties and, no less important, the ability to maintain lifelong patterns of existence not interrupted by old age and its many losses. While typical of a large segment of older people, they by no means are immune from the problems affecting those of their age-peers who are poorer, more ill, more alone, or older and more enfeebled. The second presentation is an example of the institutionalized aged.

Mr. A., a widower, is a 92-year-old retired industrial chemist who has lived in a home for the aged for the past 10 years. Like most of his fellow residents in this superb, nationally recognized geriatric care center, he came to live in the home when his only daughter could not care for him due to his increased infirmities. He can usually be seen walking around the grounds of the home or working at a crafts project in the Occupational Therapy room. Both activities not only serve to keep him active and busy, but they also help alleviate the anxieties he was previously able to repress through his compulsive, scientific work. An inventor of many well-known products, he devoted all of his energies to research, thinking, and other solitary scientific endeavors. His present mild-to-moderate memory loss of about 8–10 years duration prevents him from pursuing the kind of obsessive, detailed thinking that used to occupy him, and it has resulted in depression stemming from the awareness of the loss of the mental ability which was the focus of his identity in the past. Thus, Mr. A. walks alone, works alone (though in a group), and, when he is in a group, sits with his face downcast and arms folded over his chest in a defiant gesture of negativism to those who try to approach him. Yet when asked by staff how they might help him, he repeatedly asks them to teach him how to make friends. His solitary life-style, depression, and memory impairments make this difficult, since he has few skills in this area and has a difficult time being less than self-absorbed. His greatest amount of social interaction is with the physician at the nursing home, with whom he debates the composition and side effects of medication prescribed for him after he has thoroughly researched each drug in his personal copy of the Physician's Desk Reference. He complains most about constipation, though his major problem is the arterio-sclerotic heart disease and circulatory disturbance which has resulted in his memory impairment and overall weakness. He has been in group psychotherapy for about 18 months, and has just begun to show signs of diminished depression and the ability to engage in conversation with others for a protracted period of time.

Miss M. is quite young (69 years old) to be a resident of the same nursing home where Mr. A. resides since the average age there is 87. She was admitted following spinal surgery because she was too ill to care for herself. Her only relative, a sister, could not cope with Miss M's needs for constant attention and care. Miss M. became a problem for the staff of the home because of her endless demands for medical attention, complaints about everything from the nurses to the food, and her refusal to eat in the dining room, which she could physically do. She demanded instead to eat in the T.V. room in a part of the home far removed from her own living area.

Miss M. was referred to a staff psychiatric social worker when her demands that she "be first among others and get what I want immediately" monopolized the time of an inordinate number of staff. She complained of having no energy, no appetite, terrifying and disturbing thoughts which awoke her at night, and insomnia. All of these problems began with her spinal problems, well before her surgery. At that time, she said she was unable to concentrate on anything and that she felt intimidated by even the slightest tasks of the day. Fright incapacitated her almost all of the time, and she stated that she "had a short fuse" and should be taken care of just because she was "in the greatest pain of anybody." Her central thought was that the spinal operation had failed (which was not true) and she would request rediagnoses and medical confirmation of her hopelessness on a daily basis. Initial contacts with the social worker took place with Miss M. lying on her bed "because of my back," though she could have and indeed would have benefited from being upright or walking.

As a result of individual psychotherapy and a coordinated management regime, Miss M. was soon back on her feet and helped to understand the causes of her depression, helplessness, demands for attention, and need to manipulate others from a passive dependent, aggressive position. Within six months, she discarded her heretofore omnipresent four-legged walker and adopted a cane, which she used more to swing around in less veiled aggression than to assist with her by now excellent ambulation ability (see Ronch and Maizler, 1977, for a more detailed analysis of this case).

The two cases described above were both about a long-term care institution, and they illustrate some of the typical characteristics of persons who are found in nursing homes. Their real physical problems, complicated by psychological reactions, interacted to produce management problems which are not atypical of this population but which can be treated with some success to produce more satisfactory (to patient and staff alike) adjustments and future-oriented, rather than disease-centered, treatment. There are, of course, those who are more and less ill than the persons described above, or who suffer chronic debilitating illnesses and are in fact so physically deteriorated that they are waiting to die while in a nursing home. The point is, however, that living in a long-term care institution does not by itself eliminate the chance for growth, change, and happiness if the institution is so oriented. There are, unfortunately, not enough settings which provide such an atmosphere.

The newly de-institutionalized elderly is the third circumstance of the aged described in this chapter. There are two types of older adults who live in institutions—predominantly in mental hospitals and nursing homes. The first group, like the persons introduced above, were admitted to institutions late in life. There are also those who are admitted to mental hospitals, rather than old age homes or nursing homes, because they have developed mental illness late in life (usually diagnosed as chronic organic brain syndrome, to be discussed below). The other group currently reside in state (a few in private) mental hospitals and have grown older there. Many were admitted early in life, in their twenties or thirties, and were segregated within the institutions because the then current psychiatric treatment did not allow for return to the community with any reasonable degree of certainty that they would not harm themselves or others. This generation had the misfortune to exhibit signs of mental illness (an alarming number would not be so diagnosed today) prior to the use of major tranquilizers like phenothiazines (Thorazine, Stelazine), antidepressants, and electroshock therapy (Butler & Lewis, 1977). With the advent of these forms of treatment and the concomitant decline in overt psychiatric symptoms sometimes brought about by the effects of old age, and in response to economic and political pressure, the process of "de-institutionalization" has introduced into the community a new kind of aged—those who lived abnormal adult lives within institutions or who were shuttled in and out of institutions for a good portion of their adult lives. The following are two cases in point:

> In 1903, Mr. H. came to the United States from Hungary at the age of 2, together with his parents and brother and sister. According to spotty hospital records, he was placed in an orphanage at age 5 (probably due to his mother's ill health) where he remained for 12 years and completed his education at the 11th grade. He worked at many unskilled jobs, never holding any one for a great period of time.
>
> In 1933, Mr. H. became seclusive, antagonistic, and resistive, while suffering paranoid delusions and auditory hallucinations. Upon admission to a large state hospital, he was diagnosed as "schizophrenic—paranoid type." By 1935, he was transferred to his third and last state mental hospital, where he remained without interruption until 1977. Over the years, his paranoia, delusions, hallucinations, and "dull, apathetic" behavior gradually abated, until 1953, when he was found to be "cooperative, neat, clean and non-assaultive." He never expressed a desire to leave the hospital, and became a highly valued member of the grounds squad. With his parents and brother long since dead, his sister made no attempts to have him released. Hospital records indicate a loss of hearing at some unspecified date, prompting Mr. H. to learn to read lips and communicate via written messages.
>
> At the age of 76, he was released into the community to reside in an Adult Proprietary Care Home with a group of similar people, and was enrolled in a community aftercare program for discharged chronic state hospital patients. On admission to this program he was alert, sociable, energetic, enthusiastic, and cooperative, or in the words of the program psychiatrist, "remarkably free of the signs of chronic institutionalization." Until he was fitted with a body-type bone oscillator hearing aid, he was handicapped by a bilateral mixed hearing loss with a conductive element averaging 36 dB at the right ear and 48 dB at the left ear. That is, unless someone spoke directly to him, Mr. H. lived in a world relatively devoid of audible speech, and normal social contact. Those who worked with him wondered how long he had this problem, and imagined his years of silence in the hospital. His voice is hoarse and raspy, and ill-fitted dentures make it more difficult for him to speak so that he could be understood.
>
> When Mr. H. was given his hearing aid, and he heard our voices, his face lit up in a joyful grin, tears came to his eyes, and to most of us who watched, he radiated an intensity of happiness we had never before seen him communicate. For him, it was not too late to hear again at the age of 77. With his improved hearing ability, he could now begin to derive greater benefit from therapeutic activities at the center. Commenting on Mr. H.'s superb physical prowess, a staff member remarked, "Now when he plays soccer he can hear people telling him how good he is!"
>
> Mr. O. is actually 70 years old, but due to his original psychosis and the dementia resulting from electroshock and insulin therapy administered to treat his catatonic schizophrenic condition, he says he is 100, 108, 116, or 125 years old, "as I was born in 2008." When confronted with the logical impossibility of his calculations, he uses autistic, idiosyncratic

reasoning to explain the disparity between the present year the rest of the world recognizes and his notion of time. Hospitalized since 1940, he has recently been placed in a family care residence managed by the state hospital. After 38 years of hospitalization, he remains delusional, hears voices, and says he is "insane, like a demented person." A passive, quiet, cooperative man, Mr. O. is profoundly ambivalent about being outside of the hospital grounds, and often speaks of his fears of death and his wishes to return to the hospital.

There are, of course, many other aged persons who have been discharged into the communities surrounding state mental hospitals; very few of them are in the comparatively fine condition of Mr. H. Increasingly, accusations of "dumping" these people into the community have arisen, and a large number of old, and many younger, chronic psychiatric patients are caught in the center of an escalating controversy. In truth, no one answer will suffice to meet the multiple needs of this diverse population. The impact of de-institutionalization, as well as its wisdom as a method of treatment, will be addressed later on in this presentation. No matter what the outcome, the two people introduced above, and thousands like them, are currently attempting to cope with their old age in a society for which they are inadequately prepared and which is not sure about what to do with them.

The final discussion and presentation involves the community-based service consuming elderly. The majority of aged persons are not now, and will never be, in institutions. Unlike the well elderly, however, there are many persons who exist in the community because they are supported by a wide variety of services designed to keep them out of institutions and functioning within the supports provided by their natural environments. There are, in addition, an alarmingly large group of elderly adults who, in spite of their need for services to assist them in many areas of life, somehow survive as best they can in the absence of critically needed community resources. The following are examples of these persons:

Mr. R., when in his mid-eighties, came to the attention of an outpatient mental health clinic specializing in treating the elderly. He had become very depressed, began weeping much of the time, and could not regain his stamina or do many of the things which brought him pleasure. He lived in a "retirement hotel" where he was served his meals in a communal dining room. He otherwise existed in an atmosphere of suspicious isolation with 50 other elderly people. His physical problems included hypertension, increasing blindness, a recent stroke, progressive kidney failure, and the recent installation of his third cardiac pacemaker. His daughter, who lived in the same city, visited him weekly, but neither she nor her brother was able to care for their father because of their own life tasks and problems. Mr. R.'s wife had resided in a mental institution for the past 30 years, and he had not seen her for many of those years.

Recognizing her father's need to talk to an objective listener with whom he could share his feelings (a difficult task for this reserved New Englander), his daughter requested that her father be seen for psychotherapy, a plan which Mr. R. cautiously favored. Mr. R. tried to be optimistic and tried as hard as he could to master his environment after each physical setback. His chief source of sadness was his by now almost total blindness which severely curtailed his mobility and the death about two years prior to treatment of his lady friend, with whom he lived in "an equal 50-50 relationship." His most enthusiastic, honest, description of their relationship, after tentative attempts to characterize it was: "Well, I might as well tell you. We shacked up!"

While Mr. R. proved to be an excellent candidate for psychotherapy, his progressive physical deterioration proved frustrating to him and to his therapist, and he began to lose sufficient ground and enter a nursing home. Therapy continued so that when Mr. R. died six months later after suffering another stroke, he had come to terms with life, and death. His attempts to live in the community for as long as he could brought him great satisfaction.

If it were not for the senior adult day center Mrs. L. attends, she would have had to be placed in an institution. Unable to care for herself after she suffered a stroke at age 78, she is partially paralyzed and is mobile only through the use of a wheelchair. Mrs. L.'s daughter is happy to have her mother live with her, but she cannot give up her job to provide the constant supervision Mrs. L. requires. Now that the day care center provides round-trip transportation, gives all its participants a well-balanced hot meal and two snacks, and provides the opportunities for socialization and stimulation that Mrs. L. could not have had if she were at home even if the family could afford nursing care, she, her daughter, and her grandchildren enjoy a harmonious relationship which most likely could not have existed had Mrs. L. been a constant burden and imposition to her daughter.

Depending on the particular community, older persons have greater or fewer resources available to enhance their independent functioning and provide for the highest possible quality of life. As our society becomes increasingly aware of the numerous kinds of services required to maintain the elderly in the community, these people enjoy happier lives at less cost to families and the community than if these service-needy aged were to be prematurely or unnecessarily institutionalized.

IS THERE A TYPICAL "AGED" PERSON?

As can be gathered from the diverse cases presented above, there are as many different kinds of aging as there are aged persons on this earth. The portraits presented above are only meant to be examples of some of the styles of life and needs for service represented by the heterogeneous elderly population. There are, however, some characteristics of the aging population which merit attention so that the overall circumstances of the aged may be better understood.

The almost 23 million people over the age of 65 constitute the group typically identified as "the aged." However, this group is not homogeneous with regard to most factors, and gerontologists have found it useful to divide the aged into the younger (age 65–75) and older aged (75 years and older) (Busse & Pfeiffer, 1977). Shanas and Maddox (1976) have identified three subgroups of aged: those aged 45–64 (the "young old"), the old (age 65–74), and the "old old" who are over 75 years of age. This latter breakdown, drawn from categories used in the U.S. National Health Surveys, is indicative of the notion that there are significant differences in the life-tasks, abilities, resources, health, and other factors between a 50- or 55-year-old and someone who is 75, and a greater likelihood of similarities among 65-year-olds. It should be noted, however, that chronological age in and of itself delineates few realities of aging, except perhaps the onset of Social Security payments, and should not be taken as an indicator that all persons of the same age are experiencing aging in the same way, or that physiological, psychological, and social changes, among others, are waiting to unfold in a preprogrammed biologically determined fashion.

Dimensions of Age

Birren (1959) distinguishes three kinds of age which provide useful dimensions within which to assess a person's progress along the finite life span. These ages are

1. Biological, or the length of life in years, months, etc.
2. Psychological, which indicates the adaptation capacity of the organism
3. Social age, or the social output and performance of the person relative to his or her culture and social group

Thus, one's attention is properly diverted from chronological age as the immutable indicator of a person's "agedness" status, and we are encouraged to look at the multiple spheres in which a person grows, develops, and gains experience and satisfaction, as well as the interface of the three aspects of life. By this model it is possible to consider an individual's overall balance or imbalance in life, and thereby recognize that people of the same biological age are probably quite diverse in respect to their adaptational capacity and social accomplishments; viz. Mrs. D. and Mr. H. above.

It is therefore important to realize that the probability of looking at the aged as a homogeneous group, which represents a significant discontinuity from earlier stages of life, decreases as greater familiarity is gained with aging persons and the aging process.

Geographic Distribution

Just as the aging process is not equally manifested in every older person, neither are the aged equally distributed throughout the United States or the world. For example, the highest proportion of American elderly live in the Midwest and upper New England, although some of the so-called sunbelt states—Arizona, New Mexico, Hawaii, and Florida—are experiencing the greatest growth of elderly residents. Florida, as many would have expected, leads the nation in proportion of elderly, with 15.5 percent of its population age 65 and over. New York, California, Pennsylvania and Illinois each have over one million elderly citizens (Butler & Lewis, 1977). The American population distribution is congruent with the international picture in that the more industrialized nations, such as Germany, France, Great Britain, and the United States, have a relatively greater proportion of the world's elderly than do the industrially underdeveloped nations (Sheldon, 1960). While the correlation of industrialization and longevity is significant, it does not speak to the quality of life of the aged in the societies which possess greater technological advancement. As will be discussed in greater detail below, technological advancement seems to be bought at the price of obsolescence of the aged, among other costs. With advances in technology and medical care, those countries with populations having a greater preponderance of younger citizens should in the future more closely approximate the distribution of elderly in industrial societies (Hauser, 1976). The status of societal attitudes and concern shown toward the aging in these technologically evolving nations remains to be determined. It can only be hoped that any existing traditional respect for the aged will somehow survive economic evolution.

Without further belaboring the point, it may be concluded that each aged person must be appreciated both in terms of his or her similarity to other elders, and the lifelong patterns of individuality brought into the stage of life.

THE INTERDISCIPLINARY PERSPECTIVE

Because the elderly person is really a complex organism attempting to interact with an equally complicated environment in a dynamic, mutually demanding way, it is necessary to understand the many factors that make up the world of the older adult. Busse and Pfeiffer (1977) have remarked that no single discipline, whether it be psychiatry, sociology, biology, or economics, can claim to offer a comprehensive explanation of how aged people act, think, and feel, or what the multiple determinants of their behavior are. We agree, and believe that to obtain the maximal understanding of the whys and hows of behavior in the aged, knowledge in all fields of inquiry must be gathered and integrated into an interdisciplinary product which offers the most accurately parsimonious and powerful explanation available. In this light it becomes apparent why psychologists must know that depression in an old woman who survives on $157.50 a month cannot be alleviated simply by psychotherapy, but that treatment of social and economic realities takes primacy over delving into her childhood experiences; and that psychotic behavior in an old man can appropriately be alleviated by having a physician adjust his insulin dose rather than giving him an antipsychotic drug or writing him off as "senile." Similarly, professionals who are trained along the traditional lines of disciplinary focus must be willing and able to understand the necessity of knowing as much as possible about all of the many factors which must be in harmony if the aged person is to function well.

Stresses

One way of conceptualizing this problem is to analyze old age as a stage of life wherein multiple stresses are experienced with a dwindling number of internal and external resources available to reduce them. Eisdorfer and Wilkie (1977) define a stressful stimulus as one which is "perceived in some way as potentially harmful, threatening, damaging, unpleasant or overwhelming to the organism's adaptive capacity" (p. 252). Different events will be variably stressful depending on the time of life they are experienced (Neugarten, 1973), and the prior experience of the person with such stimuli. Many sources of stress can be perceived as consequences of the aging process and the biological, psychological, and social changes which may occur (Lawton, 1977). This can induce further stress on the individual's personality. They may be overwhelmed by feelings of helplessness because of growing old, and they panic. In examining the realities of life which in part or in total affect aging persons, it can be concluded that the period of life beginning at around age 50 or 60 and continuing for the rest of one's life is a time during which many aspects of a person's world undergo change. Typically, there are significant, stressful changes in these areas. Among others, these include:

The family of origin—parents, brothers, and sisters become ill or die
Marital relationship—death or illness of spouse, estrangement due to empty-nest syndrome, pressures due to retirement
Peer group—friends die or become separated by geographical relocation for health, family, or retirement reasons
Occupation—retirement
Recreation—opportunities become scarce due to physical limitations or unavailability

Economic—income reduced by retirement, limited income tapped by inflation or medical costs not covered by insurance
Physical condition—loss of youth, changes in physiological and biological aspects of the body causing poor health and its emotional consequences
Emotional/sexual life—loss of significant others through death, separation, and reduction in sexual activity due to societal expectations or personal preference, or death of partner

Degree of Stress

Old age is a difficult and stressful time because two things occur in a complementary and simultaneous manner. The various aspects of life, or life systems, as suggested above, are prone to stresses in greater *numbers,* while at the same time each system or aspect is the source of a greater *degree* of stress than in the past. When experienced in combination with the all-too-often limited biological, psychological, and societal resources available to alleviate stress quickly and efficiently, the organism's ability to adapt is compromised. In other words, older persons experience so much stress in so many areas of life, while internal and societal supports are not as available as they once were to promote a comfortable readaptation, that they have a greater likelihood of becoming disorganized and feeling incapable of coping. It then becomes imperative that as many sources of stress be reduced as much as possible if the older person is to successfully negotiate the potentially treacherous period of old age and still enjoy life.

The need, therefore, is to come to appreciate the whole aging person through integrated, interdisciplinary knowledge, and to understand the intricate relationship between the various things happening to a person as he or she ages and the impact of the aging process on a person's ability to competently master his or her environment and thus reduce stress. Likewise, if treatment is to be appropriate, effective, and dignified, it must be borne in mind that rarely can a person of any age, and surely not an aging person, be dealt with in a helping relationship without full cognizance of the totality of his or her life situation. It is only when the total person is addressed and understood that discrete problems may be most beneficially remediated.

THE AGING PROCESS

The Mechanism of Aging

The period of life designated as "old age" is unique in that it inevitably brings with it various declines in functioning, and the ultimate end of life. Whereas all prior life stages involved biological, social, or psychological development or maintenance and refinement of available resources, this last period of life demands that the person experience and adjust to some degree of debilitation and reduced capabilities. Even in persons who enjoy a relatively healthy, happy old age, there are decrements in abilities which are noticeable enough to produce a subjective feeling that the aging process is proceeding with some regularity. Some of the signs people have reported as indicating to them that they were growing old include nervous difficulties, deterioration of skin and hair, sense organ impairment, diminution in the ability to move about, and an increased tendency to fatigue resulting in a greater need for daytime naps (Wolf, 1963).

The mechanism of aging is not as yet totally understood, and there are a number of energetically debated positions reflected in the current literature (Shock, 1977). Busse (1977), in his excellent review of biological theories of aging, says that these theories are "often overlapping and frequently differing only in semantics, not substance" (p. 13). Two theories differ, for example, as to whether aging is a result of a breakdown in the body's immune system, thus leaving the body vulnerable to infection, disease, and eventual death, or whether by some still unknown process there is a given limitation in each cell's ability to reproduce itself. Hayflick (1977), who has demonstrated some convincing support of the latter position, has concluded that normal cells have a finite capacity for replication and function in vitro and that each species has a certain number of replications available. While even a summary of the entire spectrum of theories and findings in this fascinating area is outside the scope of this chapter, it is at least worthy of attention that there are efforts underway to understand the basis of the finite life span. Much attention has recently been devoted to cultures in which people are reputed to live well into their twelfth or thirteenth decade of life in far greater proportion than other groups. Reports of Ecuadoreans, Caucasian Russians, and Kashmiris who live to be 120 or 140 years old due to genetic, dietary, or occupational factors, while intriguing, are still short on scientific verification. Many sources of documentation have been found to be spurious, and a great deal of the validation does not stand up to rigorous scientific investigation (Medvedev, 1974).

While longevity itself may be a noble aspiration, the quality of life one experiences during an increased life span cannot be ignored. Current research findings seem to indicate that there are a number of changes which take place as a person ages, and these changes can make life less enjoyable depending on the way in which a given person ages. Some of these changes occur within the person's internal environment (the body), while others are a result of societal or intrapersonal reaction to the aging process. All of the changes, however, do not occur in a vacuum. A change in one aspect of functioning can and usually does influence many others. To appreciate more fully the reality of aging in the absence of firsthand experience, it is instructive to take a brief look at the parameters of change which influence the life of aging persons.

Change takes place in almost every aspect of a person's functioning, at a rate which varies from individual to individual and within each individual. How rapidly and in which areas physiologic and psychologic changes occur is largely dependent on a person's genetic endowment, the environment(s) in which he or she was reared and presently lives, and the total life history of the person prior to old age. Of greatest significance perhaps, are the changes in the aspects of functioning included in the following brief discussion. It should be borne in mind, however, that this is a description of what *can* happen, and that not all old persons experience all of these changes (if at all) in the same way.

Normal Aging

The normal biological and physiological changes concomitant with aging which are not due to disease are many. They include

1. Decline in heart output and blood supply, particularly to the brain
2. Reduced stomach and intestine motility, which produces digestive problems and constipation

3. Decreased vital capacity of the lungs
4. Bone decalcification leading to osteoporosis
5. Stiffening of joints and ligaments
6. Loss of teeth
7. Graying and loss of hair
8. Loss of genitourinary system efficiency
9. Reduction of subcutaneous fat
10. Decrease in oxygen utilization
11. Lowered hormonal output (especially in the adrenal glands and gonads), and more (See Wolf, 1963; Butler & Lewis, 1977)

On a cellular level, there is

1. Gradual retardation of cell division and repair
2. Retardation of tissue oxidation rate
3. Loss of water and increase of solid elements
4. Increases in cell pigmentation and infiltration of fat (Rosenwasser, 1964)

Sensory Processes in Aging

Particularly important for everyday activities are the changes in sensory processes which accompany old age. Butler and Lewis (1977) report that about 30 percent of the elderly (mostly men) suffer from significant auditory losses, although present research has indicated as many as 50 percent. Pitch discrimination, auditory acuity, and speech perception are worse among older persons (Fozard & Thomas, 1975), though the inability to understand speech among older subjects may be a function of vocabulary as well as audiometric considerations (Farrimond, 1961), and is accentuated when listening takes place under environmentally stressful conditions (Corso, 1977). There is evidence that reduced perceptual abilities in audition (and other senses as well) are more likely due to problems in central (brain) processing, than to sense organ changes. This is due to an overall decrease in the speed of central decision-making involved in many of the experimental tasks used to obtain data on age differences in sensation (Fozard & Thomas).

Research data also indicate increased thresholds of touch (leading to decreased sensitivity in this sense), decreased pain sensitivity, and a lowered ability to perceive tastes (Fozard & Thomas). Butler and Lewis (1977) report that 30 percent of people over 80 have trouble identifying common substances by smell, correlated with a loss of taste buds and reduced taste sensations. Engen (1977) concludes that one must view the evidence indicating decreases in taste and olfactory sensitivity carefully, due to spotty verification and the fact that many observed changes may be due to disease, smoking, sex differences, and other subject variables. Fozard and Thomas advise that there are serious methodological problems in such research because much evidence has been obtained by cross-sectional studies where different subjects of various ages are studied, which do not take into account "cohort effects" (Schaie, 1977) such as the health, environmental and nutritional factors that differentially affect members of each historical age group studied in a cross-sectional design. Such cohort effects can produce results that look as though they are due to differences in age alone, while in fact they are not a function of the process of aging. Culture also plays a role in the aging of sensory systems. The Mabaan tribe, found in the Sudan, appear to evidence a very slight hearing decrement in old age as compared to the best functioning samples of old people who were exposed to industrial society's noise. The Stone Age culture of these tribesmen protects them from the damaging acoustic environment of modern civilization (Rosen, Bergman Plester, El-Mofty, & Hamad Satti, 1962). They also exhibited a lower incidence of coronary thrombosis, ulcers, elevated blood pressure, and other changes concomitant with normal aging in technological societies.

The visual problems of the aged include reduced peripheral vision; greater vulnerability to glare; increased visual thresholds, yielding decreased perceptual abilities; and poorer dark adaptation, visual acuity, contrast sensitivity, accommodation, and color matching. Again, these findings are not all due to commonly seen physical changes in the eye, and are probably due to the central processing problem mentioned above (Fozard & Thomas). Cataracts, glaucoma, poor visual orientation, and visual perceptions that are frightening and resemble hallucinations are other visual problems which reduce mobility and increase the isolation of the aged (Butler & Lewis, 1977).

Brain Function

The normal brain undergoes a probable loss of neurons in older age, but this loss is not equal in all areas of the brain. Bondareff (1977) reports that lipofuscin can be found in some normal-aged brain cells, but it is not demonstrably related to any particular behaviors or syndrome. Brain weight, which normally decreases from 5 to 10 percent by age 80, is about 20 percent less in persons of the same age with Alzheimer's disease (see below) (Krauss, 1981). Most of the physiological and biological changes that occur in the aged can result in some behavioral disturbance. A striking example of the intimate relationship between physiological and behavioral changes occurs in the conditions collectively known as senile dementia.

Dementias in older persons are due to a variety of causes and are not inevitable consequences of aging. While there is an increased incidence of dementia in successive decades after age 60, there is no evidence to suggest that this is due to normal aging. Dementia is not a singular condition, but rather a group of symptoms involving decreased cognitive ability (memory loss; poor judgment; attention problems; impaired social, work, or peer relationships; disorientation; and reduced learning ability) in the absence of delerium or specific intellectual dysfunction (e.g., aphasia, anomia). There has been a historical trend (that is now changing) to consider all loss of intellectual ability as a sign of inevitable "senility." Dementias are neither confined to the aged, nor are most irreversible if treated early enough. The term *cognitive dysfunction* is much less value-laden and nihilistic, and is more specific in pointing to the actual area of deficit manifested by the individual and possible intervention (Verwoerdt, 1981).

Dementias are classified as either reversible or nonreversible, with the former constituting the majority of cases. Cognitive impairments in the aged person will present in a similar way with both etiologies, and it is crucial that an accurate diagnosis be obtained so that treatment might begin. Origins of reversible dementias in the aged include intercranial tumors, subdural hematomas, normal pressure hydrocephalus, sensory disturbances, systemic infections (e.g., pneumonia), metabolic disorders (e.g., electrolyte disturbances, thyroid disorders, diabetes mellitus, hypoglycemia and hyperglycemia, calcium supply disturbances, toxins), nutritional disorders, circulatory diseases, pulmonary diseases, medication misuse, mismanagement or interaction with other medications or foods, and psychiatric disorders (e.g., depression, anxiety, paranoia). With an error rate found to be as high as 50 percent in one study (Simon and Cahan, 1966) it is no surprise that clinicians are well-advised to consider a reversible etiology for dementing conditions in older patients before making a reflexive and ageistic assumption that cognitive dysfunction in an older person is an inevitable result of the aging process for which there is no need for treatment.

Dementias that are not reversible are categorized as Alzheimer-type or primary neuronal degeneration (involving somewhere between 50 to 70 percent of all demented individuals), multi-infarct or vascular dementia (about 15 to 25 percent of cases), and the so called "mixed" types which are a result of the combined effects of primary neuronal degeneration and vascular damage (Eisdorfer, Cohen and Veith, 1981). An older person may also be suffering from the multiple effects of irreversible dementia that is complicated by vascular disease and a reversible dementia (e.g., drug misuse).

The impact of dementia, whatever the cause, is often seen as depression, anxiety, or both in the older person with the severity of the cognitive dysfunction and emotional reaction a function of the subjective value of the lost ability, cultural, and other considerations. Thus, the degree of impact is not a simple function of a measurable amount of organic damage. In older persons with visual and/or auditory deficits and other sensory and/or motor impairments, the reaction is often withdrawal and confusion to the point of manifesting paranoid ideation. These people begin to fill the information gaps which their cognitive, sensory, and motor dysfunctions create with their own anger that is projected onto others.

PSYCHOLOGICAL CHANGES

The psychological changes in aging are usually assumed to be of two kinds. Those are 1) intellectual-cognitive changes and 2) emotional-personality alterations. To put an old myth to rest, we must recognize the evidence which indicates that in neither of these two areas is there a radical change in functioning due solely to the aging process. There are, however, a number of gradual and important processes which seem to occur in aged persons that influence their psychological functioning. Again, it must be remembered that different abilities are diversely affected by age, and that there are greater differences within age groups than between age groups in most functions (Thompson, 1973). Furthermore, all measures of performance which are used to evaluate age differences in cognitive abilities are influenced by sociocultural factors (educational experience, economic and social opportunities, work history and pertinent cultural-historical values) and physiological differences (environmental, genetic, nutritional, and health) in an interactive way (Thompson, 1973).

Memory

Memory, which is popularly assumed to deteriorate in old age (and hence is seen as yet another sign of "senility"), is a very complex process, and is still in the process of being clarified. Thus, changes in memory are described and conceptualized in terms of what memory is thought to be and according to the manner in which the available evidence seems to indicate it is structured. Far from being a singular function, memory is composed of at least three components through which information enters and is processed. Sensory memory (also referred to as very short-term memory) and long-term memory (secondary storage) are apparently not negatively influenced by the aging process, as anyone who has ever heard an older person recall the past will attest. Between these two types of memory, a holding and organizing process occurs. This form is described as short-term or primary memory, and it is within this function that decrements are evident among older persons. The nature of the deficit seems to be an inability to transfer information from short-term to long-term memory, and the inability of the short-term memory system to organize information so that it can be successfully transferred to long-term storage (Craik, 1977). This finding is in agreement with research results which implicate reduced central processing as the cause for diminished perceptual abilities (Fozard & Thomas, 1975). All voluntary responses have increasing latencies as age increases, indicating that there is a need to provide an older person more time to process and organize sensory input so that the appropriate response may be chosen (Birren, 1965). On a practical, everyday basis, these findings would suggest that many older people are unable to understand speech, for example, because the rate of presentation is too rapid, and they are unable to perceive and respond to the confusing and anxiety-inducing onslaught of stimuli.

Learning

Learning ability also is influenced by the above central processing problem. Research has shown that older persons with an average I.Q. do better at more slowly paced (or self-paced) tasks than in more rapidly paced learning situations (Eisdorfer, 1977). Therefore, it is likely that in a given situation where it is possible to have more time available, the older person's learning will be enhanced. A correlated problem is that in most learning situations, aged persons are more motivated by their fear of failure than with any achievement or success motivation (Eisdorfer, 1977). As has been demonstrated with disadvantaged children (Labov, 1970), this results in inhibition of responses which are feared to be incorrect, usually accomplished by saying "I don't know" or "I can't do it." This serves to curtail testing experiences which involve greater degrees of autonomic stress (heightened anxiety levels). Thus the aged frequently opt to avoid embarrassment and failure. Studies, therefore, tend to demonstrate unnecessarily pessimistic pictures of the cognitive abilities of aged persons.

Intelligence

Since memory and information processing are crucial functions underlying successful performance on standard tests of intelligence, information about the nature of these capacities must be taken into account when considering data on reported intellectual decline in old age. Eisdorfer (1963), using subjects from the Duke Longitudinal Study samples, found no demonstrable decline in intelligence in persons aged 60 to 94 in a three-to-four-year follow-up. Wechsler (1958) found that more rapid losses occur on measures of perceptual motor functioning as measured by the Wechsler Adult Intelligence Scale, while the ability to manipulate words and verbal symbols is maintained fairly well into old age. Schaie and his co-workers, who have conducted sophisticated studies in this area, have concluded that "decline on some dimensions, for some persons, at some historical periods can indeed be part of the picture. However, the concept of universal, inevitable and irremediable intellectual decline in adulthood and old age . . . remains a myth" (Schaie & Baltes, 1977, p. 1119). Noting once again the differences obtained using cross-sectional and longitudinal designs (the latter follows the same group of people at successive ages), Schaie and Strother (1968) found that cross-sectional designs depress the age at which maximum ability is seen.

EMOTIONAL MANIFESTATIONS

The emotional experiences of old age are in large part due to the personality one carries into the process of growing old (Butler & Lewis, 1977). Britton and Britton (1972) found in their longitudinal study of aged persons a remarkable continuity of personality, interests, and sources of emotional gratification which people maintained into very old age. There are, according to Oberleder (1966), four fairly distinct sets of emotional/psychological characteristics of old people. They are

1. The psychological characteristics which result from societal expectations about old age, to which the aged adhere to expedite conformity and acceptance (social aging)
2. The psychological reactions to the losses and deficits incurred as a result of the aging process
3. Those characteristics which are independent of age and which arise from poor health
4. The psychological characteristics which are basic to the elderly person, and have been so throughout the life-span

Running through these and other observations is the theme that old age itself brings with it no appreciable change in personality that is alien to the individual and the way he or she has traditionally felt, expressed emotion, and defended against anxiety. It is far from being a stage during which a person has no emotional life; Butler and Lewis (1977) have found a number of characteristics which describe the ''unique developmental work'' the aged have to do. These are:

1. The desire to leave a legacy and develop a feeling of continuity (through money, land, ideas, children, or students)
2. The need to serve the ''elder'' function, and to share their knowledge and experience (a task made difficult by the information explosion and rapid obsolescence of old knowledge by new technology)
3. An attachment to familiar objects (as in the case of Mr. W., who wanted to leave his awful rooming house but feared losing his books, clothes, and other treasured possessions if he couldn't find a new room of adequate size)
4. A change in the sense of time, resulting in a sense of immediacy with emphasis on the ''here and now''
5. A sense of the life cycle and its finiteness and a need for completion, resulting in a renewed emphasis on religion and culture. (In Japan, old men frequently begin to write poetry as a way of expressing their relationship to life.)
6. A renewal of curiosity, creativity, and surprise, at its height described by McLeish (1976) as the ''Ulyssean Adult, who brings with him the light of creativity retained or regained, and the surging joy of human powers confidently held and used'' (p. 11). (Note the contributions of Einstein, Picasso, Rubenstein, Tolstoi, and the Durants in their old age.)
7. A sense of consummation and fulfillment as in Erikson's (1959) sense of ego integrity, though Butler and Lewis have found that contrary to Erikson, many adults seek to ''escape their identities'' rather than fatalistically accept them (Butler & Lewis, 1977)

In summary, the older person must ''clarify, deepen and find use for what one has already attained in a lifetime of learning and adapting and ''continue to develop and change in a flexible manner of health as to be promoted and maintained'' (p. 20) (Butler & Lewis, 1977). One way in which this is accomplished is the life-review method first identified by Butler (1975) in which the aged person puts his or her ''psychological house in order'' and comes to terms with the past. Nostalgia, reminiscing, storytelling, and asking ''expert'' opinions are but some of the ways this process occurs, and in so doing the older person adapts to old age. Thus, reminiscing and talking about the past is not an ominous sign of senile deterioration, but a necessary piece of work (Ronch & Maizler, 1977) often carried out successfully with anyone who will listen.

Reasons for Emotional Problems

Emotional problems of older persons have of late undergone expert analysis, and much is known about the causes and treatment of mental illness in later life. Recent works by Busse and Pfeiffer (1977) Butler and Lewis (1977) and Verwoerdt (1981) are some of the more outstanding resources in this area and should be consulted by anyone interested in this area. Rather than attempt to distill these highly informative and superbly written texts, this writer will deal with the topic in a general way in the hope that follow-up reading will be undertaken.

The aged have the highest incidence of new mental illness (236.1 per 100,000 population, Butler, 1974), the highest proportion of hospitalized mental patients (30 percent of public and 11 percent of private psychiatric hospital patients are 65 and over) and an alarmingly low rate of community-based mental health care. About two percent of people seen in outpatient mental health clinics are age 60 and over, four to five percent of the patients of community mental health centers are over age 65, and only two percent of private psychiatric time is devoted to the elderly; typically for routine evaluations and rapid referral (Butler & Lewis, 1977, Busse & Pfeiffer, 1973). These data indicate the tragic state of affairs that confronts an older person who experiences emotional problems, because they indicate that hospitalization is all too often the treatment of choice. Among the reasons for this situation are the antipsychiatric attitudes of many elderly, the anti-aged feelings of many professionals, the incorrect notion that the aged do not respond to therapy, the tendency of the aged and the public to see manifestations of mental illness as ''a natural part of old age'' (senility once again), and the economic and logistical problems in getting the needy elderly and service providers together (Busse & Pfeiffer, 1977).

Reactions to Dramatic Change

Significantly, the aged suffer from no exotic mental illnesses, and in fact manifest a comparatively narrower range of problems than do younger patients. The most commonly seen problems of a functional nature, that is, where no organic etiology can be found and for which the origins appear to be emotional, are involutional psychotic reactions (seen in both sexes and felt more and more to be related to life events rather than to menopause), psychotic depressive reactions (usually precipitated by a serious loss or disappointment), and paranoid states (Butler & Lewis, 1977). The above are all psychotic reactions, and as such are more serious but nevertheless are treatable by psychotherapy, pharmacotherapy, and milieu supports (see Ronch & Maizler, 1977; Oberleder, 1964, 1966; Pfeiffer & Busse, 1977; Butler & Lewis, 1977). Neuroses, which represent unsuccessful attempts to resolve unconscious emotional conflicts characterized by anxiety, are chiefly manifested in the aged as depressive neuroses (the major functional psychiatric disorder in old age), anxiety neuroses, hypochondriacal neuroses, alcoholism, and transient situational disturbances (Butler & Lewis, 1977). Schizophrenia rarely begins in old age and is typically seen only in those persons who have grown old in mental hospitals, rather than in people who first experience emotional disorders in old age. ''While retaining *some* schizophrenic symptomatology, these patients are primarily manifesting the devastating impact of long-term custodial care'' (p. 196) (Busse & Pfeiffer, 1977).

Isolation

The isolation experienced by aged persons with visual and/or auditory impairments often results in hallucinations, paranoid thinking, and hostile withdrawal, which can be alleviated by proper remediation and supportive therapy. The anxiety, fear, and anger that sensory impairment generates are often alien to the older person, and in turn generate greater emotional distress.

Functional disorders are predominant in hospitalized and community elderly of ages 65 to 74 (they occur in more than half of patients seen), while those hospitalized aged over 75 are diagnosed more than one half of the time as having an organic disorder (Busse & Pfeiffer, 1977). Whether this reflects a bias among those making the diagnoses or the actual distribution of these disorders is still unclear.

One manifestation of the high prevalence of depression among the elderly is the high suicide rate among older persons—a major precipitant of which is loss, for example of a spouse. While the elderly represent about 11 percent of the population, they account for 25 percent of reported suicides in the United States (Butler & Lewis, 1977). In Miami Beach, the fabled haven for the elderly, the suicide rate among elderly is five times the national average. If loss is a trigger for depression, then the elderly are exceptionally vulnerable because of the almost endless series of losses they experience. The unreported or nonobvious suicides among the elderly would certainly inflate these already horrifying statistics.

Economic Conditions

Economic conditions under which the majority of aged must survive further compound the stress of old age. The United States devotes only 4.2 percent of its gross national product to the aged, as compared to 6.7 percent and 7 percent in England and France, respectively (Butler, 1975). In fact, the United States is the second lowest of the nine major industrialized Western nations (only Japan is lower) in the percentage of its wealth used to help the aged (Schulz, 1976). It should come as no surprise, then, that about 16 to 25 percent of the elderly in America live below poverty levels (Butler, 1975) and constitute 20 percent of America's poor. Most of these persons became poor after they became old, thereby adding another source of stress to their lives.

Not all of the elderly are poor. In 1970, of the 7.2 million families headed by persons 65 and over, 1.8 million had annual incomes of over $9,000 (Butler & Lewis, 1977). The major sources of income for the aged are retirement benefits (46%), earnings from jobs (29%), income from assets (15%), public assistance (4%), and V.A. and other sources (3% each) (Butler, 1975). The category of ''other sources'' includes monies from families (children, siblings, etc.), and while in agricultural societies ''the fate of an individual often depends upon his wealth in children'' (Goody, 1976), in technological society the amount of this proportionally small amount of support all too often depends on the wealth of a person's children—a resource that, when shared, can be had at the cost of an older person's dignity and much emotional travail. The assets of most elderly are more often than not held as equity in an owned home (Schulz, 1976), so that in order to liquify this asset older people must sustain a loss of neighborhood, familiar territory ownership, and the security gained by owning one's home.

The primary factor in producing a drastic change in economic status for the aged is retirement. While this is an event which is sometimes eagerly sought, it is regarded as an achievement in principle but dreaded as a crisis when it actually occurs (Back, 1977). There are many reasons for this, particularly in our work-oriented society. One is that retirement is actually a two-pronged process, wherein a person ''retires'' both economically and socially and loses a work role, a source of identification, and frequently the social contacts and relationships the work situation provided (Back, 1977). In addition, retirement in nonindustrial society and in those like our own involves withdrawal from production activities and the transfer of control over resources (Goody, 1976). With the latter, power is yielded to the next generation, and the formerly powerful must cope with a new degree of powerlessness.

In agricultural societies this problem is lessened because the aged tend to have high status and many satisfactions. The Palaung in North Burma and the Kaffir are examples of cultures that, because of greater food supplies and shelter to share with their aged, presence of useful auxiliary tasks for the elderly, and the use to which the greater experience and knowledge of elders are put in leadership roles, allow for smoother, less traumatic, and more integrated transition into old age. Elderly persons therefore must not only retire from something, but must have something to retire to (Wolf, 1963).

SOCIAL CHANGES

Social changes in aging are perhaps best discussed in light of the perspective of the ''disengagement hypothesis'' of Cumming and Henry (1961) which attempted to account for the withdrawal and disinterest from the physical and social environment that occurs during old age as a natural phenomenon of aging. They suggested that there was a universal mutual withdrawal process between the aged and society which was biologically and psychologically inherent in the aged, and which was correlated with and necessary for successful aging. This development, which began in the sixth decade of life, was felt to be the start of an anticipatory socialization to becoming aged (Wolf, 1963), whereby they began to assume the role society dictated to be culturally appropriate. The hypothesis suggests that as society is ready to push them out, old persons are intrinsically ready to cooperate by becoming ''out of sight and mind''.

Not all investigators have agreed with this theory, and some have demonstrated that disengagement is neither a universal process nor was it the only way to achieve satisfaction in old age (Busse, 1977). Chief among the critics of disengagement theory has been Maddox (1964), who asserts that a majority of aged do not change much in regard to their level of activity or involvement. Engagement or disengagement is more a function of past styles of life and socioeconomic factors, and successful aging usually necessitates the maintenance or development of appropriate levels of social, physical, and mental activity (see also Palmore & Maddox, 1977). It has been noted by Back (1977) that a combination of the two theories best explains what happens in almost every case of aging. Mindel and Vaughan (1978) have observed that, as in many older persons' orientation to religion, an individual can be "disengaged" on an organizational basis, that is, retired from work or a nonattender of church, but still "engaged" on an interpersonal basis (socializes with former friends at work, as does Mr. J above), or nonorganizationally engaged according to personal feelings of affiliation, such as believing strongly in God, and thereby deriving personal satisfaction and comfort in this area of life.

Rosow (1976) finds that the unique role of the aged person has five aspects. These include:

1. The loss of former roles, which excludes the older person's significant social participation and produces social devaluation
2. The experience of systematic status loss for the entire cohort, rather than the social growth which marked other periods
3. The lack of socialization in our society to the fate of aging
4. The lack of a specified "aged role" yielding socially unstructured lives with no "duties" except perhaps for disengagement
5. The deprivation of a person's social identity

This reality can lead to what Busse and Pfeiffer (1977) have termed the social pathologies which arise in some aged. Among these are social isolation as a result of losses and lack of new relationships (about one fourth of all older people live alone); loneliness, which is experienced as a feeling of exclusion from the good things which other people have available; and family conflicts around the feelings of the various generations as problems of role reversals (daughter cares for mother), living arrangements, and guilt and anger which have been brewing for years burst forth under the pressure of new stresses. These problems of social pathology can lead to psychopathology in the elderly and their children (see Silverstone & Hyman, 1977).

FAMILY LIFE

The family life of older persons does not escape change as the couple ages, and as in other aspects of life, loss is the primary outcome. Stresses take their toll on marital relationships, for example, when one spouse becomes ill and thereby creates a "disequilibrium" in the marriage and old role relationships are no longer viable. Whether it be a physical or emotional illness that is the problem, the "patient" can come to be resented for all of the demands for care (realistic or exaggerated) he or she makes on the healthier spouse, who in turn may become depressed and angry and also develop physical and/or psychiatric symptoms (Butler & Lewis, 1977). Typically, the female becomes the one "in charge" and is confronted with her own feelings about being a caretaker and decision maker. In some relationships, however, men play this role, or two friends of the same sex who share a household may assign roles based on the realities of need and not gender. The situation can become so out of balance that, as in one case seen by this author, the husband always answered inquiries addressed to his depressed wife as if their nervous systems were shared.

When a spouse is not available or capable of providing needed supports, the next most sought resource is a child. Four fifths of older people have living children (Butler & Lewis, 1977), and about 83 percent of these aged live less than an hour's distance away from one child (Sussman, 1976). Almost 30 percent of the elderly reside with their children, a phenomenon reported to be on the increase in rural areas (Sussman). Usually, it is a daughter to whom older persons turn at times of crisis, the choice of which is based on long-standing family dynamics. The one chosen may be the one who lives closest, is the wealthiest, was the most or least favored as a child, wishes to increase his or her favor with the parents, or who historically could be prevailed upon by the siblings to do almost anything.

Many older persons are now developing alternative living arrangements which involve cohabitation of unmarried men and women (because either their children or social security regulations discourage marriage), moving in with a friend of the same sex to allow for companionship and reduced expenses, or starting communal residences, which in some localities have been legally defined as families and are thus immune to hostile zoning ordinances (Sussman, 1976).

Relationships between aged parents and their children (who are usually "middle age," that is, caught in the middle of their parents and children) do not necessarily deterioriate, nor do all marriages. While some families are able to be positively and happily involved with each other no matter what stresses arise, others are fraught with tension, guilt, anxiety, and multigenerational unhappiness. In most cases, the outcome is a function of the nature of the family relationship as it had been for years, and not a result of the aging process of some of its members.

MINORITY STATUS

To be old and poor is bad enough. To be old, poor, and a member of a racial or ethnic minority (particularly if one is a female), places the aged person in "multiple jeopardy" (Butler, 1975). Blacks, Hispanics, Native Americans, Orientals, and other minority groups are overrepresented among the old poor and underrepresented among the nation's elderly. Blacks, for example, comprise 10 percent of the population but only 8 percent of the elderly population. Only 7.8 percent of all black Americans are over 65, and the life expectancy of black men is six and one-half years below the average of non-black men's life span and is decreasing (Butler & Lewis, 1977). Proportionally, there are more poor black aged (one half) than non-black aged (one fourth of whom are poor). The poorest of the poor are black women, 47 percent of whom had annual incomes under $1,000 (Butler & Lewis, 1977).

The situation is worse for elderly Hispanics who comprise only 4 percent of this population. There are about 11.2 million Hispanic elderly in the continental United States (including persons of Cuban, Mexican, Puerto Rican, and South American origin), and this number does not include the almost 8 million illegal aliens of Latin origin. Wherever they live, their life expectancy is significantly lower than their caucasian counterparts. In Colorado, for example, the average white resident lives to be about 67.5 years old, while an Hispanic lives an average of only about 56.7 years (Butler & Lewis, 1977).

Native Americans get to be old much less frequently than any other group. In 1970, there were estimated to be almost 800,000 Native American elderly, nearly half of whom lived in the western United States, although there are no reliable estimates of the number of elderly among this group. One is shocked to discover that their average life expectancy is only 47 years. Those few Native Americans who do grow old are left impoverished and cut off from traditional family supports (Butler & Lewis, 1977).

The shortened life span among minority elderly is in great part due to the higher prevalence of disease and a higher age-specific death rate that exist among lower socioeconomic groups (Shanas & Maddox, 1976). Poverty brings with it an increase in chronic disease, dental problems, poor vision, and hearing impairments, probably due to poorer medical care, and there is very likely a higher incidence of depression and overall stress in aging.

Many elderly persons speak English as their second language. As they age, they find it difficult to adjust to the differences in language and culture between themselves and the rest of society. For many, English gradually loses its effectiveness as they begin to experience difficulty in central nervous system processing and analysis of their second language (Butler & Lewis, 1977). This can be compounded in persons with organic brain syndrome whose anxiety approaches panic and terror as they are less and less able to understand what they hear and increasingly revert to their native language in an attempt to make order out of linguistic-cognitive chaos.

THE MYTH OF SENILITY

The most damaging example of popular misinformation is the myth of senility, which stresses that most old people become forgetful, confused, childlike, and inattentive as a result of aging-induced brain damage. The term "senile" is used to denote this condition, and it is overtly or covertly used to lump together and discount all older persons with these and other symptoms. In fact, much of the behavior attributed to "senility" is due to anxiety, depression, and reversible dementing conditions which are not a function of the aging process itself. To be sure, some cases of "senile behavior" are due to chronic brain damage as well, but when the inaccurate diagnostic label of senility is used it implies (and insures) hopelessness and untreatability (Butler, 1975). In too many cases of treatable neurotic depression, an older person has been diagnosed as having "senile dementia" and is tragically doomed to unnecessary deterioration and indignity in a nursing home.

Oberleder (1969), in fact, feels that anxiety is the basis of all senile symptoms and that "most senile symptoms are substitutes for frustrated impulses or buffers against inner conflict" (p. 22).

SEXUALITY

Rivaling senility as the most widely believed and damaging myth is the contention that sexuality in the aged is nonexistant, and if it does exist is surely a sign of aberrant, senile, "second childhood" regression. It is as if every person over age 50 is seen by both the public and professionals as sexually impaired (Butler & Lewis, 1977). Thirty-five percent of graduate students in counseling psychology and communication disorders curricula at a major university and 74 percent of men aged 65 and over who were in a retirement community in Florida agreed that old age brings with it declining sexual interest and decreased physical ability to engage in sexual activity (Ronch, Ronch, & Gentile, Note 1). This belief is based on many subjective feelings, such as that old people are physically unattractive, or that any sexuality is wrong and shameful for old persons, and is rooted in the anxieties young people have about the sexual activity of their parents (Butler & Lewis, 1977).

Sex is a matter of great concern in later life, and the source of many emotional problems. The research of Masters and Johnson (1966) put aside many of the incorrect impressions of the Kinsey report (which was based on extrapolations of data on younger subjects) and found that sexual response in old age diminished in speed and activity, but not in the capacity to achieve orgasm. They also found that like most aspects of the behavior of older persons, levels of sexual activity tended to be stable over a person's lifetime. Pfeiffer (1977) reports that older men are more interested and active sexually than are women (a finding consistent with the cultural values of this cohort) and that some men (20–25 percent) and a small percentage of women showed patterns of rising sexual interest and activity as they aged. The preponderance of women and lack of sexual partners among the older population as well as older people's belief in their asexuality are strong influences working against sexual satisfaction in old age.

FINANCIAL SECURITY

When older people complain about economic hardships, many people deny these reports, based on the myth that older persons are financially secure thanks to Social Security and Medicare. As we have noted above, economic stress is all too prevalent among the old. As of June 1976, monthly Social Security benefits averaged $218 for an individual and $372 for a couple, though many people received only the minimum of about $155 per month on which to live. A few desperate aged have been caught stealing dog food to eat because they had run out of food and money. These people would have faced $300 fines or 30 days in jail had some communities not initiated social service referral programs in lieu of punishment when the public outcry about these conditions became loud enough. Medicare meets only 42 percent of the net health costs of the aged, and the remainder must be paid for out of the barren pockets of a large proportion of the aged.

INFLEXIBILITY

Older people are stereotypically and inaccurately seen as inflexible (Ryan & Capadano, 1978), unteachable, and unwilling to change. If old age teaches nothing else, it instructs one in devising novel ways of coping with new problems against mounting odds. Scientific data, as reviewed earlier, indicate that the learning ability of the aged is not impaired per se, and that intellectual capacity does not decline due to aging. Much of this prejudicial myth is justified by a statement by Sigmund Freud, who said that "older people are no longer educable" (Freud, 1959), but Pfeiffer (1971) points out that this statement referred to the "old" of Freud's time who were aged 45 or 50. As has been demonstrated in psychotherapy (Oberleder, 1969, Pfeiffer, 1971, Blank, 1974, Ronch & Maizler, 1977), older people can and do learn to change their modes of adaptation, and this change is primarily a function of lifelong attitudes toward learning, changing, and ability to accept help rather than age. Characteristic inflexibility, learning difficulties, negativism, and other temperamental traits are far more important in determining a person's amenability to change than is age. If an old dog cannot be taught new tricks, who is to say the fault is not with the teacher? Perhaps the issue might rather be whether professionals, and not the aged, are "educable" (see Ronch & Maizler, 1977).

AGEISM

Butler (1975) has coined the term "ageism" to denote the "systematic stereotyping of and discrimination against people because they are old, just as racism and sexism accomplish this with skin color and gender" (p. 12). Much of this bigotry functions to distance younger generations from their own eventual aging, though ageists stand to become objects of their own prejudice (Butler & Lewis, 1977). Comfort (1977) points out that "even Archie Bunker confines his bigotry to groups he will never join" (p. 9). That statement is a telling example, for it has been found that those who had negative attitudes about the aged also tended to have more negative attitudes about the physically and mentally disabled and ethnic minorities, especially blacks (Kogan, 1961). Yet alarmingly enough, studies of medical students (Spence, Feigenbaum, & Fitzgerald, 1968) and rehabilitation counseling trainees (Rasch, Crystal & Thomas, 1977) have shown these groups to have markedly negative attitudes toward older persons. Together with the data indicating scarce devotion of psychotherapeutic time (Butler & Lewis, 1977, Weintraub & Aaronson, 1968) to the aged, we have no choice but to conclude that professionals in many fields have definite prejudices against treating elderly patients. Some of the reasons for this may be that the aged stimulate the anxiety and conflicts professionals have about their own aging and aging relatives, the belief that old people cannot be helped so professional expertise and time is wasted on "senile" or soon to be dead patients, that it is a waste of their good training, or that they are uncomfortable "giving" to an emotionally demanding older person in what is unconsciously perceived as an incongruous role reversal (Group for the Advancement of Psychiatry, 1971).

On a realistic level, many professionals find it difficult to give as much of themselves as the aged client or patient demands of their nurturing or social interaction. Many times, an older person will want to talk about his or her children, tell old stories, or do anything to hold the attention of the often too busy professional. When one does not have an audience or a responsive and regular conversation partner, the "ticket of admission" can often be a physical complaint. Usually seen as hypochondriasis, a not uncommon neurotic condition among the aged, the complaint of physical illness or other symptom can really be understood as a safe way of saying "I want to be taken care of" (Pfeiffer, 1973). These complaints are usually about a physical problem, as psychological or emotional problems are too stigmatic or threatening to talk about.

All questionable cases should be seen by a physician. Busse, Barnes, and Dovenmuehle (Note 2) found that most of their subjects who had physical complaints with both physical and neurotic bases did not seek medical care, but instead used their condition to extract sympathy, forgiveness, and help from others, and as a social crutch.

INSTITUTIONALIZATION VERSUS DE-INSTITUTIONALIZATION

Institutionalization

In the minds of many, the natural habitat of the aged is undoubtedly and inevitably the institution. To the surprise of many, only about 5 percent of this nation's aged reside in institutions (Butler & Lewis, 1977), a pattern not unlike other Western, industrialized nations (Shanas & Maddox, 1976). Furthermore, contrary to a prevalent myth and even personal experience, older persons are not "dumped" by their families, but rather represent an older, more ill and more severely impaired segment of the aged group. Shanas and Maddox report that the institutionalized aged are more likely to be women who were never married or widows, and were likely to be childless or to have one child. Taking up residence in an institution usually means that familial, economic, and health resources have become inadequate to maintain an older person in the community, the last "heroic effort" (Goldfarb, 1977) toward this end usually having taken place in the home of a relative. The process of institutionalization and its effects on the prospective resident have been well studied by Tobin and Lieberman (1976), who have found that many of the so-called institutional behaviors (apathy, depression, resignation, etc.) cited by many critics of nursing homes actually begin to appear when the decision to enter an institution is made and while the person is on the waiting list. Families of the old, institution-bound person are not immune to intense feelings of stress, guilt, anxiety, and ambivalence about the decision and ultimate reality of institutionalizing mother or dad, and they take out much of this emotional reaction on nursing home staff and their newly institutionalized relatives in thinly disguised ways.

One type of institution with which an all too great proportion of aged persons become familiar is the state mental hospital, in which older persons constitute 25 percent of new admissions and 30 percent of the residents (Shanas & Maddox, 1976). Much has been said about these facilities, most of it uncomplimentary and properly critical. Concomitant with current social, political, and economic considerations, patient care is now being viewed as psychiatrically more advantageous if it takes place outside the hospital in the "natural community."

De-Institutionalization

Notwithstanding the reasons and intensity of the debate over policies regarding institutions, we are faced with an increasing number of aged who have been de-institutionalized physically but who find it difficult to abandon the behaviors which were successful in adapting to the "total institution" (Goffman, 1961).

A great number of these newly released aged persons were quite dependent and in need of help when as younger adults they were hospitalized. Thus, they readily exhibited what has been termed "institutional dependency" (Tobin, 1969) as well as characterological dependency. In contrast, many nursing home residents become institutionally dependent but were not, historically, characterologically dependent. Goldfarb (1969) has pointed out that it is rare for a person, particularly an older one, to become independent if he or she has always been dependent on others. The greater likelihood is that if he or she does change, such a person will become increasingly less dependent in small steps, but probably never change rapidly to the other end of the scale. For the characterologically and institutionally dependent elderly, de-institutionalization offers many stresses with which they have had little or no experience at a time of life when society allows (some would say prefers) more passive adaptation to stress (viz. disengagements, retirement). In other words, while society permits or encourages dependency to their age peers, the de-institutionalized aged are being forced to adapt to a degree beyond the capability of many of them even when they were 40 or 50 years younger and probably had more resources available in every sphere.

What all of this points to is the reality of "institutional behavior" becoming part of a person's repertoire so that he or she can successfully adapt to life in such a setting, and that this occurs in younger and older persons alike. If a person is by nature a dependent person, the adjustment is less difficult, but if a person is not so inclined, becoming dependent on an institution causes stresses and anxieties which at times are seen as misbehavior but are really attempts to maintain autonomy. In observing an elderly nursing home resident, many ''senile'' behaviors are signs that the person is frustrated at not being able to maintain old satisfactions and a former level of gratification to keep his sense of self or 'ego' intact (Oberleder, 1966). Likewise, a newly de-institutionalized person may exhibit the same type of behavior as a sign that he or she wishes to return to a former, less demanding but more mastered set of environmental demands. The greatest irony is that at an age when ''normal'' aged are thinking about institutions as a possible future alternative, people of the same age group, who are in most cases less able to cope, are being de-institutionalized and being made to ''re-engage''—a demand beyond the reach of most of them at any age.

CONCLUSIONS

The aged person, though undergoing changes in almost every aspect of life, is no less like him or herself than in the past. In this period of life, as in every other which precedes it, individual differences are maintained with no reduction (Maddox & Douglass, 1974) in the dimensions or magnitude of difference. Despite myths, stereotypes, and prejudicial distortions to the contrary, people retain their essential personalities and continue to manifest most of their essential abilities to adapt and change as they become old. Major sources of interference to coping or adequate adaptation come mainly from the severe stresses and limited resources which the elderly experience in a variety of ways depending on genetics, life experiences, past and present environment, and traditional ways of dealing with life.

Knowing older persons as people who possess characteristic individuality and a lifetime of experience permits the most productive possible relationship with them. In addition, it aids in establishing fertile ground for the development of their trust and thus encourages the older person to assume an optimistic, progress-oriented approach toward treatment as well as toward life. Nothing is worse than for older persons to perceive the negative, impatient attitude of those who purport to help them but who have in fact given up hope of providing appropriate aid simply because the person in need is old. In many cases, calming reassurance and objective listening do wonders in promoting reduced anxiety and encourageing older persons to mobilize their own resources to help produce improved functioning.

Who, then, are these aging persons? The question might perhaps be rephrased to ask not only who, but what are they like, and why are they so. The answers are crucial not only to the achievement of a full understanding of the aged, but on a most personal level, to ourselves, for we are all aging persons.

REFERENCES

Back, K. W. The ambiguity of retirement, in E. W. Busse & E. Pfeiffer (Eds.), *Behavior and adaptation in late life*. Boston: Little, Brown and Company, 1977, pp. 78–98.

Beattie, W. Aging and the social services, in R. H. Binstock & E. Shanas (Eds.), *Handbook of aging and the social sciences*. New York: Van Nostrand Rheinhold Co., 1976, pp. 619–642.

Birren, J. E. Principles of research in aging, in J. E. Birren (Ed.), *Handbook of aging and the individual—psychological, biological and social aspects*. Chicago: University of Chicago Press, 1959.

Birren, J. E. Age changes in speed of behavior: Its central nature and physiological correlates, in A. T. Welford & J. E. Birren (Eds.), *Behavior, aging, and the nervous system*. Springfield, Illinois: Charles C Thomas, 1965, pp. 191–216.

Blank, M. Raising the age barrier to psychotherapy. *Geriatrics,* 1974, *29,* 141–148.

Bondareff, W. The neural basis of aging, in J. E. Birren & K. W. Schaie (Eds.), *Handbook of the psychology of aging*. New York: Van Nostrand Rheinhold, 1977, pp. 157–176.

Britton, J. H., & Britton, J. O. *Personality changes in aging*. New York: Springer, 1972.

Busse, E. Theories of aging, in E. W. Busse & E. Pfeiffer (Eds.), *Behavior and adaptation in later life,* Washington, D.C.: American Psychiatric Association, 1977.

Busse, E. W., & Pfeiffer, E. Functional psychiatric disorders in old age, in E. W. Busse & E. Pfeiffer (Eds.), *Behavior and adaptation in later life*. Washington, D.C.: American Psychiatric Association, 1977, pp. 158–211.

Butler, R. Mental health and aging. *Geriatrics,* 1974, *29,* 59–60.

Butler R. N. *Why survive? Being old in America*. New York: Harper and Row, 1975.

Butler, R. N., & Lewis, M. I. *Aging and mental health: Positive psychosocial approaches*. St. Louis: C. V. Mosby Co., 1977.

Comfort, A. Review of *Growing old in America* by D. H. Fischer. *N.Y. Times Book Review*. April 17, 1977.

Corso, J. F. Auditory perception and communication, in J. E. Birren & K. W. Schaie (Eds.), *Handbook of the psychology of aging*. New York: Van Nostrand Reinhold Co., 1977, pp. 535–553.

Craik, F. Age differences in human memory, in J. E. Birren & K. W. Schail (Eds.), *Handbook of the psychology of aging*. New York: Jan Nostrand Reinhold Co., 1977, pp. 384–420.

Cumming, E., & Henry, W. E. *Growing old: The process of disengagement*. New York: Basic Books, 1961.

Eisdorfer, C. The WAIS performance of the aged: A retest evaluation. *Journal of Gerontology*. 1963, *18*, 169–172.

Eisdorfer, C. Intelligence and cognition in the aged, in E. W. Busse & E. Pfeiffer (Eds.), *Behavior and adaptation in later life*. Washington, D.C.: American Psychiatric Association, 1977, pp. 212–227.

Eisdorfer, C., Cohen, D., & Veith, R. The psychopathology of aging, in *Current concepts*. Upjohn Company, 1981.

Eisdorfer, C., & Wilkie, F. Stress, disease, aging and behavior, in J. E. Birren & K. W. Schaie (Eds.), *Handbook of the psychology of aging*. New York: Van Nostrand Reinhold Co., 1977, pp. 251–275.

Engen, T. Taste and smell, in J. E. Birren & K. W. Schaie (Eds.), *Handbook of the psychology of aging*. New York: Van Nostrand Reinhold Co., 1977, pp. 554–561.

Erikson, E. The problem of age identity, in Identity and the life cycle, *Psycological Issues*. 1959, *1*, 101–164.

Farrimond, T. Prediction of speech hearing loss for older industrial workers. *Gerontologia,* 1961, *5,* 65–87.

Fozard, J. L., & Thomas, J. C. Psychology of aging, in J. G. Howells (Ed.), *Modern perspectives in the psychiatry of old age*. New York: Bruner-Mazel, 1975, pp. 107–169.

Freud, S. On psychotherapy, in J. Riviere (translator), *Collected papers*. New York: Basic Books, 1959, pp. 249–263.

Goffman, E. *Asylums: Essays on the social situation of mental patients and other inmates*. New York: Anchor Books, 1961.

Goldfarb, A. The psychodynamics of dependency and the search for aid, in R. A. Kalish (Ed.), *The dependencies of old people*. Ann Arbor, Michigan: The Institute for Gerontology, 1969, pp. 1–15.

Goldfarb, A. Institutional care of the aged, in E. W. Busse & E. Pfeiffer (Eds.), *Behavior and adaptation in later life*. Washington, D.C.: American Psychiatric Association, 1977, pp. 264–292.

Goody, J. Aging in non-industrialized societies, in R. H. Binstock & E. Shanas (Eds.) *Handbook of aging and the social sciences*. New York: Van Nostrand Reinhold Co., 1976, pp. 117–129.

Group for the Advancement of Psychiatry. *Aging and mental health: A guide to program development*. Vol. 8, 1971.

Hauser, P. M. Aging and world wide population change, in R. H. Binstock & E. Shanas (Eds.), *Handbook of aging and the social sciences*. New York: Van Nostrand Reinhold Co., 1976, pp. 58–86.

Hayflick, L. Cellular aging, in C. E. Finch & L. Hayflick (Eds.), *Handbook of the biology of aging*. New York: Van Nostrand Reinhold Co., 1977, pp. 159–188.

Kogan, N. Attitudes toward old people: The development of a scale and an examination of correlates. *Journal of Abnormal Psychology,* 1961, *62,* 616–626.

Krauss, I. K. The psychology of aging, in R. H.

Davis (Ed.), *Aging: Prospects and issues* (3rd ed.). Los Angeles: The University of Southern California Press, 1981.

Labov, W. The logic of non-standard English, in F. Williams (Ed.), *Language and poverty*. Chicago: Markham Publishing Co., 1970, pp. 153–189.

Lawton, M. P. Impact of the environment on aging and behavior, in J. E. Birren & K. W. Schaie (Eds.), *Handbook of the psychology of aging*. New York: Van Nostrand Reinhold Co., 1977, pp. 276–301.

McLeish, J. *The Ulyssean Adult*. Toronto: McGraw-Hill Ryerson Co., 1976.

Maddox, G. L. Disengagement theory: A critical evaluation. *Gerontologist*, 1964, *4*, 80–82, 103.

Maddox, G., & Douglass, E. Aging and individual differences: A longitudinal analysis of social, psychological and physiological indicators. *Journal of Gerontology*, 1974, *29*, 555–563.

Masters, W. H., & Johnson, V. E. *Human sexual response*. Boston: Little, Brown and Co., 1966.

Medvedev, Z. A. Caucasus and Altay longevity: A biological or social problem. *Gerontologist*, 1974, *14*, 381–387.

Mindel, C. H., & Vaughan, C. E. A multi-dimensional approach to religiosity and disengagement. *Journal of Gerontology*, 1978, *31*, 103–108.

Neugarten, B. L. Personality changes in late life: A developmental perspective, in C. Eisdorfer & M. P. Lawton (Eds.), *The psychology of adult development and aging*. Washington, D.C.: American Psychological Association, 1973, pp. 311–335.

Oberleder, M. Aging: Its importance for clinical psychology, in L. E. Abt & B. F. Reiss (Eds.), *Progress in clinical psychology*. New York: Grune and Stratton, 1964, pp. 158–171.

Oberleder, M. Psychological characteristics of older age. Presented at *United States Department of Public Health Geriatric Training Conference*. Philadelphia, 1966.

Oberleder, M. Emotional breakdowns in elderly people. *Hospital and Community Psychiatry*, 1969, *20*, 191–196.

Palmore, E., & Maddox, G. L. Sociological aspects of aging, in E. W. Busse & E. Pfeiffer (Eds.), *Behavior and adaptation in later life*. Washington, D.C.: American Psychiatric Association, 1977, pp. 31–58.

Pfeiffer, E. Psychotherapy with elderly patients. *Postgraduate Medicine*, 1971, *50*, 254–258.

Pfeiffer, E. Interacting with older patients, in E. W. Busse & E. Pfeiffer (Eds.), *Mental illness in later life*. Boston: Little, Brown and Company, 1973, pp. 5–18.

Pfeiffer, E. Sexual behavior in old age, in E. W. Busse & E. Pfeiffer (Eds.), *Behavior and adaptation in later life*. Boston: Little, Brown and Company, 1977, pp. 130–141.

Rasch, J. D., Crystal, R. M., & Thomas, K. R. The perception of the older adult: A study of trainee attitudes. *Journal of Applied Rehabilitative Counseling*, 1977, *8*, 121–127.

Ronch, J., & Maizler, J. Individual psychotherapy with the institutionalized aged. *American Journal of Orthopsychiatry*, 1977, *47*, 275–283.

Rosen, D., Bergman, M., Plester, D., El-Mofty, A., & Hamad Satti, M. Presbycusis study of a relatively noise-free population in the Sudan. *Annals of Otology, Rhinology, and Laryngology*, 1962, *71*, 727–743.

Rosenwasser, H. Otitic problems of the aged. *Geriatrics*, 1964, *19*, 11–17.

Rosow, I. Status and age through the life span, in R. H. Binstock & E. Shanas (Eds.), *Handbook of aging and the social sciences*. New York: Van Nostrand Reinhold Co., 1976, pp. 457–482.

Ryan, E. B., & Capadano, H. L. Age perceptions and evaluative reactions toward adult speakers. *Journal of Gerontology*, 1978, *33*, 98–102.

Schaie, K. W. Quasi-experimental research designs in the psychology of aging, in J. E. Birren & K. W. Schaie (Eds.), *Handbook of the psychology of aging*. New York: Van Nostrand Reinhold Co., 1977, pp. 39–58.

Schaie, K. W., & Baltes, P. B. Some faith helps to see the forest: A final comment on the Horn and Donaldson myth of the Baltes–Schaie position on adult intelligence. *American Psychologist*, 1977, *32*, 1118–1120.

Schaie, K. W., & Strother, C. R. The effects of time and cohort differences on the interpretation of age changes in cognitive behavior. *Multivariate Behavioral Research*, 1968, *3*, 259–294.

Schulz, J. Income distribution and the aging, in R. H. Binstock & E. Shanas (Eds.), *Handbook of aging and the social sciences*. New York: Van Nostrand Reinhold Co., 1976, pp. 561–591.

Shanas, E., & Maddox, G. L. Aging, health and the organization of health resources, in R. H. Binstock & E. Shanas (Eds.), *Handbook of aging and the social sciences*. New York: Van Nostrand Reinhold Co., 1976, pp. 392–618.

Sheldon, H. D. The changing demographic profile, in C. Tibbitts (Ed.), *Handbook of social gerontology, societal aspects of aging*. Chicago: University of Chicago Press, 1960.

Shock, N. W. Biological theories of aging, in J. E. Birren & K. W. Schaie (Eds.), *Handbook of the psychology of aging*. New York: Van Nostrand Reinhold Co., 1977, pp. 103–115.

Silverstone, B., & Hyman, H. K. *You and your aging parent: The modern family's guide to emotional, physical and financial problems*. New York: Pantheon Books, 1977.

Simon, A., & Cahan, R. B. The acute brain syndrome in geriatric patients, in W. M. Mendel & L. J. Epstein (Eds.), *Acute psychotic reaction*. Washington, D.C.: *Psychiatric Research Reports*, No. 16, American Psychiatric Association.

Spence, D., Feigenbaum, E., & Fitzgerald, F. Medical student attitudes toward the geriatric patients. *Journal of the American Geriatrics Society*, 1968, *16*, 967–983.

Sussman, M. B. The family life of old people, in R. H. Binstock & E. Shanas (Eds.) *Handbook of aging and the social sciences*. New York: Van Nostrand Reinhold Co., 1976, pp. 218–243.

Thompson, L. W. Psychological changes in later life, in E. W. Busse & E. Pfeiffer (Eds.), *Mental illness in later life*. Washington, D.C.: American Psychiatric Association, 1973, pp. 53–74.

Tobin, S. Institutional dependency in the aged, in R. A. Kalish (Ed.), *The dependencies of old people*. Ann Arbor, Michigan: Institute for Gerontology, 1969, pp. 85–96.

Tobin, S., & Lieberman, M. *Last home for the aged*. San Francisco: Jossey-Bass, 1976.

Townsend, P. On the likelihood of admission to an institution, in E. Shanas & G. F. Streib (Eds.), *Social structure and the family: Generational relations*. Englewood Cliffs, New Jersey: Prentice-Hall, 1965.

Verwoerdt, A. *Clinical Geropsychiatry* (2nd ed.). Baltimore: Williams and Wilkins, 1981.

Wechsler, D. *The measurement and appraisal of adult intelligence* (4th ed.), Baltimore: Williams and Wilkins, 1958.

Weintraub, W., & Aronson, J. A survey of patients in classical psychoanalysis: Some vital statistics. *Journal of Nervous and Mental Disorders*, 1968, *146*, 98–102.

Whanger, A., & Lewis, P. Survey of institutionalized elderly, in E. Pfeiffer (Ed.), *Multidimensional functional assessment: The OARS methodology—A manual*. Durham, North Carolina: Center for the Study of Aging and Human Development, Duke Univeristy, 1975, pp. 71–78.

Wolk, R., & Reingold, J. The course of life for old people. *Journal of the American Geriatrics Society*, 1975, *23*, 376–379.

REFERENCE NOTES

1. Ronch, J. & Gentile, M. A survey of graduate student and elderly beliefs in ageist stereotypes. Unpublished report, 1977.
2. Busse, E. W., Barnes, R. H., & Dovenmuehle, R. H. The incidence and origin of hypochondriacal patterns and psychophysiological reactions in elderly persons. *First pan-American congress on gerontology*. Mexico City, September 1956.

Raymond H. Hull

Chapter 15: The Impact of Hearing Impairment on Aging Persons: A Dialogue

From the information presented in Chapter 14 regarding the process of aging and its effect on the aging person, we become aware that we are dealing with very special people. The effects of aging on individuals are as unique as their response to the process. One aspect is common, however, and that is that aging in the advanced years is generally not a pleasant process. When the effects of aging begin to impact negatively upon the sensory processes which have in the past permitted efficient personal and social functioning, then aging becomes even more difficult to cope with. The sensory deficit to be discussed here, and its impact on aging persons, is presbycusis, or hearing impairment as a result of aging.

THE IMPACT

Whatever the cause of the disorder called presbycusis, the effects on the 14 million persons who possess it are in many respects the same. The frustrations they experience from an inability to understand, for example, what their children and grandchildren were saying at the last family reunion are defeating to say the least. It becomes easier to withdraw from situations where communication with others may take place, rather than face embarrassment from frequent misunderstandings of statements and inappropriate responses which may take place. To respond to the question, "How did you sleep last night?" with "At home, of course!" is unquestionably embarrassing, particularly when other misinterpretations have occurred within the same conversation and are occurring with increasing regularity. The elderly person, who may be an otherwise alert, intelligent adult, is understandably also concerned over those misunderstandings of conversations. Many elderly adults who experience such difficulties feel that perhaps they are losing their "senses," particularly when they may not know the cause for the speech discrimination problems that they are experiencing. Perhaps their greatest concern is that their family may feel that they are losing the ability to function on an independent basis and that those personal aspects of life for which they are still responsible will be taken away.

Communication is such an integral part of financial dealings, for example, that elderly persons may also question their own ability to maintain a responsible position in the family, although in the end they may not wish to withdraw from those responsibilities. The self-questionaing that may occur is frequently further aggravated by well-meaning but thoughtless comments by, for example, an elderly person's children. Such comments as, "Dad, why don't you think about selling the house and moving into a small apartment? You know this house is too much for you to care for," can be defeating. Even though an elderly family member may be adequately caring for the house, cooking nutritious meals, and looking forward to each spring so that he or she can work in the garden, a seed of doubt regarding his or her ability to adequately maintain the house and other life requirements because of age has been planted. A statement by his or her physician such as, "Of course you are having aches and pains, you're not a spring chicken any more," can bring about doubts of survival. Such doubts are the beginning of defeat among many elderly unless they are uniquely resiliant.

Compounding these self-doubts may be a growing inability to understand what others are saying as a result of presbycusis and the fear, anger, and embarrassment that result. It becomes easier, for lack of other alternatives, to withdraw from those situations where embarrassment or fear of embarrassment may occur than to enter them. If forced into such a situation, the easiest avenue is to become noncommunicative rather than to attempt responses to questions and fail, thus instilling further doubts in younger family members' minds regarding one's ability to maintain independent living. If forced into responding to a question that is not fully understood because an important word is not understood, frustration on both the part of the elderly person and the family can ensue. Anger and embarrassment on both parts is usually the ultimate result.

HOW DO ELDERLY PERSONS REACT TO THEIR HEARING IMPAIRMENT?

Embarrassment, frustration, anger, defeat, and ultimate withdrawal from situations which require communication have been mentioned with great regularity above. And those reactions are very real on both an overt and covert basis, depending upon the nature of a particular elderly hearing impaired person. When so much else is taken away from many older adults, including leadership in a family, a steady income, a spouse or friend who may have recently passed away, convenient transportation, and a more regular social life, a gradually increasing ability to hear and understand what others are saying can be debilitating. As one elderly person said, "I feel like death has arrived, but I am still alive." Many feel so agonized by their inability to understand what the minister is saying at church, what their friends are saying at the senior center, or what the speaker at a meeting they were looking forward to attending is saying, that they do withdraw as genuinely defeated shells of what they used to be. And for some, with withdrawal comes death at an earlier time than was necessary. All too many of these people are described by their family or others with whom they associate as "confused," disoriented, noncommunicating, uncooperative, and "angry, old ———," withdrawn, and most unfair of all, "senile." In some instances, a hearing aid does not provide help for the person who possesses presbycusis because of the complex nature of that auditory disorder. The inability to use amplification well further instills the fear in the older adult or his or her family that, perhaps, the disorder is mental rather than simply auditory.

It has been observed by this writer that in many instances, a portion of the depression experienced by the hearing impaired elderly is brought about by that person's feelings that the breakdowns in communication which are being experienced "are all my fault because *I* possess the hearing impairment." It does not seem to occur to him or her that the disorder of hearing may be magnified by family members who do not speak plainly, or by being thoughtlessly placed in communicative environments which are so noisy and otherwise distracting that only a person with normal auditory function would be able to hear and understand what was being said. Those, for example, may include attempting to listen to a speaker in an auditorium which possesses very poor acoustics and the only seat left when he or she arrived was toward the rear of the room, watching a 15-year-old distorting television set, or attempting to understand what his or her shy three-year-old granddaughter is saying.

Many elderly hearing impaired persons become so defeated in their attempts at communication and their reduced feelings of self-worth that it does not dawn on them that they might be better able to understand what others are saying if those with whom they are communicating would either improve their manner of speaking or improve upon the communicative environment. Most elderly persons have resigned themselves to "not be a bother" rather than assert themselves by criticizing their family's manner of speaking or the environments in which they are asked to communicate. Rather, older adults may simply visit their families less frequently, even though they desire to talk to a daughter or son and grandchildren. In the end, however, they may withdraw into isolation at home rather than attempt to maintain social or family contacts where they have felt frustration and embarrassment before.

HOW DO OTHERS REACT TO THE ELDERLY WHO POSSESS PRESBYCUSIS?

One elderly hearing impaired person has quite eloquently stated, "For every poor ear, there is at least one poor speaker." In regard to the reactions of others to the hearing impaired elderly person, he may be quite accurate.

As stated earlier, many elderly persons have placed themselves in a position of "not being a bother," perhaps not realizing that at least a portion of their difficulties in communication with others may be the result of attempting to talk to persons who do not speak clearly, or being asked to communicate in environments which may cause even a person with normal hearing to have difficulty. Even though, for example, an elderly person's adult son may not possess good speech skills, the blame for miscommunication or misunderstanding by his elderly parent is placed on the parent and his or her hearing deficit, and not the speaker. Again, the interpretation of the disorder all too often includes "confusion as the result of age," without attempting to analyze the problems of communication per se.

Generally, the initial *visible* frustration at the elderly person's inability to understand what is being said is observed in the listener. Any other lesser reaction may have resulted in a simple request for repetition or rephrasing of the statement for clarification. When the elderly hearing impaired listener fails to understand a statement after several repetitions of a difficult word, it is usually he or she who first notices the apparent frustration, rather than the speaker. Increased self-imposed pressure to succeed in understanding the problem word within the speaker's sentence tends to increase anxiety and heighten the probability of failure to ultimately understand the word. One of two reactions generally follow. The most frequent on the part of the elderly listener is to become equally frustrated, apologize, and withdraw from the situation. The second probable response is a feeling of anger coupled with frustration and embarrassment, and either an inner or overt expression of "Why don't you speak more plainly!" Withdrawal from that frustrating situation may occur rather suddenly.

Who initiated this trying situation? In all probability it was the speaker rather than the elderly listener. The speaker's initial unspoken display of frustration at the elderly listener's inability to understand the statement or question caused heightened anxiety on the elderly person's part. Anxiety, in that situation, breeds failure, failure breeds frustration, frustration breeds further failure, and on and on, until some resolution to cease the conversation, leave the situation, or continue to display anger and frustration is reached. Did the initial attempt at the conversation prompt this less-than-tolerable situation? Probably not. The elderly person who has experienced frustrating attempts at holding a conversation on prior occasions usually develops an immediate awareness of signs of anxiety or frustration or concern which are reflected in the speaker when a nonunderstood word or phrase causes a delay in the conversation. After failure in various communicative environments has occurred on other occasions, and perhaps is now occurring with greater regularity, the elderly person begins to anticipate the speaker's response, perhaps in some instances prematurely in anticipation of a *possible* negative response.

In any event, a speaker at some time has planted the seed of suspicion that he or she was frustrated, concerned, and perhaps even angry at that elderly person's failure to understand or interpret what he or she was saying.

The second party's negative response to the older hearing impaired person's obvious difficulty in understanding what he or she is saying may be the result of either an unanticipated interruption in the flow of a conversation, a lack of desire to really communicate with the elderly person, a lack of tolerance for a disorder that is not readily visible and therefore disconcerting to the nonimpaired person, or a lack of knowledge regarding ways in which the situation could be made more comfortable for both the impaired listener and the speaker. A nonimpaired person will typically react to assist a physically handicapped person across a busy street, or guide a visually handicapped person through a maze of chairs. In those situations, however, the impairment and the manner in which assistance can be offered are both obvious to a person who may, in fact, know little about the handicapping effects of those disorders. But verbal communication, which is generally experienced as an ongoing set of events, when interrupted by a nonvisible disorder such as hearing impairment, is usually disconcerting to the nonimpaired person. This is particularly true when a hearing aid is not worn or otherwise displayed. This generally occurs when the speaker suddenly realizes that his or her verbal message was misunderstood. Communication for that brief instant no longer exists. The normal hearing person is suddenly perplexed regarding what to do at that point. The misunderstood word or phrase is repeated, but perhaps to no avail. The hearing impaired person still misinterprets the verbal message. A natural response is to repeat the word or phrase once again in a louder voice, perhaps with emphasis and facial expression that reveals at least some frustration, since the speaker may have not yet determined why the listener is having such great difficulty. The evident frustration may, in turn, concern the hearing impaired listener, and communication is thus at a stalemate.

It appears that if the impaired auditory system of the hearing handicapped listener were as noticable as impaired limbs of the paraplegic or the eyes of the blind, perhaps the perplexing frustrations that occur could at least have been softened. The disorder of presbycusis is so complex, however, that simply raising the intensity of one's voice may do little to ease the difficulty. In fact, in some instances, the misinterpretations actually increase. In other words, the frustrations experienced by persons who communicate with any age of hearing impaired persons do exist, and thus also exist among the hearing impaired persons themselves.

HEARING IMPAIRED ELDERLY PERSONS VERSUS HEARING IMPAIRED OTHERS

Why do family members, friends, or spouses of elderly persons who possess the disorder of presbycusis appear to experience greater frustrations than those persons who, for example, must communicate with hearing impaired children? Adults and children, perhaps, tend to be more compassionate toward children and young adults who have difficulty communicating as the result of hearing impairment. That is not to say that there are not instances where attempts at getting a message across to a hearing impaired child fail in frustration for both the hearing impaired child and the speaker. Accommodations by nonimpaired children and adults, however, appear to be made willingly in most instances because they know that the child is likely to have difficulty understanding their verbal message, either because of the hearing impairment per se or as the result of language delay. On the other hand, the nonimpaired person who is frustrated at attempts to communicate with a hearing impaired elderly person may rationalize the reason as being because the person is simply "old" and generally less accommodating.

Are the frustration and resulting tension expressed because the listener is simply an older person? Perhaps in a few instances this may be true, but probably not as a general rule. The frustration experienced by those persons who may have known the elderly person for some time prior to the onset of the auditory difficulties, may arise from the fact that this person "was always quite alert and could 'hear a pin drop.' " For reasons unknown to them, however, frustrating and failing attempts at "communicating with Dad" are causing friction within their family. "Dad's mind seems to be failing. I told him yesterday to get the safety inspection sticker for his car renewed, and he replied, 'Who was safe?' Maybe we should get him a hearing aid, or take his car away from him." When a hearing aid is perhaps, purchased for him by a well-meaning son or daughter, but he refuses to wear it because, as he says, "it doesn't help," he may be then described by his family as stubborn. Or they may feel that "he refuses to do anything to improve himself," when in all probability the hearing aid made listening even more difficult because of the complex neurologic nature of presbycusis.

So how do others who associate with the elderly person who possesses presbycusis react to him or her? As one family member said to this writer,

> We are concerned about Dad. We used to have a good time talking about "the good old days," and about what he wanted to do after he retired. Now that he can't seem to hear us, or understand what we say, we all get angry. He can't understand what we are saying no matter how loud we talk, and all he does is get mad because no matter how many times we repeat what we say, he still can't get it. We tried a hearing aid, but he won't wear it. He says it doesn't help. For $400, it *should* do something for him, but we all feel that he just can't get used to something new. Besides, he's just stubborn, we think. Our whole lives

> have changed since this hearing problem has gotten worse. We don't communicate anymore. We don't even like to have him over anymore, and no one goes to visit him. He just sits. We are embarrassed to take him out to restaurants because he can't understand the waiters and then becomes angry when we try to interpret what they are saying. So we just let him sit at his house. We told him to sell the house and move into an apartment complex where older persons live. He says that if we try to sell his house he'll lock the doors and windows and never come out until the hearse takes him away. His hearing problem has changed all of our lives for the worse. We really are at our wits' end.

The above statements are made many times over by concerned and frustrated children, friends, and spouses of elderly hearing impaired persons. But many of these persons can be helped if those who serve them take the time to listen to their responses to the auditory disorder and their state in life. From this information, viable service programs can be developed, not only for the hearing impaired elderly, but also for those who most closely associate with them.

REACTIONS OF ELDERLY PERSONS TO THEIR HEARING IMPAIRMENT: A DIALOGUE

How do elderly persons who possess hearing impairment react to the disorder and the difficulties they experience while attempting to communicate with others? The following statements regarding clients' feelings about their state in life are taken from initial pretreatment interviews with ten older hearing impaired clients. All were recorded on videotape by this author. The statements will be presented individually. This type of personalized information provides important insights into the feelings and desires of elderly clients that are not only important in the counseling process, but also in developing their treatment programs.

The Interviewees

All but one of the persons presented in this section are from northern Colorado, immediately north of Denver. One client is from Albuquerque, New Mexico. All of these persons are of an average socioeconomic level.

Occupational History

Two women were teachers at the elementary and high school level. One man managed a grain elevator in a small town. He acquired no education past the sixth grade. One man is a retired agricultural agent for Weld County, Colorado. One man was a farmer, with no education past the third grade. Four women still consider themselves to be housewives and not retired. One man is a retired missionary. Four of these clients presently reside in a health care facility, and the remainder are living in the community in their own homes.

State of Health and Mobility

The six clients interviewed who reside in the community all describe themselves as being well. They feel that they are mobile, although only one of the women drives a car. All of the men who do not reside in a health care facility drive their own car. The women who do not drive a car said that transportation was occasionally a problem, but that bus service was generally adequate. All clients interviewed, except one man who was troubled with the gout, stated that they sometimes walked where they needed to go, mostly for health reasons.

No clients interviewed who resided in health care facilities drove a car. Transportation was stated as being generally adequate through local bus service or by the health care facility's "ambulo-bus" service. The clients who reside in health care facilities generally described the reason for placement there as health reasons, except for one who felt that she was simply deposited there. Physical problems among those confined persons include heart problems, kidney dysfunction, Parkinson's disease, cataracts, and hearing loss. Walking was described by all as difficult. Two clients were confined to wheelchairs—one due to Parkinson's disease, and one due to arthritis.

Age

Ages of the clients included in this description ranged from 66 to 95 years. The mean age was 75 years.

Reason for Referral

All persons interviewed for this discussion had been referred for aural rehabilitation services, or had sought out the service. All had consented to participate in aural rehabilitation treatment on an individual or group basis after an initial hearing evaluation and counseling.

The Dialogue

The following are the above persons' descriptions of themselves and the impact of their hearing impairment on them. The dialogue is taken from videotaped responses by each client to the question, "How do you feel about yourself at this time, and your ability to communicate with others?" Such videotaped interviews are held with each client seen by this author prior to aural rehabilitation services, and again at their conclusion. The purpose for all pre and post videotaped interviews is to allow clients to confront themselves and their feelings about their ability to cope in a communicating world. Changes in their opinions of themselves and their ability to function auditorily are thus more easily mapped. Clients are, further, allowed the opportunity to note changes in themselves and their opinions of their ability to communicate with others by watching and listening to their own statements. The following are the brief but descriptive exerpts of statements by these clients.

Case No. 1

Age: 70 years Sex: Female
Residence: Community—in own house
Marital Status: Never married
Prior Occupation: Elementary educator
Health: Good
Mobility: Good

Dialogue:

I try to say, "What did you say?" but sometimes they begin to appear angry.

I become frustrated— so— so frustrated that I then become angry at myself because I have become angry at those with whom I am talking.

Do other people have problems where they cannot understand what people are saying? Am I the only one?

. . . I didn't realize why I had begun to dislike going to meetings until I realized I was not understanding what they were saying. I had been blaming my friends—and they had been secretly blaming me. I hope I can retain their friendship after I explain to them that the problems weren't all their fault.

Comment: This woman's comments indicate concern over the difficulties she is experiencing in her attempts at interacting with others. She is, however, not resigned to the fact that she will continue to fail. She is still striving to retain friendships with others. Further, she is still enrolled in aural rehabilitation treatment and making satisfactory progress.

Case No. 2

Age: 72 years Sex: Female
Residence: Health care facility
Marital status: Widow
Prior Occupation: Housewife
Health: Arthritis, renal disease
Mobility: Confined to wheelchair. Mobility severely limited.

Dialogue:

I feel handicapped. Anymore, I don't know what the demands are, or what capabilities I have.

. . . I try so hard to hear that I become so very tired.

I may pass away any day. . . . Is there hope for me? I want to talk to my children more than anything else, but they are so busy and can't come to see me very often. I want to hear what the minister here is saying at the chapel. Church means a great deal to me now.

. . . I feel so alone when I can't participate in things I want to do. I can't weed out what I want to hear from the noises around me.

. . . The most important thing is communication. I desperately want it. My grandchildren— I pray that I can someday spend a pleasant afternoon with them.

Comment: This woman feels defeated. She is, however, an alert person and desires that her life situation improve. She is enrolled in an aural rehabilitation treatment program, but her state of depression has not improved significantly. She says that if her family would visit her, it would help. Most important, she desires to have someone to communicate with.

Case No. 3

Age: 76 years Sex: Male
Residence: Community—in own house
Marital Status: Widower
Prior Occupation: Grain elevator manager

Health: Generally good. Has known cardiovascular problems. Some dizziness noted on occasion.
Mobility: Good. Drives own car and is physically mobile. He is mentally alert and always seems to have a joke for the occasion. But, in most respects, he is a man of few words.

Dialogue:

It's embarrassing. When people find out that you have trouble hearing, they don't seem to want to talk to you anymore. If you ask them to speak up—sometimes they look angry.

. . . I feel that time is lost when I go to a meeting I have looked forward to going to, and I can't understand a word they are saying. Most people do not seem to have good speech habits. On the other hand, my poor hearing doesn't help a bit either.

. . . My main goal in coming here is to learn to hear a woman's voice better—maybe a woman's companionship won't be so hard to come by. . . . As they say, a woman's voice may not be as pretty as the song of a bird, but it's awful darn close.

Comment: This man possesses a significant speech discrimination deficit, and strongly desires that aural rehabilitative services be of help to him. He feels that he has much to live for and is willing to work to improve upon his auditory problems. Assertiveness training and manipulation of his communicative environments has supported those efforts.

Case No. 4

Age: 95 years   Sex: Female
Residence: Health care facility
Marital Status: Widow
Prior Occupation: "Housewife"
Health: Parkinson's disease
Mobility: Severely limited. Is confined to a wheelchair. Effects of Parkinson's disease are progressing rapidly.

Dialogue:

I would like to be free—to drive—to go visit children and friends. I would like to get away from confinement.

I would like to be able to hear again—to be able to be a part of the conversations that take place in this home. It would be pleasant to hear the minister again, or to talk to my children. They live far away, though, and can't come often.

My main concern is death right now. I know that the infirmity I have will end in death. I don't know if I'm ready. If I could hear the minister, maybe I would know.

Comment: These comments are tragically typical of many elderly persons who are confined to the health care facility. They feel so many needs, but few can be fulfilled. This woman is alert, however, and can respond to aural rehabilitation treatment. If, for example, accommodations can be made in the chapel so that she can better participate in those services, then one of her desires would be fulfilled. Further, if learning to manipulate her more difficult communicative environments can be achieved so that she can function better within the confines of the health care facility, then her last years will become less isolating.

Case No. 5

Age: 72 years Sex: Male
Residence: Health care facility (post-hospitalization)
Marital Status: Married
Prior Occupation: County extension agent
Health: Intestinal blockage. Arthritis. Otherwise in generally good health.
Mobility: Generally good. Drives own car on occasion. Walks to many places.

Dialogue:

I feel lost sometimes. If I look at people right straight in the eye, then sometimes I get what they say.

. . . I get angry sometimes, but I've finally figured out that for every poor ear, there's a poor speaker!

It's rough to have poor ears. I have trouble hearing women's voices. I wish I could hear them since I'm around women more now than ever before.

Maybe it's me—maybe I don't have good attention.

I wish I could hear my preacher. I go to church every Sunday, but I don't get much out of it.

I wish I could understand what people are saying in a crowd—like when our children and our grandchildren come back home.

If I'm talking to only one person, sometimes I do OK.

Comment: This man expresses a great many "wishes," but so far has not extended himself a great deal in aural rehabilitation treatment. In other words, he desires to improve, but seems to feel that either he does not possess the capability to regain greater communication function, or simply does not want to put forth the effort. He appears to have great communicative needs, but does not yet seem to be convinced of their importance.

Case No. 6

Age: 71 years Sex: Male
Residence: Community—in own house
Marital Status: Widower
Prior Occupation: Farmer
Health: Excellent, except for gout, which restricts his mobility.
Mobility: Not as mobile as desired due to the gout. Drives own car. Is an avid fisherman.

Dialogue:

In a crowd—I have my worst trouble. Riding in a car drives me crazy!

. . . People don't talk with their mouth open.

My ears 'hum,' and that hurts too—in terms of my ability to understand what people are saying.

Some people talk with their hands in front of their mouth—that is very disturbing.

I don't think that my children understand that my problem is my hearing—not my mind.

. . . It just seems like the voice don't come through.

I went to the doctor and he says my hearing is ruined.

My hearing is my only handicap. My minister has an English brogue and I can't understand a word of what he is saying.

Groups sound kind of like a bee hive. I feel embarrassed. Someone speaks to you and you give them the wrong answer. I like to go to social gatherings, but I still get embarrassed. I certainly am not going to give up.

Comment: This man represents the almost ideal elderly client for aural rehabilitation services. He is alert and active, and desires to maintain himself as an active social person. He has also found a female companion who is also an avid fisherman. What an ideal motivational factor for success in aural rehabilitation!

Case No. 7

Age: 81 years Sex: Male
Residence: Community—in own house with his spouse
Marital Status: Married
Prior Occupation: Missionary. Still functions as part-time minister for a local church. He receives many requests to serve on community and church committees.
Health: Excellent
Mobility: Excellent. Walks a great deal and drives own car.

Dialogue:

My greatest concern is my inability to participate in council meetings at church. In some cases, I am in charge of the meeting, but if I cannot understand what the members are saying, then my participation is made almost impossible. It distresses me tremendously that in some instances I cannot perform my duties.

Maybe it's me? Maybe my concentration wanders. Maybe my mind is not working as well now—although I feel that it is.

I have 20–30 members in the Sunday School class that I teach. I find that I have terrible problems determining what their questions are. If I do not know what their questions are, how can I respond to their needs?

Comment: These statements are made by an obviously frustrated man. "How can I respond to their needs?" This man has a great deal to offer his community and church, but is beginning to feel defeat. The audiologist must consider this type of older client as a high priority and intervene as a strategist to aid the person to function more efficiently in those prioritized communicative environments.

Case No. 8

Age: 72 years Sex: Female
Residence: Community—in own house with spouse
Marital Status: Married
Prior Occupation: Nonretired housewife
Health: Excellent
Mobility: Excellent, but has never learned to drive a car. Depends upon husband or bus for transportation. Walks a great deal.

Dialogue:

My hearing loss has been a handicap to me. I ask people to speak up, and they sigh and sometimes I feel terribly embarrassed.

Sometimes they shout at me, which hurts in more ways than one.

I do wish people would talk more distinctly.

Even with my family—they sometimes forget to speak up "for Mom."

On the telephone—I tell people that I'm wearing a hearing aid whether I am or not. They usually speak up more after that.

My husband says I am a different person in this later age. I used to be full of fun, but now I don't even want to go to church. I don't like to go because I don't understand what others are saying.

. . . It isn't all peaches and cream to be this way.

It hurts more than anything when people laugh at you when you give the wrong answer to something they say. I just go home and cry.

People mumble—mumble when they talk.

I just sometimes want to get out of people's way. I don't want to be a bother to anyone—be a nuisance. I've lost my self-confidence and I don't know if I'll ever get it back.

Comment: This otherwise vital woman was on the verge of giving up. Further, her husband was talking about placing her in a nursing home. After 30 weeks of individual aural rehabilitation treatment, she has learned to manipulate the majority of those communicative environments which were most difficult for her. Further, she has rejoined a women's social group from which she had previously resigned membership. The gradual progression from a depressed woman to one with renewed hope has been rewarding to observe.

Case No. 9

Age: 66 years Sex: Female
Residence: Community—in own house
Marital Status: Single
Prior Occupation: Elementary educator
Health: Excellent
Mobility: Excellent

Dialogue:

I was feeling concerned in as much as when people would ask me a question, I would know they were speaking, but I couldn't make sense out of it. I was afraid that my mind was going. I felt closed in, not comfortable, —like I could hear, but little of it made sense—like I was losing my mind.

I think sometimes that people want me to go away.

When I found out that my problem was with my hearing and not my mind—the relief was wonderful. Now I feel that I have something I can try to handle, where before I didn't think I had a chance again.

If people will bear with me, I'll be able to talk with them. I'm going to stay in there just as long as I can.

Comment: This hearing impaired woman benefited greatly from an initial counseling session regarding her auditory problem and some reasons for the difficulties she was encountering. After she found that the communicative problems she was experiencing were not so much the result of her mind, but rather her hearing, she was a ready candidate for a formal aural rehabilitation treatment program.

Case No. 10

Age: 79 years Sex: Female
Residence: Health care facility. Stated that she thought her daughter was looking for an apartment for her, but found herself there.
Marital Status: Widow
Prior Occupation: Housewife (nonretired)
Health: Generally excellent except for broken hip two years ago
Mobility: Somewhat restricted due to fear of falling. Otherwise excellent. She takes the bus to those places she desires to go.

Dialogue:

I used to blame others for my inability to hear, but one the other day told me it was my fault—me and my inability to hear.

A speaker at a concert meeting the other evening spoke for 45 minutes and I did not understand what she was saying. The disturbing thing was that she refused to use the microphone!

I was in a car with two friends the other day—I rode in the back seat. They were talking in the front seat. They were talking about a person I had not seen for quite a while. I heard them say something about a ball game, something about Omaha, and something about someone becoming very ill. I finally felt that I had to say something, so I asked, "She *is* well, isn't she?" Well, what they had said was that my friend had died! She became very ill during a ball game in Omaha and died while being taken by ambulance to the hospital.
It was terribly embarrassing, but they don't become angry with me.

It is *so* frustrating to try to do well, but continually fail. I try not to be irritable. I think I can overcome it.

Comment: This is an example of an alert older woman who, because of factors beyond her control, fell and found herself unable to provide for her physical needs. She was thus placed in a health care facility—hopefully for a relatively short period of time. She has accepted such placement because of the evident short stay. She is responding well to aural rehabilitation treatment services, particularly in regard to learning to cope within her most difficult environments. She has analyzed the reasons for her communicative difficulties well, and is aware of her limitations.

Conclusion

Auditory deficits as the result of presbycusis are as real as the people who possess that frustrating disorder. The disorder, however, affects each person in unique ways. One common denominator is evident, however, and that is that the resulting communication problems can be terribly frustrating, and in many instances debilitating. The most common strain among the confessions of these elderly persons, however, is the pain caused by the isolation and loneliness they experience as the result of their inability to communicate with other human beings.

Jerome G. Alpiner

Chapter 16: The Role of the Audiologist in the Aural Rehabilitation of Aging Persons

HISTORICAL TRANSITION BY AUDIOLOGISTS TO INTEREST IN GERIATRIC AUDIOLOGY

When is one old? When does old age begin? The process of aging is a relative matter. Sheldon (1958) considers aging and old age as a composition of many contributing factors affecting individuals in different ways and degrees at different times. There are individual differences in the rate of growing old. One individual may be physically, mentally, and emotionally "old" at an earlier age than another person who may be chronologically older. Unfortunately, most of the data reported in the literature regarding geriatric aural rehabilitation have referred simply to the age of 65 and above to describe procedures, methodologies, characteristics, and results of clinical studies, rather than such information pertinent to those hearing impaired clients who are indeed aged. With that limitation in mind, a summary of audiologic efforts in the remediation process will be discussed. Reviewing past efforts may allow us to project future directions for aural rehabilitation for older adults.

EARLY EFFORTS

Early efforts in geriatric audiology in this country appeared to focus on changes in auditory threshold sensitivity accompanied by aging rather than on rehabilitative procedures (Bunch, 1929; Beasley, 1938; Corso, 1959; Glorig, Wheeler, Quiggle, Grings, & Summerfield, 1957; Goetzinger, Proud, Kirks, & Embrey, 1961). The data from these studies have helped to verify that hearing sensitivity tends to diminish as a function of age, resulting in communication problems for many individuals.

Early data created a greater awareness among audiologists that individuals with presbycusis had considerable need for aural rehabilitation services. Although need had been established historically, there was little interest in providing therapy for this population. The general feeling seemed to be that the effort might not be worth the results obtained through the therapy process. Additionally, audiologists and students in training programs were, for the most part, more interested in audiologic assessment and hearing aid evaluation. Some audiologists felt that it was too depressing to work with older persons, particularly those living in extended care facilities.

This writer's initial contact with older adults in an extended care facility was as a graduate student (Alpiner, 1978). The assignment was to develop a therapy program for the residents in a home for the aged. A tour of the facility indicated that a number of persons were sleeping in their rooms or in front of a television set in the lounge. Conspicuous was the lack of communication among residents in the home. During one hour of observation, not one exchange of conversation took place between any of the people seated in the lounge. The home was quiet except for conversation and work noises created by the nursing, maintenance, and dietary staffs. The same day, a physician conducting an in-service for all staff stated that medical science had given more years to life and we had a responsibility to put more life into the years of these elderly persons. The question that came to mind was how to accomplish this.

A review of the literature indicated little information regarding rehabilitative audiology procedures for the older population. As far as specific information on therapy procedures was concerned, the usual "lipreading" books were available but they had no emphasis on methods for working with older adults. Attempts to use traditional lipreading procedures usually ended in failure. There appeared to be no relationship between lipreading instruction and improvement in communication ability.

PRESENT STATUS OF THE AUDIOLOGIST IN GERIATRIC REHABILITATIVE AUDIOLOGY

The American Speech and Hearing Association (1971) has indicated that there are at least 2.5 million citizens in the over age 65 population with significant bilateral hearing impairment. The ASHA estimate projects more than three million with hearing loss by 1980. As early as 1967, Chaffee stated that 90 percent of individuals living in extended care facilities had significant hearing impairment. The Senate Committee on Aging ("Senate Aging Committee launches investigation," 1968) indicated that hearing loss affects between 30 and 50 percent of the population over 65 years. Most recently, Hull and Traynor (1977) stated that hearing loss is present in about 60 percent of all persons over the age of 65. The differences in the data regarding the numbers of older adults with hearing loss may be due to difficulties experienced in sampling this population.

When one compares the incidence of handicapping hearing impairment in the elderly in the United States to persons being served, it is apparent that our service delivery system is inadequate. These persons reside in thousands of extended care facilities and private residences throughout the country, in both rural and urban areas. No formal national incidence study has been conducted to date, but we are undoubtedly addressing ourselves to the fact that several million older adults possess hearing loss resulting in a breakdown in their communication process. The population of elderly persons within the United States is not as easily identified as the school age population. It is this writer's opinion that if it were not for university training programs that attempt to expose students to the problems of presbycusis, rehabilitative services would be even more minimal. Realistically we have been meandering in the unknown regarding those elderly persons who need the rehabilitative assistance of the audiologist.

Let us consider present remediation processes. These include, first, the aspects which make up the rehabilitation process; and second, the individuals who provide therapy to minimize the difficulties encountered by senior citizens. These categories may apply to hearing impaired individuals whether they reside in extended care facilities or in private residences (their own homes or with family or friends).

Aspects of the Rehabilitation Process

Hearing rehabilitation has been considered synonymous with lipreading for many years. It is unfortunate that this concept, in part, lingers. Numerous clients continue to come to us to learn how to lipread, i.e., how to perceive spoken communication by relying totally on the visual modality. It is strongly contended that lipreading is only one aspect of a total rehabilitative process. Emphasis should be directed toward methods which help individuals become better communicators, not better lipreaders.

Changes regarding various aspects of the rehabilitation process are occurring. A significant model has been developed by Hull and Traynor at the University of Northern Colorado (1977). They describe seven essential ingredients for a geriatric aural rehabilitation program. The first is screening and diagnostic evaluation for the determination and type of hearing loss. Procedures include pure-tone audiometry, speech audiometry, and impedance audiometry. Evaluation of these data leads to initiation of motivational counseling if aural rehabilitation seems appropriate. A hearing aid evaluation for those clients who may benefit from amplification is the second step. Hull and Traynor recommend a conservative approach to amplification, with strong consideration given to the actual benefits received from the use of a hearing aid. Their approach seems to be realistic in avoiding what this author has labeled "the dressed drawer syndrome." The third aspect consists of speechreading and auditory training. This approach combines visual cues and residual hearing to allow the client to piece together verbal information when not all of it is heard. Analytical approaches to speechreading instruction are not recommended due to difficulties in phoneme recognition and the questionable worth of this method.

Fourth is motivation counseling, regarded as one of the most vital aspects of a geriatric aural rehabilitation program. Extensive emphasis in this approach is assisting the client to achieve self-confidence in the communication activities of everyday living. Obviously there must be a need to communicate in the client's environment. Hull and Traynor state that the audiologist should have a real desire to work with this age group, or risk a resultant disservice to clients. Clients must have confidence in those persons who provide service to them.

The fifth aspect deals with carryover of the aural rehabilitation process by the family. To facilitate carryover, it is recommended that family counseling be conducted to orient them to the ramifications of hearing loss. In-service training for retirement center staffs and all persons who have responsibility for working with senior citizens is the sixth aspect. An understanding of the aging process is imperative if the best possible service is to be provided. Too often, for example, we have observed staffs in retirement centers who know little about the aspects of aging. Frustration on the part of the resident results. For example, clients with hearing aids have made such comments as, "There is not one person in this nursing home who knows how to help me place this ear mold in my ear."

The seventh aspect is teaching sign language to clients who have lost all measurable hearing bilaterally and are otherwise noncommunicating elderly persons. In this situation, the use of manual language allows people at least to express basic needs without having to write messages. It is useful only if others in a client's environment are taught sign language and if the client has the physical capability to sign.

It may be observed that the rehabilitative process is multifaceted and that more is involved than traditional lipreading. As more audiologists become involved in geriatric rehabilitative audiology, further changes in methodology and philosophy undoubtedly will occur. We will have the opportunity to build on both past and present methods. Harless and Rupp (1972) have stated that it is important for hearing centers to incorporate more effective programs of aural rehabilitation for the elderly population.

Personnel Involved in Rehabilitative Management

The older client with a hearing impairment must first be considered a person with the same basic needs as anyone. Due to the complexities of the aging process, the impact of hearing loss may be a secondary consideration. We need to be cognizant of the ways in which hearing loss may affect an individual emotionally relative to other problems. Certain concomitant problems extending beyond the training of the audiologist may occur. Other individuals, both professional and nonprofessional, may assume roles in the remediation process. It has been stated by Williams (1961) that the hearing impaired need to be understood, to be treated as individuals, to achieve social maturity, and to replace attitudes of apathy. If an individual's basic needs are to be fulfilled, we must be aware that the audiologist is only one part, although a major part, of the rehabilitation process. The purpose of this section is to discuss other personnel who may be involved in client management.

Who should assume the responsibility to make certain that clients receive all necessary services? Depending on the nature of the problem and its manifestations, it is possible that audiologists, physicians, psychologists, social workers, nurses, nursing home administrators, and others may be involved in remediation. Alpiner (1978) has indicated that as long as all needed rehabilitative services are provided and medical clearance is given by the physician, it is probably incidental who assumes primary case management for the client. The responsibility, however, must be assigned and should be designated at the point of client entry into the rehabilitation process. Cooper (1971) has stated that delayed and inadequate service has been compounded at all levels. Physicians have been slow to refer or to follow up on referral to hearing and speech centers. Hearing and speech centers have delayed referrals for other services. No single discipline has the competence to provide total service for a client. The issue, therefore, may be not who provides a given service but rather who assumes the responsibility to verify that all required services are received. There is a need to improve the present system.

Many individuals are involved in the remediation process. The physician evaluates the overall medical condition of the client and provides necessary treatment. The otologist is involved in the medical management of ear pathology. The audiologist is concerned with evaluation of hearing function and subsequent rehabilitative audiology, including, in many instances, hearing aid evaluation and hearing aid dispensing. Social workers may deal directly with clients and their families, helping to determine appropriate assistance. Social workers may provide emotional support to both the client and the family. They can evaluate the client's way of life, his or her day-to-day environment, and general emotional strength. This member of the team may obtain significant information to help in therapy planning. Psychologists may use tests and measurements, interviews, therapy and evaluation. This provides another way for observing human behavior to permit greater understanding of clients. The expertise of the psychologist may add a dimension for dealing with the complex and sometimes frustrating problems possessed by the acoustically handicapped client. For clients residing in extended care facilities, both nurses and nursing home administrators usually have direct responsibility for residents on an ongoing basis. They assume responsibility to ensure that the needs of their residents are met.

Family members also are an extremely important part of the team. Not unlike the roles parents assume in understanding the problems of their children with hearing loss, the families of elderly persons may be effectively involved in enhancing the total rehabilitation process. Certain basic principles which spouses and children need to be aware of include:

1. Accepting the existence of hearing loss in the member of the family
2. Understanding the ramifications of the hearing loss as it affects members of the family
3. Providing emotional support for the family member with hearing loss
4. Training family members as to how they can help in the remediation process as a follow-up to formal therapy

Hopefully, we now have an increased awareness that there are individuals, in addition to the audiologist, who may contribute to successful therapy. The important point is that appropriate referrals be made when necessary and that audiologists become aware of when to utilize these other resources. Even though case management of the elderly adult may be assumed by someone else, the audiologist is still an integral part of the team. The team approach to rehabilitation has not yet been fully accepted and implemented, even though most of us agree that it is desirable. We are in a position to help effect positive change in the relationships between professionals and individuals.

PAST AND PRESENT REHABILITATIVE EFFORTS WITH ELDERLY PERSONS

Formal aural rehabilitation programs for the elderly are still in their infancy. Kleemeier and Justiss (1954) indicated that while clients tended to make satisfactory adjustment to hearing aids, these individuals seemed to be restricted socially and suffered more from personality maladjustment than did a matched group of normal hearing persons. Grossman (1955) investigated the use of hearing aids in a home for the aged. His results indicated that only 6 of 181 residents were wearing hearing aids when 21 might have profited from the use of amplification. Gaitz and Watshow (1964) engaged in an audiometric screening program in an extended care facility. Fourteen of the 40 residents had serious hearing impairment according to the authors, with only 3 accepting recommendations for amplification. Those residents who rejected amplification indicated the following reasons for not purchasing hearing aids:

1. Lack of money (even though the home agreed to pay for the aids)
2. Denial of hearing impairment
3. A feeling that they were too old to learn to use hearing aids

Gaitz and Watshow (1964) stated that lack of motivation was the major reason why clients rejected amplification. They indicated further that hearing testing should not become a part of the routine examination in homes for the aged. Their position was that hearing evaluation should be reserved for residents who asked for assistance or members of the facility staff requested testing for an individual. These programs emphasized hearing and hearing aid evaluations exclusive of a complete hearing rehabilitation program.

PROGRAMS IN HEALTH CARE FACILITIES

Alpiner (1964) administered hearing conservation programs in two residential extended care facilities as well as in a Golden Age Center. The emphasis in these programs was audiologic evaluation, hearing aid evaluation, and aural rehabilitation therapy (primarily lipreading instruction and hearing aid orientation). The primary purpose of this testing aspect of the programs was to identify residents needing therapy, whether or not amplification was recommended. Of 80 clients who were candidates for hearing aid evaluation, only five percent were interested in participating in the evaluation process. It should be noted that all these clients were in good physical and mental health. Subjectively, it appeared that clients lack motivation either to wear hearing aids or engage in therapy. Three client attitudes emerged in this study:

1. A denial that a hearing problem existed
2. An attitude of hopelessness (residents indicated that therapy should be reserved for younger persons—they were going to die soon)
3. An acceptance of hearing loss but no desire for rehabilitation

It appears that the early efforts in the 1950s and 1960s emphasized hearing and hearing aid evaluations. Initial attempts were made to provide more comprehensive services but evidence indicates these efforts were not successful. Clients lacked motivation for audiologic services. We know that lack of motivation, in part, was due to various physiological and psychological problems that accompanied the aging process.

This writer's experiences with previously cited and ongoing programs undertaken as part of university training subjectively indicate that many extended care facilities in the United States do not offer environments that make communication a necessity for existence. Consequently, therapy programs are "dead-ended" because there are not always effective communication environments which make therapy meaningful and allow for carryover from aural rehabilitation. Despite these apparently negative prior conditions, renewed efforts may lead to more successful rehabilitation for older adults. In essence, the early programs were at the grass roots level, leading to later innovations in the rehabilitation process.

PROGRAMS FOR THE ELDERLY IN THE COMMUNITY

Harless and Rupp (1972) reported on a program at the University of Michigan designed to reach the elderly in the Ann Arbor community for hearing conservation. This program included hearing screening, speechreading practice, review of tips and helpful hints, group discussion, overview of service availability, and a summary report to each participant. For hearing screening, each person received an abbreviated hearing test including air- and bone-conduction thresholds in the frequency range of 500–4000 Hz.

If significant hearing deficits were found, one or more of the following suggestions were made:

1. *Ear specialist's review*—a careful medical evaluation constituted the first step. All otologists in the Ann Arbor community were listed, and the elderly person was encouraged to make an appointment with the physician of his or her preference.
2. *More complete audiological review*—the audiologic evaluation provided knowledge not only about the nature and degree of hearing impairment, but also about the communicative disability of the individual. In every case this recommendation accompanied the first suggestion.
3. *Investigation into purchasing a hearing aid*—if the otologic and audiologic findings indicated the need for a hearing aid, the elderly person was encouraged to make an appointment at the clinic for a hearing aid evaluation.
4. *Speechreading instruction*—this recommendation was for a 10-week class, suggesting that such training could help to improve listening and attending abilities.

Other highlights of this program included a review of helpful hints for overcoming the hearing handicap. Pamphlets and other materials were distributed to each class member to read, and these articles were discussed at subsequent sessions. Group discussion enabled the members of the class to consider aspects of hearing impairment and the special problems it posed. The intent was for the client to achieve greater insight regarding his or her hearing problem and to learn to cope with it. Another unique factor of this program was three satellite locations, alleviating some of the transportation problems encountered by the elderly. The fee for the 10-week program was $10.

Colton and O'Neill (1976) describe a cooperative outreach program for the elderly. They indicated that hearing problems of older adults have long been neglected, with services almost nonexistent. Initially, this program was implemented at the University of Illinois in conjunction with the Champaign County Office on Aging. Funding was received through a grant from the Older Americans Act, Title III. After grant monies were discontinued, the program was maintained. Hearing screening centers were established in six different locations throughout the county. Public health nurses, trained by the university audiology staff, conducted the screenings. Client failure to respond at any two (octave) frequencies to a 30 dB tone (re: ANSI, 1969), resulted in recommendation to the rehabilitation program. After initial recommendation, a series of lectures was presented by the audiology staff at various senior citizens' meetings. The topics were:

1. Discussion of the basic parts and function of the ear
2. Types and causes of hearing loss
3. Remedial approaches that might be recommended (medication, surgery, amplification, and aural rehabilitation)

Concurrent with the lecture series for the senior citizens was the training of individuals from the community who would serve as instructors for the lipreading classes. They had been recommended as potential teachers by the Office on Aging. Their training consisted primarily of lectures and demonstrations dealing with the following topics:

1. Historical perspectives of lipreading
2. Basic approaches to lipreading
3. Basic organization of a lipreading lesson
4. Lesson plans

5. Sources of materials
6. Types of materials

At least one graduate student from the university's aural rehabilitation practicum was assigned to each aide. Their responsibilites included teaching every third lesson, providing additional resource material for the lay teacher, conducting one-to-one therapy sessions for individual clients with particular problems, and conducting audiological and hearing aid evaluations. Some of the strengths and weaknesses of this program were outlined by the authors. Weaknesses included the inability of university personnel to be at each meeting of the lipreading class, transiency of lay teachers, emphasis of a unisensory approach, lack of funds for the purchase of hearing aids, and inability to conduct complete audiologic evaluations on many of the senior citizens, resulting in some therapy groups which were heterogeneous in terms of problem severity. The advantages of this program were the opportunity for students to be exposed to the hearing problems of the elderly, to become involved in a grass roots community project, and to provide a needed service to the community while socialization opportunities were provided for senior citizens.

McCartney, Maurer, and Sorenson (1974) reported on a mobile audiology service for the elderly called Project ARM (Auditory Rehabilitation Mobile) serving three counties in the Portland, Oregon, area. This project utilized an interdisciplinary team including staff members from the Portland State University Speech and Hearing Program, the Institute on Aging, and the Department of Audiology. Services included evaluation and rehabilitation. In reflecting on two and one half years of service, the authors presented the following comments about the program.

The program would not have been possible without college or university support in terms of funding, staff, and graduate students. Project ARM consisted of two audiologists, one part-time audiologist, five audiology and speech pathology students, one student research assistant, one secretary, and additional student clerical help.

The senior author felt the age of the urban mobile audiology clinic might have already come and passed, due primarily to economic and ecological considerations. Funds for operation of the mobile unit could have provided considerable money for transportation of clients to an established audiology center.

The single most effective and substantial contribution of Project ARM was public education through hearing screenings and handout materials.

The best responses to hearing screenings were obtained at senior adult centers where hot meals were served. The meal program provided a captive audience for hearing screening and a climate for socialization and participation in other activities.

Perhaps the most important result of the project was a need for better professional publicity on who an audiologist is and more effective communication between hearing aid dealers, audiologists, and otologists.

The programs discussed in this section are representative of past and current rehabilitative efforts with the elderly. It would appear that we have progressed from screening clients for hearing and hearing aid evaluations to attempts to reach more individuals for subsequent rehabilitation. The audiologists working with older adults are to be commended for their efforts to increase awareness of the audiologic needs of the elderly. Even though much remains to be accomplished, several points can be made. First, without university training programs in audiology and speech pathology, services for senior citizens would be even more meager than they are. Second, funding for hearing conservation programs is inadequate; the present system seems to be financially carried as a commitment by universities with some exceptions in terms of grants and volunteer workers. Third, the provision of services seems to be a hit and miss situation, depending on resources available to audiologists, whatever their employment environment. Put another way, there is no model available today that can be nationally adopted and/or modified. The University of Northern Colorado model is an excellent one to consider, but most facilities in the United States do not have the resources to implement such a program. Fourth, it would appear that the dilemma regarding public awareness of who audiologists are and what they do still exists. Fifth, the relationships between audiologists and ancillary professionals has not been solidified, although we tend to agree that co-operative efforts are necessary for an effective rehabilitation process. We may now consider some of the directions to follow in our commitment to serve older Americans.

FUTURE DIRECTIONS AND RESPONSIBILITIES OF AUDIOLOGISTS IN THE REHABILITATION PROCESS

This writer views four basic areas of concern with regard to future development of rehabilitative audiology for older adults. They are public awareness, development of therapy methodologies, student training program directions, and program financing. The audiologist must serve as a facilitator in all of these areas. O'Neill (1977) has stated that by observing current efforts at providing service to the aging population, it is obvious that one of the first professions to move into this area and still active is the speech and hearing profession. It appears this pattern was brought on by training needs. A symbiotic relationship developed between speech and hearing training programs and aged populations. So far, according to O'Neill, it has been a relationship beneficial to both groups.

PUBLIC AWARENESS

A community may be inspired to develop programs if an audiologist can create awareness of the problems encountered by its hearing impaired senior citizens. Since so many worthy projects compete for community participation and funding, it may no longer be assumed that all of them can be supported. Porter and Smith (1973) have stated the community must decide which projects will be of greatest benefit. How can individuals and groups within a community be motivated? The audiologist needs to be familiar with ways to approach a community for support for its older adults. Porter and Smith cite examples:

One may become interested in program development because he or she is personally involved with the particular problem.

Another person may be sincerely interested in making his or her community a better place to live, so civic pride may be the basis of motivation for encouraging programming. These persons often are members of service organizations such as Kiwanis, Lions, and Rotary.

Some individuals may be motivated for economic reasons. They would prefer citizens to remain productive and contributors to the community in terms of purchasing power rather than have citizens be recipients of welfare funds.

Some individuals feel a moral and spiritual need to help persons with handicapping conditions.

Newman (1970) stated there is no comprehensive approach to providing services for persons with communicative disorders. Lack of organization appears characteristic at the community level. We must know what community resources are available before attempting to contact those who may help in the development of programs for older adults.

In reviewing university training programs in speech pathology and audiology, one will not be surprised to find a lack of course work and practicum in public relations. This important aspect is crucial in development of public awareness. It would appear that we have entered an era in which the audiologist is involved in not only the narrow aspects of evaluation and rehabilitation but also as a legitimate participant in community affairs.

Development of community interaction is time consuming and can be frustrating, especially in the early stages of our involvement. We need to be cognizant of the fact that, for the most part, activity in this area is relatively new to us. Erickson (1977) cites misconceptions made by audiologists.

1. Not understanding or taking into consideration the culture of the geriatric client.
2. An attitude that everyone feels aural rehabilitation is important. Clients with increased communicative competence are the best public relations source, both to their geriatric peers and to professionals such as physicians.
3. Thinking that the public knows what aural rehabilitation is. Public media announcements should use public-oriented terminology.

These comments can be of value to us in approaching the community for geriatric rehabilitative audiology programs. It is important that we do not assume the profession is understood by all persons. For too many years we have invested considerable time and energies selling ourselves to ourselves. We now need to go beyond this concept. The audiologist has a new responsibility—he or she is also a public relations person. A course has been suggested by Erickson (1977), using an outline developed by one of her students (Pamela Ford). Hull (1979) has developed a course entitled, "The Administrative Aspects of Communication Disorders." It not only stresses the financial and legal aspects of program function, but also the process involved in public relations.

DEVELOPMENT OF THERAPY METHODOLOGIES

Two significant aspects appear to be developing regarding remediation approaches utilized for the elderly. The first deals with the objectives and implementation of therapy. The second is the development of assessment procedures to determine communication function. Both aspects represent a sharp contrast from the early programs of the 1950s and 1960s in that they allow us to become more "total therapy" oriented rather than only lipreading or hearing aid oriented.

The first aspects appear to have been well presented by Hardick (1977). Hardick's procedures were used on more than 400 clients. He cites specific characteristics of this program.

1. The program must be client centered.

2. The program must revolve around amplification and/or modifying the communication environment.
3. All programs consist of group therapy with some individualized help when necessary.
4. The group must contain normal hearing friends or relatives of the hearing impaired person.
5. Aural rehabilitation programs are all short-term programs with no intermediate or advanced courses.
6. The program is consumer oriented.
7. The program emphasizes an outreach aspect to make the services of aural rehabilitation better known to colleagues and other professionals.
8. The program attempts to utilize successful clients as resource people in group activities whenever feasible.

This program appears to fulfill the total needs of the hearing impaired older adult. It is a client-centered program emphasizing improvement in communication, involvement of family and friends in the process, utilization of ancillary personnel, and counseling clients regarding problems which have emerged.

The second significant aspect in the remediation process emerged from the frustrations and limitations imposed on audiologists regarding communication function. If one of our major attempts was to improve communication and minimize the associated problems caused by hearing impairment, there was a need to devise communication assessment inventories. Three major efforts have been made. They are identification of Communicative Competence in the Geriatric Population (Garstecki, 1977), a Feasibility Scale for Predicting Hearing Aid Use (FSPHAU) with Older Individuals (Rupp, Higgins, & Maurer, 1977), and the Denver Scale of Communication Function for Senior Citizens Reading in Extended Care Facilities (DSSC) (Zarnoch & Alpiner, 1978). The DSSC for identification and evaluation of problem areas resulting from hearing loss is an example. It was designed for presentation through individual interviews with residents. Client input from the DSSC permits us to identify areas of difficulty and plan more realistic therapy. Since client input is an important part of the therapy process, it appears that assessment scales will become increasingly more sophisticated and used as a routine part of the total remediation process.

DIRECTIONS IN UNIVERSITY TRAINING PROGRAMS

As interest in geriatric audiology increases, there undoubtedly will be additions to the curriculum in university training programs. Past training has emphasized general aural rehabilitation courses and children's rehabilitation courses. Historically, students appear to be most interested in providing therapy for children. It is anticipated that this trend will continue, but increasing numbers of students also will be interested in all age groups with some wishing to emphasize geriatrics.

Kaplan and Rickerson (1977) have described competencies that should be developed by student clinicians by the end of their semester practicum experience. These include:

1. The ability to evaluate the communicative needs of the geriatric hearing impaired clients using proper interview and discussion techniques and appropriate audiological testing.
2. The ability to prepare and conduct group speechreading and auditory training lessons.

3. The ability to prepare lecture-discussion material and present that material in a form understandable to clients.
4. The ability to recognize and deal with problems relating to the use and care of the hearing aid.
5. The ability to recognize and appropriately refer problems not within the realm of communication. Such referrals might be for medical problems, financial assistance, family problems, or hearing aid purchase.
6. The ability to write appropriate progress and final reports, using proper format and proper English. The final report must be written in such a way that it may be submitted to the client, if so desired.

In addition to this course and knowledge of public relations, other courses should be required in psychology, sociology, anatomy, physiology, and neurology which would include information on geriatrics. It is essential that students receive training to allow them to better understand the complexities of the aging process.

PROGRAM FINANCING

At this writing, the most unknown factor regarding comprehensive aural rehabilitation programs for the elderly is monetary. Unfortunately, rehabilitative services for hearing impairment are not usually reimbursable, except with some private insurance companies. Audiologic evaluation is reimbursable by Medicare and Medicaid. With greater interest by the federal government, favorable changes may occur which will allow the provision of rehabilitative services for elderly persons. The American Speech and Hearing Association is working to facilitate change for increased financial coverage for services by audiologists. It is felt that if sufficient numbers of individuals, both professionals and clients, make their feelings known to appropriate governmental officials, the situation can change. When change occurs, we will be able to implement urgently needed aural rehabilitation programs for the elderly in the United States.

REFERENCES

Alpiner, J. G. Audiologic problems of the aged. *Geriatrics,* 1964, *18*, 19–26.

Alpiner, J. G. Diagnostic and rehabilitative aspects of geriatric audiology. *Journal of the American Speech and Hearing Association,* 1965, *7*, 455–459.

Alpiner, J. G. Rehabilitation of the geriatric client, in J. G. Alpiner (Ed.), *Handbook of adult rehabilitative audiology*. Baltimore: Williams & Wilkins, 1978, pp. 141–171.

1971 White House conference on Aging. *Journal of the American Speech and Hearing Association,* 1971, *13*, 14–17.

Beasley, W. Generalized age and sex trends in hearing loss, in *Hearing study series bulletin no. 7*. Washington, D.C.: National Health Survey Public Health Service, Department of Health, Education & Welfare, 1978.

Bunch, C. Age variations in auditory acuity, *Archives of Otolaryngology,* 1929, *9*, 625–636.

Colton, J. C., & O'Neill, J. J. A cooperative outreach program for the elderly. *Journal of the Academy of Rehabilitative Audiology,* 1976, *9*, 38–41.

Cooper, L. Z. Deafness: One physician's view, in D. Hicks, (Ed.), *Medical aspects of deafness*. Atlantic City, New Jersey: Council of Organizations Serving the Deaf, 1971.

Corso, J. Age and sex differences in pure tone thresholds. *Archives of Otolaryngology,* 1959, *77*, 385–405.

Erickson, J. G. Pragmatics of the development of community resources. *Journal of the Academy of Rehabilitative Audiology,* 1977, *10*, 23–30.

Gaitz, C., & Watshow, M. F. Obstacles encountered in correcting hearing loss in the elderly. *Geriatrics,* 1964, *19*, 83–86.

Garstecki, D. C. Identification of communicative competence in the geriatric population. *Journal of the Academy of Rehabilitative Audiology,* 1977, *10*, 36–45.

Chaffee, C. E. Rehabilitation needs of nursing home patients—A report of a survey. *Rehabilitation Literature,* 1967, *18*, 377–389.

Glorig, A., Wheeler, D., Quiggle, R., Grings, W., & Summerfield, A. *1954 Wisconsin State Fair hearing survey* (Monograph). American Academy of Ophthalmology and Otolaryngology, 1957.

Goetzinger, C. P., Proud, G. O., Dirks, D. D., & Embrey, J. A study of hearing in advanced age. *Archives of Otolaryngology,* 1961, *73*, 662–674.

Grossman, B. Hard of hearing persons in a home for the aged. *Hearing News,* 1955, *23*, 11–12, 17–18, 20.

Hardick, E. J. Aural rehabilitation programs for the aged can be successful, *Journal of the Academy of Rehabilitative Audiology,* 1977, *10*, 51–67.

Harless, E. L., & Rupp, R. R. Aural rehabilitation of the elderly. *Journal of Speech and Hearing Disorders,* 1972, *37*, 267–273.

Hull, R. H. Implications for training programs. *Journal of the Academy of Rehabilitative Audiology,* 1979, *12*, 74–77.

Hull, R. H., & Traynor, R. M. Hearing impairment among aging persons in the health care facility: Their diagnosis and rehabilitation. *American Health Care Association Journal,* 1977, *3*, 14–18.

Kaplan, H., & Rickerson, C. Geriatric aural rehabilitation: Student training. *Journal of the Academy of Rehabilitative Audiology,* 1977, *10*, 13–18.

McCartney, J. H., Maurer, J. F., & Sorenson, F. D. A mobile audiology service for the elderly: A preliminary report. *Journal of the Academy of Rehabilitative Audiology,* 1974, *7*, 25–36.

Newman, E. the future for rehabilitation. *Hearing and Speech News,* 1970, *38*, 16–17, 20.

O'Neill, J. J. Background and information of training and service for the geriatric client. *Journal of the Academy of Rehabilitative Audiology,* 1977, *10*, 19–22.

Porter, E. B., & Smith, J. H. Hearing loss, a community loss, *Hearing and Speech News,* 1973, *41*, 20–21, 28.

Rupp, R. R., Higgins, J., & Maurer, J. F. A feasibility scale for predicting hearing aid use (FSPHAU) with older individuals. *Journal of the Academy of Rehabilitative Audiology,* 1977, *10*, 81–104.

Senate Aging Committee launches investigation of hearing aids with two days of hearings before consumer interest subcommittee. *Washington Sounds.* House of Representatives Publication 2, July 22, 1968.

Sheldon, H. D. *The older population of the United States.* New York: John Wiley and Sons, Inc., 1958.

Williams, B. R. Basic needs of persons with impaired hearing, in *Proceedings of the rehabilitation of the deaf and hard of hearing.* Stowe, Vermont: University of Vermont College of Medicine, 1961.

Zarnoch, J. M., & Alpiner, J. G. The Denver scale of communication function for senior citizens living in retirement centers, in J. G. Alpiner (Ed.), *Handbook of adult rehabilitative audiology.* Baltimore: Williams and Wilkins, p. 157.

Section 2: Presbycusis

Lennart L. Kopra

Chapter 17: The Auditory–Communicative Manifestations of Presbycusis

That many elderly persons have difficulty understanding speech because they cannot hear well is common knowledge. However, the reasons for this difficulty and the nature of the difficulty are not readily available.

Observations that hearing loss accompanies the aging process were documented before the turn of the century. Clinical and large field studies have more recently been conducted, and from these studies some information about the effect of aging on hearing has become available. The applications of distorted tests of hearing which were originally developed for differential diagnostic test batteries have also been used with elderly persons. Data from these studies have provided new insights into the nature of the deterioration of hearing that accompanies aging. The search for improved methods of quantifying the degree to which hearing loss imposes a social handicap on hearing impaired persons has continued over the past 35 years, and methods for the assessment of social adequacy of hearing have been developed. This chapter summarizes information on hearing loss and aging, types of presbycusis, and auditory performance and aging, including social adequacy of hearing.

HEARING LOSS AND AGE—HISTORICAL BACKGROUND

Current knowledge of the effect of age on auditory sensitivity is based on a number of laboratory and field studies that have been conducted by various investigators over the past 90 years. The following section summarizes most of these studies.

1891—Zwaardemaker

The first documented and historically important effort to examine the relationship between hearing and aging was conducted by Zwaardemaker (1891). In his classic article he relates the length of the air column of the Galton whistle to the hearing ability of five age categories: infant, adolescent, adult, old person, and senility. Subsequently, Zwaardemaker (1894) elaborates on the use of the Galton whistle and describes what he calls "The Presbycusic Law." Although his procedures were admittedly crude by today's standards, his insightfulness is revealed by his observation that hearing sensitivity for high-pitched tones begins to deteriorate in the fourth decade of life. More recent field studies and well controlled laboratory studies in the United States and abroad have corroborated Zwaardemaker's keen observation.

1894—Bezold

In another early study, Bezold (1894) used whispered voice tests at distances ranging from 16 meters to 6 cm and closer and examined 100 people (200 ears) ranging from 50 to 70 years and older. His results clearly indicate that hearing loss for whispered speech increases as a function of age, and he stated that "in the decades following that from the fiftieth to the sixtieth years there is therefore not only a successive decrease in the number of those with nearly normal hearing, but there is also a successive increase in the degree of deafness" (p. 221).

Bezold also observed that males have poorer hearing than females, a fact that has been documented in a number of studies during the twentieth century. He stated, "The explanation is to be sought *in the many hurtful influences of their calling,* noisy occupations, detonations, trauma, alcohol, nicotine, etc." (p. 222; author's emphasis) and he concluded that the higher incidence of hearing loss in males in contrast to females results from the noxious elements he cited. He also generalized that diseases of the middle ear are anomalies of childhood, not of old age. Finally, on the basis of Rinné tests, he concluded that reduced "hearing power of the aged" results from an affected inner ear and not from disease of middle ear structures.

1929—Bunch

In the United States, the most notable study that first called attention to the relationship between hearing and aging was carried out at the Johns Hopkins Hospital and was reported by Bunch (1929). He examined 353 patients who had no subjective indication of hearing impairment. A Western Electric 1A audiometer was used to test frequencies ranging from 32 to 16,384 Hz. Hearing test data were analyzed for each of five decade-age groups—20-year-olds through 60-year-olds. Bunch's data indicate (1) that for all groups, pure-tone sensitivity is more variable in the high frequencies than in the low frequencies, and (2) that primarily for high frequencies above 1024 Hz there is a progressive deterioration in auditory sensitivity as a function of age.

1935–36 National Health Survey (NHS)

The first large-scale field study on auditory sensitivity was carried out in conjunction with the National Health Survey (NHS) conducted by the United States Public Health Service in 1935–36. Results of the survey are reported in a series of reports (National Institute of Health, 1938). Beasley (1940) describes the characteristics and distribution of impaired hearing in the population of the United States.

A sample of 9324 individuals was chosen from the National Health Survey for a hearing examination. Pure-tone air-conduction threshold tests for frequencies 128 Hz through 8192 Hz and bone-conduction tests at frequencies 256 Hz through 4096 Hz were administered to 9324 persons. Tests were administered in moderately controlled acoustic environments.

Although methodological differences between the NHS and subsequent surveys resulted in rather large discrepancies in estimated incidence of significant hearing impairment, the NHS data do indicate that there is an exponential increase in hearing loss with advancing age. According to Beasley's data, the age group 65 years to 74 years has an incidence of significant hearing loss about 20 times greater than the 15- to 24-year-old group. The incidence is slightly greater for males when older females are compared to the younger group of females. Finally, Beasley's report indicates that for all age groups, from under 25 to 65 and over, the incidence of hearing loss is less as family income increases.

1939 World's Fair Survey

A large-scale hearing survey was conducted at the 1939 World's Fair in New York and San Francisco. Results are reported by Steinberg, Montgomery, and Gardner (1940). Test results of about 550,000 listeners were obtained for a recorded phonograph test which had tones of 440, 880, 1760, 3520, and 7040 Hz. At each of nine progressively attenuated levels, a listener was required to hold a single earphone to the ear and to indicate whether a tone was presented once, twice, or three times. The range covered was 62 dB for the first four frequencies and 48 dB for 7040 Hz. From the total number of records, 35,589 test scores were randomly chosen for statistical analysis by sex and by five age groups: 10–19 years through 50–59 years. Although the authors caution us not to generalize their results to groups that vary in socioeconomic status and educational level, they give additional evidence that hearing sensitivity declines with age and that, for the higher frequencies, reduction in auditory sensitivity is greater for males than for females. Furthermore, as has been indicated from other studies, variability of auditory sensitivity increases as a function of frequency and age.

1948 San Diego County Fair Hearing Survey

At the San Diego County Fair in 1948, a phonographically recorded test of the ability to hear pure-tones was given to 3666 persons (Webster, Himes, & Lichtenstein, 1950). Absolute thresholds were established at five frequencies (440, 880, 1760, 3520, and 7040 Hz), and masked thresholds were measured at two frequencies (880 and 3520 Hz). Results were analyzed according to the age, sex, musical training, and past noise exposure of the listeners, and according to whether or not they said they experienced difficulty in hearing. Results showed that auditory sensitivity decreased with age; women had better hearing than men in the higher test frequencies; and men with history of noise exposure had higher thresholds (more loss) than normal at the higher test frequencies. The data also showed that musically trained men and women had better hearing sensitivity than individuals without such training. Finally, the 20- to 29-year-old men tested at the San Diego County Fair appeared to have a greater amount of hearing loss at the higher test frequencies than did men of the same age group who were tested in surveys before World War II.

1954 Wisconsin State Fair Hearing Survey

The most comprehensive field study on hearing and its relation to a number of factors is the 1954 Wisconsin State Fair Hearing Survey reported by Glorig, Wheeler, Quiggle, Grings, and Summerfield (1957). Additional information on this survey is also provided by Glorig (1957) and by Glorig and Wheeler (1955).

The 1954 Wisconsin State Fair Hearing Survey was directed by the staff of the Research Center of the Subcommittee on Noise in Industry of the Committee on Conservation of Hearing of the American Academy of Ophthalmology and Otolaryngology in cooperation with the Wisconsin Manufacturers' Association. The survey was organized as a means of studying the relationship between noise exposure and hearing loss, particularly for obtaining audiometric data in a large sample of an industrialized population.

About 3,500 fairgoers (1,741 males and 1,724 females) participated in the hearing survey at the State Fairgrounds in Milwaukee, Wisconsin. The interviewing and testing procedures were well controlled and were conducted by professionally and technically competent personnel.

First, a medical history was obtained and an otological examination was administered. Then each participant completed a personal history form, which included general noise-exposure information. Third, each person responded to an interview on occupational life and provided specific information on military service and farm or factory noise exposure. Finally, auditory tests were administered. Pure-tone thresholds were measured at 500, 1000, 1500, 2000, 3000, 4000, and 6000 Hz. Spondee thresholds were measured with the CID Auditory Test W-1.

In addition to a basic question regarding the relationship between hearing and aging in males and females, the Wisconsin State Fair Hearing Survey data were analyzed to determine relative hearing levels (1) in urban versus rural groups, (2) in persons who reported their hearing ability as good, fair, and poor, (3) of persons who worked on farms, in offices, and in factories, (4) of men working in noises of various levels, (5) of men who had had exposure to gunfire noise, and (6) of men with military service.

Consistent with findings of previous studies, auditory sensitivity decreased with age, with the rate of decrease being greater in the higher frequencies. The median hearing level at 6000 Hz increased 10 dB with each decade in males, and the corresponding increase at 500 Hz was 3 dB. The hearing sensitivity of females was consistently better than that of the males, even in younger age groups which are not subject to the effects of aging. For the decade-age groups 40 to 49, 50 to 59, and 60 to 69 years, the spondee thresholds of the women were significantly better than those of the men.

In the older age groups, farm workers showed significantly higher hearing levels than office workers at the higher test frequencies. The hearing levels of individuals who worked in noisy jobs (such as drop hammer, riveting, chipping activities, and construction) showed that the hearing of the workers who were exposed to higher levels of noise was significantly poorer than the hearing of workers whose jobs were less noisy. Men who had often shot a gun had significantly more hearing loss in the high frequencies than those who had not often shot a gun. The hearing levels of men with military service experience showed that men who had served in the Navy had the least amount of hearing loss in the high frequencies, and men who had served in the Marines had the most loss.

The data from the 1954 Wisconsin State Fair Hearing Survey corroborate some of the findings of earlier investigations on hearing and aging. This study provides us with additional evidence of the effects of noise on hearing and highlights the need for considering the possible effects of noise exposure when we attempt to identify the effect of aging on hearing.

1960–62 Health Examination Survey

The most recent large-scale survey of hearing levels in a sample of the population of the United States was carried out in conjunction with the Health Examination Survey conducted in 1960–62, as reported by Glorig and Roberts (1965). Hearing levels of 6672 individuals were measured at 500, 1000, 2000, 3000, 4000, and 6000 Hz with calibrated audiometers (ASA 1951) by trained technicians in controlled acoustic environments. In addition, otoscopic examinations were made by a staff physician. Malformations of the external ear, exudate, and perforations and scarring of the tympanic membrane were recorded. A history of noise exposure was not obtained.

In contrast to the results of the Wisconsin State Fair Hearing Survey (Glorig et al., 1957), hearing levels for the right and left ears were similar for the majority of adults. However, the median data presented by Glorig and Roberts (1965) show that hearing levels for right and left ears of men are consistently different by a few dB for frequencies 2000 Hz and above, with the right ear showing better sensitivity. This tendency is not apparent in the median thresholds of females, irrespective of age.

In the lower frequencies from 500 to 2000 Hz, the median levels of the right and left ears of males are equivalent to those of females. However, for all age groups, females show better sensitivity than males at 3000 Hz through 6000 Hz.

When median hearing levels are examined in terms of age groups, there is a progressive decrease in sensitivity as a function of age, with the most decrease occurring in the higher frequencies. Although the differences are small, the effect of age reveals itself when the 25- to 34-year-old group is compared to the younger 18- to 24-year-old group. The effect of age on auditory sensitivity is more marked in males than in females.

1962 Mabaan Tribe Study

In an effort to examine the effects of aging on hearing in a group of people who are exposed to no noxious levels of noise, Rosen, Bergman, Plester, El-Mofty, and Satti (1962) examined 541 Mabaans in the Republic of Sudan, "a pre-nilotic, pagan, primitive, tribal people whose state of cultural development is the late Stone Age" (p. 727). The Mabaans are a peaceful and quiet people. They use no drums in singing and dancing but pluck a five-string lyre and beat a log with a stick. They have no guns but use spears for hunting and fishing.

Medical history information was obtained from each of 541 unselected subjects ranging in age from 10 to 90 years. The status of the ear, nose, and throat and history of skull trauma, loss of consciousness, and previous diseases were noted. General physical and neurological examinations were administered, and systolic and diastolic blood pressures were measured for each patient.

Transistorized battery-powered audiometers were used for the audiometric tests. Experimental conditions were carefully controlled.

Rosen et al. compared the median hearing levels of the 10- to 70-year-old Mabaans to the hearing levels of corresponding age groups who were tested in the 1954 Wisconsin State Fair Hearing Survey (Glorig et al., 1957). In contrast to the results of the Wisconsin

State Fair Hearing Survey, where the median thresholds for men show a sharply decreasing sensitivity in hearing, especially at the high frequencies, all Mabaan decade-age groups had median hearing levels that fell within the first two decade median levels of the Wisconsin group. Although the differences between hearing levels of the Mabaan females and the Wisconsin females were not as dramatic as those for the males of the two samples, the data show that the Mabaan females do not experience deterioration of hearing as a function of age to the same degree as the sample of women examined in the Wisconsin study. Rosen et al. compared the results of the Mabaan study with those of three other American studies (Bunch, 1929; Steinberg et al., 1940; Webster et al., 1950), and the comparisons dramatically demonstrate the retention of auditory sensitivity among the Mabaans in contrast to the American samples examined.

What might account for the superior auditory sensitivity of the middle and upper age groups of the Mabaans in contrast to older individuals in American and other industrial societies? The following characteristics suggest some reasons for this superiority:

1. The Mabaan's acoustic environment is dramatically quieter at all times than the environments in those societies from which normative hearing data have been accumulated.
2. Vascular hypertension, coronary thrombosis, duodenal ulcer, ulcerative colitis, acute appendicitis, and bronchial asthma are unknown in the Mabaans.
3. The systolic and diastolic blood pressures of the Mabaans remain essentially unelevated from childhood to old age, whereas in the American population of apparently healthy individuals the blood pressure increases progressively with advancing age, especially in the fourth decade.
4. In addition to the effects of noise in modernized industrialized societies, high blood pressure and atherosclerosis of the small blood vessels to the inner ear may contribute to the deterioration of auditory sensitivity in the natural course of aging. Rosen et al. (1962) suggest that "Possibly the improved status of the non-atheromatous capillaries nourishing the cochlea, supports and maintains the structural integrity of the cochlea and prevents presbycusis with aging in the Mabaans. . . . Diet, climate, racial differences, genetic factors, etc., must also be considered (p. 741)."
5. The stress and strain experienced by individuals in modern complex societies are significantly less in the Mabaan people.
6. The diet of the Mabaans is monotonous by American standards and consists of carbohydrates, smaller amounts of protein, and very little fat. Rosen et al. state that the Mabaans eat fish cooked with okra and an oil extracted from the kernels of wild dates. They seldom eat citrus fruits, but they do eat nuts, corn, and dry, wild dates. The Mabaans appeared healthy and showed no signs of malnutrition, vitamin or protein deficiency.

1966 Mabaan Tribe Follow-up

In a subsequent report, Bergman (1966) examined the data from the original Mabaan study (Rosen et al., 1962) and compared the auditory sensitivity of several age groups in the Mabaans to the auditory sensitivity of equivalent age groups in four surveys conducted in the United States: Glorig et al. (1957), Eagles and Wishik (1961), Glorig and Nixon (1962), and Corso (1963a). A comparison of the median audiometric thresholds of the youngest Mabaans (10 to 19 years) with the median thresholds of 2175 otologically normal Pittsburgh children (Eagles & Wishik, 1961) revealed that the Pittsburgh children (ages 3 to 17) had better average sensitivity than the Mabaan children at all test frequencies. The median thresholds of the older Mabaans were compared to older subjects' thresholds in the United States surveys. Comparisons revealed that, as a function of age, the median thresholds of the older Mabaans did not increase as rapidly as the median thresholds of older subjects in the United States studies. However, the thresholds of the best hearers (top 10 percent) in the United States studies were equivalent to the best hearers in the Mabaan group. On the other hand, the poorest hearers (bottom 10 percent) in the United States studies showed a more rapid decrement in hearing with aging than the poorest hearers of the Mabaans. Bergman concludes that the greater stability of hearing thresholds in the aging Mabaans results from this group's marked population homogeneity.

Conclusion

Prior to the development of the pure-tone audiometer, the first empirical methods used to examine the relationship between auditory sensitivity and aging were carried out before the turn of the century by European researchers who showed keen insight into the relationship between hearing and aging. The first major study in the United States was in 1929 by Bunch, who used a pure-tone audiometer. Later, field studies were first conducted to examine the state of health of representative samples of the United States population. Subsequently, after World War II, most investigations of hearing sensitivity were motivated to a significant degree by the need for more information concerning the noxious effects of noise on hearing.

Data on hearing and aging gleaned from field studies reveal that:

1. Measurable changes in auditory sensitivity for high-frequency pure tones (4000–8000 Hz) occur by the fourth decade of life for men and women.
2. The variability in pure-tone thresholds, especially in the higher test frequencies, is greater for the older age groups than in the younger age groups.
3. Men lose auditory sensitivity in the higher frequencies more rapidly as a function of age than women do.
4. The noxious elements in our culture and the unique life-styles that people lead have a significant effect on the degree to which hearing sensitivity changes as a function of age.

TYPES OF PRESBYCUSIS

There is a considerable body of literature on presbycusis, its causes and effects. Either by explicit definition or by implication, writers have referred to presbycusis as *old-age deafness, the aging ear,* or as a decrease in auditory sensitivity that accompanies the normal course of living. The American National Standard Psychoacoustical Terminology defines *presbycusis* as "the natural loss in hearing sensitivity especially at high frequencies that results from the physiological changes that occur with age" (American National Standards Institute, 1973, p. 38).

The positive identification of presbycusis as a sole cause of loss of hearing sensitivity is difficult. The problem lies in what constitutes a "natural loss." It is well known that a variety of infectious diseases can destroy portions of the sensorineural system. Ototoxic drugs, noise, head trauma, and hereditary factors, among others, can result in loss of sensorineural sensitivity. The problem of establishing a precise cause-effect relationship between hearing loss and aging is epitomized by Fowler (1959):

> Severe strains, especially recurrent and continuing strains from emotional episodes, such as fright, grief and frustration, poisonous drugs such as quinine and the salicylates, some alkaloids, antibiotics (dihydro-streptomycin), over-exertions, bacterial and virus infections, acoustic, psychic and other traumas, electric shock, endocrine and metabolic disorders (hypothyroidism or hypometabolism), pregnancy, vitamin deficiencies, hyperoxia, hypoxia, exposure to cold, allergies, thromboses and vaso-spasms and many other disorders, have been observed to precede the onset of presbyacusis and for that matter other types of neural deafness, even total deafness. With few exceptions my presbyacusis patients give a history of somatopsychic strains correlated with the subsequent onset of their presbyacusis. (p. 766)

There is no doubt about the relationship between auditory sensitivity and aging. As has been pointed out, several laboratory and field studies have submitted conclusive evidence which shows that auditory sensitivity among individuals in "civilized" societies declines with age. However, Rosen et al. (1962) and Jarvis and van Heerden (1967) have indicated that the aging process, by itself, does not account for what is called presbycusic hearing loss in elderly people. Rosen et al. (1962) suggest that, in modern industrialized and technologically developed societies, there are factors in addition to age that must be considered. Among these factors is exposure to noise. Perhaps the effects of common drugs like nicotine, alcohol, caffeine, and over-the-counter pain remedies have an insidious effect on the well-being of the total neurophysiological system. Rosen, Olin, and Rosen (1970) suggest that diet and overall nutrition have an effect on the cardiovascular integrity of the system and that diet is related to loss of auditory sensitivity in old age. We know that loss of auditory function is not an inevitable accompaniment of the aging process. All of us are acquainted with elderly persons, even in their eighties or older, who have normal sensitivity for pure tones and normal processing for speech. However, the fact remains that there is a significantly larger proportion of elderly persons than younger persons who have socially significant hearing loss.

On the basis of histopathologic studies of the ears of several cats and humans with high-frequency hearing loss, Schuknecht (1955) concluded that there are two types of presbycusis: *epithelial atrophy* and *neural atrophy*. Epithelial atrophy is characterized by degenerative changes beginning at the basal end of the cochlear duct and proceeding toward the apex. These changes affect almost equally and simultaneously the various structures within the duct, including afferent and efferent nerve fibers. The audiometric correlate of epithelial atrophy is a sloping curve, similar to the presbycusic curves reported in the literature. Schuknecht states that neural atrophy is characterized by degeneration of spiral ganglion cells beginning at the basal end of the cochlea. There is also a decrease in the population of neurons in the pathways of the auditory nervous system. The audiometric correlate of neural atrophy is high-frequency hearing loss and a disproportionately more severe loss in speech discrimination than can be accounted for by the audiometric configuration.

In a subsequent report, Schuknecht (1964) summarized histopathological studies of the temporal bones of aging individuals and identified two other types of presbycusis. In addition to *sensory presbycusis* (previously called epithelial atrophy) and *neural presbycusis* (previously called neural atrophy), Schuknecht's third type is *metabolic pres-*

bycusis. This type results from atrophy of the stria vascularis, which is essential for the maintenance of bioelectric and biochemical properties of the endolymph. Alterations of these properties have a deleterious effect on the functional capacity of the cochlea. The entire scala media is affected, and the audiometric correlate is a flat audiometric curve, much like the one that characterizes Meniere's disease. More recently, Schuknecht (1974) has used the term *strial presbycusis* to identify the site of the morphological change in the aging person's auditory mechanism. The fourth type is *mechanical presbycusis,* which may be due to stiffening of the basilar membrane or some other mechanical disorder. The audiometric correlate is a descending audiometric curve. For this type of disorder, Schuknecht (1974) has proposed a substitute term, *cochlear conductive presbycusis,* which may result from a disorder in the motion mechanics of the cochlear duct. Although the cochleae of many individuals exhibit a rather pure atrophy of one of the types he has described, Schuknecht states that there are some cochleae that show a combination of these types. In these cases, the functional deficits appear to be additive.

Recently, two other categories of presbycusis have been described by Johnnson and Hawkins (1972). The first is *vascular presbycusis,* which is characterized by a loss of the minute blood vessels that supply the spiral ligament, stria vascularis, and the tympànic lip. The second is *central presbycusis,* in which there is a loss of neurons in the cochlear nucleus and in other sites in the central auditory system. Although categorization helps us understand the pathogenesis of presbycusis, Corso (1976) points out that the various types of presbycusis rarely, if ever, occur separately.

Not all of the ten terms that have been used above to identify types of presbycusis are mutually exclusive, and of those that are, two or more types may coexist. The degree of the neurological deficit in the auditory system determines to what degree the elderly person can perform on auditory tests and to what extent he or she can function adequately in oral communication environments.

AUDITORY PERFORMANCE AND AGING

The field studies reviewed thus far have established that deterioration of hearing accompanies aging. All of these studies have reported results of pure-tone tests applied to samples of the population. Since non-age-related variables such as prior noise exposure and otologic disease have not been controlled in these studies, other investigators have attempted to control for these variables in their study of hearing and aging.

Other tests of auditory performance include suprathreshold tests of speech discrimination (phonemic differentiation) in undistorted test conditions. Distorted tests of speech perception have also been used. Studies related to how the aged person processes undistorted and distorted speech have shed light on the nature of the deterioration in the aging auditory system.

Pure-Tone Sensitivity

If one wanted to identify age effects on hearing, one should isolate such effects from hereditary, environmental, and disease effects. Such a task is extremely difficult and has not been accomplished to date (Glorig, 1977). However, Glorig and Nixon (1960) attempted to control for some of these effects and screened 328 men from approximately 2000 professional and office-type employees. These 328 men had no presence or history

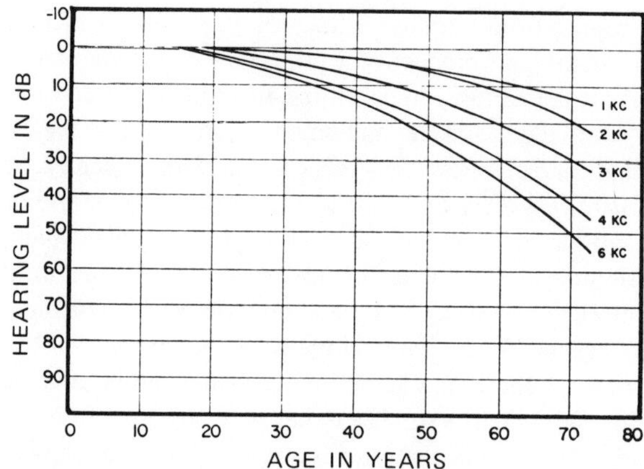

Fig. 17-1. Average hearing levels as a function of age of 328 males who reported negative otologic history and no exposure to high-level noise. (Reproduced with permission from Glorig, A., & Nixon, J. Distribution of hearing loss in various populations. *Annals of Otology, Rhinology, and Laryngology*, 1960, *69*, 502.)

of otological disease and no history of having been exposed to gunfire or noise levels high enough to make conversation difficult. Figure 17-1 shows the effect of age on hearing levels for several different frequencies within that study. The aging process reveals itself by changes in auditory sensitivity at 1000 Hz beginning at age 30. On the basis of these data, the rate of decrease in auditory sensitivity for 1000 Hz is about 3 dB for every 10 years of age through 70 years. For 6000 Hz, the decrease is approximately 10 dB for every 10 years through 70 years.

Much of the research on the effects of aging on hearing has been motivated by a need for identifying the presbycusic component in noise-induced hearing loss (Corso, 1976). In an effort to describe the presbycusic effect on auditory sensitivity for pure tones, Spoor (1967) analyzed the results of eight studies on pure tone thresholds as a function of age including those by Beasley (1938); Johansen (1943); the Z24-X-2 report of the American Standards Association (1954); Glorig et al. (1957) report of the 1954 Wisconsin State Fair; Hinchcliffe (1959); Jatho and Heck (1959); Glorig and Nixon (1962); and Corso (1963b). Because these studies reported hearing levels based on reference threshold levels (SPL) in effect prior to ANSI 1969, Lebo and Reddell (1972) applied corrections to Spoor's 1967 data in order to show presbycusic curves relative to the ANSI 1969 standard (American National Standards Institute, 1970). These curves are shown in Figure 17-2 for males and in Figure 17-3 for females. These curves show that reduction of auditory sensitivity as a function of age is frequency dependent. Pure-tone sensitivity for 250, 500, and 1000 Hz is approximately equivalent for males and females across decade-age groups, but males experience a more rapid decline in sensitivity than females for frequencies 2000 Hz and higher.

In interpreting the difference between the Lebo and Reddell (1972) and Glorig and Nixon (1960) data, some precautions are necessary. First, note that the Lebo-Reddell data are based on a number of studies where control for previous noise exposure was not consistently applied and that the hearing levels are re ANSI 1969. Second, the Glorig-Nixon hearing levels are based on thresholds measured with audiometers calibrated to

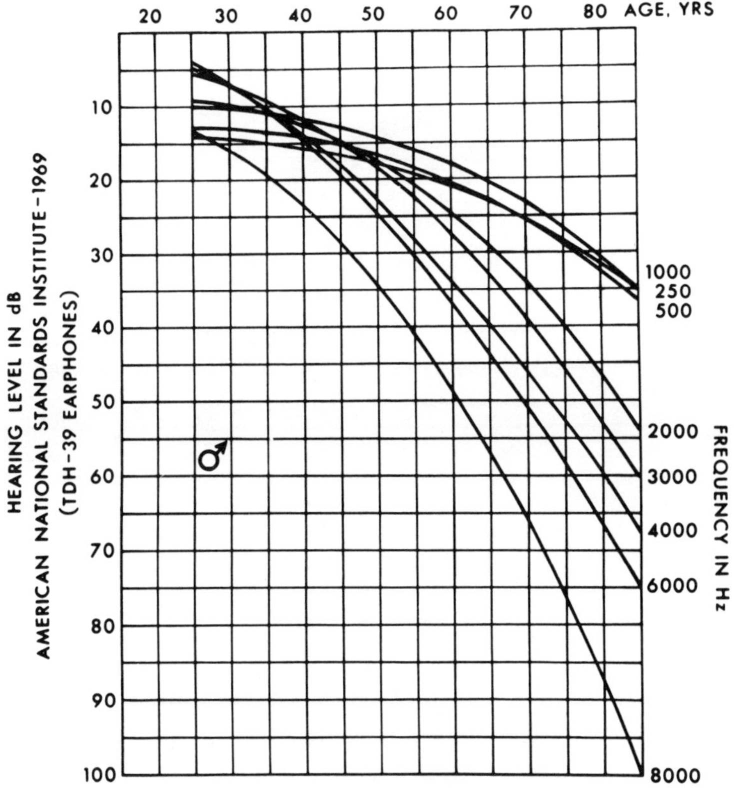

Fig. 17-2. Spoor's (1967) composite male presbycusic curves modified to conform to the ANSI 1969 standard. (Reproduced with permission from Lebo, C. P., & Reddell, R. C. The presbycusis component in occupational hearing loss. *Laryngoscope,* 1972, *82*, 1402.)

ASA 1951 reference threshold levels (American Standards Association, 1951). Nonetheless, if one were to apply corrections to the Glorig-Nixon data to account for the ASA 1951–ANSI 1969 differences in reference threshold levels, the superiority of the hearing of the non-noise-exposed males with negative history of otopathology would be even more marked than is evident from a comparison of Figures 17-1 and 17-2. The differences in the Lebo-Reddell and Glorig-Nixon data on hearing levels as a function of age highlight the effect of noise and other contaminating variables that exist in field studies of pure-tone sensitivity.

Most studies on the effects of aging and hearing have been cross-sectional studies. In contrast, Eisdorfer and Wilkie (1972) report on a seven-year follow-up study on 92 individuals initially seen at ages 60 to 79 years. Auditory sensitivity decreased during the seven-year period. The amound of decrease for the group that advanced in age from 67 to 74 years was equivalent to the decrease observed for the 75- to 82-year-old group. Women had better hearing than men at the higher frequencies. In contrast to the findings in the National Health Survey of 1960–62 (Glorig & Roberts, 1965), Eisdorfer and Wilkie (1972) found that blacks, and particularly black men, had more sensitive hearing than their white counterparts at the low as well as the high frequencies. Bunch and Raiford's (1931) pure-tone threshold data for white and black males and females show equivalent hearing for white and black females but older black men have better mean

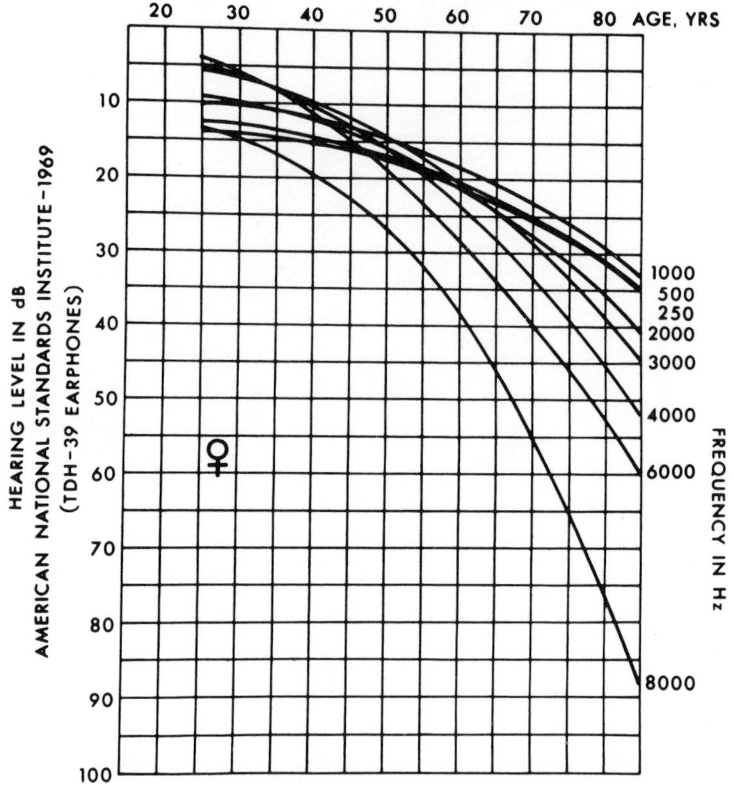

Fig. 17-3. Spoor's (1967) composite female presbycusic curves modified to conform to the ANSI 1969 standard. (Reproduced with permission from Lebo, C. P., & Reddell, R. C. The presbycusis component in occupational hearing loss. *Laryngoscope,* 1972, *82*, 1403.)

thresholds than older white men at test frequencies 4096 Hz and higher. The statistical significance of these differences is not reported by Bunch and Raiford. Eisdorfer and Wilkie (1972) suggest that the differences they observed probably reflect differences in previous history of exposure to noise. More definitive exploration of racial differences in hearing and aging is needed.

Examining the audiometric results of individual elderly hearing impaired persons highlights the obscuring effect of statistical estimates of central tendency. Although some audiometric findings reveal the classic presbycusic configuration, there are many exceptions. In examining a group of audiometric results of elderly people, one sees all types of configurations and all degrees of severity. The histories of these individuals also indicate a variety of possible etiologies, i.e., otitis media, administrations of quinine for malaria, mumps, mycin drug therapy, typhoid fever, noise exposure, physical trauma to the head, hearing loss in members of the family or in relatives, and so on.

Figures 17-4, 17-5, and 17-6 show sensorineural hearing loss in three elderly individuals. The pure-tone configurations as well as the degree of loss differ. Results of speech audiometry reveal that their ability to hear and process speech differs widely.

Patient A's results (Figure 17-4) indicate a marked degree of sensorineural hearing loss for high frequencies. Results of speech audiometry reveal that he has extreme difficulty in phonemic discrimination when tested with PB-K-50 word lists at suprathreshold

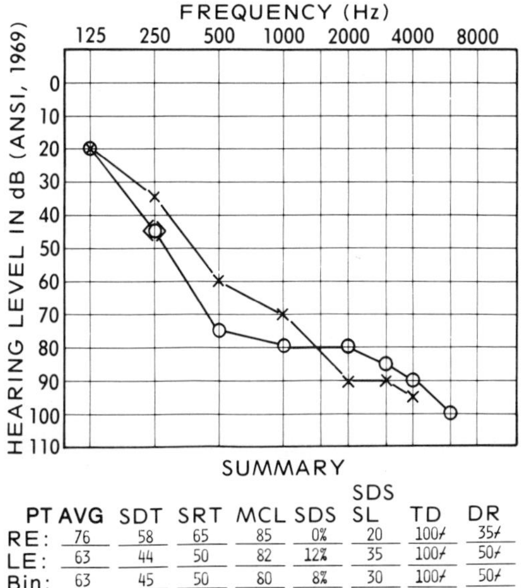

	PT AVG	SDT	SRT	MCL	SDS	SDS SL	TD	DR
RE:	76	58	65	85	0%	20	100+	35+
LE:	63	44	50	82	12%	35	100+	50+
Bin:	63	45	50	80	8%	30	100+	50+

Fig. 17-4. Audiometric results of Patient A, an 82-year-old male whose history includes noise exposure, vertigo, and recently, diabetes mellitus.

levels. Other test results indicate very poor speechreading ability and limited success with hearing aid use.

Patient B's audiometric results (Figure 17-5) show the characteristic presbycusic-type curve sloping downward from the low frequencies to the high frequencies. Speech audiometry shows speech-detection thresholds in the middle 20s, speech-reception thresholds in the middle 30s, and speech-discrimination scores (%NU-6) in the 60s. Although this patient had a lower-than-average threshold of discomfort, she had moderately good success with a hearing aid and a program of aural rehabilitation.

Patient C's results (Figure 17-6) show a flat, pure sensorineural audiometric contour. She reported a long-standing hearing loss, with onset prior to 40 years of age. Results show much usable residual hearing. Although she had tried to use two hearing aids during the past 10 years without success, she adjusted well to a hearing aid which was systematically used in a program of aural rehabilitation.

The audiometric results of the patients referred to in Figures 17-4, 17-5, and 17-6 demonstrate a number of things. First, the audiometric configuration of an elderly person may or may not resemble the classic presbycusic curve. The auditory sensitivity is dependent on a number of factors, including etiology and site(s) of lesion. Second, the degree of usable residual hearing will vary considerably among elderly hearing impaired persons. Carefully administered audiometric tests should reveal the amount of usable residual hearing. Third, the potential for success from aural rehabilitation is highly variable. Fourth, the degree of social handicap is related not only to auditory sensitivity but to suprathreshold performance with hearing aids.

Speech Discrimination

A major contribution to the literature on speech perception by elderly persons was made by Gaeth (Note 1). He examined the speech-discrimination (PB-50) ability of 27 subjects ranging in age from 43 to 79 years with a mean age of 65 years. His results

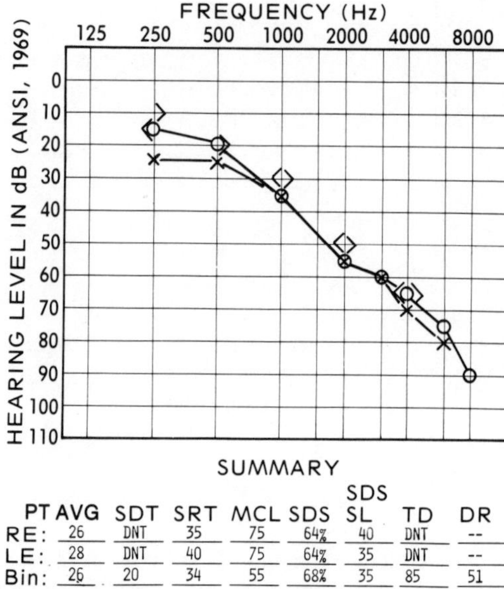

SUMMARY

	PT AVG	SDT	SRT	MCL	SDS	SDS SL	TD	DR
RE:	26	DNT	35	75	64%	40	DNT	--
LE:	28	DNT	40	75	64%	35	DNT	--
Bin:	26	20	34	55	68%	35	85	51

Fig. 17-5. Audiometric results of Patient B, an 81-year-old female whose history includes suppurative nephritis at age three or four years, typhoid fever as a teenager, and mastoidectomy at about age 50.

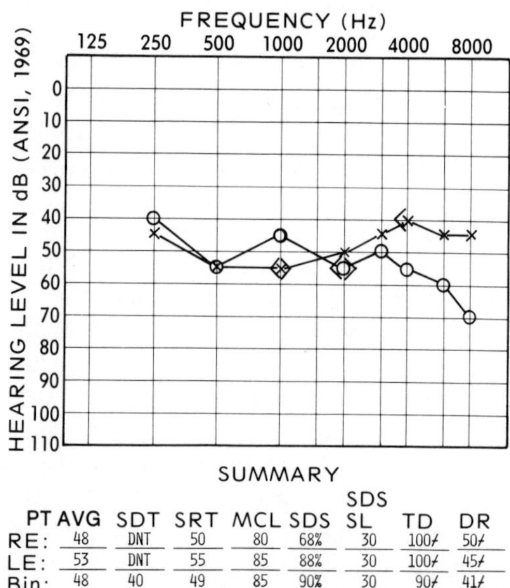

SUMMARY

	PT AVG	SDT	SRT	MCL	SDS	SDS SL	TD	DR
RE:	48	DNT	50	80	68%	30	100/	50/
LE:	53	DNT	55	85	88%	30	100/	45/
Bin:	48	40	49	85	90%	30	90/	41/

Fig. 17-6. Audiometric results of Patient C, a 67-year-old female whose significant history includes quinine therapy during childhood and quinine for malaria at age 35.

indicated that there are elderly individuals who have a more severe speech-discrimination difficulty than one would expect on the basis of the pure-tone threshold configuration. He termed this syndrome *phonemic regression.* The wisdom of the choice of the term has been argued by some writers. However, what Gaeth intended by the term related to problems in phoneme perception—a reduced ability in phonemic differentiation not accounted for by pure-tone threshold sensitivity.

Gaeth found that the differences in speech-discrimination performance were not related to age, duration of loss, educational or socioeconomic background, intellectual level, reaction-time scores, or accuracy and speed of performance on a cancellation test. He concluded that "phonemic regression may be related to a breakdown in the ability of the hearing mechanism to resolve the elemental aspects of sound."

Jerger's (1973) data show that when pure-tone threshold averages for 500–2000 Hz (presumably also SRT) are held constant, there is a systematic decrease in speech-discrimination scores as a function of age. His average scores vary from better than 90 percent for the 20- to 29-year-olds in a nonlinear fashion to about 60 percent for the 80- to 89-year-old group. This observation highlights the difference between two different dimensions of hearing—auditory sensitivity on the one hand and suprathreshold processing of speech on the other.

The aging auditory mechanism in an individual for whom there is no documentable otopathology undergoes subtle neurophysiological changes which may not be revealed by simple auditory detection tasks. Nor may these changes be revealed by significant difficulties in standard suprathreshold tasks of phoneme differentiation which are basic to speech-discrimination testing.

Discrimination of Distorted Speech

Elderly individuals who have close-to-normal sensitivity for continuous discourse often state that they have no problem in understanding speech in quiet situations, in one-to-one conversational situations, and when a talker speaks clearly. They state that when there is noise, when they are in groups, or when speakers have smoking apparatus in their mouths or otherwise speak inarticulately, they have difficulty understanding. These subjective reports have their corollary in audiologic test results. Pure-tone test results may show some mild degree of loss with slightly higher thresholds in the high frequencies. Speech-discrimination test results in quiet may reveal moderately good to good ability in phoneme differentiation. However, when the listening situation is made more difficult, that is, when noise is added to the speech signal, the older listener's performance deteriorates to a much greater degree than is observed for his or her younger counterpart.

Suprathreshold tests of speech perception examine a listener's ability to appreciate the linguistic significance of a sample of speech. Given a sufficiently high intensity of the signal, and given that the listener is linguistically competent for the task, speech materials can be used to examine the degree to which the auditory system transduces, conducts, and integrates the message for comprehension by the listener. The ability of the auditory system to deliver the message to the cortex is dependent on the integrity of the entire system. Fortunately, the normal auditory system has an overabundance of neuronal connections, a state which Bocca (1967) calls *neural redundancy* or *intrinsic redundancy*. Thus, a speech signal may be considerably distorted acoustically and yet it may be understood by the normal listener because the message is processed by a neurally redundant system and because the message has linguistic redundancy.

Linguistically, redundancy refers to ''that part of the message that can be eliminated without significant loss of information,'' (Sanders, 1971, p. 31) or, as Carroll (1964) states it, ''Redundancy is the property of texts that allows us to predict missing symbols from the context'' (p. 56). Miller (1951) accounts for three rules of language that can lead to redundancy: semantic, syntactic, and pragmatic. Bocca (1967) refers to linguistic redundancy as *extrinsic redundancy,* in contrast to *intrinsic* (neural) *redundancy*. Both intrinsic and extrinsic redundancy affect how well a listener, normal or hearing impaired, will understand a speech message. These redundancies allow a normal hearing person to understand a speech message even though it is considerably distorted from poor articulation of the speaker, grammatical inaccuracy, high levels of ambient noise, and so on. It follows, then, that to the degree that the aging auditory system has lost some of its intrinsic redundancy, reducing linguistic redundancy of speech messages should have a more deleterious effect on speech intelligibility of aging persons than on younger normal hearing persons. This is the implicit underlying hypothesis that has been tested in studies where distorted speech has been used in the examination of auditory performance of elderly persons.

The use of distorted speech as a stimulus for examining the integrity of the central auditory nervous system is described by Bocca and Calearo (1963). The kinds of distortion used for examining the integrity of the peripheral and central auditory system as a function of age have included broad-band white noise, competing messages (including simultaneous and overlapping speech), frequency filtering, temporal interruption, reverberation, time compression and expansion, and high levels of presentation. The effect of the articulation of the talker on the discrimination performance of older listeners has also been examined. The first application of distorted tests was in investigations of central lesions of the auditory system. Since the aging ear undergoes deterioration along all parts of the mechanism, a number of investigators have applied distorted speech tests to examinations of auditory performance as a function of aging.

Phoneme Perception in Noise

Smith and Prather (1971) tested phoneme perception in a group of subjects older than 60 years and in another group of younger subjects between 18 and 30 years. Both groups had normal hearing for the speech frequencies. Test stimuli included consonants in a CV context in six sensation levels of noise over four signal-to-noise ratios. Results showed that the older listeners performed significantly more poorly in all listening situations. However, there was no difference in the relative performance between the two groups as either the sensation level of the noise was increased or as the signal-to-noise ratio became poorer. This latter finding may relate to Bocca's observation that the use of nonmeaningful stimuli examines the integrity of the peripheral auditory mechanism and linguistically meaningful stimuli require processing by the central auditory mechanism.

Competing Messages

The effect of a competing message on the speech perception of older listeners is demonstrated by Orchik and Burgess (1977). They administered synthetic sentence (SSI) materials (Speaks & Jerger, 1965) to children, young adults, and older adults. The synthetic sentences were presented at 40 dB sensation level at five message-to-competition (MCR) ratios. The oldest listeners performed significantly more poorly than the two groups of younger listeners. The Orchik-Burgess data reveal the reduced ability of elderly persons to perceive sentences when competing speech is delivered at MCRs that are relatively innocuous for younger adults.

Frequency Filtering

The effect of frequency filtering on speech discrimination by elderly persons has been investigated by a number of authors (Kirikae, Sato, & Shitara, 1964; Harbert, Young, & Menduke, 1966; Frager (Note 2); Korsan-Bengsten, 1968; Palva & Jokinen, 1970; Marston & Goetzinger, 1972).

The following observations of these investigators are pertinent: (1) older listeners perform significantly more poorly than younger listeners under low-pass filter conditions; (2) when a low-band-pass signal is delivered to one ear and a higher-band-pass signal is fed to the other ear, deterioration in binaural synthesizing ability is evident by the fourth decade of life; (3) listeners who have experienced sensorineural (cochlear) hearing loss early in life perform better in binaural integration tasks than their older counterparts; and (4) elderly listeners with presbycusis perform much more variably on filtered speech tests than young listeners.

It is apparent from studies on binaural integration of speech signals that older persons vary widely in their performance. This variability suggests that the nature of the deterioration at the several levels of the central auditory system also varies in a correspondingly variable way.

Periodically Interrupted Speech and Reverberation

Periodically interrupting speech reduces the amount of information contained in the message. The degree to which such speech remains intelligible is related to the redundancy of that speech. Theoretically, if the intrinsic redundancy of the central auditory mechanism of a listener is reduced, such a listener should perform more poorly than a listener whose central auditory pathways are intact. This theoretical position has been supported by a number of authors.

Marston and Goetzinger (1972) administered periodically interrupted (eight times per second with a 50 percent duty cycle) CID Everyday Sentences to a group of subjects under 40 years of age and another group over age 40. The older subjects performed more poorly on the interrupted speech material than the younger group. Similar findings are reported by Bergman (1971), who used interrupted speech with subjects ranging in age from 20 to 89 years. These subjects had been screened so that none of them had pure-tone thresholds in excess of 35 dB (ISO 1964) for 500, 1000, and 2000 Hz or poorer than 40 dB at 4000 Hz. Bergman's interrupted speech resulted in decreases in scores of about 12 percent per decade-age group. Although the use of reverberated speech (reverberation time of 2.5 seconds) and overlapping speech (staggered spondees—Katz, 1962) also resulted in significantly poor performance among older listeners in contrast to younger listeners, interrupted speech showed the most deleterious effect on speech intelligibility by elderly listeners.

Effect of Rate and Precision of Articulation

It is often observed that older persons can understand our speech better if we slow down our rate of speech. These individuals apparently need more processing time. Calearo and Lazzaroni (1957) obtained speech intelligibility scores from young and elderly subjects when the rate of speech was 140 words per minute and 350 words per minute. The younger listeners maintained good intelligibility for the faster rate although a higher signal intensity was required. On the other hand, the aged listeners' intelligibility scores did not exceed 50 percent when the rate of 350 words per minute was used, irrespective of increases in signal intensity.

In addition to the effect of rate of speech on the speech perception of elderly persons, poor articulation by a talker affects speech intelligibility. Goetzinger, Proud, Dirks, and Embrey (1961) administered the CID W-22 test and the Rush Hughes recording of the PB-50 word lists to 90 subjects ranging in age from 60 to 90 years. The precision of articulation of the talker and the quality of the W-22 test are much better than the Rush Hughes recording. In effect, the Rush Hughes recording possesses distortion. Goetzinger et al. found that the difference scores between the W-22 test and the Rush Hughes recording increased as a function of age of the listeners. This finding is another example of the effect of reduced intrinsic redundancy of the older listeners' central auditory mechanisms.

Time Compression

Time compression is another method for distorting speech for the purpose of examining processing of speech as a function of age (Luterman, Welsh, & Melrose, 1966; Korsan-Bengsten, 1968; Sticht & Gray, 1969; Antonelli, 1970; Berruecos, 1970; Schon, 1970). Time-compressed speech reduces the amount of information conveyed by the message. The fact that normal listeners can maintain over 90 percent intelligibility for monosyllabic words when the words are time-compressed by as much as 50 percent (Beasley, Schwimmer, & Rintelmann, 1972) is additional evidence of the highly redundant nature of the normal auditory mechanism. Consistent with the application of other forms of distorted speech, time-compressed speech is perceived significantly more poorly by older listeners with auditory sensitivity considered to be "normal" for their age than by young normal listeners and by younger individuals with sensorineural hearing loss.

Speech Discrimination at High Presentation Levels

In routine clinical practice, it is customary to measure suprathreshold speech discrimination performance at some relatively high level—30 or 40 dB sensation level or at the most comfortable loudness level. Such a measurement provides us with a maximum discrimination score, that is, a score at a presentation level where the performance-intensity function (P-I function) has reached its asymptote. However, for listeners with certain retrocochlear lesions, the P-I function reveals a decrease in speech-discrimination scores when speech is presented at levels higher than the intensity at which the asymptote of the P-I function is reached (Jerger & Jerger, 1971). This reduction in performance has been referred to as the roll-over phenomenon.

Gang (1976) explored the presence of the roll-over phenomenon with a group of 32 male veterans aged 60 years and older. His subjects had pure-tone averages (500 to 2000 Hz) close to within normal range based on normative data proposed by Glorig and Roberts (1965). Data for the P-I functions were obtained by presentation of the CID Auditory Test W-22 at as many suprathreshold levels as possible until the maximum output of the speech audiometer was reached or until the subject's uncomfortable loudness level was reached. The P-I functions for these elderly listeners show that (1) the maximum discrimination score was not achieved until the presentation level was 50 dB SL, in contrast to Carhart's (1965) results that showed that normal listeners achieve PB Max at 25 dB SL; (2) the degree of roll over in the P-I function was significantly correlated with age—the older subjects demonstrating more severe roll over; and (3) of the subjects who demonstrated the most roll over, none had abnormal tone decay (interpreted as their not having retrocochlear pathology). In terms of communicative efficiency of elderly persons, Gang's (1976) results indicate that given increases in the intensity of monosyllables do not result in as much of an increase in intelligibility as is observed for younger normal listeners. Also, when the intensity of speech is increased beyond the point where maximum scores have been achieved, the intelligibility may decrease with increases in presentation levels.

As just described, the auditory performance of elderly hearing impaired persons is manifested in a variety of ways. However, it should be pointed out that reduced speech discrimination is not an inevitable accompaniment of aging. For example, Melrose, Welsh, and Luterman (1963) tested the hearing of 52 relatively healthy Spanish-American War veterans ranging in age from 74 to 89 years, with a mean age of 82 years. Three ears in this group had pure-tone thresholds within normal limits, and 30 percent of the ears yielded speech-discrimination scores (CID W-22 test) in excess of 90 percent.

RECENT FINDINGS ON CENTRAL AUDITORY FUNCTION IN AGING

Recent studies of higher auditory function and aging reveal new information that alters the manner in which auditory behaviors are being assessed in older adults, and which also alters our approaches to aural rehabilitation. As noted earlier, research on hearing and aging has demonstrated differences between younger and older persons in their responses to altered auditory stimuli. This has led to the conclusion that the ability to deal successfully with more difficult listening tasks declines with age. The locus of the decline appears to be the higher auditory centers of the brainstem and brain.

Recent studies by McCroskey and Davis (Note 3) and McCroskey (1979) have demonstrated that the amount of time required for temporal fusion becomes shorter as children age from 3 to 10 years. Temporal fusion appears to reach maximum efficiency at about 10 years of age and remains relatively constant through age 40. Beyond age 50, however, that ability steadily declines through the seventh decade. That is, more time is required for auditory fusion to occur. Their research revealed that at age 70 the length of time required for successful completion of auditory fusion tasks was identical to that required by three-year-old subjects (Kasten, 1981).

McCroskey and Kasten (1980) also examined the amount of time required for auditory fusion among elderly subjects, learning disabled children, and young normal subjects. Their results revealed that, for auditory fusion, the young normal subjects required the least amount of time, the learning disabled children required a significantly greater amount of time, and the elderly subjects required a significantly greater amount of time than the learning disabled subjects. This result led Kasten (Note 4) to hypothesize that some elderly persons, who demonstrate problems in auditory communication, process auditory signals in ways similar to those demonstrated by learning disabled children. As stated by Kasten (1981), it was interesting to note that Hull (Note 5)—drawing from a different data base—arrived at the same conclusion at the same time.

As stated earlier in this chapter, Bergman (1971)—and most recently in his 1980 text—has also concluded that the compounding factors in auditory function that lead to greater than expected problems in communication among the elderly involve a decline in function in the higher auditory pathways. These findings and those by Jerger (1973), and Hayes (1977), Feier and Gerstman (1980), and others also confirm a decline of central auditory function that accompanies aging. These findings lead one to conclude that changes may be warranted in the methods used for assessing communication function of older hearing impaired adults, in evaluation for the use of hearing aids, and in the processes involved in aural rehabilitation treatment of persons with this type of deficit. The aural rehabilitation aspect is discussed in Chapter 26. Bergman (1980) stated that it is the central functions of speech perception that attract those who would investigate age-related changes in the ability to communicate. Since the understanding of speech involves an intricate process—including expectancy, synthesis, selective attention, and many others—the fields of research in this area indeed are rich and include the anatomic, physiologic, assessment, and treatment aspects.

EVALUATING SOCIAL ADEQUACY OF HEARING

Simply stated, social adequacy of hearing refers to how well a hearing impaired person hears and understands speech in the everyday oral-communication situation. Granted, there are nonspeech sounds that enhance the aesthetic value of our acoustic environment and there are sounds that alert us to impending danger, but speech remains the single most important sound to which humans react and respond.

The social adequacy of hearing in the hearing impaired person is influenced by a number of interrelated characteristics in the listener. Perhaps the most obvious one is the sensitivity of the auditory system as measured by pure tones and by speech materials like spondees and conversational discourse. Given equivalent auditory sensitivity for speech, two hearing impaired listeners may have significantly different ability in speech discrimination or phonemic differentiation. Consider two hearing impaired persons. One has a mild degree of hearing in the low frequencies and an abrupt precipitous drop in the audiometric configuration after 1000 Hz. The other has equivalent loss in the low frequencies accompanied by relatively good hearing in the high frequencies. This person may have significantly better speech discrimination ability than the first person. Or, going one step further, another person may have good sensitivity for all pure tones from 250 Hz through 4000 Hz, but understanding suprathreshold level speech may be very poor because of central auditory-processing problems.

Further complicating the task of identifying the social adequacy of a given hearing impaired person are the innumerable characteristics that make that person unique. Hearing impaired persons differ in their need for oral communication. Life styles differ. Some are gregarious and some are loners. Motivation to listen, to attend, and to concentrate varies among individuals. Some people have excellent innate abilities to integrate and to synthesize nonverbal clues that accompany a speech-communication act. Others have limited ability. The adjustment of individuals varies widely. Some are able to take the hearing loss and its consequences in their stride. Others are affected emotionally to the point where ability to communicate is severely altered.

Efforts to assess social adequacy of hearing and to designate it by some type of statistical index have been made over the past 35 years. These efforts have been directed toward assessing the social adequacy of postlingually hearing impaired adults. Only recently has attention been given to elderly individuals' degree of hearing handicap. The following section summarizes some of the attempts that have been made to quantify social adequacy of hearing. Generally, these attempts have used questionnaires of one type or another, with the questions exploring the relative difficulty the respondent has in a variety of listening situations.

Early Attempts to Quantify Social Adequacy of Hearing

Hearing Attitude Scale

The first attempt to objectify the effect of hearing loss on adjustment (one aspect of social adequacy) was by Bronfenbrenner (1945) as reported by Levine (1960). The Bronfenbrenner Hearing Attitude Scale consists of 100 simply worded statements which describe possible reactions to situations involving hearing loss. The patient simply responds by circling either *agree* or *disagree*. Attitudes sampled by the statements include self-appraisal, depression, overoptimism, tension, reaction to rehabilitation, job worry, sensitivity, cover up, withdrawal, and eccentric reactions. The scale can be used as a clinical probe and interview guide, but is not appropriate in its present form for quantifying the attitudes of hearing impaired persons toward their hearing loss.

Although the Bronfenbrenner Hearing Attitude Scale does not constitute a measure of social adequacy of hearing, it does represent an early effort to examine one aspect of social adequacy—adjustment to hearing loss.

Performance-Intensity (P-I) Function

In an effort to predict and evaluate the social adequacy and inadequacy of patients on whom fenestration surgery was performed for otosclerosis, Walsh and Silverman (1946) proposed the application of the articulation function, i.e., the performance-intensity (P-I) function. These authors used the Harvard Psychoacoustic Laboratory PB-50 lists and administered them at three levels relative to the normal PB threshold: 20 dB (soft), 35 dB (conversational level), and 50 dB (loud). An average of these three discrimination scores provided a score or an "index" of the person's social adequacy. They suggested that an index of 50 (the 50 percent point on the P-I function) or better would represent restoration of the patient to social adequacy. It should be pointed out that in current practice we are not accustomed to making reference to "PB threshold" which, according to Davis (1948), occurs at 33 dB SPL for normal listeners.

Threshold of Social Adequacy

In a follow-up study of 161 patients on whom a fenestration operation had been performed, Silverman, Thurlow, Walsh, and Davis (1948) mailed questionnaires to obtain each patient's impression of the benefit of the surgery. The questionnaire included items on various oral-communication settings like person-to-person communication ability in quiet and in noisy situations and communication in noisy group settings and in large audiences such as lectures, movies, and church. On a five-point scale, respondents were asked to estimate their ability to understand speech prior to fenestration surgery and at periodic intervals through one year after the operation.

Other items in the questionnaire related to each patient's subjective reaction to surgery, information about hearing aid use, tinnitus, vertigo, and quality of speech during the first two months after the operation. The questionnaire ratings were analyzed to derive a *threshold of social adequacy,* a concept introduced earlier by Walsh and Silverman (1946). The threshold of social adequacy was that "value of the SAI (Social Adequacy Index) below which the patient would experience a serious social handicap from his deafness in half or more of his everyday situations.'' (Silverman et al., 1948, p. 612). As described by Davis (1948), the SAI is the average score of PB-50 words correctly identified at three presentation levels: 55 dB SPL (faint), 70 dB SPL (average), and 85 dB SPL (loud).

Later Scales and Indices

Other scales which have value in assessing social adequacy and communicative function are found in other chapters of this text. Among those are the Hearing Handicap Scale (HHS) by High, Fairbanks, and Glorig (1964). That scale has been extensively evaluated by Speaks, Jerger, and Trammel (1970), who found that the HHS scores did not correlate with measures of speech-discrimination ability. Blumenfeld, Bergman, and Miller (1969), however, did find that the HHS scores of a group of elderly subjects correlated with speech discrimination measured with the Rhyme Test (Fairbanks, 1958).

Scales which also appear to provide information relative to social adequacy of older hearing impaired persons include the Hearing Measurement Scale (Noble & Atherley, 1970), the Social Hearing Handicap Index (Ewertsen & Birk-Nielsen, 1973). The Ewertsen and Birk-Nielsen Index requires simple yes and no responses to 21 questions which query whether the respondent can or cannot understand speech in a variety of conversational situations. Other scales include the Denver Scale of Communication Function (Alpiner, Chevrette, Glascoe, Metz, & Olson, 1971), the Profile Questionnaire for Rating Communicative Performance (Sanders, 1975), the Denver Scale of Communication Function for Senior Citizens Living in Retirement Centers (Zarnoch & Alpiner, 1977), and the Nursing Home Hearing Handicap Index (Schow, Christensen, Hutchinson, & Nerbonne, 1978). The majority of these scales are discussed in detail in other portions of this text.

The most recent and most comprehensive effort to assess social adequacy of hearing has been reported by Giolas, Owens, Lamb, and Schubert (1979). Their Hearing Performance Inventory, in its experimental form, examines six categories of an individual's response to sound, including understanding speech, intensity, response to auditory failure, social, personal, and occupational. These categories are described as follows:

1. *Understanding speech* examines a person's ability to understand the speech of various talkers (men, women, and children) in a variety of communication situations.
2. *Intensity* explores a person's awareness (detection) of social and nonsocial sounds in the environment.
3. *Response to auditory failure* seeks to identify compensatory behavior when there is lack of understanding in a variety of talker-listener situations.
4. *Social* effects examines the person's ability to participate conversationally in a group of more than two persons convened primarily for recreation, including dining, conversing, playing games, and so on.
5. *Personal* seeks to determine how the respondent feels about his or her hearing impairment as it influences self-esteem and social interaction.
6. *Occupational* covers some of the dimensions within an occupational context. The questions are appropriate for persons who are currently employed or recently employed, and others who may be participating in activities similar to an occupational assignment, such as a student or a volunteer aide. If the questions are not relevant to a person's activities, the items are simply omitted.

Experimental Form II of the Hearing Performance Inventory consists of 158 items and, according to Giolas et al., can be administered in 30 to 45 minutes. The client responds to a written question, for example, "You are with a male friend or family member in a fairly quiet room. Can you understand him when his voice is loud enough for you and you can see his face?" The response sheet provides six alternatives: (1) practically always, (2) frequently, (3) about half the time, (4) occasionally, (5) almost never, and (6) does not apply. Although all of the items appear to be unambiguous, a clinician should be available to answer the respondent's questions and to elaborate on a given item, if necessary.

A revision of the Hearing Performance Inventory (HPI) was prepared in mimeographed form by Lamb, Owens, Schubert, and Giolas (Note 6). The lines of inquiry in the revised version are the same as in the 158-item form, but it has been reduced to 90 items. Because of its reduced length and shortened administration time, it is much more usable than the Experimental Form II of the HPI.

The inventory can be applied in several ways. First, a client's responses to items can be used as starting points for discussion. Second, responses by the hearing impaired person can be compared to those of a significant other person (spouse, friend, etc.). Third, the benefits of hearing aid use can be assessed by before and after measurements. Fourth, effects of aural rehabilitation therapy can be assessed over time.

COMMON FEATURES AMONG SCALES OF SOCIAL ADEQUACY OF HEARING

An analysis of the various attempts to describe or assess the social adequacy of hearing impaired persons reveals many common features among these assessment or measurement scales. The primary type of sound for which hearing performance is evaluated is, of course, speech. However, it is instructive to note the other kinds of sounds and listening experiences that are included in the several formalized scales and questionnaires that have been developed. The adequacy of auditory performance is related to ability to hear and understand:

1. Speech in a one-to-one situation in quiet
2. Speech in a one-to-one situation in noise
3. Speech in a group situation where there is relative quiet
4. Speech in a group situation where there is noise
5. A single talker in a theater, church, auditorium, or lecture hall
6. As distance between talker and listener varies
7. In a car, train, or bus
8. In varieties of noise
9. And recognize a speaker by his or her voice
10. Without speechreading (lipreading)
11. When precision of articulation of the talker varies
12. When a man versus a woman versus a child is the talker
13. Phone conversation
14. A radio, TV, or record player

The assessment of social adequacy of hearing is multifaceted and complex but it is imperative that such an assessment be made. An understanding of the unique characteristics of the social adequacy and inadequacy of the hearing impaired person can help the clinician to plan and to carry out more relevant and meaningful aural rehabilitation.

REFERENCES

Alpiner, J. G., Chevrette, W., Glascoe, G., Metz, M., & Olsen, B. The Denver Scale of Communication Function. Unpublished study, University of Denver, 1971. (Cited in Alpiner, J. G. Evaluation of communication function, in J. G. Alpiner (Ed.), *Handbook of adult rehabilitative audiology,* Baltimore: Williams & Wilkins Co., 1978, pp. 30–66.)

American National Standards Institute. American national standard psychoacoustical terminology, ANSI S3.20-1973. New York: American National Standards Institute, 1973.

American National Standards Institute. American national standard specifications for audiometers, ANSI S3.6-1969. New York: American National Standards Institute, 1970.

American Standards Association. American standard specification for audiometers for general diagnostic purposes, Z24.5-1951. New York: American Standards Association, 1951.

American Standards Association. Exploratory subcommittee Z24-X-2; The relations of hearing loss to noise exposure. New York: American Standards Association, 1954.

Antonelli, A. R. Sensitized speech tests in aged people, in C. Røjskjaer (Ed.), *Speech Audiometry.* Second Danavox Symposium, Odense, Denmark, 1970, pp. 66–78.

Atherley, G. R. C., & Noble, W. G. Clinical picture of occupational hearing loss obtained with the Hearing Measurement Scale, in D. W. Robinson (Ed.), *Occupational hearing loss.* New York: Academic Press, 1971, pp. 183–206.

Beasley, D. S., Schwimmer, S., & Rintelmann, W. F. Intelligibility of time-compressed CNC monosyllables. *Journal of Speech and Hearing Research,* 1972, *15,* 340–350.

Beasley, W. C. Characteristics and distribution of impaired hearing in the population of the United States. *Journal of the Acoustical Society of America,* 1940, *12,* 114–121.

Beasley, W. C. Hearing study series bulletin no. 7, National Health Survey. National Institute of Health, United States Public Health Service, 1938.

Bergman, M. Hearing and aging: Implications of recent research findings. *Audiology,* 1971, *10,* 164–171.

Bergman, M. Hearing in the Mabaans. A critical review of related literature. *Archives of Otolaryngology,* 1966, *84,* 411–415.

Bergman, M. *Aging and the perception of speech.* Baltimore: University Park Press, 1980.

Berruecos, P. Jr. Binaural temporal integration in presbyacusis. *International Audiology,* 1970, *9,* 309–313.

Bezold, F. Investigations concerning the average hearing power of the aged. *Archives of Otology,* 1894, *23,* 214–227.

Blumenfeld, V., Bergman, M., & Millner, E. Speech discrimination in an aging population. *Journal of Speech and Hearing Research,* 1969, *12,* 210–217.

Bocca, E. Distorted speech tests, in A. B. Graham (Ed.), *Sensorineural hearing processes and disorders.* Boston: Little, Brown and Co., 1967, pp. 359–370.

Bocca, E., & Calearo, C. Central hearing processes, in J. Jerger (Ed.), *Modern developments in audiology.* New York: Academic Press, 1963, pp. 337–370.

Bronfenbrenner, U. The psychological program in the Army Hearing Center at Borden General Hospital. Unpublished study, 1945. (Cited in Levine, E. S. *The psychology of deafness.* New York: Columbia University Press, 1960, pp. 258–265.)

Bunch, C. C. Age variations in auditory acuity. *Archives of Otolaryngology,* 1929, *9,* 625–636.

Bunch, C. C., & Raiford, T. S. Race and sex variations in auditory acuity. *Archives of Otolaryngology,* 1931, *13,* 423–434.

Calearo, C., & Lazzaroni, A. Speech intelligibility in relation to the speed of the message. *Laryngoscope,* 1957, *67,* 410–419.

Carhart, R. Problems in the measurement of speech discrimination. *Archives of Otolaryngology,* 1965, *82,* 253–260.

Carroll, J. B. *Language and thought.* Englewood Cliffs, New Jersey: Prentice-Hall, Inc., 1964.

Corso, J. F. Aging and auditory thresholds in men and women. *Archives of Environmental Health,* 1963, *6,* 350–356 (a).

Corso, J. F. Age and sex differences in pure-tone thresholds. Survey of hearing levels from 18 to 65 years. *Archives of Otolaryngology,* 1963, *77,* 385–405 (b).

Corso, J. F. Presbycusis as a complicating factor in evaluating noise-induced hearing loss, in D. Henderson, R. P. Hamernik, D. S. Dasanjh, & J. H. Mills (Eds.), *Effects of noise on hearing.* New York: Raven Press, 1976, pp. 497–524.

Davis, H. The articulation area and the social adequacy index for hearing. *Laryngoscope,* 1948, *58,* 761–778.

Eagles, E. L., & Wishik, S. M. A study of hearing in children. I. Objectives and preliminary findings. *Transactions of the American Academy of Ophthalmology and Otolaryngology,* 1961, *65,* 261–282.

Eisdorfer, C., & Wilkie, F. Auditory changes in the aged: A follow-up study. *Journal of the American Geriatrics Society,* 1972, *20,* 377–382.

Ewertsen, H. W., & Birk-Nielsen, H. Social hearing handicap index. Social handicap in relation to hearing impairment. *Audiology,* 1973, *12,* 180–187.

Fairbanks, G. Test of phonemic differentiation: The Rhyme Test. *Journal of the Acoustical Society of America,* 1958, *30,* 596–600.

Feier, C. D., & Gerstman, L. J. Sentence comprehension abilities throughout the adult age span. *Gerontology,* 1980, 35, 722–728.

Fowler, E. P. Presbyacusis—the aging ear. *Annals of Otology, Rhinology and Laryngology,* 1959, *68,* 764–776.

Gang, R. P. The effects of age on the diagnostic utility of the roll-over phenomenon. *Journal of Speech and Hearing Disorders,* 1976, *41,* 63–69.

Giolas, T. G., Owens, E., Lamb, S. H., & Schubert, E. E. Hearing performance inventory. *Journal of Speech and Hearing Disorders,* 1979, *44,* 169–195.

Glorig, A. Auditory processing and age, in Proceedings of a conference at the Dallas Geriatric Research Institute, Sensory Processes and Aging. Denton, Texas: University Center for Community Services, North Texas State University, 1977, pp. 39–60.

Glorig, A. Some medical implications of the 1954 Wisconsin State Fair Hearing Survey. *Transactions of the American Academy of Ophthmology and Otolaryngology,* 1957, *61,* 160–169.

Glorig, A., & Nixon, J. Distributions of hearing loss in various populations. *Annals of Otology Rhinology and Laryngology,* 1960, *69,* 497–516.

Glorig, A., & Nixon, J. Hearing loss as a function of age. *Laryngoscope,* 1962, *72,* 1596–1610.

Glorig, A., & Roberts, J. Hearing levels of adults by age and sex. United States 1960–62. Public Health Service Publicaion No. 1000, Series 11, No. 11. USGPO, Washington, D.C., 1965.

Glorig, A., & Wheeler, D. E. Historical record of the Wisconsin State Fair Hearing Survey—1954. *Noise Control,* 1955, vol. 1, no. 6, 18–25.

Glorig, A., Wheeler, D., Quiggle, R., Grings, W., & Summerfield, A. *1954 Wisconsin State Fair survey—Statistical treatment of clinical and audiometric data,* (Monograph). American Academy of Ophthalmology and Otolaryngology, 1957.

Goetzinger, C. P., Proud, G. O., Dirks, D., & Embrey, J., A study of hearing in advanced age. *Archives of Otolaryngology,* 1961, *73,* 662–674.

Harbert, F., Young, I., & Menduke, H. Audiologic findings in presbycusis. *Journal of Auditory Research,* 1966, *6,* 297–312.

High, W., Fairbanks, G., & Glorig, A. Scale of self-assessment of hearing handicap. *Journal of Speech and Hearing Disorders,* 1964, *29,* 215–230.

Hinchcliffe, R. The threshold of hearing as a function of age. *Acustica,* 1959, *9,* 303–308.

International Organization for Standardization. ISO Recommendation R389—Standard reference zero for the calibration of pure tone audiometers, ISO/R 389-1964 (E). Switzerland: International Organization for Standardization, 1964.

Jarvis, J. F., & van Heerden, H. G. The acuity of hearing in the Kalahari bushmen. *Journal of Laryngology and Otology,* 1967, *81,* 63–68.

Jatho, K., & Heck, K. H. Schwellen audiometrische Untersuchungen Uber die Progredienz und Charakteristik der Alterschwerhörigkeit in den verschiedenen Lebensabschnitten. *Zeitschrift* fuer Larngologie, Rhinologie, Otologie und Ihre Grenzgebiete, 1959, *38,* 72. (Cited in Spoor, A. Presbycusis values in relation to noise induced hearing loss. *International Audiology,* 1967, *6,* 48–57.)

Jerger, J. Audiological findings in aging. *Advances in Oto-Rhino-Laryngology,* 1973, *20,* 115–124.

Jerger, J. F., & Hayes, D. Diagnostic speech audiometry. *Archives of Otolaryngology,* 1977, *103,* 216–222.

Jerger, J. F., & Jerger, S. Diagnostic significance of PB word functions. *Archives of Otolaryngology,* 1971, 93, 573–580.

Johansen, H., Den Aldersbetingede Tunghørhed, Munksgaard, Kobenhavn, 1943. (Cited in Spoor, A. Presbycusis values in relation to noise induced hearing loss. *International Audiology,* 1967, *6,* 48–57.)

Johnsson, L. G., & Hawkins, J. E., Jr. Sensory and neural degeneration with aging, as seen in microdissections of the human inner ear. *Annals of Otology, Rhinology, and Laryngology,* 1972, *81*, 179–193.

Kasten, R. N. The impact of aging on auditory perception, in R. H. Hull (Ed.), *The communicatively disordered elderly.* New York: Thieme-Stratton, Inc., 1981.

Katz, J. The use of staggered spondaic words for assessing the integrity of the central auditory nervous system. *Journal of Auditory Research,* 1962, *2*, 327–337.

Kirikae, I., Sato, T., & Shitara, T. A study of hearing in advanced age. *Laryngoscope,* 1964, *74*, 205–220.

Korsan-Bengtsen, M. The diagnosis of hearing loss in old people, in G. Liden (Ed.), *Geriatric Audiology.* Stockholm: Almquist & Wiksell, 1968, pp. 24–36.

Lebo, C. P., & Reddell, R. C. The presbycusis component in occupational hearing loss. *Laryngoscope,* 1972, *82*, 1399–1409.

Levine, E. S. *The psychology of deafness.* New York: Columbia University Press, 1960.

Luterman, D. M., Welsh, O. L., & Melrose, J. Responses of aged males to time-altered speech stimuli. *Journal of Speech and Hearing Research,* 1966, *9*, 226–230.

Marston, L. E., & Goetzinger, C. P. A comparison of sensitized words and sentences for distinguishing non-peripheral auditory changes as a function of aging. *Cortex,* 1972, *8*, 213–223.

McCroskey, R. L. Some characteristics of temporal auditory behavior among elderly persons, in M. A. Henoch (Ed.), *Aural rehabilitation of the elderly,* New York: Grune & Stratton, 1979.

McCroskey R. L. & Kasten R. N. Assessment of central auditory processing, in R. R. Rupp & K. Stockdell (Eds.), New York: Grune & Stratton, in press.

Melrose, J., Welsh, O. L., & Luterman, D. M. Auditory responses in selected elderly men. *Journal of Gerontology,* 1963, *18*, 267–270.

Miller, G. A. *Language and communication.* New York: McGraw-Hill Book Co. Inc., 1951.

National Institute of Health. Hearing Study Series Bulletins 1–7, The National Health Survey, 1935–36, preliminary reports. Public Health Service, Washington, D.C., 1938.

Noble, W. G., & Atherley, G. R. C. The Hearing Measurement Scale: A questionnaire for the assessment of auditory disability. *Journal of Auditory Research,* 1970, *10*, 229–250.

Orchik, D. J. & Burgess, J. Synthetic sentence identification as a function of age of the listener. *Journal of American Audiology Society,* 1977, *3*, 42–46.

Palva, A., & Jokinen, K. Presbyacusis. V. Filtered speech tests. *Acta Otolaryngologica,* 1970, *70*, 232–241.

Rosen, S., Bergman, M., Plester, D., El-Mofty, A., & Satti, M. H. Presbycusis study of a relatively noise-free population in the Sudan. *Annals of Otology, Rhinology, and Laryngology,* 1962, *71*, 727–743.

Rosen, S., Olin, P., & Rosen, H. V. Dietary prevention of hearing loss. *Acta Otolaryngologica,* 1970, *70*, 242–247.

Sanders, D. A. Aural rehabilitation. Englewood Cliffs, New Jersey: Prentice-Hall, 1971.

Sanders, D. A. Hearing aid orientation and counseling, in M. C. Pollack (Ed.), *Amplification for the hearing-impaired.* New York: Grune & Stratton, 1975, pp. 323–372.

Schon, T. D. The effects on speech intelligibility of time compression and expansion on normal-hearing, hard of hearing, and aged males. *Journal of Auditory Research,* 1970, *10*, 263–268.

Schow, R. L., Christensen, J. M., Hutchinson, J. M., & Nerbonne, M. A. *Communication disorders of the aged: A guide for health professionals.* Baltimore: University Park Press, 1978.

Schuknecht, H. F. Further observations on the pathology of presbycusis. *Archives of Otolaryngology,* 1964, *80*, 369–382.

Schuknecht, H. F. *Pathology of the ear.* Cambridge, Massachusetts: Harvard University Press, 1974.

Schuknecht, H. F. Presbycusis. *Laryngoscope,* 1955, *65*, 402–419.

Silverman, S. R., Thurlow, W. R., Walsh, T. E., & Davis, H. Improvement in the social adequacy of hearing following the fenestration operation. *Laryngoscope,* 1948, *58*, 607–631.

Smith, R. A., & Prather, W. F. Phoneme discrimination in older persons under varying signal-to-noise conditions. *Journal of Speech and Hearing Research,* 1971, *14*, 630–638.

Speaks, C., & Jerger, J. Method for measurement of speech identification. *Journal of Speech and Hearing Research,* 1965, *8*, 185–194.

Speaks, C., Jerger, J., & Trammell, J. Measurement of hearing handicap. *Journal of Speech and Hearing Research,* 1970, *13*, 768–776.

Spoor, A. Presbycusis values in relation to noise induced hearing loss. *International Audiology,* 1967, *6*, 48–57.

Steinberg, J., Montgomery, B., & Gardner, M. Results of the World's Fair Survey. *Journal of the Acoustical Society of America,* 1940, *12*, 291–301.

Sticht, T. G., & Gray, B. B. The intelligibility of

time compressed words as a function of age and hearing loss. *Journal of Speech and Hearing Research,* 1969, *12*, 443–448.

Walsh, T. E., & Silverman, S. R. Diagnosis and evaluation of fenestration. *Laryngoscope,* 1946, *56*, 536–555.

Webster, J. C., Himes, H. W., & Lichtenstein, M. San Diego County Fair hearing survey. *Journal of the Acoustical Society of America,* 1950, *22*, 473–483.

Zarnoch, J. M., & Alpiner, J. G. The Denver Scale of Communication Function for Senior Citizens Living in Retirement Centers. Unpublished study. University of Denver. (Cited in Alpiner, J. G. Rehabilitation of the geriatric client, in J. G. Alpiner (Ed.), *Handbook of adult rehabilitative audiology,* Baltimore: Williams & Wilkins Co., 1978, pp. 141–171.)

Zwaardemaker, H. Der Verlust an hohen Tönen mit zunehmendem Alter. Ein neues Gesetz. *Archiv für Ohrenheilkunde,* 1891, *32*, 53–56.

Zwaardemaker, H. The presbycusic law. *Archives of Otology,* 1894, *23*, 228–234.

REFERENCE NOTES

1. Gaeth, J. H. A study of phonemic regression associated with hearing loss. Ph.D. dissertation, Northwestern University, Evanston, Illinois, 1948.
2. Frager, C. R. Auditory integration in geriatrics. Masters thesis, Colorado State University, Fort Collins, Colorado, 1968.
3. McCroskey, R. L., & Davis, S. M. Auditory fusion-developmental trend. Scientific exhibit at the American Speech and Hearing Association, Houston, 1976.
4. Kasten, R. N. Differential diagnosis of language based factors in presbycusis. Paper presented at the Aspen Symposium on Aging, Colorado, July, 1980.
5. Hull, R. H. Aural rehabilitation treatment for the older adult: A new look at an old subject. Paper presented at the Aspen Symposium on Aging, Colorado, July, 1980.
6. Lamb, S. H., Owens, E., Schubert, E. D., & Giolas, T. G. *Hearing Performance Inventory, revised form* (mimeo). San Francisco State University, 1979.

James F. Maurer

Chapter 18: The Psychosocial Aspects of Presbycusis

THE EQUIVOCAL NATURE OF AGING

The typical masthead of an audiological assessment form calls for the client's name, address, and birth date or age. These data serve to identify the individual. They also represent the individual in the sense that certain information tends to take the client's place during report writing and rehabilitation planning. Age is a prime example. Decisions are made about the person because he or she is elderly. Even the diagnosis of "presbycusis" is inextricably associated with numbers representing longevity. Reaching the seventh decade of life evokes categorical assumptions about the hearing impaired person.

Consider for a moment a revised masthead which not only reflects chronological age, but biological, experiential, and psychosocial age as well. Mr. Smith has a chronological age of 76 years, but in all other respects he is 55 years old. How would this additional information alter our assumptions and attitudes about this "elderly" client? What courses of action might be changed insofar as direction and prognosis of intervention are concerned?

The relationship between chronological age and factors that produce aging is, at best, a disparate one. Although systemic changes do occur with advancing years, they are not invariably associated with longevity; moreover, the capacity to adapt to these changes is highly individual (Atchley, 1972; Birren, 1959). An older person is the summed products of *biological aging* (which is forged by genetic programming), *experiential aging* (shaped by lifestyle and environmental forces), and *psychosocial aging* (as reflected by adaptive behaviors and social output). The interaction of these three forces across the population spectrum of persons 65 years of age and older is complex and infinitely variable. Some individuals advance into their seventies with all the good health and perspicacity of young adults; others seem to resemble the stereotype of "old age" in their fifties. The variables associated with such extreme individual differences are well worth considering, since by the year 2000 one in eight persons in the United States will be a member of the "aging society," (i.e., 65 and older) (U.S. Bureau of

Census, 1976). In addition, they provide a foundation for understanding the consequences of hearing impairment on this heterogeneous population.

Biological Aging

Human aging occurs at the biological level as a result of decreased cellular functioning. Certain cells may be programmed to cease functioning within a specific genetic time frame, or they may fail to divide because of a gradual accumulation of waste products which impair their function. Entire body systems are affected. For example, the nervous system experiences a gradual attrition of brain cells (Brody, 1973), which may account for the slowing of neuron discharge speed and for short-term memory problems; the endocrine system becomes increasingly inefficient, affecting rate of metabolism and lowering resistance to stress and disease (Rockstein, 1975).

Experiential Aging

Experiential aging refers to the lifetime of abuses that have become cumulative in the older person. Injuries, toxic exposures, and disease processes all contribute to physical deterioration in later life. Body systems fail to sustain the recuperative proficiency of youth and are more prone to dysfunction because of insults acquired during earlier years. Long-term exposure to intense levels of noise, for example, precipitates a sensory hearing disability that is compounded by the deafness of old age.

Psychosocial Aging

Psychosocial theories of aging, which have generated considerable research among gerontologists, recognize the immutable forces of physiological decline that mark senescense. They also probe in other directions, however, in order to account for individual adaptations to longevity.

It seems likely that aging is a multidimensional phenomenon in which biological, experiential, and psychosocial forces interact in unique ways with the later stages of human chronology. Some illnesses occurring during later life—atherosclerosis, for example—seem to have a genetic/experiential basis (Goldstein, Schrott, Hazzard, Bierman, & Motulsky, 1973), whereas others, such as duodenal ulcers, exhibit both hereditary and psychosocial determinants (Mirsky, 1958). Some psychosocial states, such as disengagement, can be traced to experiential factors, such as poverty, but without ignoring the biological capacity of the individual to maintain relationships. While the process of growing older is inevitably accompanied by degenerative physical changes, environmental influences also play a prominent role. Life satisfaction indices reported by the elderly support the concept that perceived health status, financial conditions, and activity level of the individual are the three most important factors relating to self-fulfillment (Edwards & Klemmack, 1973; Neugarten, Havighurst, & Tobin, 1961). These three correlates of life satisfaction should be kept in mind as we focus on some of the sensory experiences that undergo change with advancing years.

THE INTERACTION OF HEARING IMPAIRMENT WITH LIFE FORCES

A hearing handicap experienced during the later years of life represents more than an imposition on the ability of the individual to communicate receptively. For many, it represents the superimposition of degraded auditory reception on a small galaxy of concomitant problems, ranging from other sensory deficits to necessary changes in life style. Presbycusis compounds the consequences of coexisting physical and social limitations. Psychiatrist Robert Butler describes it as "potentially the most problematical of the perceptual impairments, (because) it can reduce reality testing and lead to marked suspiciousness, even paranoia." (Butler & Lewis, 1973, p. 30). Stress factors that interface with this handicap may be allocated to one of three categories: co-existing health problems and impairments, environmental stimulation, and financial status and mobility. Specific psychosocial problems arising from presbycusis together suggest that these categories are, more often than not, interrelated.

Coexisting Health Problems and Impairments

Nearly 35 percent of the population 65 years of age and older have disabilities which hamper their capacity to work, keep house, or engage in other major activities (Riley & Foner, 1968). The incidence of multiple handicaps is highest within this aging segment. As one elderly woman stated with resignation after putting on her hearing aid for the first time, "Well, I suppose this thing will go along with my dentures, glasses, and support brace. It's getting so it takes me *half* the morning to make myself *whole*!" (Maurer, 1976, p. 72). Each new physical problem that the older person encounters is another grim reminder that the body system is failing and that remaining years are numbered.

Reporting on the intervention needs of aged persons in a chronic disease hospital, Smith (1977) noted that current health status was of major importance in the success or failure of aural rehabilitation and that other physical limitations seemed to carry more importance than the severity of the auditory problem. An unfortunate paradox exists among a number of elderly people who have suffered traumatic interruptions in expressive communication due to stroke or laryngectomy, and whose auditory skills have not even been investigated. The interaction between hearing impairment and disabling conditions that are nonauditory is often ignored.

> The daughter of a hearing impaired elderly woman, who had just undergone earmold impressions, was overheard announcing to the clinic office staff, "Be sure and call her when the earmolds are returned from the laboratory, and let the phone ring at least seven or eight times. She usually sits in the living room of her apartment, and it takes her that long to get there."

It never occurred to either of them to move the telephone!

Health concerns are very close to the surface among the elderly. One old gentleman with an arrhythmic heart condition and severe loss of hearing sensitivity returned his body-type aid to the clinic in a state of stress; it was amplifying his irregular heartbeat. Fortunately, the auditory contribution to his anxiety could be solved with postauricular hearing aids. Another elderly man, however, related the effects of coexisting visual and hearing problems: "I used to watch TV until my eyes went bad, then I took to listening to the ball games on the radio until my ears started to fail. Now, about all I can do is sit and think."

Environmental Stimulation

Location

No environment is a conducive one for persons with hearing impairments, some are simply better than others. The institutionalized aging (which comprise approximately 5 percent of the entire population) reside in environments that would seem to be basically antagonistic to human communication. However, many senior adult centers also fall into this category. Moriarity (Note 1) surveyed 25 group-living environments for the elderly, including nursing homes, high-rise apartments, extended-care facilities, and senior adult centers. He concluded that

1. Most of the facilities were located in high-traffic areas, where average outside noise levels exceeded that of normal conversational speech
2. Most were poorly insulated against the intrusion of outside noise
3. Only 4 of the 25 facilities were adequately equipped with acoustic tile, drapes, and carpeting to dampen inside noise
4. Nearly half of the buildings contained inside noise-producing sources, such as vibrating fans and kitchen and laundry appliances, which were in close proximity to both recreation and meeting areas

Too few places of worship have been architecturally designed to accommodate individuals with presbycusis.

> Vaulted ceilings, resonating walls, and a general absense of acoustical treatment can create a pandemonium of unintelligibility for the hearing impaired, one that may be enhanced by too distant, wall-mounted speakers. Sanctuaries that provide pew speakers which are energized directly from the pulpit microphone provide some assistance, as do certain closed-loop amplification systems which, operating in conjunction with the telephone coil on individually worn hearing aids, also eliminate some of the background noise. Fortunately for most elderly worshippers, the familiarity of the message content may be the greatest blessing (Maurer, 1976, p. 69).

Private residences of low-income, aging persons often are located in heavily populated urban areas where intrusion from outside noise sources is common. A sample of 100 such residents who moved from private dwellings to quality high-rise apartments were questioned about changes in the extent of unwanted sound. Fifty-one percent reported quieter sound levels in their new apartments, and nearly all indicated increased life satisfaction (Note 2).

Social Interactions

The nucleus of individuals associated with the handicapped older person in the living environment is a key ingredient in psychosocial adjustment. What Comfort (Note 3) described as "childrenization" of the elderly all too frequently occurs within family constellations in private residences and among staff members in collective environments. That is, there is a tendency to regard the older person from the standpoint of his or her age—elderly—rather than what he or she needs. This attitude, when associated with ignorance about the problems of hearing impairment, may lead to dangerous misconceptions about individuals and social communicative potential. As Hull (1973) has observed,

> Hearing impairment, as seen by the "lay person," is often mislabeled as senility because the elderly person will often times respond to questions or statements with wrong or inappropriate answers. Senility is, without question, seen among geriatric patients, but non-senile hearing impaired patients often seem to demonstrate similar symptoms with inappropriate responses to questions, depression, anxiety, suspiciousness, and withdrawal (p. 298).

In some environments there is virtually a collusion of anonymity operating against the handicapped person. Although collectively sharing in his or her general welfare, no member of the nursing staff or family accepts personal responsibility for the older individual's auditory difficulties. Such a milieu has a powerfully negative effect on his or her frequency of social interaction. People communicate less with those individuals because he or she does not understand them and because of their lessening interest. They reciprocate by ignoring his or her social presence. The elderly person adjusts to this deprivation by interacting more often with him- or herself through thoughts and imageries that are intrinsically more reinforcing than the social environment.

Financial Status and Mobility

The financial status of older Americans was discussed in detail in an earlier Chapter. Aging persons who are more financially self-sufficient, albeit equal in other respects, seem to be better adjusted to their hearing handicaps than those who have fewer means (Note 4). More alternatives for psychosocial adjustment are available to those who are more affluent. The cost of clinical and medical services, hearing aid purchases, and special equipment, such as telephone amplifiers, are within their financial means. While auditory impairment may dampen their enthusiasm for some activities, a sounder economy creates more options for compensating for the loss. The case is reversed among low-income persons, who have fewer alternatives available to them.

Aging individuals who are economically more sufficient also tend to be more mobile. They can travel to community clinics for weekly lessons in speech reading. They can seek immediate adjustments for a hearing aid in need of repair. They can turn to others, friends and family members in distant places, who can provide therapeutic understanding of their problem.

Financial restrictions and lack of mobility create a cul de sac around the hearing impairment. Compensatory behaviors engaged in to avoid the stress of faulty communication become increasingly entrenched. As Miller (1963) has observed, when given an opportunity to extricate themselves from this situation, "some older persons would rather not 're-enter the world of sound' because, apart from their hearing problem, they feel rejected by their environment" (p. 3).

ATTITUDINAL CHARACTERISTICS OF PRESBYCUSIS

How do most older persons feel about their hearing impairments? As suggested earlier, if the loss of sensitivity is first recognized during the aging years, it is likely to be negatively viewed as a reminder of senescense. There are, however, other factors that account for its rejection. The present generation of elderly is not far removed from the stigmatic association of deafness and dumbness that prevailed only a century ago. They are in an age bracket in which a number of friends and relatives have tried hearing aid prostheses, often with marginal success. Such word of mouth experiences can become powerful deterrents to their accepting their own problem. Until recently, hearing aid manufacturers emphasized the concealable aspects of their devices, a strategy that both paid homage to and abetted negative popular opinion.

Middle aged (the young-old) persons, on the other hand, appear to better accept the problem and are less resistant to intervention. One reason for this is that therapeutic gains generally are significantly greater for these individuals than for very old persons. Another reason is that amplification is gaining in popular acceptance, and these younger old individuals are more likely to move with the tide of public sentiment than individuals who are psychosocially older.

Nonetheless, stress factors do operate to a greater or lesser extent among all persons with presbycusis handicaps, whether they realize the source of their difficulty or not. Even a mild loss of hearing sensitivity or a mild degeneration in central processing would manifest itself in situations where the normal hearing mechanism could respond with accuracy. The gradational nature of most presbycusic losses is the very antithesis of their detection. It is not surprising, therefore, that some older persons might not report hearing difficulties. Powers and Powers (1978) examined a sample of 172 aging individuals whose self-reported absence of hearing difficulties did not change substantially over a 10-year period. Although hearing threshold levels were not given, the losses were presumably mild enough to go unnoticed by the respondents. However, unnoticed losses are not necessarily inconsequential problems.

One must question why, for example, a most common method of adjustment to stresses associated with presbycusis seems to be projection (Maurer & Rupp, 1978). Older persons commonly attribute their own problems with faulty registration to the failure of others to speak clearly. This seems to be particularly true for mild-loss cases, in which hearing sensitivity is most depressed in the high frequencies. Thus, perhaps it is the low-frequency information that sustains the individual in the belief that he or she is still hearing normally and that the distortion belongs to someone else. The Powers and Powers (1978) study, however, did question psychosocial problems and aging.

Stress associated with hearing impairment does reveal itself clinically through intensive counseling of older adults. It surfaces in the adjustment techniques employed to relieve anxiety and is therefore of more than passing interest to the audiologist who is interested in patient management. Methods of adjustment are acquired early in life as mechanisms for defending against or escaping from stressful situations (Cameron, 1947). Since they are employed to relieve tension, the audiologist may rightfully question what factors or events in the geriatric environment are discriminative for their appearance. A more detailed discussion on this topic may be found in *Hearing and Aging: Tactics for Intervention* (Maurer & Rupp, 1979).

PSYCHOSOCIAL ADJUSTMENT TO PRESBYCUSIS: SOME CASE STUDIES

Defending against the Hearing Impairment

> Mr. J. arrived at the clinic dressed for a dinner party and accompanied by his wife. The audiologist was prompted by his appearance to compliment him on his attire. Mr. J. beamed, exhibiting some au courant head and torso movements, while proclaiming, "Well, this should go smoothly. What do you want me to do?"
>
> Mrs. J. stared at her husband in disbelief. Later, she acknowledged, "I don't know what got into him this morning. He hasn't worn that suit since we took an ocean voyage 4 years ago."

Comment: Since Mr. J.'s impeccable dress and youthful behaviors were inconsistent with his usual attire and demeanor, one might justifiably raise the question of whether these efforts were designed to reduce stress by drawing attention away from the real problem. Later, when the positive test results for a hearing deficiency became known, he appeared deflated and the youthful mannerisms were no longer evident.

> Mrs. R. listened patiently while the audiologist gave instructions regarding pure-tone testing. Then she announced, "I didn't sleep well last night, so I doubt if you will get very good results on me today." After the examination, she reflected, "I'm not sure I pushed the button every time I heard the sound. Those earphones pressing on my head really bothered me."

Comment: Mrs. R. presented some very good reasons for not performing well in the test suite. However, the validity of her excuses is highly questionable. The real message in her rationalizing might be summed up as, "My hearing is quite normal, I'm just having a bad day."

Attention-getting and *rationalization* are defense techniques used to avoid the stress or anxiety of a perceived problem. In the above cases they represented mechanisms for drawing attention away from or denying the possible existence of a hearing impairment. They are avoidance behaviors in the sense that they are aimed at preventing the occurrence of a potentially distasteful consequence. Other defense techniques employed to similar ends are identification, compensation, and projection.

Identification relieves stress in the individual who temporarily assumes other roles or attributes. For example, a 74-year-old woman about to undergo a hearing test announces that she has "the ears of a cat." A 61 year old, about to start a hearing aid evaluation, irrelevantly indicates that he has just completed a thorough physical examination, and the diagnostician told him he had "the arteries of a 40 year old."

Compensation avoids stressful encounters by substituting less distasteful activities in their place. A 74-year-old retiree rejects the need for amplification because, "I don't go out much anymore. I mostly just watch television."

Projection defends the individual against the problem by referring it to others. Clinically, it seems most commonplace to hear variations on the statement, "I can hear others fine, but my wife doesn't speak clearly."

Escaping from the Impairment

> Mrs. O. was asked, during the counseling session which followed the hearing tests, "What changes in your life have been necessary because of your reduced hearing?"
>
> "Quite honestly," she began, "the only change I deeply regret is church attendance. Our pastor has a soft voice and the services always contain a lot of music. And there's something about that building . . . the sanctuary . . . that makes it very difficult to hear. I reached the point where I would spend most of my time sitting there, thinking about other things." She shook her head. "Finally, I just gave up on it."

Comment: Mrs. O. seems to recognize that, in this situation, she has insulated herself from her problem by avoiding certain stimuli which produce it. *Insulation* represents a retreat from situations that interact negatively with the impairment. A positive aspect of her conversation is that she has not insulated herself from her clinician; she is willing to discuss her actions. Moreover, her possessive description of "our pastor," and her use of present-tense verbs suggest that she really hasn't "given up on it."

Another example of insulation was observed in the behavior of a hearing impaired woman who was seated at a group dining table in a nursing home. In the midst of conversations around her she maintained a stereotypical expression on her face, avoiding any eye contact with others at the table. Her expression seemed to convey the message, "I am thinking about something terribly important and do not wish to be disturbed."

Negativism, on the other hand, reduces stress by opposition. Older persons may argue that they can not learn to lip read, or they can not endure any object in their ears. One 62-year-old woman, returning after a 2-week trial period with amplification, unleashed a veritable avalanche of invectives, including references to an unmanageable and uncomfortable earmold, a heavy, bulky, and poorly concealed hearing aid, and a number of negative environmental factors, ranging from disturbing wind noise to confusion with hearing in groups. Having relieved her stress during the counseling session, her response to the closing question, "Do you want to continue wearing a hearing aid?" was an automatic, "Of course I do. I need it!"

Some potentially stressful situations or events are simply eliminated from the elderly person's repertoire. At least momentarily, *repression* reduces anxiety by excluding the problem. The individual may selectively forget to wear the hearing aid, although the eyeglasses are never forgotten. In addition, auditory experiences which have not been perceived in a number of years may be inhibited. One elderly man was asked, "How long has it been since you heard a whisper?" The question provoked a smile, and then shaking his head incredulously, he replied, "A whisper! I've never even thought of it until you mentioned it. Why, it's been years!"

Regression is a mechanism that permits the client to retreat from a problem by assuming a dependent role—one that contraindicates participation in the conflict. The "childrenization" of some older persons by others in their environments would seem to contribute toward dependency. Two sisters, both in their early nineties, characterize this point. One sister, who had relatively normal hearing for her age, had assumed the dominant, caretaking role over the other, who had a more significant hearing impairment. During the interview, the first sister persisted in answering all questions, even though they were directed at the other woman. In fact, the handicapped sister frequently turned from the examiner's question, as if pleading with her companion to respond for her. Not until the two women were separated was it learned that the sister with the hearing impairment was quite capable of conversing in her own right.

As a method of adjustment to stress, *fantasy* is often equated with daydreaming. Although this behavior is not reported to be more frequent in the aging population than in younger age groups, its frequency has not been studied among the hearing impaired elderly (Note 5). Clinically, fantasy is manifested in the older person who, frustrated by not being able to keep up with or comprehend a group conversation, simply tunes it out and permits thoughts to wander to other topics.

> The individual feels disengaged from group interaction and apathy ensues, the product of the fatigue which sets in from the relentless effort of straining to hear. Frustration, kindled by begging too many pardons, gives way to subterfuges that disguise midunderstandings. The head nods in agreement with a conversation only vaguely interpreted. The voice registers approval of words often void of meaning. The ear strives for some redundancy that will make the message clearer. Finally, acquiescing to fatigue and frustration, thoughts stray from the conversation to mental imageries that are unburdened by the defective hearing mechanism (Maurer, 1976, p. 60).

It should be emphasized that engaging in methods of adjustment is a normal reaction to stress. The behaviors become clinically significant only when they interfere with the intervention of the handicapped person. Furthermore, although the defense and escape techniques are segregated into categories of responses, the observed behaviors that represent them are often overlapping. Detecting them in an aging person is measureably more important than labeling them.

It also seems apparent that many of the psychosocial problems associated with hearing impairment among the aging are not singular to the elderly. This is to be expected, since they are not, except for chronological age, a uniquely defined group. It is, however, the very lack of singularity which should command our attention. No other segment of the population is more challenging, when one considers the diversity of biological, experiential, and psychosocial variables that are expressed within this group. The superimposition of a hearing handicap on the remarkable changes that occur during senescense may range from subtle to profound. Similarly, the adjustive behaviors expressed may vary from minor irritation to self-imposed isolation. If there is one thread of professional continuity between such extremes, it must be the discipline of audiology.

It was in this spirit that the following open letter to an older person who has hearing difficulties was written. It is entitled "You Don't Listen to Me."

> Dear Grandperson,
>
> Your problems are very real. They are witnessed a thousand times in countless places where people are talking to you. Their mouths move and sounds reach your ears, but somehow they don't say what they are talking about; or their message arrives on a slow train, and you respond too late to avoid the flashing signal of concern. Sometimes they frown, their voices kindling with a spark of exasperation that attracts everyone's attention to your dilemma. Too often they take the path of least effort, and oblivious to the strain of your forward head movements and raised eyebrows, they continue to mouth their sounds to others. The space you occupy is disregarded.
>
> Is it any wonder that you seek an occasional rendezvous with yourself? At least your inner thoughts are not burdened by speakers that mumble and patchwork conversations that have no meaning.
>
> Your complaints are altogether familiar. The television newscaster seems bent on cramming as many words into a minute as is humanly possible. The musical background gets in the way of the actor's voice. Everyone talks at once on that show. Who decided that woman should appear on national TV? And when did they take the tick out of watches?

Places are annoying, too. The city transit service is a foreign country, where people seem to speak in tongues against the drones and hisses of spasmodic motion. Restaurants . . . couldn't we find a quiet place where the dishes don't clatter, the music doesn't swell, and the waitress was once a state elocution champion? Churches . . . the architect who designed them must have borrowed the plans from the Tower of Babel. The open banking system . . . whatever happened to the dignity of discussing one's fixed income in the quiet confines of a private office?

People . . . those teenage children who converse in short, accelerated bursts of unintelligible enthusiasm. Conversation stoppers, such as "Don't you remember?" Heart stoppers, such as the voice that appears suddenly at your elbow or the bicycle that materializes on soundless tires. Whisperers . . . their secrets are well guarded, since you don't have the remotest idea what they are talking about.

Your complaints are very reasonable, and the communication problems that you are experiencing extend well beyond your diminishing hearing ability. They are your listeners' responsibility as well. But how do you tell them to speak slowly and clearly without shouting; to call your name before addressing you so that your attention can surface; to turn the noise down so you can understand? How do you tell them without exposing the "old person" in you? How do you project your difficulties on a society that is one or two generations away from sharing your experiences? If only for a moment they could listen to their future through your ears!

Unfortunately, they cannot. However, there are a number of things they can do. They can learn to speak to you more slowly and clearly. They can select quiet places to communicate with you. They can turn off distracting noises before addressing you. They can touch you to gain your attention and look at you when they talk. And they can pause in their conversation long enough for your train of thoughts to catch up with their meaning. These things they can do for you if you will muster the courage to step outside of your older person and assert yourself. Your problem must be shared with your listener.

You must not give up. You must not relinquish one listening experience that contains a shred of satisfaction. You must not withdraw from one conversation that invites your participation. Communication must be regarded as your personal invitation to learning, your private insulation against mental aging.

Finally, you will need to adopt the attitude that the emotional cost of trying to hear again is miniscule compared to the depersonalizing experience of disengagement. Once you have resolutely determined to master your handicap, you will find that you are no longer a helpless spectator in the traffic of language, but a willing participant in the wonderful word transaction that is human communication.

And the next time someone says, "You don't *listen* to me," try responding with a smile and the gentle reminder, "Perhaps you were not *talking* to me."

REFERENCES

Atchley, R. C. The psychological foundations of behavior, in R. C. Atchley (Ed.), *Social forces in later life: An introduction to social gerontology*. Belmont: Wadsworth Publishing Co., 1972, pp. 116–126.

Birren, J. E. Principles of research in aging, in J. E. Birren (Ed.), *Handbook of aging and individual psychological and biological aspects*. Chicago: University of Chicago Press, 1959.

Brody, H., in M. Rockstein, & M. L. Sussman (Eds.), *Development and aging in the nervous system*. New York: Academic Press, 1973, pp. 121–133.

Butler, R. N., & Lewis, M. I. *Aging and mental health*. St. Louis: C. V. Mosby Company, 1973, pp. 30–46.

Cameron, N. Basic adjustive techniques, in N. Cameron (Ed.), *The psychology of behavior disorders*. Boston: Houghton-Mifflin, 1947, pp. 141–186.

Edwards, J. N., & Klemmack, D. L. Correlates of life satisfaction: a re-examination. *Journal of Gerontology,* 1973, *26,* 497–502.

Goldstein, J. L., Schrott, H. G., Hazzard, W. R., Bierman, E. L., & Motulsky, A. G. Hyperlipidemia in coronary heart disease. *Journal of Clinical Investigation,* 1973, *52,* 1544–1568.

Hull, R. H. *Preface to the workshops on geriatric rehabilitation: Hearing aids and the older american.* Hearings before the Subcommittee on Consumer Interests of the Elderly of the Special Committee on Aging, United States Senate. Washington, D.C.: U.S. Government Printing Office, 1973, p. 298.

Maurer, J. F. Auditory impairment and aging, in B. Jacobs (Ed.), *Working with the impaired elderly.* Washington, D.C.: The National Council on the Aging, Inc., 1976, pp. 59–84.

Maurer, J. F., & Rupp, R. R. *Hearing and aging: Tactics for intervention.* New York: Grune & Stratton, 1979.

Miller, M. H. Audiological rehabilitation of the geriatric patient. *Maico Audiological Library Series,* 1963, *II,* Report 1, 3.

Mirsky, I. A. Physiologic, psychologic and social determinants in the etiology of duodenal ulcer. *American Journal of Digestive Diseases,* 1958, *3,* 285–314.

Neugarten, B. L., Havighurst, R., & Tobin, S. The measurement of life satisfaction. *Journal of Gerontology,* 1961, *16,* 134–143.

Powers, J. K., & Powers, E. A. Hearing problems of elderly persons: Social consequences and prevalence. *Journal of the American Speech and Hearing Association,* 1978, *20,* 79–83.

Riley, M. W., & Foner, A. *Aging and society: An inventory of research findings,* vol. 1. New York: Russell Sage, 1968, p. 309.

Rockstein, M. The biology of aging in humans: An overview, in R. Goldman, & M. Rockstein (Eds.), *The physiology and pathology of human aging.* New York: Academic Press, 1975, p. 6.

Smith, C. R. A program of auditory rehabilitation for aged persons in a chronic disease hospital. *Journal of the American Speech and Hearing Association,* 1977, *19,* 417–420.

U.S. Bureau of Census. *Current population reports.* Special Studies (series P-23), No. *59,* 1976.

REFERENCE NOTES

1. Moriarity, M. *A survey of noise levels in senior adult environments.* Unpublished paper presented to the Speech and Hearing Sciences Program, Portland State University, Portland, Oregon, 1974.
2. Cain, L. D., Fine, M. A., & Maurer, J. F. *Responses of the elderly to socialization demands in the move to public high-rise housing.* Paper presented at the 27th Annual Scientific Meeting of the Gerontological Society, Portland, Oregon, November 1, 1974.
3. Comfort, A. *Keynote address.* Presented at the 24th Annual Meeting of the Western Gerontological Society, Tucson, April 9–12, 1978.
4. Maurer, J. F. Unpublished report to the Oregon State Program on Aging. Oregon: Portland State University, 1974.
5. Giambra, L. Personal communication, 1978.

Robert M. Traynor

Chapter 19: Implications of Aging on the Feasibility of Rehabilitating Elderly Hearing Impaired Persons

In today's predominantly youth-oriented society where being old has been considered more of a liability than an asset, health-related services for the elderly have received a low priority. This low priority has not only existed within the field of audiology, but also within medicine and other allied health professions. Those attitudes have inadvertently promoted some misconceptions regarding the rehabilitative capabilities of older individuals. Some of these misconceptions have been perpetuated even among older clients themselves. This low self-concept regarding their ability to benefit from health-related services, however, may have been prompted by a lack of interest in providing those services among professionals. As a result, elderly clients often do not seek rehabilitative or other restorative services since they feel that the probability of their successful response to treatment is only slight. Thus, the prevailing attitude among some potential elderly clients and professionals alike has traditionally been that, "You can't teach an old dog new tricks."

The intent of this chapter is to facilitate an awareness of the rehabilitative capabilities possessed by aging clients and provide audiologists with information that will aid them in making intelligent decisions regarding the provision of services to older clients. Aging clients will be presented as being individualistic in their capability to respond to aural rehabilitation services.

THE AGING INDIVIDUAL

In an effort toward achieving a greater understanding of hearing impaired older clients and their capabilities to respond to aural rehabilitation treatment, it is necessary to examine the variables which manifest themselves in later life.

What Age Is Old?

Being "old" is an abstract, often socially generated misconception that as people grow older, they no longer respond to restorative services. In truth, however, Botwinick (1973) indicates that the capabilities of older people are as variable and individualistic as those of any younger age group. In fact, they appear to be more so. As a group, older persons demonstrate trends toward greater differences in capability.

The onset of old age certainly varies from person to person. Tibbitts (1960) identifies three stages of advanced adulthood: middle age, later maturity, and old age. Atchley (1977) offers realistic definitions of these three stages to facilitate an understanding of the hearing impaired elderly client in terms of biological and social stages of life, not merely age as a chronological measure of potential. These are presented below.

Middle Age

People are generally aware of the fact that they are becoming older during the period called middle age. Although the correlation is not perfect, this phase of life generally occurs during the forties and fifties. During this time, individuals may become aware that they have less energy than they used to, and they often begin to seek intellectual activities to replace more physical pursuits as a source of satisfaction. Chronic illness becomes more prevalent. In the fifties, vision and hearing may begin to decline. Work careers often reach a plateau, and children may have left home by the time most couples reach their early fifties. Some women go back to work, while others remain in their house wondering what to do with themselves or what is to become of them. This period can be frustrating for both sexes as it marks the close of childrearing, work careers, and the satisfaction of both of these activities. However, middle age can also mark a new beginning for a marriage or a new occupation, and so provide new sources of satisfaction. Finally, middle age is the time when many people are forced to come to grips with the fact that death is real, and not just something that happens to someone else.

Later Maturity

The period of life noted as later maturity is marked by an even greater awareness of the fact that aging is a reality. Some persons experience difficulty in orienting themselves toward the future. Chronologically, later maturity usually occurs correspondingly in the sixth and seventh decades of life. There is a drastic reduction in physical energy during this period, and people become very aware of failing eyesight, hearing, and other sensory modalities. Long-term chronic health care problems begin to limit activity during this period. Retirement and the accompanying reduction of income (sometimes combined with poor health) reduce personal/social contacts. Death of relatives or friends and movement of children also may reduce the size of the social environment. Some women are widows by the time they reach their mid sixties. Later maturity, however, can be a pleasant period. Most people retain a fair measure of physical vigor which, when coupled with freedom from responsibilities, can make later maturity one of the most open and free periods in the life cycle, for those prepared to take advantage of it.

Old Age

The period of old age is described by many as the "beginning of the end." It generally is characterized by frailty, disability, or invalidism, and mental processes generally slow to some extent. People tend to dwell on themselves rather than others, concentrating on past experiences in an effort to find some meaning for their life. At this point, the individual knows the end of life may be near. As activity becomes restricted, loneliness and boredom are common. The onset of old age often does not occur until the late seventies. On the other hand, as is often observed, many people in their eighties show few symptoms of old age. The onset of this period of life varies greatly among persons, and appears to generally be related to health, genetic, and social/personal factors.

The above description of the stages of advanced age and their great variability among individuals explains why some audiologists, such as Alpiner (Note 1), have stated that they have observed 45-year-old clients who act as if they were in their seventies (later maturity or old age) and, conversely, 70 year olds who seem much younger, particularly in their response to rehabilitative treatment. Possibly these chronologically older clients may still be in the stage of Middle Age in terms of their physical and mental capabilities, whereas the chronologically younger clients may be functioning prematurely in the stages of later maturity or old age.

THE AGING POPULATION

General demographical data on the aging population have been compiled by several investigators (Atchley, 1977; Botwinick, 1973; Butler & Lewis, 1977; Cutler & Harootyan, 1975; Moss & Halamandaris, 1977) on the aging population in the United States. In terms of discussing the potential of elderly clients to achieve successes in aural rehabilitative treatment, information regarding typical aging persons in the United States is critical. A summary of those research findings reveals that 22.5 million Americans are over age 65 years, 10 million are over age 73, 1 million are over age 85, and 106,000 are over age 100. These older people make up 10 percent of the total U.S. population and comprise 12.5 million females and 10 million males. Most of these elderly men are married whereas most elderly women are widows. Of these individuals over age 65 years, 95 percent are living independently in their community. Thus, only 5 percent of individuals over age 65 reside in geriatric health care facilities, mostly in the south, particularly, the south Atlantic region.

The lifestyles of these elderly U.S. residents also have been reviewed. Seventy-three percent live in urban areas, and 30 percent live in substandard housing. In 1971 it was found that 50 percent of the elderly in the U.S., or approximately 10 million people, lived on less than $10.00 per day. In 1976, social security benefits were $218.00 per month for an individual and $372.00 for a couple; older individuals earn only 29 percent of their own income. Chronic health problems afflict 86 percent of the older population, only 6 percent are college graduates, and no more than 50 percent have completed elementary school.

Additional information on residents of geriatric health care facilities indicate that most are in the "older" range of elderly, with a mean age of 82 years; most are nonambulatory people who came to the health care facility after leaving their own home; and most are widows or widowers. Their average length of stay is 2.4 years. Only 20 percent will leave the facility for reasons other than death, and 27 percent will expire within the first month of residence. Fifty percent of these "facility" residents have no close living relatives; 60 percent have no visitors. The average resident takes 4.2 drugs per day.

REACTIONS OF OLDER PERSONS TO AN AUDITORY DEFICIT

In light of the social-psychological variables presented above, hearing impaired older adults offer some often typically repeated reactions to the added isolation resulting from their auditory deficit. Although the following do not exhaust the reactions to this problem, they do present those most often encountered by professionals who work with the hearing impaired.

Denial of the Hearing Impairment

Often, older individuals neither recognize nor deny that they have a problem. In their opinion, it is not their inability to hear, but "that people mumble these days," "speak too fast," or are otherwise "inconsiderate speakers." The first task of the rehabilitative audiologist is to facilitate the client's recognition of the hearing impairment. Such recognition often occurs during or just after the initial audiometric evaluation. In many cases, a simple explanation of the evaluation in layman's terminology is sufficient. An example of this type of explanation is as follows.

> Now, I would like to discuss the results of your hearing evaluation with you. These graphs represent the right and left ears. The numbers along the top represent the various "pitches" of sound, while those along the side are "how loud" each sound was made before you could hear it. Normal hearing on this graph is usually between 0 and 20 on this scale. As you can see you are below that level. Have you noticed difficulty hearing? . . . The words I asked you to repeat were an evaluation of how well you understand speech. Have you had any difficulty understanding speech, particularly when there are other noises around you?

The responses to these questions certainly will vary from individual to individual. However, a skilled audiologist usually can demonstrate, when it is the case, that there is an existing auditory impairment that is of sufficient degree to interfere with that person's ability to communicate. Further, it is the duty of the audiologist to facilitate discussion regarding the possible rehabilitative alternatives which may facilitate remediation of the communication problems.

Feelings of Hopelessness

"Go help someone who is worth the time," "I'm just going to die tomorrow anyway," or "maybe a younger man" are common reactions by elderly persons when the audiologist suggests rehabilitative intervention for auditory impairment. This is particularly true among residents of geriatric health care facilities. Older persons with such attitudes, of course, present a real dilemma to the audiologist. The clinician must be ever aware that a person's uncooperativeness may be the result of, or enhanced by, the frustrating auditory deficit. Houston and Royse (1954) have drawn some conclusions regarding the relationship between deafness and negative psychological involvement. For example, not knowing what others are saying may cause the person to become doubtful of their ability to respond adequately in any way, although they may not know the reason for such inadequacy. They may misinterpret auditory sensations which have been distorted by central auditory dysfunction, and may, in some cases, turn away from possible aural rehabilitation treatment. In most instances, however, elderly persons do hope that services by the audiologist will benefit them. In other cases, though, repeated defeat at attempts toward rehabilitation in other areas of their life may prompt the opinion that there is no real reason to try. Efforts must be made to reach these people, who are—in their own way—asking for assistance.

Recognition of the Problem, but no Rehabilitative Treatment Needed

These clients are, quite possibly, the best adjusted of all those mentioned. They generally recognize the hearing problem, and may be compensating for it in some way. One characteristic of these individuals is that they are generally more assertive than others. They often demand to know what is being discussed in a conversation. They watch the speaker and/or utilize other communication alternatives, which have been acquired on their own, to facilitate communication. Although some of these people may be ineffective communicators, they do possess the necessary assertiveness to facilitate treatment. These individuals are sometimes better assisted in their auditory impairment without formal aural rehabilitation programs. It has been found, in some cases, that bringing undo attention to their problem may depress their positive attitude toward the hearing loss and the delicate balance between withdrawal and their present outgoing personality.

PSYCHOPHYSICAL CAPACITY FOR AURAL REHABILITATION

For the aural rehabilitation process to be successful, the client must possess the psychophysical capacity to utilize other senses as a means of circumventing the impaired auditory system. There may be, however, some psychophysical limitations which the client can work around to some degree if he or she is sufficiently motivated.

Ocular Limitations

Very often the ocular mechanism is utilized to offset the loss or partial loss of the use of the auditory modality, i.e., speechreading. It is apparent, of course, that the client possessing significant ocular dysfunction will experience special difficulties in learning to utilize visual clues in communication. Furthermore, the audiologist usually will find the provision of services for these multiply handicapped clients more difficult.

There are three ocular disorders that occur most frequently among elderly people. According to Atchley (1977), these are: macular degeneration, which is found in 48 percent of persons over age 65 years; cataracts, found in 33 percent; and glaucoma, afflicting 5 percent. Only 14 percent of all persons over age 65 years possess normal uncorrected vision.

Macular Degeneration

This disorder is the most common cause of visual problems of the elderly and usually involves both eyes. It is thought to be secondary to changes in the choroid layer of the eye. The result is a dramatic loss of the central visual field. These clients often cannot respond to visual stimuli except within their peripheral visual field, as opposed to a normal/total (and central) visual field.

Cataracts

These affect the opacity of the ocular lens, the consequence being similar to a smudge on a pair of glasses. In other words, the visual field is clouded in one spot. Fortunately, this disorder may not have much of an effect upon the use of visual clues in the aural rehabilitation process because current surgical procedures generally provide good results.

Glaucoma

Ninety percent of all cases of glaucoma occur among individuals over 40 years of age (Atchley, 1977). Symptomatically, the client usually experiences halos or rainbows around lights during the early stages, and a slow, progressive loss of peripheral vision. These individuals can utilize visual clues best if spoken to from a direct face-to-face position. Clients are best instructed in speechreading from this position, as it concentrates on the use of central vision rather than peripheral.

In general, the effects of ocular disorders on elderly clients' ability to participate in the aural rehabilitation process are highly individual. Butler and Lewis (1977) have stated that about 80 percent of older people have reasonably good sight until age 90 years and beyond, thus limiting the magnitude of this problem. If, however, disorders of ocular acuity are known among specific clients, the effect of the impairments often can be circumvented.

There are many clients for whom the use of visual clues in aural rehabilitation will not be beneficial. In these cases, the audiologist may choose to assist the person by concentrating on auditory training to make the best of the client's residual hearing.

Perception

Rabbitt (1965) has concluded that older individuals take longer to discriminate between relevant and nonrelevant stimuli. For example, a watermelon might appear smaller than normal, slightly different in color, or unusually shaped, but the watermelon is still perceived as a watermelon. As the aging process continues, one may be less able to accurately perceive part of an object as being a part of a whole object. In addition, whole objects may appear distorted. Furthermore, the ability to deal with specific items within a class of objects may become more difficult. These categorization difficulties include, for example, a woman looking at a sign on a bathroom door which says "Men" and wondering why the sign was placed on that door, rather than responding appropriately by going to the correct door. As a result of these difficulties, the older person may have a reduced ability to evaluate stimuli and take appropriate action relative to them.

One method of circumventing this problem in the aural rehabilitation process is by utilizing a more synthetic approach to the teaching of speechreading, discussed in Chapter 26. Such an approach capitalizes upon the perceptual strengths of the client and minimizes the confusion offered by analytic methods. Synthetic approaches should be considered particularly, for those clients confined to the limits of a geriatric health care facility as categorization problems are more often observed among that population.

Psychomotor Performance

Psychomotor ability refers to a complex chain of events that begins with a sensory mechanism and ends with a reaction, usually through an effector such as a muscle. It involves sensory input, attachment of meaning through perception, integration incorporating this information with other information, a decision regarding action to be taken, and appropriate instructions to be sent to the proper effector. In general, older people demonstrate slower psychomotor performance than younger people. Atchley (1977) has indicated that there is a 45 percent reduction in effector strength between ages 20 and 70 years.

Further, among older individuals, nerve impulse conduction is slower, endurance is reduced, and coordination may have declined. Increases in reaction time tend to be less for simple tasks but greater for more complex tasks. Within the audiologist's realm, simple tasks may include responses to standard audiometric evaluations, but more importantly refers to the responses required in special tests for site of lesion. Complex tasks, further, could include rehabilitative procedures in speechreading/auditory training and the effective use of amplification.

Although much psychomotor slowing is thought to be due to central degeneration, some has been traced to a cognitive need for increased accuracy among aging persons. Botwinick (1973) has indicated that older individuals often wait to respond until they are very sure that they will be responding correctly. The audiologist, therefore, must be aware that there may be both a physiological and psychological basis for slower responses during diagnostic and rehabilitative evaluations and treatment among older clients. It is important, however, to be aware of the fact that when the responses to the given task are obtained, they are often more accurate than those among their younger counterparts.

Intelligence

Overall, intelligence scores are lower among older people than among an average mix of younger population. This is logical since most investigations of intelligence utilize tests which are standardized to younger adult populations. These evaluations often emphasize timed responses to questions which are considered general knowledge among the standardization sample. As described in other sections of this chapter, reduced perceptual, psychomotor, and other sensory modalities inhibit the older person's ability to perform on these examinations. Although IQ scores among the elderly population are often lower than for younger clients, when these scores are corrected for the age factor by considering the aforementioned variables, they may be the same or higher as when tested at a younger age. Botwinick (1973) has suggested that there is not yet a completely appropriate intelligence test, either in content or interest level, for the elderly. Current IQ tests tend to emphasize contemporary skills and, therefore, deemphasize the skills of people educated in earlier years.

Atchley (1977) has stated that at least a part of what appears to be the decline in intelligence of older people is actually a change in the emphasis of skills being assessed. He further has indicated that probably the most important variable affecting intelligence is health. Changes in health status may seriously affect not only the individual's ability to perform on such tests, but also his or her participation in rehabilitative treatment. The audiologist must, as suggested by Alpiner (1965), consider the physiological and psychological well-being of the patient first and communication problems second. On the other hand, it must be realized that at times, communication deficits appear to contribute to the physiological/psychological and health problems incurred by the elderly. Clients who demonstrate more severe levels of intellectual deficiency may not be good candidates for aural rehabilitation.

Memory and Learning

Memory is intimately related to the learning process. There is a direct correlation between the level of acquisition of knowledge or skills and the ability to store and recall information. Memory consists of three stages: registration, retention, and recall. *Registration* is similar to the recording of information on a tape recorder. Neurologically, the material is recorded for later utilization. *Retention* is the ability to retain the registered information over an indeterminate period of time. *Recall* refers to the ability to cognitively retrieve information that has been registered and retained. Failure of this interrelationship at any of the stages interrupt the accuracy of memory.

The ability to remember often is divided into types, based on the period of time lapse between registration and the instance designated for recall. These are referred to progressively as short-term memory, recent memory, remote memory, and "old" or long-term memory. *Short-term memory* is the recalling of information after very little delay, usually 5 to 30 seconds. *Recent memory* involves the recall of information after a brief period of time, usually about 1 hour to several days. *Remote memory* is the recall of events over the course of a lifetime. Lastly, "old" or *long-term memory* refers to the recall of events which may have occurred a long time ago and have not been thought of or rehearsed since.

The practicing audiologist is familiar with older clients who forget the directions given for a hearing evaluation even before it begins, or clients who do not recall when their appointment is, or, further, may not recall what occurred during the last counseling session. Concurrently, however, these same patients may be able to tell you about the time their husband was driving the family Model-T Ford when it had a flat tire on the way to the Presbyterian Church by the little red gas station with two pumps on the corner of 9th Avenue and 10th Street, and the fact that the tire already had five patches on it because of conservation measures during the great depression, and on and on. Obviously, this is a demonstration of breakdown in the retention and recall stages of short-term and recent memory. Additionally, there appears to be some enhancement of remote and long-term retention and recall with age. Memory deficits are very real obstacles which must be surmounted if rehabilitative treatment is to be successful. It may be necessary to present some or all of the information in a repetitive format to allow for these retention-recall difficulties. Although the memory problems described above are observed in many older clients, audiologists must be aware that these are deficits which vary from one person to another.

Generally, the audiologist should remember that even though short-term and recent memory may be somewhat reduced, older people generally can learn as well as those who are younger. It may take them longer to learn, but if the information is presented in an unambiguous format, older clients generally will have little difficulty.

WHAT DOES AURAL REHABILITATION ACCOMPLISH FOR THIS POPULATION?

Weston (1964) describes two types of aging: *primary aging*—the inevitable act of becoming older—and *secondary aging*—which is often the result of a debilitating condition such as a chronic health problem. Symptoms of secondary aging can also result from disorders such as hearing impairment. An auditory deficit can lead to complete withdrawal from communication with others, which may lead to other problems. The goals of the aural rehabilitation program for active individuals is, obviously, to keep them communicating and ambulatory. The program assists these individuals in coping with the hearing impairment as it progresses, with the aim of preventing the communication deficits which may have resulted otherwise.

The purpose of a program for individuals confined to the limits of a geriatric health care facility is not usually to integrate them back into the community, although that desire always exists. Indeed, all but about 20 percent of the confined clients will remain in the health care facility, even if they are successful in the aural rehabilitation program. The goal of the audiologist is to slow the secondary aging process by facilitating the client's ability to function within the limits of the institution and to enable the client to interact better on a social basis.

CONCLUSIONS

In determining the feasibility of providing services to individual clients, probably the most important variable is the person's health. Unfortunately, the audiologist cannot hope to provide services to clients where particular combinations of problems cannot be circumvented, i.e., hearing impairment, blindness, memory/learning problems. It is a wise clinician who admits defeat when it is obvious. Despite their ocular, perceptual, psychomotor, and memory limitations, however, most older people can be assisted through aural rehabilitation treatment. The clients who have uncircumventable problems are a very small percentage of the total aging population.

Earlier in this chapter, an attitude was presented which, unfortunately, has prevailed among clients and professionals that, "You can't teach an old dog new tricks." If an old dog is given ambiguous directions, it will get the new trick mixed up with other previously learned tricks. It is probable, however, provided the trainer knows the animal's limitations, likes and dislikes, etc., that the teaching of the trick, although perhaps not an easy task, is feasible.

The provision of rehabilitative services to the elderly demands extreme patience, as progress may be slower than among other age groups. Conversely, serving the elderly population does offer a real challenge to the resourceful professional who is able to circumvent certain limitations and make modifications in his or her technique.

REFERENCES

Alpiner, J. G. Diagnostic and rehabilitative aspects of geriatric audiology. *Journal of the American Speech and Hearing Association*, 1965, *7*, 455–459.

Atchley, R. C. *Social forces in later life*. Belmont, California: Wadsworth Publishing Company, 1977.

Botwinick, J. *Aging and behavior*. New York: Springer Publishing Co., 1973.

Butler, R. N., & Lewis, M. I. *Aging and mental health*. St. Louis: C.V. Mosby Co., 1977.

Cutler, N. E., & Harootyan, R. A. Demography of the aging, in D. Woodruff, and J. E. Birren (Eds.), *Aging: Scientific perspectives and social issues*. New York: D. Van Nostrand and Co., 1975, pp. 31–69.

Houston, F., & Royse, A. B. Relationship between deafness and psychotic illness. *Journal of Mental Sciences*, 1954, *100*, 990–993.

Moss, R., & Halamandaris, V. *Too old, too sick, too bad*. Germantown, Maryland: Aspen Systems, 1977.

Rabbitt, P. M. A. An age decrement in the ability to ignore irrelevant information. *Journal of Gerontology,* 1965, *20,* 233–238.

Tibbits, C. *Handbook of social gerontology*. Chicago: University of Chicago Press, 1960.

Weston, T. E. T. Presbycusis: A clinical study. *Journal of Laryngology and Otolaryngology,* 1964, *78,* 273.

REFERENCE NOTE

1. Alpiner, J. G. *Feasibility of rehabilitating the hearing impaired older person* (Workshop in Geriatric Aural Rehabilitation). Unpublished manuscript, Greeley, Colorado: University of Northern Colorado, 1973.

Section 3: Toward Rehabilitation: Assessment of the Elderly Adult Client

Rick L. Bollinger

Chapter 20: Nonauditory Communication Disturbances Resembling Presbycusis

In an endeavor to accurately identify and treat hearing impairment among elderly patients, the audiologist must be aware of other communication disorders which are common among those persons. It is particularly important that the audiologist be aware of other disorders which manifest physical, psychological, emotional, and social behaviors that might be confused with similar behaviors often precipitated by reduced auditory sensitivity. The task confronting the audiologist working with a geriatric population is that of differential diagnosis of auditory sensitivity; that of assessing the impact of the hearing loss relative to any other communication problem that may be present; and that of managing the effects of the hearing problem based on the patient's communicative strengths and weaknesses. The liability that audiologists face, however, is that other disorders of communication may resemble presbycusis, but, in fact, are not auditory problems. The alert audiologist must be aware of those disorders, how they are manifested, and how they can be differentiated from true auditory disorders.

Consequently, the purpose of this chapter is to provide the audiologist with information concerning the different types of communication disorders common to the geriatric population. Information is provided which describes and compares the various types of atypical behaviors resulting from the different communication disorders most prevalent in the elderly. In keeping with the intent and philosophy of this text, this chapter attempts to provide the audiologist with information that is discriminating and practical.

COMMUNICATION DISORDERS COMMON AMONG THE AGED

The predominant communication disorders encountered among the elderly include chronic brain syndrome (organic psychosis or confusion), aphasia, apraxia, dysarthria, dysphonia, apathy, and presbycusis. In the following section, the primary features for each of the diagnostic groups will be described. For each disorder, those descriptive characteristics which serve to differentiate nonpresbycusic from presbycusic patients will be emphasized.

CHRONIC BRAIN SYNDROME

Chronic brain syndrome is a common diagnostic entity among patients in nursing homes, extended-care facilities, and hospitals. Fox, Topel, and Huckman (1975) related studies suggesting that senile dementia (one type of chronic brain syndrome) is a very common problem among the elderly—with an estimated incidence of 10 percent for those patients over 65 years; another investigator found an incidence of 21 percent in individuals over the age of 80 (Arie, 1973).

The term chronic brain syndrome is also called organic psychosis, confusion, and senility. Generally, the diagnostic label—chronic brain syndrome—indicates a clinical category descriptive of patients having a gradual history of intellectual and/or personality disorganization. Characteristic symptoms include disturbances in comprehension, memory, orientation, and emotional response. More specifically, patients with an organic psychosis may present disorientation to person, place, and time; reduction in immediate, day-to-day, and remote memory; reduction in level of consciousness and attention; poor socialization behavior; confabulation and hallucinations; and poor awareness of monitoring of personal grooming (Wolff, 1963).

Signs and Symptoms

Chronic brain syndrome may be caused by senile brain disease, arteriosclerosis, alcoholic brain disease, central nervous system (CNS) trauma, convulsive disorder, idiopathic Parkinson's disease, CNS syphilis, and brain disease of undetermined origin (Simon & Neal, 1963). The most prevalent chronic brain syndromes among the aged are multi-infarct dementia* and senile dementia. These types of brain dysfunction affect the cortex diffusely and subsequently yield a wide range of cognitive, emotional, and communicative behaviors.

The generalized brain involvement, which is the etiology for chronic brain syndrome disorder, causes a number of nonlanguage brain injury behaviors. These include intermittent attention to a given task, difficulty in shifting from one task to another, distractability, and visual and/or auditory hallucinations (Allison, 1962). These generalized brain injury behaviors also are responsible for the use of the label "confused" when discussing chronic brain syndrome patients. That label suggests that a patient may not remember having met you before even if he has, in fact, seen you on a number of occasions. A confused individual may forget what the nature of a task is, where his room is, when he was admitted to the hospital, etc. He may very well be able to articulate memories from remote past experience and yet not be able to tell you what he had for breakfast, what the weather was like yesterday, or what day it is. Of note will be the confused patient's lack of or reduced ability to monitor his or her activities. For additional information with regard to this population, the reader is referred to Ginzberg (1955) who has presented added relevant observations on communicative behaviors among organic psychoses.

---

*The label multi-infarct dementia is used in favor of arteriosclerotic dementia since it implies a broader base of vascular disorders (Selzer & Sherwin, 1978).

Capabilities

Barring a specific language deficit, the chronic brain syndrome patient should be able to comprehend and follow short commands and instructions. In a study completed by Bollinger (Note 1) it was noted that chronic brain syndrome patients required frequent repetitions of instructions during the completion of a given task. Their pattern of response was such that it suggested the patients comprehended the input but were unable to retain it over successive items. The confused patient's limited attention span may require the use of louder voice and an accompanying physical contact to establish attention during instruction giving. If such instructions are not followed correctly, the causal factor is usually inadequate or inaccurate registration of the information rather than a lack of comprehension per se. For example, one patient being screened audiometrically by this author responded appropriately to the first pure-tone presented at 25 dB at 1000 Hz. When a second and third tone were presented at the same intensity and frequency, the patient did not respond. When asked if he heard the signal, he nodded, smiled, and said "yes." When asked if he remembered what to do when he heard the sound, he said "no." When tones were presented at even higher intensities and the patient was given repeated instructions to raise his hand when he heard the sound, the patient did not respond as requested though he did give indication that he had heard the sound by blinking his eyes or raising his eyebrows.

Bollinger (Note 1) found that verbal output skills of chronic brain syndrome patients were characterized by lengthy and recognizable responses which frequently were unrelated to the task. That is, speech was generally intelligible but not semantically relevant. Such unrelated verbalizations appeared more frequently during unstructured tasks and when subjects were unsure of the desired performance. When individual patients did present unintelligible or muffled speech, they were able to increase intelligibility for brief periods when their attention was refocused and they were told to speak clearly.

In general, confused patients will be able to repeat strings of words or sentences modeled by the clinician. The clinician must be cautioned, however, that even in the presence of such imitative abilities, these patients may fail to understand the information because of lack of registration.

Assessing the Patient

The clinical audiologist must be very skillful in observing the listening-speaking behaviors of the chronic brain syndrome patient. Some patients will make it very clear that they understand auditory input and utilize the spoken word in their customary environment. Such apparent use of the auditory signal will be evidenced by (1) the repetition of words presented at a conversational speech level; (2) the completion of simple, concrete, directional commands; (3) the incorporation of words or sentences used by the clinician although in an inappropriate manner (such as repeating in a sing-song fashion, incorporating the words in a dialogue about a past event, etc.); and (4) attending to sounds in the environment which are obviously at levels compatible with those of conversational speech. In severe cases, confused patients will be difficult to rouse. For example, even when physically touched or shaken, they will avoid or not attend to the clinician's face. These same individuals may speak aloud when no one is present, may laugh or cry inappropriately, and may evidence visual and auditory hallucinations.

APHASIA

Aphasia is a familiar diagnostic term in the fields of audiology and speech/language pathology. However, that diagnostic label—like chronic brain syndrome—encompasses a number of different behavioral patterns and various degrees of adequacy with respect to linguistic understanding and production.

Aphasia is a result of brain injury to the dominant language hemisphere in the brain. In the majority of cases, this means a left-hemisphere lesion with a probable right-sided paralysis or paresis. In addition to the language problem, the aphasic individual may present additional nonlanguage brain-damaged behaviors such as perseveration, visual field cuts, and attention span reductions. In most cases, however, those behaviors will be much less handicapping than the speech-language problem.

Depending on the specific region in the left hemisphere of the brain that is affected, an aphasic individual may present verbal production behaviors that may be labeled either fluent or nonfluent (Geschwind, 1971). In addition to this very apparent discriminating factor, there are additional language behaviors and non-language behaviors that separate these two groups (Goodglass & Kaplan, 1972).

Fluent Aphasia

Signs and Symptoms

Immediately subsequent to a stroke, a fluent aphasic may show some disorientation and confusion. As the length of time from onset extends, however, he or she will begin to show appropriate orientation to surroundings and accurate memory for events which have occurred. Herein lies the discriminating characteristic between the confused patient and the fluent aphasic. The confused patient (chronic brain syndrome) will show short- and long-term memory deficits, orientation problems, and will have verbal output that is most often grammatically correct and comprehendable in that it relates to a topic. That topic, however, may not be the topic being discussed. The fluent aphasic, on the other hand, will present strings of articulated words or "pseudo-words" (neologisms—words idiosyncratic to the individual) but there will be little or no content to the verbalization. Furthermore, the fluent aphasic individual will generally take advantage of environmental cues, something a confused individual rarely does. Also, the socioenvironmental types of behavior such as eating, toileting, and dressing will all be satisfactorily performed by the fluent aphasic though may not be by the confused patient.

Capabilities

The majority of aphasic individuals will have some difficulty with auditory comprehension (Schuell, Jenkins, & Jimenez-Pabon, 1965). In many instances, these listening difficulties may appear to the audiologist as a hearing loss. Fluent aphasics oftentimes will ask the clinician to "speak up" or "talk louder so I can hear you." They may go so far as to suggest, in their rambling and rather vague speech, that an operation or hearing aid might assist them to hear better. In fact, the difficulty is primarily one of auditory association—not auditory sensitivity. In a study assessing auditory attention, Bollinger and Hedrick (Note 2) found that fluent aphasics who had bilateral hearing sensitivity within normal limits, performed markedly inferior to normal adults and nonfluent aphasics on a test of auditory attention—diotic listening ability. This would suggest that the fluent aphasic is less able to screen out nonmeaningful auditory stimuli and perhaps has a "noise build-up" in the auditory association area. Such inability to screen out unwanted auditory distractions might, in part, account for fluent aphasics' often observed difficulty in comprehending the nature of their auditory–input problems.

In contrast to their appropriate syntax and articulate verbal output, the fluent aphasic may have severe auditory comprehension problems—even to the point of being unable to understand single words and/or simple directions. It is not uncommon, moreover, to find fluent aphasic adults who deny having any difficulty with their comprehension and, rather than appearing depressed, present an almost euphoric affect (Geschwind, 1971). Their somewhat personable and socially appropriate nonlanguage behaviors, combined with their flowing and articulate verbal output, may mislead the clinician into overestimating the individual's comprehension abilities.

The fluent aphasic presents speech that is characterized by accurate articulation, appropriate intonation, and a fairly rapid rate. There may be many circumlocutions in evidence, paraphasias (either words that sound like the words intended—foy for boy—or words of related meaning—chair for table). Social interactive speech is generally well preserved and appropriate. However, some fluent patients are so severely involved that even when their verbal output is flowing and well articulated, it is surprisingly lacking in any semantic content. This type of fluent output, when observed in the patient who has minimal paralysis and other physical problems, make such patients difficult to discriminate from the confused patient.

Nonfluent Aphasia

Signs and Symptoms

The second type of aphasic, categorized on the basis of verbal output, is the nonfluent aphasic. In general, the nonfluent aphasic patient is appropriate in social interactions, is generally cautious and slow in his approach to any given activity, and will present a right-sided paralysis or paresis. The somewhat impulsive response mode that characterized the fluent aphasic is not characteristic of the nonfluent aphasic. Most frequently, the nonfluent patient will be well oriented to his surroundings, may appear somewhat depressed, and be somewhat reticent about becoming involved in activities (Geschwind, 1970). He or she will, however, appear to monitor activities of daily living and generally will be socially and emotionally appropriate.

Capabilities

The nonfluent aphasic presents better auditory comprehension than might be assumed on the basis of the rather limited verbal output. When something said is not understood, the nonfluent aphasic generally will ask for or give indication that it was not understood. This somewhat ready admission of nonunderstanding is in contrast to the fluent aphasic's tendency to deny comprehension problems. The nonfluent aphasic, as well as the fluent aphasic, will make maximal use of any nonlanguage visual or auditory environmental cues to assist in comprehension of auditory input.

The nonfluent aphasic will present speech that is halting, frequently lacking in verbs and function words, and composed primarily of content words—speech which gives the impression of telegraphic style. Frequently, articulation of the words employed will be accurate. However, there will be instances of word-finding difficulty, many pauses, and a slower-than-normal rate. To most people, the nonfluent aphasic most closely epitomizes the condition labeled aphasia. He or she usually presents a right-sided weakness and a halting anomic style of speech most frequently assumed to typify an aphasic disorder. In contrast, the fluent aphasic may evidence no paralysis and produce lengthy, rambling, clearly articulated utterances that appear to be appropriate to the situation but somehow miss the primary intent.

The nonfluent aphasic and the confused patient are usually easy to differentiate. The nonfluent aphasic is a "sensible" individual. Even in the presence of a somewhat devastating communicating problem, he or she most often attempts to maximize the ability to get along the best as possible. He or she will be oriented, in touch with the environment, and socially and emotionally appropriate. Any apparently inappropriate behaviors will probably be the result of inaccurate comprehension of instructions or conversation. The confused patient's inappropriate behaviors on the other hand, are the result of his lack of attention to, registration of, and/or interest in the messages from his environment.

APRAXIA

A speech disorder that is very similar to that presented by the nonfluent aphasic is verbal apraxia. Some writers suggest that these two disorders are, in fact, the same (Goodglass & Kaplan, 1972). There would appear, however, to be sufficient clinical observational difference to justify the two conditions and labels (Darley, 1970; Halpern, Darley, & Brown, 1973).

It is believed that the lesion responsible for apraxia is more localized than that responsible for the aphasias. As such, the apraxic patient may present a motor speech formulation disturbance in the absence of any other significant brain injury behaviors. That is, this particular patient may show no disorientation, attention disturbances, memory deficits, or inappropriate emotional behaviors.

The apraxic individual will generally show good response to basic audiometrics. His or her comprehension of directions and conversational speech should be intact. In contrast to the confused patient and the aphasic patient, the apraxic individual will also show fair to good reading comprehension and make good use of written directions.

When apraxia is uncomplicated by specific language disorder, the apraxic individual will present a marked disturbance in voluntary control of the speech mechanism. He or she will exhibit a disturbance in the ability to voluntarily imitate and spontaneously produce sounds and words in the presence of good swallowing and vegetative muscle function. Such an individual will also evidence awareness of the problem and, during speaking, will make frequent attempts to correct articulation errors. If the apraxia is severe, and the patient has not had formal and appropriate treatment, he or she may be very reticent to talk. In contrast to the disturbed speech skill, the apraxic patient may be capable of written response, or at least able to write words to assist his or her disturbed verbal output.

It is important to note that apraxia is commonly accompanied by an aphasic disturbance. If the aphasia is of sufficient severity to compromise basic auditory comprehension, written output, and reading comprehension, then the label of apraxia may be irrelevant with regard to management. When apraxia is uncomplicated by aphasia, however, the individual will show only a form of motor formulation disturbance—an inability to program the muscle movements in a manner to appropriately articulate the spoken word.

DYSARTHRIA

The term dysarthria implies a motor-speech disorder which is the result of trauma or disease processes in the central or peripheral nervous system (Darley, Aronson, & Brown, 1975). Such disorders may be characterized by spastic, flaccid, and/or ataxic disturbances in the strength, mobility, and coordination of the speech musculature. Dysarthria may occur in isolation or may be a part of a generalized condition such as amyotrophic lateral sclerosis (ALS), Parkinson's disease, or choreic disorders.

The dysarthric individual may present nonlinguistic brain-damaged behaviors as a result of the specific nervous system impairment. That is, in addition to the speech–voice disorder, the dysarthric patient may present memory problems, perceptual problems, and attentional deficits. These additive brain injury behaviors are particularly apparent in those individuals who have sustained more than one stroke or who manifest a generalized cortical dysfunction as in anoxia, encephalitis, and diseases like Huntington's chorea.

In the absence of specific auditory and language disorders, the dysarthric individual will present intact comprehension. The nonlanguage brain injury behaviors, such as attention deficits and reduced memory span, must be considered to assure that such behaviors are not linguistic or sensitivity problems. A dysarthric patient may have a very slight articulation disturbance with generalized imprecision of the sibilants and blends, or may evidence such severe involvement that he or she is totally incapable of moving the oral–peripheral musculature to achieve speech. In either case, the dysarthric individual knows what he or she wants to say, and how to produce the sounds, but the involved muscles do not respond appropriately and/or sufficiently. Severe dysarthric patients will most frequently manifest a swallowing and chewing disorder immediately post stroke. That disorder may extend well into the post-stroke recovery period if attention is not provided and swallowing management undertaken. All activities which use the muscles of the lips, tongue, palate, and larynx will be involved.

The dysarthric individual may be differentiated from the confused, aphasic, and apraxic patients on the basis of his or her intact language abilities and the paralysis or incoordination of his or her articulators. In most cases, the reason for the patient's speech difficulty will be obvious—paralyzed muscles with drooling and weakness of the facial muscles apparent.

DYSPHONIAS

While it is not anticipated that the audiologist would assume dysphonias to be the result of a hearing loss, a discussion of voice disorders may help in clarifying the speech–language problems previously discussed. That is, dysphonias, or voice disorders, are much more specific than the speech–language problems discussed heretofore. Generally speaking, with the exception of dysarthria—which might include both articulatory and voice-resonance disturbances as the result of a neurologic disorder—a voice disorder occurs in the presence of appropriate articulation and intact language skills. An individual presenting the voice complaint well may be able to whisper or mouth words and, if necessary, should be able to write complete sentences to express him- or herself.

The voice problems most commonly encountered among the geriatric population include dysphonia secondary to paralysis or paresis of the vocal cords, absence of voice following laryngectomy, and weakness of the vocal cords, secondary to general physical debility (1974). Less common disorders might include vocal cord granuloma secondary to intubation procedures for the administration of anesthesia, weakness of the vocal cords following prolonged tracheostomy, and vocal cord polyps and nodules. The effect of any pathological vocal cord condition upon voice production may range from a mild, almost imperceptible hoarseness to complete aphonia (voice loss).

The patient presenting a voice disorder in the absence of any other psychological or neurological problem may be differentiated from the confused, aphasic, apraxic, and dysarthric individual in that his or her only problem is that of abnormal voicing. In all other respects, he or she will behave as any other individual in similar circumstances. It might be noted, that in instances where the individual appears unaware of the voice problem, such as a mild-to-moderate hoarseness, it is not unreasonable that such an individual might present a hearing loss. Such a loss would act as a high-frequency filter that would cut out the high-frequency aperiodicity that characterizes hoarse voice.

APATHY

A disorder of neurological and/or psychiatric etiology that may be apparent in the nursing home, extended-care facility, or hospital environment is that of the patient with a "lack of drive to communicate" (Grewel & Greene, 1968). Such patients present a deterioration in the urge to speak and withdraw almost completely from interaction with those around them. The withdrawing response could be thought of as the erection of a barrier of silence wherein the individual attempts to protect himself from future changes: a strategy which serves only to maintain the severity of the disorder. Such individuals will usually maintain appropriate activities of daily living and basic self-care though they often need verbal and gestural directions to facilitate their activities. However, they rarely interact verbally with those around them and frequently do not care to watch television or listen to the radio. If left to their own devices, they will withdraw further into themselves. When such depression progresses to the point where the individual no longer maintains self-care, he or she is difficult to differentiate from the advanced chronic brain syndrome patient. The patient described as apathetic presents no speech, language, or hearing disorder, per se. When such disorders are present, they are generally unobserved because of the patient's lack of communicative interaction.

PRESBYCUSIS

The presbycusic individual who exhibits no specific linguistic or psychological disorder will maintain adequate contact with his or her environment and evidence none of the atypical behaviors associated with the brain-damaged individual. The aged individual with presbycusis, as the reader is aware, will present a number of typical auditory–communicative behaviors. These include a diminished sensitivity for high-frequency tones, a concomitant reduction in the ability to hear speech sounds, a diminished ability to understand (discriminate) speech that is disproportionate to the severity of the pure tone hearing loss, and a lack of understanding of the nature of phonemic regression. Willeford (1971) and Kopra (1981) present excellent reviews of the research into and the auditory behaviors characteristic of the presbycusic adult. In addition to those auditory behaviors which may be revealed by formalized audiometric assessment, there are several communicative behaviors that appear with regularity among the presbycusic population.

These include the individual's use of a louder-than-needed voice when speaking; the individual's admonishment to his or her speaking partner to "talk louder" and/or not to "yell"; statements inferring that people do not talk clearly; inattention to social speaking distance; and a degree of monopolizing of conversation.

DIFFERENTIATING BETWEEN COMMUNICATION DISORDERS OF THE AGING

When attempting to differentiate the hearing-related communication disturbed patients from those whose disorder is not related to hearing, it is helpful to observe the patient's communication behaviors in terms of the language modalities used. Those modalities include auditory input (listening), visual input (reading), verbal output (speaking), and graphic output (writing). As an example, presbycusis will affect primarily the auditory input channel with a secondary and much less handicapping verbal output problem, e.g., the misarticulation of certain high-frequency sounds. The involvement of the auditory input channel can be determined on the basis of the individual's responses to conversational speech and standardized audiometric tests and his or her reports of hearing difficulty, particularly in understanding the speech of others. To determine whether the disorder is only of auditory input, it is helpful for the clinician to observe the other modalities.

The typical presbycusic adult should be able to read, write, and speak commensurate with his educational level. There should be few word-finding errors, word-choice errors, or grammatical errors. While there may be some disturbance of articulation and/or intensity, the linguistic message should be semantically and syntactically appropriate. The patient with a very mild dysarthria, however, may present a speech problem very similar to that of the patient with a long-standing presbycusic disorder. Because of weakness of the muscles of the tongue and mouth, or because of a mild coordination disturbance, a dysarthric individual may present a mild generalized imprecision of articulation which may be greater for the sibilants and blends. In this case, however, the individual may be able to comprehend and respond accurately to pure tone assessment and to conversational speech, is able to read and write, and presents only an output modality problem, i.e., the inability to accurately articulate because of paralyzed muscles.

Some presbycusic individuals who for some reason are unable to cope with the hearing loss, may withdraw from situations which require verbal communication with others. Such individuals communicate less rather than risk the inaccurate interpretation of a message. Such misinterpretations in the past may have lead to embarrassment, confusion, and danger for that person. This withdrawal from communication differs from that presented by the apathetic patient *only* with respect to degree. The differentiating characteristics between the hearing impaired and the apathetic patient will be apparent again via the language modalities. The hearing impaired individual will continue to take advantage of visual input in that he or she will be aware of individuals walking into his room, will take advantage of signs and directional clues, and generally will utilize communicated input that is necessary for daily living. The patient defined as "apathetic" generally will not respond via any modality unless some stimuli are forced upon him.

Table 20-1 presents characteristics of the communication disorders previously discussed. This table is provided to assist the audiologist in differentiating the hearing impaired and non-hearing impaired communication disturbances. It must be emphasized

Table 20-1
Behavioral Indices of Communication Disorders Among the Elderly[a]

	Aphasia	Apraxia	Dysarthria	Voice	Confused	Apathy	Hearing Impaired
Auditory Input (Listening)							
Understands single words though may require repetition or increased loudness	+/−	+	+	+	+	+	+
Understands short simple instructions accompanied by gestures or when repeated or when loud voice is used	+/−	+	+	+	*	+	+
Understands short simple instructions with no modification or gestures	+/−	+	+	+	*	+	+/−
Understands conversational speech when modifications in loudness, repetition, or written cues provided	+/−	+	+	+	*	+	+
Understands conversational speech with no modification	−	+/−	+	+	−	*	−
Visual Input (Reading)							
Understands single printed words, short sentences and phrases	+/−	+	+	+	+/−	+	+
Newspapers, magazines, letters	−	+/−	+	+	−	−	+
Verbal Output (Speaking)							
Spontaneous Speech:							
Jargon	+/−	−	−	−	−	−	−
Telegraphic meaningful	+/−	+/−	−	−	−	−	−
Fluent but little meaning	+/−	−	−	−	*	−	−
Expresses basic wants	+/−	+/−	+	+	+/−	+/−	+
Uses grammatically correct sentences	−	+/−	+	+	+	+	+
Grammatically correct but irrelevant	−	−	−	−	+	−	−
Elicited Speech							
Repeats words	+/−	+/−	+	+	+	+	+/−
Repeats phrases and sentences	−	−	+	+	+	*	+/−
Automatic speech (days of week, counting, etc.)	+/−	+/−	+	+	+	+	+

Articulation (Speech)							
Intelligible	+	−	−	+	+	+	+/−
General slurring	−	−	+	−	−	−	+/−
Unintelligible	−	+/−	+/−	−	−	−	−
Voice							
Appropriate	+	+	+/−	−	+	+/−	+/−
Excessively loud	−	−	−	−	−	−	+/−
Weak, soft	−	−	+/−	+/−	+/−	+/−	−
Hoarse	−	−	+/−	+	−	−	−
No voice, whisper	−	−	−	+/−	−	−	−
Graphic Output (Writing)							
Name	+/−	+	+	+	*	+	+
Single words	+/−	+	+	+	*	+/−	+
Short phrases	−	+	+	+	*	*	+
Sentences	−	+/−	+	+	−	−	+
Gestures							
Uses simple appropriate gestures	+	+	+	+	+/−	*	+
Uses complicated gestures	−	+/−	+	+	−	−	+
Memory							
Immediate	+	+	+	+	−	+/−	+
Day-to-day	+	+	+	+	+/−	+/−	+
Remote	+	+	+	+	+/−	*	+
Level of Consciousness							
Alert	+	+	+	+	+/−	+	+
Intermittent "tuning out"	−	−	−	−	+	−	−
Unresponsive	−	−	−	−	+/−	+	−
Orientation							
Appropriate	+	+	+	+	−	+/−	+
Confused	−	−	−	−	+	+/−	−
Hallucinates/confabulates	−	−	−	−	+/−	−	−

[a] + = Present; − = absent; +/− = present or absent, depending on severity; * = intermittent performance.

that these disorders are presented as if each occurred in isolation, while in fact, it is not uncommon for two or more communicative disorders to appear together (e.g., aphasia and apraxia, aphasia and dysarthria, hearing loss and aphasia).

THE AUDIOLOGIST'S ROLE IN DIFFERENTIAL DIAGNOSIS

Increased attention and concern on the part of governmental and social agencies has significantly expanded the role of health care providers in nursing homes, extended-care facilities, and geriatric day-care centers. Increasingly, the audiologist is becoming a member of the health care delivery team in those special geriatric settings. In that role, he or she must be capable of

1. Identifying those patients who have hearing-related communication disorders
2. Differentiating the hearing disordered patient from the non-hearing disordered patient
3. Determining the presence of a hearing disorder in addition to a nonhearing-related communication deficit
4. Establishing appropriate management targets for the hearing impaired
5. Making appropriate referral of the non-hearing impaired communication disturbed
6. Educating the staff and the patient's family and friends

All of the preceding duties will necessitate a much greater reliance upon the audiologists' observational skills than upon the utilization of standardized audiometric tests. That is not to say that such tests are not necessary or effective, but only to emphasize that responses to those tests will need to be considered in relation to the patient's overall communicative abilities and disabilities.

Formal Observations

The audiologist who has taken the responsibility of casefinding, diagnosing, and managing hearing disorders among the geriatric population (inclusive of aural rehabilitation) must have highly structured observational skills. Such structured skills may be categorized as formal (as in audiometrics) and informal (discerning the patient's mode of relating to others). The first, formal, includes those routine and highly specialized audiometrics that utilize equipment and procedures designed to identify and define a given hypacusis. The informal observations include patient behaviors that occur with specific relevance to the environment and the self. Both types of structured observational skills must be practiced by the audiologist working in geriatric settings, particularly, because the audiologist often enters into such settings with an educational bias—the bias being that hearing sensitivity decreases with age. Therefore, a large proportion of the elderly patients observed will have a hearing disorder. Such a bias, having prima facie validity, may result in the misdiagnosis and mismanagement of patients having other communicative disorders which resemble presbycusis.

During formal assessment, the audiologist must give special consideration to the "overcautiousness" that characterizes the aged adult's response behavior. That characteristic is achieving some research confirmation. With particular reference to audiometric assessment, Rees and Botwinick (1971) pinpoint some of the unique testing behaviors exhibited by the aged adult. The investigators first carefully documented the hearing thresholds for groups of aged and younger adults. Both groups were then presented with a decision-making task wherein they were to affirm the presence of auditory inputs of given intensity. It was found that the younger adults made significantly greater decisions affirming the presence of low intensity inputs which corresponded to their tested hearing thresholds, while the aged adults, even though their performance on detection assessment affirmed their sensitivity to the stimulus, would not affirm the presence of low-intensity input. The conclusion of the examiners was that the determination of ''absolute threshold audiologically'' confounds criterion and sensory effects; that is, audiologically, one might overestimate the magnitude of the sensory deficit because the aged individual is overcautious or overcareful in his or her response.

The overcautiousness of responding among aged adults has been reported as an age-related behavioral style (Botwinick, 1973). Okun and Di Vesta (1976) reported that older individuals, as compared with younger individuals, were more cautious in their response mode and were less shapeable by positive or supportive encouragement to attempt more difficult or challenging task performances. The authors concluded that in some situations, the aged adult would rather not respond where there is some risk of failure. This type of behavior certainly would influence any type of standardized communication testing and, specifically, would influence audiological assessment. Practically speaking, one might attempt to define or modify assessment tools in such a way that there is a high chance of successful performance with the greatest amount of information obtained.

Informal Observations

The audiologist in settings such as a nursing home consciously or unconsciously uses many of his or her own clinical observations to assist in developing a diagnosis of hearing impairment. The use of such informal observation requires that the audiologist pursue a logical analysis of a given behavior. That is, if the audiologist observes a patient using loud voice, he or she must analyze the use of that loud voice in relation to background noise, specific situation, the patient's emotional attitude, any vocal pathology which necessitates increased volume, and the individuals per se with whom he or she is speaking.

A further example where the astute observer will back-step from a behavior to determine the precipitating factor, is when an individual appears to respond positively to the use of loud voice. Such behavior would make one tend to think that the increased intensity is compensating for some type of hearing impairment. However, loud voice not only means increased intensity, but tends to reflect shorter input. As we increase loudness, there is a tendency to abbreviate our comments to include only the salient features and omit nonessential elements (Fordyce & Fowler, 1972). Also, louder voice (shorter input) can gain attention from confused and/or disoriented patients. That is, the individual who appears not to hear until loudness is increased, could, in fact, be unreactive to the stimulus until the intensity is such that it can draw his or her thinking from reverie to the environment.

Another instance where the audiologist's clinical presupposition that greater intensity leads to better reception must be questioned, is that of the moderate aphasic patient's apparent better reception when intensity is greater. Here, as was described in a preceding paragraph, the use of greater intensity will tend to telegraph or abbreviate the clinician's verbal output. This telegraphing will, in fact, facilitate comprehension on the part of the aphasic patient. For example, when instructing a patient to respond to pure tone testing, the audiologist might well say, "Listen for the tone. When you hear it, raise your hand on the same side as the ear that you hear the sound." Those instructions, when presented in loud voice might become, "When you hear the sound, raise your hand," with accompanying gestures. Such input tends to cut the message to the bare essentials, i.e., a telegraphing of words that attempts to evoke gestures on the part of the speaker and similarly tends to facilitate comprehension of the meaning on the part of the language-disturbed patient.

A given patient's request for increased volume during on-the-ward conversations can be very misleading with respect to differentiating the hearing impaired from the non-hearing impaired. The confused patient may routinely request a repetition of some input during a conversation, as will an aphasic, a hearing impaired individual, or a non-communication disturbed aged individual. One reason for the frequent request for loud voice use is that, in a relatively noisy ward environment, ambient noise may be distracting. An aged adult, further, may make very poor use of the speaker's gestures, facial expression, and other visual cues, tending instead to rely upon the spoken word. Thus, responses to and requests for loud voice may be a poor indication of hearing status unless the patient is in a quiet environment under optimal conditions.

Formal Assessment

The conventional standardized measures employed to determine audiological function may include pure tone hearing assessment, determination of speech reception threshold (SRT), and speech discrimination ability (articulation). For the non-brain injured or the non-psychologically disturbed aged adult, these auditory tools can contribute meaningful information. However, prior to measuring the auditory sensitivity and auditory discrimination of communication disturbed elderly patients, the audiologist must initially make some basic determinations with respect to the given individual's level of consciousness, attention span, ability to profit from instruction, and intactness of the response modalities. In emphasizing this requirement to make careful analysis of patients' abilities, one might consider the aphasic patient who performs in an accurate and responsive manner to pure tone testing and shows significant and marked differences between that performance and SRT as measured by ability to repeat spondaic words and/or speech discrimination as measured by ability to repeat phonetically balanced (PB) word lists. If an audiologist is unaware of the nature of the aphasic involvement, he might interpret the results as one indicator of a possible presbycusic involvement.

It is important that the audiologist attempt to use the most objective measures of auditory function possible. The majority of aged nursing home residents can be tested via conventional pure tone audiometrics (Schow & Nerborne, 1980). There will be many situations, however, when modification in presentation, stimulus, response mode, and response criterion will be required to achieve a practical, reliable, and valid measure of hearing discrimination among the communication disturbed aged. In general, the audiologist, when assessing the aged communication disturbed patient, should consider the following suggestions:

1. The task directions should be presented slowly, carefully, and in as concise a manner as possible. Gestures should accompany the verbal instructions, and a demonstration should be provided whenever possible. In some cases, written instructions should accompany the verbal instructions.

2. The interstimulus interval should be longer than that provided for non-communication disturbed individuals. Such intervals will account, to some degree, for the aged patient's cautiousness, the brain injured patient's slower shifting from one stimulus or response to the next, the relatively greater time required by aged and brain injured for the responses to be formulated, and perseveration that is often characteristic of the brain injured.
3. The number of stimuli presented during a given test may need to be substantially reduced to account for general physical fatigue, perceptual fatigue, attention span limitation, and what has been described as "noise build-up" in the system (Porch, 1967).
4. The response mode should be determined according to each patient's abilities. If a confused patient blinks his or her eyes each time he or she hears a tone and does not change this behavior upon repeated instructions, such a response, if consistent, should be accepted. Similarly, during speech discrimination testing, the aphasic, apraxic, and dysarthric patient should not be expected to respond verbally. The dysarthric might write his or her responses, as might the mild apraxic patient. Newby (1972) suggested writing as the method of choice when factors such as illiteracy or fine motor control disturbance do not prohibit such. In those cases, a gestural response to pictures might be devised.
5. The audiologist must determine that the patient is attending to the task. In many cases, this will mean that he or she stops the assessment to readminister the instructions, perhaps to touch the patient and point to the earphones, or to give a brief reminder, such as "Remember, raise your hand when you hear the sound."

As mentioned, the modifications that may be required to achieve optimal auditory performance from a communication disturbed aged patient are few but very important. Table 20-2 presents suggested modifications the hearing specialist may wish to consider when evaluating patients having a specific communication disturbance.

When evaluating communication disturbed adults, the audiologist must clearly determine what he or she is attempting to achieve. If the goal is to differentiate the hearing impaired from non-hearing impaired, then diagnostic procedures may only need to be modified in the ways previously suggested. On the other hand, if the evaluation target is that of assessing the patient's listening skills in order to determine if the patient can benefit from amplification, then the audiologist must make every attempt to carefully define hearing levels, speech reception threshold, and speech discrimination abilities as accurately as possible. This seemingly routine assessment is a most imposing task when it must be accomplished with an aged patient presenting other communication disturbances.

Finally, the audiologist must be able to determine the reliability and validity of common audiological procedures employed with the communication disturbed aged. The information presented in Table 20-3 is a guide for the professional to consider when analyzing various audiometrical responses from a patient manifesting one or more of the disorders specified.

In most instances, diagnostic measures other than pure tone air and bone conduction measures will be conducted outside the communication disturbed aged adult's place of residence. With the exception of the hospitals and large rehabilitation centers, other geriatric settings such as nursing homes, extended-care facilities, and geriatric day-care centers may not have the necessary facilities for sophisticated assessment procedures. In

Table 20-2
Suggested Audiologic Assessment Modifications when Assessing Elderly Persons who Possess Communication Disorders

	Pure Tone	SRT	Discrimination (PB Lists)
Aphasia	Simplify instructions; gesture; demonstrate	Use only with mildly involved; simplify instructions; increase stimulus interval	Use only with mildly involved; questionable reliability
Apraxia	Simplify instructions; gesture; demonstrate	All above, plus allow graphic responses that approximate spellings	Reliable only with mildly involved; allow graphic responses and spelling errors; increase stimulus interval
Dysarthria	Simplify instructions	Increase stimulus interval; allow consistent speech distortion or written response	Increase stimulus interval; allow consistent speech distortion or written response
Voice	None	Allow whisper or written response for aphonic	Allow whisper or written response for aphonic
Confused	Simplify instructions; demonstrate; gesture; reduce number of stimuli; frequently confirm attention and retention of task. Low intensity stimuli unreliable	Simplify instructions; demonstrate; gesture; reduce number of stimuli; frequently confirm attention and retention of task. Low intensity stimuli unreliable	Simplify instructions; demonstrate; gesture; reduce number of stimuli; frequently confirm attention and retention of task. Low intensity stimuli unreliable
Apathy	Same as for Confused	Same as for "Confused"	Same as for "Confused"
Hearing Impaired	Simplify; demonstrate	Simplify; demonstrate	Simplify; demonstrate

Table 20-3
Response Reliability* of Communication Disturbed Aged to Certain Auditory Assessment Procedures

	Pure Tone	SRT	Discrimination (PB Lists)
Aphasia	1	2–3	3–4
Apraxia	1	2 (written response)	2 (written response)
Dysarthria	1	1 (optional written)	1 (optional written)
Voice	1	1	1
Confusion†	2–3	3	2–3
Apathy†	3	2	3
Hearing Impaired	1	1	1

*1 = Good; 2 = fair; 3 = poor; 4 = unreliable.

†Confused and apathetic patients usually will not respond if the tone or word is not presented at a level that will draw their attention. They are usually not vigilant to stimuli.

most cases, the audiologist will have a high degree of control over the testing environment. However, he or she usually will not have access to the ward information that is so critical to understanding the patient's auditory and communicative behaviors. That is, the audiologist may not know if the environment is noisy, if the patient generally stays by him- or herself, or if he or she will be dependent on others for assistance. The use of the Hearing Status Questionnaire (discussed in the appendix section of this chapter) can be of great benefit to the audiologist when the nursing staff, speech–language pathologist, or audiologist him- or herself has completed the questionnaire prior to the patient's audiological evaluation.

The astute audiologist is aware that both formal or informal assessment during the patient's first 1 or 2 weeks of residence in a nonhome environment will yield equivocal results. It is advised that the hearing and speech professional utilize the initial contact to make the patient familiar with him or her and to describe procedures which will be conducted at a future time. Such nontesting contacts are very important. They are important even to the presbycusic individual who presents no other significant communication or psychological disorder, maintains adequate contact with his or her environment, and usually makes appropriate attempts to adapt for his or her hearing loss. It has been this author's experience that, not infrequently, the individual who has a history of hearing loss suddenly presents greater symptoms of that loss upon entry into a nursing home or extended-care facility. This appears to be a reaction to the increased stress in changing from home environment to the institution. In such a circumstance, the individual must utilize all of his or her psychological resources to adapt to the new environment. This organismic adaptation frequently leaves little energy or motivation for the patient to maintain whatever auditory coping skills he or she had previously established.

After an individual has had sufficient time to become adjusted to his surroundings, the observing clinician must determine how well the patient handles or copes with sensory inputs. A hard-of-hearing adult will have predictable problems in certain situations but, in general, his or her behavior will be compatible with the situation. He or she will attempt to compensate through a number of avenues. These might include (1) asking the speaker to increase intensity, (2) being more careful to observe the speaker's lips and gestures, (3) asking for written or increased visual input, (4) telling the individual "I can't understand you" and terminating the attempted conversation to avoid faulty or "interfering" input, or (5) monopolizing the conversation to minimize the involvement in subsequent auditory confusions. All of those behaviors are adaptive and are in keeping with the individual's attempt to maintain overt and covert stability. Such behaviors give indication to the clinical audiologist that those individuals are attempting to adapt to their disability. This suggests that they have an awareness on either a conscious or unconscious level—an awareness that would be a positive factor with respect to use of amplification and/or aural rehabilitation. These types of adaptive behaviors would rarely be observed in a patient manifesting chronic brain syndrome and/or psychiatric disorders.

Once it is determined that a patient manifests a hearing disorder, regardless of concomitant speech–language disorders, the clinical audiologist must carefully define his or her responsibility and level of commitment. Individuals in special geriatric settings will generally require more consistency, more attention, and more structure if rehabilitative efforts are to succeed. This is particularly true relative to auditory training. The audiologist must consult with other members of the staff to determine, first, if the patient will have someone in his or her environment who might be able to fit the aid and to be sure it is functioning properly on a daily basis, and second, if it is possible for the patient to be included in activities which would improve his or her orientation skills as well as facilitate better reception and integration of the auditory signals.

Relevant Preassessment Considerations

In the special geriatric setting, the majority of patients will be referred to the audiologist by nurses and/or physicians. The referral may be motivated by an inability on the part of the staff to explain certain patient behaviors, by questioning behaviors that do, in fact, appear to be hearing related, or by the family requesting the nurse to make such a referral. The nursing home or extended-care facility staff may or may not be of assistance in determining a given patient's communication status. That is, the pressures of the nursing home are such that too frequently there is insufficient time for staff and patients to know one another well. Also, the aide population has a very high turnover in a given year. However, any information that the staff can provide with respect to a suspected hearing impaired patient should be obtained. Such information can be obtained via the Hearing Status Questionnaire (see appendix section of this chapter). The Hearing Status Questionnaire should be useful to the hearing professional in that it enables him or her to make basic determinations about the patient's ability to be tested. That is, (1) whether the patient can respond to sophisticated audiometrical procedures, (2) whether certain types of audiometrical procedures (pure tone but not spondaic words) are practical, or (3) whether informal ward observation is required. Such initial information also provides the audiologist with a litany of behaviors that may enable him or her to more effectively counsel the patient's family and the staff. Such environmental–disability interactions are critical considerations for effective management (Bollinger, Waugh, & Zatz, 1977).

REFERENCES

Allison, R. S. *The senile brain*. Baltimore, The Williams and Wilkins Company, 1962, p. 288.

Arie, T. Dementia in the elderly: Diagnosis and assessment. *British Medical Journal,* 1973, *4,* 540–543.

Bollinger, R. L. Geriatric speech pathology. *The Gerontologist,* 1974, *14,* 217–220.

Bollinger, R. L., Waugh, P. F., & Zatz, A. F. *Communication management of the geriatric patient*. Danville, Illinois: The Interstate Press and Publishers, Inc., 1977, p. 45

Botwinick, J. Cautiousness in advanced age. *Journal of Gerontology,* 1966, *21,* 347–355.

Botwinick, J. *Aging and behavior: A comprehensive integration of research findings*. New York: Springer Publishing, 1973.

Darley, F. L. Presentation 8, in A. L. Benton (Ed.), *Behavioral change in cerebrovascular disease*. New York: Harper and Row, 1970, pp. 51–71.

Darley, F. L., Aronson, A. E., & Brown, J. R. *Motor speech disorders*. Philadelphia: W. B. Saunders Company, 1975.

Fordyce, W. E., & Fowler, R. S. Adapting care for the brain damaged patient, parts I and II. *American Journal of Nursing,* 1972, *10,* 1832–1835, *11,* 2056–2059.

Fox, J. H., Topel, J. L., & Huckman, M. S. Dementia in the elderly: A search for treatable illness. *Journal of Gerontology,* 1975, *30,* 557–564.

Geschwind, N. E. Current concepts—aphasia. *New England Journal of Medicine*. 1971, *284,* 654–656.

Ginzberg, R. Attitude therapy in geriatric ward psychiatry. *Geriatrics,* 1955, *3,* 445–462.

Goodglass, H., & Kaplan, E. *The assessment of aphasia and related disorders*. Philadelphia: Lea and Febiger, 1972, p. 210.

Grewel, F., & Greene, M. C. L. Diagnosis and treatment of speaking and language disorders following cerebral injury in old age. *Psychiatria, Neurologia, Neurochirurgia,* 1968, *71,* 469–482.

Halpern, H., Darley, F., & Brown, J. R. Differential language and neurologic characteristics in cerebral involvement. *Journal of Speech and Hearing Disorders,* 1973, *37,* 162–173.

Kopra, L. L. The auditory/communicative manifestations of presbycusis, in R. H. Hull (Ed.), *Rehabilitative audiology, part II: the elderly client.* New York: Grune and Stratton, in press.

Newby, H. A. *Audiology, 3rd Ed.* New York. Appleton-Century-Crofts Educational Division, Meredith Corp., 1972.

Okun, M. A., & Di Vesta, F. J. Cautiousness in adulthood as a function of age and instructions. *Journal of Gerontology,* 1977, *31,* 571–576.

Porch, B. E. *The Porch Index of Communicative Ability.* Palo Alto: Consulting Psychologists Press, 1967, p. 115.

Rees, N. J., & Botwinick, J. Detection and decision factors in auditory behaviors of the elderly. *Journal of Gerontology,* 1971, *26,* 133–136.

Schow, R. L., & Nerborne, M. A. Hearing levels among elderly nursing home residents. *Journal of Speech and Hearing Disorders, 45*(1), 124–132.

Schuell, H., Jenkins, J., Jimenez-Pabon, E. *Aphasia in adults: Diagnosis, prognosis, and treatment.* New York: Harper and Row, 1965, p. 428.

Selzer, B., & Sherwin, I. Organic brain syndromes: An empirical study and critical review. *American Journal of Psychiatry,* 1978, *135*(1), 13–21.

Simon, A., & Neal, M. W. Patterns of geriatric mental illness, in R. H. Williams, C. Tibbitts, & W. Donahue (Eds.), *Processes of aging: Social and psychological perspectives, vol. 1.* New York: Atherton Press, 1963.

Willeford, J. A. The geriatric patient, in D. Rose (Ed.), *Audiologic Assessment.* Englewood Cliffs, New Jersey: Prentice Hall and Co., 1971.

Wolff, K. *Geriatric psychiatry.* Springfield, Mo.: Charles C Thomas Publishers, 1963, p. 108.

REFERENCE NOTES

1. Bollinger, R. L. *Communication abilities of "chronic brain syndrome" patients* (Unpublished doctoral dissertation). Seattle, Washington. University of Washington, 1970, p. 94.
2. Bollinger, R. L., & Hedrick, D. L. *Diotic listening abilities of brain-injured adults.* Paper presented at the American Speech and Hearing Association Convention, Las Vegas, November 5–8, 1974.

APPENDIX: HEARING STATUS QUESTIONNAIRE

Patient's name__________ Room no. _____Health no. _____
Staff person__________Date _____Facility _____
Physician________ Date of admission _____Patient's age ___Yrs. ___Mo. ___
Family member __________Assistive devices: Glasses _____
Hearing aid _____Braces _____Other __________
Medical problems__________
Medications__________

Patient-Staff Interaction—Circle the number(s) that best describe patient.*

Talking

1. Staff can understand with no difficulty.
2. Staff understands most, but some slurring and/or garbled words.
3. Patient tries to tell what he wants but must use gestures or writing to get point across.
4. Patient tries to talk but cannot be understood.
5. Patient makes no attempt to talk to staff.

Listening

1. Patient listens and follows directions.
2. Patient listens but I have to repeat and/or talk louder for him to understand.
3. Patient seems to listen, but does not really understand.
4. Patient listens but does not do what is asked or does nothing.
5. Patient does not listen—does not do what I tell him.

Relevance

1. Patient talks about subject or activity in progress.
2. Patient responds appropriately to conversation, directions, or schedule.
3. Patient often talks about things that have nothing to do with what I said or was doing for him.
4. Patient talks about things that are fantasy.
5. Patient does not talk or act in a way that shows he knows or cares what is going on around him.

Patient–Environment Interaction

1. Patient talks and listens to other patients, watches television, and/or listens to radio.
2. Patient attempts to talk with others and participates even when he cannot be understood or has trouble understanding others.
3. Patient is hostile to others.
4. Patient does not relate to other patients.
5. Patient talks to himself, does not interact.

Dressing/Hygiene/Feeding

1. Patient is independent—needs very little help.
2. Patient does what he can for himself but needs some help because of physical problems.
3. Patient is completely dependent because of physical problems.
4. Patient does most things for himself but forgets small things like zipping pants, flushing toilet.
5. Patient must be reminded to dress, brush teeth, etc.

Orientation
1. Patient knows his way around facility and is usually aware of time, day, etc.
2. Patient knows his way around but sometimes needs reminders for meals, bedtimes, routine activities.
3. Patient sometimes cannot remember where dining room or activity room is and forgets where personal articles are located.
4. Patient needs frequent reminders for dressing, meals, etc.
5. Patient requires constant supervision.

Personality/Emotions
1. Patient shows emotions that are appropriate to given situations.
2. Patient seems depressed, does not laugh or cry, or has no emotions (bland look on face; does not get excited or upset).
3. Patient gets upset easily and cries a lot.
4. Patient switches quickly from being happy to sad and vice versa; sometimes inappropriate emotions.
5. Patient is resentful of staff and other patients, suspicious, and maybe hostile.

*Generally, characteristics numbered 1 and 2 reflect nonlanguage problems where hearing loss might be suspected and routine assessment possible. Characteristics 4 and 5 usually reflect severe neurological or psychological disturbances. The purpose of the tool is not to make a diagnosis, but to assist or direct the clinician in asking appropriate questions for clinical assessment and management.

Lennart L. Kopra

Chapter 21: Modifications of Traditional Techniques for Assessment of the Elderly Client

The elderly client may arrive at the audiological evaluation for any number of several reasons. He or she may have been brought in by a well-meaning spouse or relative, or the client may have requested the evaluation because he or she recognizes that a hearing problem is evident and a professional audiologist's evaluation is the proper recourse. The client's motivation to participate in the audiological evaluation may range from exuberant anticipation to downright disgust.

Even if the elderly person recognizes that he or she is having difficulty hearing and that there are audiologists and otologists who can evaluate the problem and provide good counseling for possible alleviation of the problem, some elderly individuals lack motivation to seek assistance. Many rationalize that, because they are old or because the examinations and a possible hearing aid cost too much money, they do not need and, therefore, do not want an audiological evaluation. Some elderly hearing impaired clients cite their acquaintances' experiences with hearing aids: these friends have had no success with hearing aids; the hearing aids have been a nuisance, have given headaches, and have only amplified noise with the result that their hearing problem has not been helped.

Elderly clients also differ in other ways. Obviously, their age may vary from the sixties to the nineties or older. Their intellectual level may be as functional as it was in their younger years, or so much cortical degeneration may have occurred that they have limited ability to function intellectually. Their physical condition also may vary from confinement to a wheel chair to spry mobility. Similarly, their ability to attend and to concentrate may extend from a few moments to fairly long periods of time common in audiological evaluations.

Life styles vary widely. Some elderly hearing impaired persons are completely self-sufficient and live by themselves or with spouses or with relatives. Others are confined to extended-care residential facilities. As these life styles differ, so does the need for social interaction and oral communication. Thus, the individuals we see for audiological

Grateful acknowledgment is made to David J. Thompson, Ph.D., Audiology/Speech Pathology Service, Olin E. Teague Veterans' Center, Temple, Texas, for his contribution of the section on acoustic impedance–admittance battery.

evaluation vary widely in their motivation to participate in the audiological evaluation and in their perception of the possible benefits they might derive from such an evaluation. They also differ in their physical, intellectual, and psychological adjustment.

The present chapter describes some methods for modifying standard audiological procedures for elderly individuals who, for one or more of several reasons, cannot respond reliably to standard procedures. In part, these procedures are based on established methods that have a scientific base; others are based on clinical intuitive methods that have been successful.

PRELIMINARIES TO AUDIOLOGICAL MEASUREMENT

It is axiomatic to say that we should conduct the audiological assessment of the client as expeditiously and reliably as our clinical know-how allows. However, the need for an initial conference can be de-emphasized or compromised by us sometimes in favor of expediting auditory measurement procedures. The importance of a thorough pre-measurement conference needs to be highlighted.

Talking to the Patient

It is a relatively common experience to observe a professional person raising his or her voice level inordinately or even shouting when talking to an elderly person. When speaking to hearing impaired individuals, especially older persons, even professionals tend to forget that we can improve our listener's chance of understanding without raising the level of our voices. There are some relatively simple ways of improving the oral communication situation for the hearing impaired person:

1. We should at all times talk to our patient at eye level.
2. The level of our voice should be raised only a small amount, if at all.
3. It is helpful to slow the rate of our speech by a small amount.
4. We can articulate a little more precisely without exaggerating.
5. We can provide many visual clues.
6. There are times when we can choose words that are more visible than others without changing the meaning of our message.
7. If our patient fails to understand, even after repeated trials by us, we must at all times try to control our impatience and look for alternative methods of communicating.

Let the patient speak for him or herself. The interview should be directed to the hearing impaired person and not to family members or friends accompanying him or her. Accompanying persons should be asked to participate in the interview only if, after repeated attempts, the information cannot be obtained from the hearing impaired person.

Gather Pertinent Information

The initial interview of the client provides an opportunity for the audiologist to gather several different kinds of information (Tables 21-1 and 21-2). (Perhaps equally important is the opportunity to allay any fears or trepidations the patient may have and to attempt to set him or her at ease.) In addition to gathering or confirming basic

Table 21-1
Information to be Explored during Initial Interview with Elderly Patient

Hearing Status

- Does the patient believe he or she has a hearing loss? If so, is it in the right ear, left ear, or both ears?
- How long ago did the patient first notice the hearing loss? Has the hearing loss become worse? If so, suddenly or gradually over a period of time?
- Has the patient been examined by an otologist or other physician? If so, when? Identify the physician by name and address. What did the physician tell the patient about the hearing loss?
- Has the patient ever had a hearing test? If so, when, where, and by whom? What was the patient informed about the results?
- Has the patient ever worn a hearing aid or does he or she wear one now?
  —If one is worn now, when did the patient obtain the hearing aid and over what period of time has he or she worn it?
  —How many hours on the average does he or she wear the hearing aid every day?
  —What are the manufacturer and model of the hearing aid?
  —Was the patient satisfied with the performance of the hearing aid?
  —If the patient was dissatisfied, what problems did he or she encounter which made performance unsatisfactory?
  —Has the patient had any aural rehabilitation, i.e., hearing aid orientation, speechreading instruction, auditory training, or counseling for adjustment to the hearing loss?
- What degree and frequency of difficulty does the patient experience in communicating with others or in understanding what is being said? Provide examples such as hearing and understanding
  —speech in a one-to-one situation in quiet.
  —speech in a one-to-one situation in noise.
  —speech in a group situation where there is relative quiet.
  —speech in a group situation where there is noise.
  —a single talker in a theater, church, auditorium, or lecture hall.
  —as distance between talker and listener varies.
  —in a car, train, or bus.
  —in varieties of noise.
  —and recognize a speaker by his/her voice.
  —without speechreading.
  —when precision of articulation of the talker varies.
  —when a man versus a woman versus a child is the talker.
  —phone conversation.
  —radio, TV, record player.
  —in other situations unique to the person's life style.
- What is the patient's reported reaction to the difficulties reported in situations described in the preceding section?
- Does the patient have any visual problems? If so, describe them. Does he or she wear glasses? What is his or her corrected vision with glasses?
- Are there any obvious problems such as poststroke hemiplegia, emotional problems, or multiple handicapping conditions that might affect the patient's ability to participate in an audiological evaluation or in follow-up aural rehabilitation?
- To the degree that it is relevant, occupational and educational history should be obtained.
- What are the patient's hobbies and other avocational activities?

Table 21-2
Medical History to be Considered during Initial Interview

- Ear infections and/or ear surgery. Type of medical treatment—when, where, and by whom?
- History of hearing loss in the patient's family.
- Record of diseases, serious infections, diabetes, mumps, etc.
- Serious illnesses such as malaria, encephalitis, stroke, heart attack, arthritis, etc.
- Serious accidents involving concussion or other head injury.
- High-level noise exposure for prolonged periods of time: when and under what circumstances?
- Tinnitus: if so, when experienced (provide qualitative description)?
- Vertigo, dizziness, fainting spells.
- Physical complaints.
- Medications currently being taken.
- Use of ototoxic drugs, past and present.
- Visual problems such as glaucoma, cataracts (if visually impaired, identify corrected vision with glasses).

identifying information, the audiologist can elicit the patient's own perception of the relative difficulty he or she has in hearing. The patient's statements concerning understanding of the onset, duration, cause, and handicapping nature of the hearing loss can help the clinician identify some aspects of the aural rehabilitation needs of the patient.

If the patient's hearing loss is so severe that he or she cannot understand well enough to respond appropriately during the interview, a portable auditory training unit with earphones should be used. If the patient is a hearing aid wearer, the listening experience will provide an opportunity to make quality judgments between hearing with his or her own aid and hearing with a relatively high-fidelity amplifying device. If the patient is not a hearing aid wearer, this experience can introduce the patient to amplified sound. The introduction of amplified sound should be done cautiously, i.e., the volume control should be adjusted carefully so as not to exceed the patient's comfortable listening level. Arbitrary adjustments of the volume control should not be made by the clinician.

The behavioral reactions of the patient during the interview can give the clinician some clues about the patient's need for speechreading. If the patient obviously is not relying on speechreading and has no difficulty understanding, this behavior suggests that the hearing loss is not severe. The average sound level of a talker's speech at a distance of 1 meter is about 65 to 70 dB sound-pressure level (SPL).

Since sound levels of various talkers vary considerably, prior to the interview it is well for the clinician to measure the sound level of his or her own speech with a sound level meter at the approximate position of a person being interviewed. Since the absolute threshold for speech for normal listeners is about 20 dB SPL, the level above normal threshold can be approximated at the position of the patient being interviewed. For example, if the binaural hearing level of the listener is 30 dB (50 dB SPL), then the speech of a talker with an average sound level of 65 dB SPL would be received by the patient at 15 dB sensation level. Given that the patient has some speechreading ability, such a level should allow him or her to understand much of conversational discourse. On the other hand, if the patient's binaural hearing level for speech were 45 dB (65 dB SPL), then the 65 dB (SPL) sound level of a talker's speech would be at the threshold

(0 dB sensation level [SL]) for the patient. In this condition, a patient's ability to understand the clinician's speech would generally be reduced and would depend to a large extent on the patient's speechreading ability.

The initial interview provides the clinician with some idea of the language ability of the patient. This is, if the patient is having difficulty understanding even with amplification via the portable auditory-training unit, then instructions for the several audiologic tests will have to be modified appropriately. During the interview, it should become obvious that attention should be paid to the physical comfort of the patient. For instance, air-conditioned audiologic booths are sometimes too cold for elderly people, or frequent rest periods may be necessary if the patient tires easily or has more frequent toilet needs than the average patient.

The modus operandi varies from one clinical facility to another. However, no matter how time-consuming these procedures may be, it is imperative that this information be obtained from the client and/or from a well-informed acquaintance (spouse, friend, nurse, etc.).

Since many elderly persons fatigue quickly and cannot pay attention for periods of time required for interviewing and for audiologic tests, this process may have to be scheduled for two or more sessions. Lack of transportation for the patient is frequently cited as a reason why he or she cannot be seen more than once or twice. Some arrangement for travel must be made. The simple fact remains, that if a sufficiently thorough inquiry is not made either prior to and/or immediately following the audiologic evaluation, the results of the assessment will be less relevant to the total rehabilitation process.

MODIFICATION OF TRADITIONAL TECHNIQUES

It is obvious that all alternatives to traditional methods of measurement cannot be described here. Only some suggested alternatives are included. The underlying principle in modification of traditional techniques is that, if a listener is not able to respond reliably to a given auditory task, progressively simplify the task until the listener is able to respond reliably. Simplifying the task includes changing the type of stimulus being used and also, as appropriate, changing the method of response. For example, if a listener cannot reliably identify the presence of a randomly presented pure tone because he or she has tinnitus, using a periodically interrupted tone or a warble tone would simplify the listener's task in differentiating the stimulus from a background of tinnitus. In speech audiometry, if a person is unable to respond reliably to spondees, then the use of a more redundant unit like numbers (paired digits, for example) might allow the listener to respond reliably to the task. In this case, the interpretation of "speech threshold" would, of course, have to take into account the difference between absolute thresholds when different types of speech material are used.

Reiterating, *the basic principle in using modifications of traditional techniques in auditory measurement is to simplify progressively the listening task and the method of response until a reliable series of responses can be obtained from the listener*. The interpretation of the results of a particular modified procedure must take into account the type of stimulus used, the measurement procedure, and the type of response obtained from the listener.

MEASUREMENT OF AUDITORY FUNCTION

Standard methods used for measurement of air- and bone-conduction pure-tone thresholds and for speech audiometry are described in several audiology texts (Martin, 1975; Newby, 1979; Rose, 1978). Additional descriptions of standard methods in audiometry are provided by the ASHA Committee on Audiometric Evaluation (1978) and by the American National Standards Institute (1978).

Modifications of standard audiometrical techniques are necessary when the listener is not able to appreciate or process the signal being used, and/or to respond behaviorally in a meaningful and reliable way to the listening task. First, we need to identify what kind of processing is required of the listener when various kinds of signals are being used. Second, we need to consider what kinds of behavioral responses usually are used for which some alternate response mode might result in a more valid and reliable response. The pure-tone threshold is a detection threshold and simply calls for a yes–no response. As such, the pure-tone threshold is a reflection of the sensitivity of the auditory system. Therefore, if we use any sound (pure tone, speech, bands of noise, etc.) and ask our listener to respond, we are asking him to judge the presence versus the absence of sound—a simple task. The listener's response to this task can vary from pressing a button or holding up a finger or hand to a verbal response such as, "Now I hear it a little bit." If pure tones are introduced via monaural earphones, then auditory sensitivity can be measured as a function of frequency. If some complex sound like speech or noise is used, then the detection threshold for that sound will depend not only on the distribution of hearing loss across test frequencies but also on the spectral distribution of the energy in that sound. The application and interpretation of detection thresholds for complex sounds will be discussed later in this chapter.

In contrast to simple auditory detection tasks characteristic of pure tone audiometry, in speech audiometry the listener is required to identify a word or words and to respond verbally to them. This task, therefore, requires linguistic processing. The listener's response is a spoken word which means that the auditory system was sufficiently sensitive to transduce the acoustic signal, the central auditory mechanism's processing allowed identification of the word(s), and the listener's expressive language was sufficiently intact to provide for a meaningful verbal response. If any one or more of these functions does not occur, the listener will not respond appropriately to speech signals.

The Audiological Test Battery

The audiological test battery has a number of tests, the results of which can contribute to the medical diagnosis of the site of lesion. Some audiological tests contribute little or no information to the medical diagnosis but are interpreted primarily for their nonmedical rehabilitative implications.

Pure-Tone Threshold Test

Although a general description of the tests and methods of response was given to the patient during the initial interview, it is important to instruct the elderly person immediately prior to the test. If the pure-tone threshold test is administered in a two-room suite with a patient's room and a control room, the clinician should give the directions directly to the patient in the patient's room. Older individuals are likely to be cautious and conservative in acknowledging their perception of pure tones at very faint levels (Rees and Botwinick, 1971). They should be encouraged to guess, and instructions should be given in a manner that will provide them confidence in the listening task. If the patient has any difficulty understanding what is expected of him or her, a face-to-face communication situation is necessary. Examples of a low-frequency pure tone (500 Hz is good) should be introduced at a sufficiently high level to be audible to the patient via a hand-held earphone close to his ear. If the test proper is to be conducted in a two-room suite, the demonstration of the test tone, its on period and its off period, can be more easily accomplished with a single portable audiometer in the patient's room.

When testing an elderly person whose attention span is short and who may fatigue quickly, the traditional order in which frequencies are tested should be changed. Usually, we begin with 1000 Hz and then progress to 6000 Hz or higher. Then 1000 Hz is tested again for an intratest reliability check, followed by 500 Hz and 250 Hz. This procedure is completed for one ear and then the other ear. For the person whose attention span is limited, the frequencies should be tested in the following order: 500, 1000, 2000, 3000, 250, 4000, 6000 Hz. Each frequency should be tested in each ear, before testing the next frequency in the sequence. That is, 500 Hz is tested in the right ear and then in the left ear; 1000 Hz is tested next in the right ear and in the left ear; and so on. The rationale for this order is that the thresholds for 500 Hz and 1000 Hz provide us the best estimate of the speech reception threshold. Each additional frequency in the sequence after 1000 Hz provides us the next most important amount of information about pure-tone sensitivity.

Traditional procedures in air-conduction audiometry have eliminated testing at 125 Hz. However, in some patients who have marked hearing loss in the mid frequencies and profound loss in the high frequencies, a threshold measurement at 125 Hz can provide useful information and so is recommended. The fundamental frequency of the adult male voice is in the neighborhood of 125 Hz, and residual hearing at this frequency may provide information for a hearing aid wearer, at least in terms of recognizing the presence or absence of the human voice.

The pure-tone threshold is arbitrarily defined as that hearing level at which the listener responds correctly fifty percent of the time to a series of tone presentations (method of constant stimuli). If the elderly listener has any problem of attending or distinguishing a randomly presented tone against a background of tinnitus, some modification is necessary. Hochberg and Waltzman (1972) found that the use of pulsed tones and continuous tones yielded equivalent thresholds and that pulsed tones appeared to facilitate patient responsiveness. To effect a better foreground–background differentiation, it is usually helpful to present a series of pulses either with the automatic pulse switch of the audiometer or by manually presenting a series or train of pulses. The patient should then be asked to respond (in some interpretable behavioral way) to the train of pulses and to continue responding as long as the train of pulses is minimally audible. The audiologist's task here is to increase the signal intensity so that positive suprathreshold responses are noted and to decrease the intensity until the patient consistently does not respond to subthreshold levels of intensity. A bracketing procedure is used for final adjustments of the intensity until a 50 percent correct response is observed for a given presentation level.

In testing by bone conduction, the usual procedures for masking apply. However, when noise is used to counteract the effects of lateralization, the elderly person may find it difficult to distinguish the foreground signal (test tone) from the background signal (noise). Prior to the bone-conduction test, it is usually helpful to administer the Weber test. With a tone of 500 Hz set at 40 or 50 dB hearing level (HL), the clinician should hold the bone-conduction oscillator and place it on various locations on the head—forehead, right mastoid process, left mastoid process, and external occipital protuberance. If lateralization occurs, this procedure helps the patient understand that the tone may be perceived in the ear opposite from the side where the oscillator is placed when mastoid-process placement is used. Forehead placement of the bone-conduction oscillator is a good alternative to the mastoid process. However, more intensity is required to reach threshold than when the mastoid process is used. Of course, calibration differences between thresholds for the mastoid process versus the forehead must be taken into account when interpreting results. The difference between thresholds obtained at the forehead versus the mastoid process may be as much as 15 dB at 250 Hz. This difference diminishes as a function of frequency and may be in the neighborhood of 5 dB at 4000 Hz (Dirks, 1978).

Since more precise diagnostic information about the conducting mechanism can be obtained by the acoustic impedance–admittance battery, a minimum amount of time should be spent on bone-conduction testing with the elderly person.

Acoustic Impedance–Admittance Battery

Few investigations have been conducted on acoustic impedance–admittance measures among older adults. Data on static values of ears of individuals past 50 to 60 years of age have suggested increased impedance (Jerger, Jerger, & Mauldin, 1972). Beattie and Leamy's (1975) report indicated increased admittance for subjects over 60 years of age. For a group of subjects 70 years and older, Blood and Greenberg (1977) reported a significant decrease in admittance. On the other hand, Thompson, Sills, Recke, and Bui (1979) reported no significant variation in admittance as a function of age. The issue is unresolved at present.

Information on the relationship between the acoustic reflex and age is also incomplete, but better agreement exists among acoustic-reflex data than for static values. There are several reports of no significant variation in thresholds of the acoustic reflex as a function of age. Acoustic-reflex growth has been investigated to some extent. Beedle and Harford (1973) suggested that the growth of the acoustic reflex is slower in older ears. Thompson, Sills, and Bui (1976) found a systematic decrease in growth of the acoustic reflex from the second through the seventh decades of life. The clinical implications of these data are not clear since measurement of the acoustic-reflex growth is not yet a common clinical tool.

The clinician should be aware of several special considerations when acquiring acoustic impedance–admittance measurements from older persons. Excessive cerumen accumulation, common in our experience, must be removed before insertion of the probe tip. Removal may be difficult, however, because the cerumen of older persons tends to be a dense, compact substance that may adhere to the skin of the ear canal. It should be removed only by a competent medical technician or an otologist. Following removal of the cerumen, the audiologist should take care to insert the probe tip gently, since the canal may be quite tender. Hirsute ear canals are another practical problem. Excess hair must be trimmed or insertion of the probe may be painful. Finally, the choice of probe cuff is different for older persons. A size or two larger than would appear necessary will often be needed. The cartilaginous portion of the canal into which the probe is inserted tends to be more elastic in older ears, thus requiring a larger cuff for an air-tight seal.

Speech Reception Threshold (SRT)

Recorded tests have the distinct advantage of a standardized method from one test presentation to another. On the other hand, in the live-voice method, carefully presented spondees have the advantage of flexibility. For many older hearing impaired individuals, a recorded test will not suffice. The time interval between the recorded words is constant (about 5 seconds), and the elderly hearing impaired person may not respond in this time interval. The monitored live-voice method provides for flexibility of time between presentations of words. In order to increase intratest reliability, the use of children's spondees (Utley, 1950) is helpful.

If a listener has a severe speech discrimination problem (phonemic differentiation problem), even at suprathreshold levels he or she may not be able to identify spondees, a relatively redundant (linguistically) speech unit. In such a case, the intratest reliability is so poor that it is difficult for the examiner to identify a 50-percent-correct response level for the spondee threshold. Since the primary objective of the speech reception threshold test is the measurement of auditory sensitivity for speech, then some more redundant form of speech should be used. The vocabulary chosen for this purpose should be familiar to the listener. Numbers (paired digits, for example) or other common words can be used. If such words are used, the resultant threshold (50-percent-correct response level) should not be confused with the spondee threshold. However, for practical, clinical purposes, the difference in decibels between these two measurements will not be large.

If simple words like numbers cannot be used because of the severity of the speech-discrimination problem, then a speech-detection threshold can be measured. In this test, the task of the listener is simply to identify when speech is either present or absent. The speech-detection threshold is that hearing level where the listener can detect or is aware that speech is present 50 percent of the time (arbitrarily defined).

The speech detection threshold will usually be 5 to 10 dB lower than the 50 percent intelligibility level for spondees. However, this relationship will vary, depending on the pure-tone sensitivity in the lower frequencies (125 Hz to 1000 Hz) where most of the vowel energy in speech lies. Since the measurement of the speech reception threshold is an effort to identify auditory sensitivity for speech, the speech detection threshold is a good alternative. In the same way that the pure-tone threshold average has corroborative value when compared to speech reception thresholds, the speech detection threshold corroborates the pure-tone sensitivity in the lower frequencies. Usually, the speech detection threshold will fall within a few dB of the lowest (best) threshold at 125 Hz and 500 Hz in cases of high-frequency loss.

Speech Discrimination

Among elderly persons, a speech discrimination problem might be primarily the result of a peripheral (cochlear) problem or peripheral in addition to a problem of processing by the central auditory nervous system. Or, the problem may be mostly the result of poor processing by the central auditory nervous system. In these cases, we have what Gaeth (Note 1) termed phonemic regression—a disproportionately larger problem of phoneme perception than can be accounted for by hearing loss for pure tones. Elderly persons with even mild degrees of hearing loss may report, "I can hear others talking, but I cannot understand them." This statement reflects a problem of phonemic differentiation or speech discrimination in the presence of relatively good sensitivity for pure tones.

Traditionally, speech discrimination has been measured with monosyllabic words. The initial development of PB-50 word lists was described by Egan (1948). Further developments for clinical purposes were described by Hirsh, Davis, Silverman, Reynolds, Eldert, and Benson (1952). The American National Standards Institute (1960) provides lists of PB-50 words that can be used for speech discrimination testing. Other monosyllabic tests were developed by Lehiste and Peterson (1959) and were adapted for clinical use in the form of Northwestern University Auditory Test No. 6 (Tillman and Carhart, 1966).

The preferred method of response in speech discrimination testing is a written response for each item. The relatively poor fidelity of talk-back systems, the variability in articulatory precision of patients' speech, the inherent bias of the clinician, and the probability of auditory imperception by the clinician make it desirable that the speech discrimination test responses be written by the patient. However, for the elderly person who may be slow in responding and who may have problems of writing legibly, an oral response is an acceptable alternative.

If relatively standard tests of speech discrimination can be used with the elderly person then, in addition to tests in quiet, tests in noise should be administered. Tests in noise are important. Elderly hearing impaired persons frequently state that they understand speech well in quiet but have significant difficulty in noisy situations. Although broad-band white noise and electronically generated speech noise have been the primary types of noise used, the application of multitalker speech babble should be explored with elderly persons. There is some evidence that a three-talker speech babble provides an efficient competing or masking signal.

If the patient's speech discrimination problem is so severe that the use of standard monosyllabic word lists is not valid, then the patient's task should be simplified by the use of easier items like the PB-K-50 word lists of Haskins (Note 2). If the PB-K-50 lists do not yield meaningful results, then a simpler task is sought. Larsen's (1960) Sound-Discrimination Lists offer an alternative. The task of the listener in this case is to differentiate between minimal pairs like lease-leash and pour-four. These lists contain consonant sounds paired with vowels in a consonant–vowel (CV) or in a consonant–vowel–consonant (CVC) context. The listener can simply be asked if, for example, lease-leash sound the same or different. The number of consonants included is sufficient to test consonant discrimination in a CVC format. However, in terms of Bocca and Calearo's (1963) observation, the ability to identify phonemes in words out of context may not be related to the ability to appreciate the linguistic significance of a meaningful sentence. That is, the ability to identify phonemes in words, highly nonredundant units of speech, may not be related to the ability to identify words in sentences that have semantic redundancy.

Another alternative to the examination of speech discrimination is the use of the WIPI test designed for children (Ross and Lerman, 1971). In this test, the listener's task is to identify in a multiple-choice format, a picture which represents the word presented by the examiner.

If standard methods for testing speech discrimination do not yield meaningful results, some effort to examine phonemic differentiation should be made with modified techniques just described. The results of such tests should be interpreted in light of the person's reported difficulty in everyday oral communication situations. If hearing aids are evaluated for the elderly hearing impaired person, the results of modified speech discrimination tests in the unaided condition may be compared to performance in the aided condition.

Speech Discrimination with Visual Clues

Obviously, everyday oral communication does not take place in a sound-controlled audiological suite nor does it take place void of visual clues we obtain from speechreading. Therefore, we should examine the contribution that speechreading makes to the elderly person's understanding of everyday speech. Since no standardized materials have been developed for this purpose, we must first examine the types of speech materials to which our elderly patient can respond meaningfully. For example, if PB-50 word lists have been used in the monitored live-voice measurement of speech discrimination and apparently reliable scores have been obtained, then these lists can be used in the following way. Having obtained a suprathreshold speech discrimination score at 30-dB sensation level, the clinician then administers a PB-50 list via the visual mode only. The two-room audiological test suite can be used for this purpose. The clinician should have ample and uniform light on his or her face while he or she uses voice and speaks the words. The attenuation between the control room and the patient's room should be adequate so that no audible sound reaches the patient. The patient views the clinician from the patient's room and responds to each word either by writing or by saying the word. The result of this test is a speechreading score for a given PB-50 list.

The next step in this procedure is for the clinician to present another list of PB-50 words at the same sensation level used for the auditory discrimination test and simultaneously to allow the patient to look at the clinician while the words are being spoken. The resultant performance for this presentation provides a bisensory score, i.e., auditory plus visual score.

For patients who have a severe speech discrimination problem, the use of unisensory (auditory alone and visual alone) plus bisensory (simultaneous auditory and visual) presentations provides some meaningful information about how auditory and visual aspects of speech are integrated by the patient. In interpreting auditory and speechreading performance, it is instructive to examine the synergistic effect resulting from the simultaneous use of the auditory and visual modalities. I have termed this effect the *bisensory synergistic gain* (BSG). BSG equals the bisensory discrimination score (Bis DS) minus the sum of the unisensory scores for audition (Aud DS) and vision (Vis DS), i.e., BSG = Bis DS − (Aud DS + Vis DS). For example, if a patient's auditory discrimination score were 46%, if the visual discrimination score were 16%, and if the bisensory score were 80% (an entirely reasonable outcome), then the bisensory synergistic gain would be 80 − (46 + 16) = 18%. Binnie's (1973) data on sensorineural hearing impaired listeners clearly showed a synergistic gain at low sensation levels when the bisensory mode was used at sub- to suprathreshold levels. Superficially examined, probable reasons for positive BSG may be accounted for by the fact that some speech sounds that are quite audible are relatively obscure visually and other sounds that are quite visible are relatively inaudible. Hence, when both auditory and visual modes are operating, auditory–visual closure allows identification of the stimulus.

The concept of BSG is a useful one. It highlights the notion that, in the everyday oral communication situation when people are talking to each other, they are not only hearing each other, but they are viewing each other. Even normal listeners under severe masking effects of environmental noise profit from BSG. It seems appropriate, therefore, that, if we attempt to estimate the oral communication efficiency of a hearing impaired person, we should examine the beneficial effects of bisensory stimulation. The need for examining BSG in the elderly person is even more important than in the younger hearing impaired person because frequently the speech discrimination ability of the older person is severely impaired. Thus, if we are going to examine speech discrimination ability of the elderly hearing impaired person, we should examine that ability via both auditory and visual modalities.

Most-Comfortable Loudness Level (MCL)

The most-comfortable loudness level (MCL) has been operationally defined as the level, usually expressed as the hearing level dial setting in dB, at which a listener would feel comfortable in listening to a particular sound for an extended period of time. The MCL can be expressed in terms of sound-pressure level as well as sensation level (re SRT). The term *range of comfortable loudness* has also been used in reference to a comfort aspect of listening (Martin, 1975; Watson & Tolan, 1949). O'Neill and Oyer (1966) described a procedure in which range of comfortable loudness is defined as the difference between the uncomfortable loudness level and the most-comfortable loudness level. However, the term range of comfortable loudness is ambiguous because it suggests some lower limit of comfortable loudness and some upper limit of comfortable loudness, not uncomfortable loudness.

Both normal listeners and hearing impaired listeners probably do not have a single sound level that they would choose for all listening experiences—conversational speech, drama, music, noise, pure tones, etc. What is more likely is that they would choose a range of intensities within which they would accept sounds as comfortable. Loftiss (Note 3) had listeners judge soft-comfortable levels, most-comfortable levels, and loud-comfortable levels. Such an approach would allow one to designate a range of comfortable loudness, that is, a range from an intensity designated as soft-comfortable to an intensity designated as loud-comfortable. Presumably, intensities lower than soft-comfortable would be uncomfortably soft and intensities higher than loud-comfortable would be uncomfortably loud. Additional application of this method seems warranted.

The MCL measurement was first proposed for use in clinical evaluation of amplification for hearing impaired persons (Carhart, 1946). Its use has also been proposed for diagnostic purposes (Bangs & Mullins, 1953; Jerger & Jerger, 1974). Only recently has research been directed toward an examination of the variables in MCL measurement. However, research conducted on the MCL apparently has been limited mostly to young normal hearing listeners and to some young hearing impaired listeners. Documented research on the MCL of elderly normal hearing and hearing impaired persons is lacking.

The notion of most-comfortable listening level has good face validity. When we listen to radios and watch TV, we adjust volume controls to what we consider comfortable loudness either in appreciating music or in perceiving speech intelligibly. In theaters and auditoriums, we are likely to place ourselves where we feel sound will reach us at comfortable listening levels. Hearing impaired persons adjust volume controls of their hearing aids to levels that are perceived by them as comfortably loud. Frequently, we are told by hearing aid wearers, especially older ones, that minor advances of the volume control setting result in changes from too soft to too much loudness. Such reports deserve our attention in the aural rehabilitation process, but before we can offer constructive advice to the hearing aid wearer, we need to be much more knowledgeable about comfortable loudness levels than we currently are.

The MCL is best measured with continuous discourse. The MCL of continuous discourse for young normal listeners is, on the average, about 65 dB SPL (Hochberg, 1975; Kopra & Blosser, 1968).

For elderly persons, instructions must be adapted to their level of understanding. Personalizing the live-voice presentation helps to keep the attention of the listener and expedites the measurement procedure. During the examiner's conversation with the patient, the level of the speech is raised so that it obviously exceeds the MCL and it is lowered so that it similarly is lower than the MCL. A bracketing approach is helpful. If the listener has difficulty in stating his or her preference for a particular level, a forced-choice technique may help. For example, "Is this loudness (65 dB HL) more comfortable than this loudness (75 dB HL)," and so on.

The MCL measurement should be accomplished as expeditiously as possible, but sufficient time should be taken to allow the examiner to judge the intratest reliability. That is, several approaches from below and above the MCL should be made so that the reliability of the measurement can be identified.

Uncomfortable Loudness Level (UCL) or Maximum-Intensity Level for Tolerance (MILT)

The terms used for designating the upper limit of intensity beyond which listeners will not accept higher presentation levels are less than precise. In the literature, the terms used to identify this limit are uncomfortable loudness level (UCL), loudness discomfort level (LDL), threshold of discomfort (TD), tolerance threshold (TT), and tolerance level (TL). This author prefers to call the upper limit of intensity acceptable to a listener the *maximum-intensity level for tolerance* (*MILT*). This term identifies more accurately the ceiling of the dynamic range. By definition, the dynamic range is the difference in dB between the tolerance level and the speech reception threshold.

The terms used for designating the upper limit of intensity acceptable to a listener apparently are not synonymous since a presentation level that results in discomfort may indeed be tolerable, at least for periods of time usually used for audiologically measuring this aspect of hearing. On the other hand, a presentation level that is intolerable will surely result in discomfort. Since several nonsynonymous terms have been used for designating the upper limit of the dynamic intensity range of hearing, there have been differences in the kinds of instruction given to subjects serving in experiments. Different types of stimuli have also been used. These differences probably account for the variation in the upper limit of intensity reported by a number of authors. Davis (1948) indicated that discomfort for speech begins when the sound-pressure level is around 120 dB. Dirks and Kamm (1976) reported loudness discomfort levels for speech (spondees) between 98 and 100 dB SPL. Similar levels for pure tones were reported by Hood and Pool (1970). Berger's (1976) data on uncomfortable loudness levels for five frequencies between 500 Hz and 4000 Hz ranged from 105 to 109 dB SPL.

Documentation of MILT of elderly normal hearing and hearing impaired listeners is lacking. However, clinically we observe that frequently the MILT of older persons with sensorineural hearing loss is much lower than normal. Whether these MILTs differ from MILTs of younger individuals with sensorineural hearing loss is not known.

The procedure for examining the MILT (UCL, LDL, TD, TT, TL) is not standardized, but the following procedure has been clinically useful. A live-voice method is preferable for the elderly person. Continuous discourse should include a discussion of the operational procedure. For example, "I am going to gradually increase the loudness of my speech from this level which, as you indicated earlier, is a comfortable listening level. I want you to pay attention to the clarity of my speech as it becomes louder and louder. Now I have increased the loudness quite a bit. How does this speech sound to you now?'' At this point, the hearing-level dial is returned to the previously established MCL and the patient's reaction to loud speech, at a hearing-level dial setting of 80 dB, for example, is discussed. Then the level of the speech is increased gradually to 80 dB HL, and higher and higher levels are introduced with the following comments, ''I am going to continue increasing the loudness of my speech until it becomes very, very loud. Please pay careful attention to the clarity of my speech. Now I reached the loudest speech you will hear (maximum output of the amplifier). How clearly do you hear me now?'' At this point, the hearing-level dial is returned to the previously established MCL and the patient's reaction to very loud speech is discussed.

It is advisable to avoid terms like tolerance, discomfort, and uncomfortable. The statement concerning clarity of speech in the instructions is purposeful. The question, ''How clearly do you hear me now?'' is used to call the listener's attention away from the ''discomfort'' aspects of the listening experience.

The MILT is an important measurement. Identifying this maximum intensity provides us with information about the desirable saturation sound-pressure level (SSPL) of hearing aids being considered for the hearing impaired person. Since many individuals' lack of success appears to stem from hearing aids with SSPLs that exceed their tolerance level, measurement of the tolerance level is critical.

Dynamic Range (DR)

The dynamic range (DR) is defined as the usable intensity range of hearing and is traditionally calculated by subtracting the SRT from the UCL, that is, from the MILT. Thus if a person's SRT was 70 dB HL and the MILT was 95 dB HL, his or her dynamic range would be 25 dB. Theoretically, conversational speech at a sensation level of 25 dB should be entirely intelligible to a listener. However, for older persons with hearing loss, the degree of intelligibility would depend on a host of factors, including, the person's speech discrimination ability—related to peripheral and central processing of speech, the fidelity of the amplifying device, and effects of environmental noise.

Measurement of the MCL, the MILT, and the derived DR are important audiological data that have not received sufficient emphasis in audiological procedures. More information is needed about these measures, especially with respect to elderly hearing impaired persons. We need clarification of terminology, consistency in instructions given to listeners, and specification of signals to be used (pure tones and speech, continuous discourse versus single words). We also need to give attention to the method of measurement.

SUMMARY

The assessment of the elderly client begins with an in-depth interview which should provide information on the social and medical aspects of the hearing loss. Behavioral reactions of the patient during the interview also alert the clinician to probable problems that may develop when standardized audiological procedures are used. To the degree that the elderly hearing impaired patient cannot respond reliably to standard audiological procedures, the test procedures should be modified.

Modification of traditional methods of auditory measurement call for simplifying the task by changing the type of stimulus and, if necessary, by changing the type of response required of the patient. If auditory tests have been modified, interpretation of the results must take into account the ways in which the modification affects the inferences made about the auditory dimension being measured.

An examination of auditory function involves threshold measurements of sensitivity and suprathreshold measurements which require linguistic processing. These tests include measurements of pure-tone thresholds, speech detection thresholds, speech reception thresholds, speech discrimination, most-comfortable loudness levels, and maximum-intensity levels for tolerance.

Elderly patients who understand the concept of the presence and absence of sound can respond to listening tasks involved in auditory detection tests. However, some modifications of the test signal and type of response may be necessary for some patients. Suprathreshold tests of speech discrimination require that the listener be able to process linguistically symbolic stimuli. If this ability is deficient or lacking in the elderly person, standard procedures for speech reception threshold and for speech discrimination must be modified.

Since speech discrimination test results vary widely in any group of patients with sensorineural hearing loss and because elderly patients may have central auditory processing problems, it is advisable to test speech discrimination at several sensation levels so that complete performance-intensity functions can be plotted for the client. An assessment of visual communication (speechreading) ability under unisensory and bisensory conditions is important for exploring the need for and nature of aural rehabilitation for the elderly hearing impaired person.

Measurement of most-comfortable loudness levels and maximum-intensity level for tolerance have important rehabilitative implications and should be included in procedures designed to explore a patient's potential benefit from hearing aid use.

REFERENCES

American national standard method for measurement of monosyllabic word intelligibility (USAS S3.2-1960). New York: American National Standards Institute, 1960.

Standard methods for manual pure-tone threshold audiometry (ANSI S3.21-1978). New York: Acoustical Society of America, American National Standards Institute, 1978.

American Speech and Hearing Association Committee on Audiometric Evaluation. Guidelines for manual pure-tone threshold audiometry. *Journal of the American Speech and Hearing Association,* 1978, *20*, 297–301.

Bangs, J., & Mullins, C. J. Recruitment testing in hearing and its implications. *Archives of Otolaryngology,* 1953, *58*, 582–592.

Beattie, R. C., & Leamy, D. P. Otoadmittance: Normative values, procedural variables, and reliability. *Journal of the American Audiological Society,* 1975, *1*, 21–27.

Beedle, R. K., & Harford, E. R. A comparison of acoustic reflex and loudness growth in normal and pathological ears. *Journal of Speech and Hearing Research,* 1973, *16*, 271–281.

Berger, K. W. The use of uncomfortable loudness level in hearing aid fitting. *Maico Audiological Library Series,* Maico Hearing Instruments, Inc., Minneapolis, Minnesota. Vol. *15*, No. 2, 1976.

Binnie, C. A. Bi-sensory articulation functions for normal hearing and sensorineural hearing loss patients. *Journal of the Academy of Rehabilitative Audiology,* 1973, *6* (2), 43–53.

Blood, I., & Greenberg, H. J. Acoustic admittance of the ear in the geriatric person. *Journal of the American Audiological Society,* 1977, *2*, 185–187.

Bocca, E., & Calearo, C. Central hearing processes, in J. Jerger (Ed.), *Modern developments in audiology*. New York: Academic Press, 1963, pp. 337–370.

Carhart, R. Volume control adjustment in hearing aid selection. *Laryngoscope,* 1946, *56*, 510–526.

Davis, H. The articulation area and the social adequacy index for hearing. *Laryngoscope,* 1948, *58*, 761–778.

Dirks, D. D. Bone-conduction testing, in J. Katz (Ed.), *Handbook of clinical audiology*. Baltimore: Williams & Wilkins, 1978, pp. 110–123.

Dirks, D. D., & Kamm, C. Psychometric functions for loudness discomfort and most comfortable loudness levels. *Journal of Speech and Hearing Research,* 1976, *19*, 613–627.

Egan, J. P. Articulation testing methods. *Laryngoscope,* 1948, *58*, 955–991.

Hirsh, I. J., Davis, H., Silverman, S. R., Reynolds, E. G., Eldert, E., & Benson, R. W. Development of materials for speech audiometry. *Journal of Speech and Hearing Disorders,* 1952, *17*, 321–337.

Hochberg, I. Most comfortable listening for the loudness and intelligibility of speech. *Audiology,* 1975, *14*, 27–33.

Hochberg, I., & Waltzman, S. Comparison of pulsed and continuous tone thresholds in patients with tinnitus. *Audiology,* 1972, *11*, 337–342.

Hood, J. D., & Poole, J. P. Investigations bearing upon the upper physiological limit of normal hearing. *International Audiology,* 1970, *9*, 250–255.

Jerger, J., & Jerger, S. Diagnostic value of Bekesy comfortable loudness tracings. *Archives of Otolaryngology,* 1974, *99*, 351–360.

Jerger, J., Jerger, S., & Mauldin, L. Studies in impedance audiometry. *Archives of Otolaryngology,* 1972, *96*, 513–523.

Kopra, L. L., & Blosser, D. Effects of method of measurement on most comfortable loudness level for speech. *Journal of Speech and Hearing Research,* 1968, *11*, 497–508.

Larsen, L. L. The Larsen sound-discrimination lists, in H. Davis & S. R. Silverman (Eds.), *Hearing and deafness*. New York: Holt, Rinehart & Winston, 1960, pp. 542–544.

Lehiste, I., & Peterson, G. E. Linguistic considerations in the study of speech intelligibility. *Journal of the Acoustical Society of America,* 1959, *31*, 280–286.

Martin, F. N. *Introduction to audiology*. Englewood Cliffs, N.J.: Prentice-Hall, 1975.

Newby, H. A. *Audiology*. Englewood Cliffs, N.J.: Prentice-Hall, 1979.

O'Neill, J. J., & Oyer, H. J. *Applied audiometry*. New York: Dodd, Mead & Co., 1966.

Rees, J. N., & Botwinick, J. Detection and decision factors in auditory behavior of the elderly. *Journal of Gerontology,* 1971, *26*, 133–136.

Rose, D. E. (Ed.), *Audiological assessment*. Englewood Cliffs, N.J.: Prentice-Hall, 1978.

Ross, M., & Lerman, J. *Word intelligibility by picture identification*. Pittsburgh: Stanwix House, 1971.

Thompson, D. J., Sills, J. A., & Bui, D. M. *Acoustic reflex growth in aging ears*. Paper presented at the convention of the American Speech and Hearing Association, Houston, November 1976, 19–23.

Thompson, D. J., Sills, J. A., Recke, K. S., & Bui, D. M. Acoustic admittance and the aging ear. *Journal of Speech and Hearing Research,* 1979, *22*, 29–36.

Tillman, R. W., & Carhart, R. *An expanded test for speech discrimination utilizing CNC monosyllabic words—Northwestern University Auditory Test No. 6* (Tech. Rep. SAM-TR 66-55). Brooks Air Force Base, Texas: USAF School of Aerospace Medicine, 1966.

Utley, J. *What's its name?* Urbana, Illinois: University of Illinois Press, 1950.

Watson, L. A., & Tolan, T. *Hearing tests and hearing instruments*. Baltimore: Williams & Wilkins, 1949.

REFERENCE NOTES

1. Gaeth, J. H. A study of phonemic regression associated with hearing loss. Doctoral dissertation. Evanston, Ill.: Northwestern University, 1948.
2. Haskins, H. A phonetically balanced test of speech discrimination for children. Master's thesis. Evanston, Ill.: Northwestern University, 1949.
3. Loftiss, E. W. An evaluation of the effects of selected psychophysical methods and judgmental procedures upon comfortable loudness judgments of connected speech. Doctoral dissertation. Urbana, Illinois: University of Illinois, 1964.

Roger N. Kasten
William E. Miller

Chapter 22: Considerations for the Use of Amplification among Elderly Clients

What an ideal time to be alive. Finally, the older individuals have reached that point in life where they no longer have to be tied to a day-to-day work schedule. They may have the time to engage in social, recreational, avocational, and helpful activities without restriction. Assuming they have adequate finances, they now have the time to travel and do the things they have always talked about doing. They have the opportunity to engage in volunteer services or helpful activities and contribute to the well-being of their fellow man as they have always wanted to do. They have the chance to engage in part-time work activities, which may provide them with just enough additional income to make the rest of their desired lifestyle feasible. It is also likely, however, that they will have impaired hearing.

When we couple hearing loss with the other maladies associated with advancing age, we come to the realization that this might be an ideal time of life, but in that respect, certainly may not be a perfect time. Older individuals must, if for no other reason than financial considerations, be cautious in their advancing age and their opportunity to enjoy this period of life. Hearing loss is simply one of many possible physical problems which may affect these persons, and it is frequently downgraded because it has been judged as having little importance on the extension of life. While this statement may be true, for many older individuals hearing loss can have a major impact on the extension of a truly enjoyable and meaningful life. Also, for many older individuals, a properly fitted and properly used hearing aid will allow a closer touch with the environment and an ability to interact more freely and more enjoyably in their social and personal world.

Amplification has never been and probably never will be of equal value to all hearing impaired clients. This fact is especially true for the hard of hearing elderly population. In the first place, selection of hearing aids to meet specific hearing deficiencies is less precise than is the fitting of glasses for visual impairments. Amplification might be classified as the use of a mechanical device to meet a physiological need. Since the hearing mechanism functions in ways quite different from that of vision, a prosthetic device cannot correct the defect with the precision achieved by optical prescription. However, it is remarkable how successful amplification can be in many cases. Even so, there are factors of great importance which affect the use of amplification among the older population. These factors will be considered below.

FACTORS AFFECTING SUCCESSFUL HEARING AID USE AMONG THE ELDERLY

Motivation

Rupp, Higgins, and Maurer (1977) consider motivation as being the most important factor in their feasibility scale for predicting hearing aid use. They point out that if individuals develop their own high level of desire for obtaining help in the use of amplification, it is most likely that they will be successful. They also point out that, in a continuum of individuals who seek help in the use of amplification, those who show less and less personal motivation and depend more and more on the urging of others have a corresponding reduction in the likelihood of successful use of amplification. Likewise, the individual who has a great desire to continue to lead a mentally, physically, and emotionally active life and to participate in the affairs of society is likely to be one who is a successful hearing aid user. On the other hand, those who have lost interest in their surroundings and are willing to withdraw from society have little motivation or desire to be successful in the use of amplification. Thus, the probability of these persons being successfully rehabilitated becomes correspondingly less.

Adaptability

One of the more important factors concerning use of amplification is the expectations of the individual. Until the person becomes hearing impaired and finds that he or she may need some type of amplification, or until he or she deals with a hearing impaired spouse or friend, it is most unlikely that the person will have a clear-cut idea regarding what might be expected from the use of a hearing aid. Average potential new hearing aid users are sometimes quite surprised when they become aware of what it is like to hear with amplification. It is likely that some people expect a hearing aid to restore their hearing to the efficiency that it had many years previously, while others probably expect it to be nothing but a nuisance and something of very little value. It is almost certain that neither of these levels of expectation is realistic or correct. If an individual has a level of aspiration that is too high and expects essentially complete correction of the hearing deficiency, he or she almost certainly will be disappointed. Conversely, if the individual has so little optimism as to think that the hearing aid will be of no help at all, then he or she is likely to be unwilling to put forth the effort necessary to become oriented to and consequently wear the instrument. In other words, he or she may simply be unwilling to give it a chance. If a person is unwilling to try something that is new or unusual, then major changes in attitude are necessary before successful use will be noted.

Personal Appraisal

The individual's personal assessment and emotional feelings about his or her communication problems are extremely important factors with respect to degree of success in the use of amplification. Rupp et al. (1977) approached this matter with the attitude that audiological assessment data are correct in determining the true degree of communication handicap, but it is their feeling that the self-assessment is also important and should be carried out by means of one of the available scales including those by High, Fairbanks, and Glorig (1964), Noble and Atherley (1970), or Berkowitz and Hochberg (1971). Another possibility would be to use one of the abbreviated scales designed by

Shotola and Maurer (Note 1) or Allen and Rupp (Note 2). It seems to be the opinion of Rupp et al. (1977), that hearing impaired older adults are very likely to minimize the handicapping effect of their hearing loss and, therefore, may be unwilling to do anything to alleviatc the condition. On the other hand, the problems of pseudohypoacusis or emotional hearing loss, where the individual views his or her communication difficulties as being much more severe than can be justified on the basis of audiometrical data, are well known. However, many cases exist where there is good agreement between the degree of handicap as determined by audiological data and also by a self-inventory using one of the self-assessment scales. It is the conviction of Rupp et al. (1977) that successful use of amplification is most likely when there is good agreement between the two sets of information, i.e., audiometrical data and client self-assessment. It seems reasonable that those authors are correct in that assumption. It also seems evident that one who is able to appraise his or her personal handicap objectively and with accuracy is in a position to understand the resulting problems in communication and comprehend a realistic approach to the possibilities, as well as to the specific procedures needed in rehabilitation.

Money

The financial status of a person certainly can have a profound effect on his or her interest or lack of interest in a hearing aid. For many older people the words "hearing aid" have the same connotation as the words "Rolls Royce" have for most of us. For the majority of potential users, however, the purchase of a hearing aid is probably not as nearly impossible as this example would indicate. On the other hand, the hearing aid still may be in the category of a luxury or near luxury and would probably be purchased only if the hearing impaired person were quite convinced that it would meet his or her needs. Many people are aware that their friends, and perhaps they themselves, have spent several hundred dollars for one or more hearing aids which proved to be unsatisfactory and were relegated to some dresser drawer or closet shelf. Thus, many people are unwilling to spend the money necessary to obtain a hearing aid. When an individual is living on a fixed income derived from a pension plan which is only meeting living expenses, then the matter of hearing aid purchase can become overwhelming. It is true that those who are eligible for Medicaid assistance can sometimes obtain help from that source in buying a hearing aid (if their state Medicaid laws provide for hearing aids), or there may be other possibilities for financial assistance by certain civic organizations. However, these sources also sometimes have restrictions which present problems in carrying out the purchase.

Even when there is no real financial problem, many older people fear that they might have a severe illness or be involved in some other calamity at a later time that would require all the money they have at their disposal. They may be unwilling to spend their money for purchase of a hearing aid in the first place and then, further, may be reluctant to purchase batteries or have repairs to keep it in operation. Thus, either real or imagined financial problems can be a deterrent to successful use of amplification among older persons.

Social Awareness

The hearing impaired elderly client, as any other hearing person, may fit anywhere along a continuum from one who is socially active to one who is extremely withdrawn. Those who are active in various aspects of social life are ones who are likely to desire to maintain contact with other people and may be able to communicate actively. Those who are withdrawn, on the other hand, may have lost interest in such contact. It seems reasonable to assume that those who are engaged in social activities would be the ones most likely to be successful in rehabilitation utilizing hearing aids. At least they would have the desire and motivation for this type of achievement. Conversely, those who are withdrawn or who lack social awareness would be the ones least likely to be successful in rehabilitation utilizing hearing aids. The large remaining group are those who are neither extremely active socially nor completely withdrawn. They are, in fact, the ones who are in the process of losing their interest in social contact because there is too great an effort needed to maintain communication with their friends. Although their lagging interest in social affairs would make them less than ideal candidates for the use of amplification, it is also highly possible that satisfactory selection of amplification and use of all rehabilitation procedures would improve their opportunity for reentry into social activities if they so desire.

Milieu

The attitudes, interests, and activities of the friends of the hearing impaired elderly client can certainly have a great deal of influence upon the attitudes and desires of that person. If the person is still employed or active in volunteer or avocational activities which involve him or her with communications, and if the people who are associated with the hearing impaired person are sympathetic, understanding, and also stimulating in their conversations, then it will enhance the desire of the elderly person to utilize amplification to its fullest. Conversely, if the living situation and the individuals involved in the life process of the older person lack stimulating ingredients, then the hearing impaired individual is likely to have little reason for wanting to try to obtain or adjust to the use of amplification.

Mobility

The ability of the hard of hearing person to move about and be involved in daily activities has a great effect on the elderly client who might desire to use a hearing aid. For example, if the individual is able to go to various functions including church, theater, musical concerts, and favorite social clubs, then he or she is likely to be a good candidate for the use of amplification. On the other hand, those who are limited in mobility and who rarely leave their living area for social or business contacts have less desire or apparent need for communication and, therefore, less obvious need for amplification. There are those who live essentially alone and seem to have little desire for communication with others. They may feel a great deal of loneliness, and yet they are unable or unwilling to make the effort to maintain contact with other human beings. These people have a great need for the help and communication which might be available through amplification, yet they often are physically and emotionally limited in their ability and/or desire to become involved in social activities. They might be victims of arthritis, a cardiac condition, or some other type of debilitating problem in addition to the hearing impairment, yet they *could* participate in social activities if properly motivated. However, the hearing problem presents an additional barrier and the combination results in greater physical isolation, which means that they are less likely to be successful from the standpoint of use of amplification than others.

Vanity

This is an aspect of human nature that can have a great effect upon a person's interest in trying to adjust to a hearing aid. The use of eyeglasses can be considered to illustrate how a prosthetic appliance can be accepted or rejected by various individuals. Most of our population would prefer not to wear eyeglasses but, nevertheless, a large majority of our society eventually need to wear some type of visual correction. In fact, most people accept corrective lenses quite readily at some time in their lives. Once an individual has accepted the necessity of eyeglasses, he or she may go to the ultimate of extremes by purchasing large and gaudy eyewear, which definitely call attention to themselves. On the other hand, based on their own opinions of appearance of self or the opinions of others, they may try to use contact lenses to conceal the problem as completely as possible. A similar situation occurs in the use of hearing aids but with one exception. It is most unlikely that anyone would buy an overly large or conspicuous hearing aid to call attention to this item in the same way that some people buy large pairs of glasses. In general, people are interested in getting hearing aids that are as small and inconspicuous as possible. This seems to be true for all people, regardless of their age or life style.

There are numerous occasions when elderly people would be far better off with a body-type hearing aid which can be readily handled and whose controls are large and easy to manipulate. However, it is rare, indeed, when an elderly person is willing to accept this type of instrument. Many older people feel that the body-type aid calls greater attention to their handicap and makes it more obvious that they are wearing a hearing aid than if they had an ear-level instrument. Even a behind-the-ear instrument is oftentimes rejected in favor of an all-in-the-ear model simply because the person feels that this would be less conspicuous. Some older persons state strongly that they might accept an ear-level instrument but would not even consider a body-type aid even though it might provide them better hearing. Problems involved with the presence of a cord undoubtedly contribute to the dissatisfaction, but general appearance is undoubtedly the major factor for making people dislike or reject the use of the body aid. Regardless of whether a person might use a body-type or ear-level aid, many are unwilling to wear an instrument of any kind because they do not wish to advertise that they have a hearing problem. They would prefer to try to "get by" and try to conceal their problem. An attitude of this type certainly presents a large barrier in acceptance of amplification.

Dexterity

Beginning with the first instruments that were built, hearing aids and their controls have become smaller. This reduction in size has made hearing aids far more acceptable to a large number of people than ever before. For the vast majority of our population, this reduction in size has presented no great problem, since many of them are able to make proper placement of the instruments and set the controls with little difficulty. However, with advancing age, the reduction in the dimensions of the instruments and the resulting decrease in the size of the controls frequently present a serious problem.

With age people lose their acuity of touch, and they find it difficult to know precisely whether they are or are not getting the hearing aid into the proper location and the ear mold seated correctly into the concha. Many an elderly person may be seen with a hearing aid hanging precariously from his or her ear or with an ear mold which is far from being seated properly. In most cases the individual is completely unaware that this situation exists even though he or she has just completed the act of putting on the hearing aid. Likewise, the older person may have such a poor sense of touch that he or she is unable to find the gain control or the off–on switch with his or her finger. When an effort is made to move one of them to a desired location, the elderly person is not certain whether or not he or she actually has been able to make such a motion. In addition, it is frequently the case that these people have reduced mobility of their fingers because of poor muscle control or arthritis. They find it very difficult to manipulate the controls even if their sense of touch is such that they can be made aware of what they need to do. Thus, good manual dexterity and good sense of touch can aid a great deal in the successful use of amplification, while reduced dexterity and sense of touch can be a strong deterrent to success and almost certainly requires the aid of some relative or other assistant to overcome this difficulty. A mandatory portion of every hearing aid fitting with an older individual should include a dexterity check to determine whether the person can use the controls, fit the aid to the ear, and actually handle and change batteries.

ASSESSING THE POTENTIAL SUCCESS OF HEARING AID USE

The above factors are by no means unique. It was mentioned previously that in 1977 Rupp et al. proposed "A Feasibility Scale for Predicting Hearing Aid Use with Older Individuals." Their scale incorporated eleven prognostic areas or factors which should be taken into consideration when dealing with aged persons. The scoring sheet used with this feasibility scale is shown in Figure 22-1, while a guide for use in scoring the feasibility scale is presented in Figure 22-2. One should note that their prognostic areas are not only listed and explained, but they are also weighted according to their relative importance as determined by Rupp et al. One should also note similarities between the prognostic areas associated with the feasibility scale and the factors listed earlier in this chapter. The important consideration for all individuals who deal with hearing aid fittings with older persons is the realization that complex and interactive issues must be dealt with to ensure successful, or partially successful, hearing aid use.

To a large extent, those of us who work with the older potential hearing aid user must be able to examine his or her probable success within the various factors or prognostic areas. We must also learn to accept certain guideline factors as they relate to successful hearing aid use. Many older individuals view themselves as being in a position where they have completed the most active phases of their lives and they are now living out the remainder of their natural existence according to their own prescribed rules. Many view themselves as having made it through the rigors and difficulties of adult life, and they therefore feel that they have an insight into life that is far more complete and comprehensive than their younger counterparts. They have established their own game plan for the coming years, and they feel strongly that the game plan should not or must not be modified. They look back on their previous years as authority figures, either in occupations or in families, and realize that oftentimes their existing authority is only an

PROGNOSTIC FACTORS/DESCRIPTIONS (continuum, high to low)	ASSESSMENT 5-High: 0-Low	WEIGHT	WEIGHTED SCORE (Possible) Actual	
1. Motivation and referral (self . . . family)	5 4 3 2 1 0	×4	(20)_____	1.
2. Self-assessment of listening difficulties (realistic . . . denial)	5 4 3 2 1 0	×2	(10)_____	2.
3. Verbalization as to "fault" of communication difficulties (self caused . . . projection)	5 4 3 2 1 0	×1	(5)_____	3.
4. Magnitude of loss: amplification results				4.
A. Shift in spondaic threshold: _____	5 4 3 2 1 0	×1	(5)_____	
B. Discrimination in quiet: _____at _____BB HTL	5 4 3 2 1 0	×1	(5)_____	
C. Discrimination in noise: _____at _____dB HTL	5 4 3 2 1 0	×1	(5)_____	
5. Informal verbalizations during Hearing Aid Evaluation Re: quality of sound, mold, size (acceptable . . . awful)	5 4 3 2 1 0	×1	(5)_____	5.
6. Flexibility and adaptability versus senility (relates outwardly . . . self)	5 4 3 2 1 0	×2	(10)_____	6.
7. Age: 95 90 85 80 75 70 65 ≦ (0 0 1 2 3 4 5)	5 4 3 2 1 0	×1.5	(7.5)_____	7.
8. Manual hand, finger dexterity, and general mobility (good . . . limited)	5 4 3 2 1 0	×1.5	(7.5)_____	8.
9. Visual ability (adequate with glasses . . . limited)	5 4 3 2 1 0	×1	(5)_____	9.
10. Financial resources (adequate . . . very limited)	5 4 3 2 1 0	×1.5	(7.5)_____	10.
11. Significant other person to assist individual (available . . . none)	5 4 3 2 1 0	×1.5	(7.5)_____	11.
12. Other factors, please cite				12.

Client ________________

Age ________________

Date ________________

Audiologist ____________

FSPHAU:		
Very limited	0 to 40%	Total Score: _____ %
Limited	41 to 60%	
Equivocal	61 to 75%	
Positive	76 to 100%	

Figure 22-1. A feasibility scale for predicting hearing aid use: An analytic approach to predicting the probable success of a provisional hearing aid wearer. (Reprinted with permission from Rupp, R. R., Higgins, J., & Maurer, J. F. A feasibility scale for predicting hearing aid use (FSPHAU) with older individuals. *Journal of the Academy of Rehabilitative Audiology*, 1977, *10*, 95.)

1. Motivation/Referral	5. Completely on own behalf 4. Mostly on own behalf 3. Generally on own behalf 2. Half self; half others 1. Little self; mostly others 0. Totally at urging of others
2. Self Assessment	5. Complete agreement 4. Strong agreement 3. General agreement 2. Some agreement 1. Little agreement 0. No agreement
3. Verbalization as to "fault" of communicative difficulties	5. Clearly created by hearing loss 4. Usually by loss 3. Loss and others 2. Environments and others 1. Mostly of others 0. Others totally at fault

4. Magnitude of loss; and results of amplification*

	ST shift	in quiet at —dB HTL	in noise at —dB HTL
5.	30 + dB	90%	70%
4.	25	80–88	60–68
3.	20	70–78	50–58
2.	15	60–68	40–48
1.	10	50–58	30–38
0.	5	48	28

5. Informal verbalizations during hearing aid evaluation re: quality of sound, mold, size, weight, look	5. Completely positive 4. Generally positive 3. Somewhat positive 2. Guarded 1. Generally negative 0. Completely negative
6. Flexibility and Adaptability A. Questionnaire and observation B. Raven's Progressive Matrices C. Face/Hand Sensory Test	5. 90th percentile 4. 70 3. 50 2. 25 1. 10 0. 5
7. Age	5. 65 years 4. 70 3. 75 2. 80 1. 85 0. 90+
8. Manual/Hand Dexterity via Purdue Peg Board and Symbol Digit Modalities Test	5. Superior 4. Adequate 3. Slow but steady 2. Slow and shaky 1. Slow and awkward 0. "Arthritic"

9. Visual Ability (with glasses)	5.	Very good—no problems
	4.	Corrected, adequate
	3.	Adequate but safeguarded
	2.	Limited visibility
	1.	Very limited
	0.	Blind
10. Financial Resources	5.	Unlimited resources
	4.	Generally unrestricted
	3.	Adequate
	2.	Adequate but close
	1.	Dipping into savings
	0.	Poverty level, on assistance
11. Significant other person	5.	Always available
	4.	Often
	3.	Sometimes
	2.	Occasionally
	1.	Seldom
	0.	Never

*Alternate scoring scheme for factor 4 in cases where the ST shift was minimal due to loss in high frequencies only.

(Average threshold shift at 2000 and 3000 Hz)	5.	25 + dB
	4.	21–25 dB
	3.	16–20 dB
	2.	11–15 dB
	1.	6–10 dB
	0.	0–5 dB

Figure 22-2. Scoring the FSPHAU factors. (Reprinted with permission from Rupp, R. R., Higgins, J., & Maurer, J. F. A feasibility scale for predicting hearing aid use (FSPHAU) with older individuals. *Journal of the Academy of Rehabilitative Audiology,* 1977, *10*, 97.)

honorary award. More specifically, they acknowledge that very many of their aged counterparts exhibit difficulties with hearing, and this particular deficit is one that simply should be accepted and tolerated. Most importantly, however, they frequently know or have heard of any number of individuals who have invested sizeable amounts of money from their generally limited resources in the unsuccessful search for improved hearing through amplification. It is relatively easy to visualize the effects that some of these circumstances can have upon the outlook of the older individual toward the successful use of amplification.

Frequently they lack motivation because of their first-, second-, or third-hand knowledge of unsuccessful experiences of their counterparts. They frequently lack a natural inclination toward adaptability since they have spent their entire lives with one psychological set and they see little reason to change at this time. They frequently show limited insight in their personal appraisement since they have been able to get along for a period of time and they can readily verbalize the affairs of others who, in their view, are in worse condition but also are able to get along. They are extremely hesitant to commit themselves to an expenditure of money for a commodity that ranks in their minds as an item of possible help but of dubious success. They frequently hesitate in their belief that a prosthetic device can allow them to change their life style and social awareness, and are not fully certain that a change will really be beneficial to them. They not uncommonly feel that a device that small can only be of limited benefit to them, but at the same time appear firmly convinced that this small device will call undue attention to the fact that yet another physical affliction has taken its toll. In short, the aged individual very often has a sizeable number of apparently logical arguments against the use of amplification, and these arguments must be successfully countered before they totally negate any potential for successful hearing aid use.

Obviously, no two hearing impaired aged individuals will be the same. Each will enter the arena as a potential hearing aid user with his or her own unique biases and beliefs. Unless the audiologist and/or hearing aid dispenser make themselves aware of the individual's beliefs regarding the factors affecting successful hearing aid use, and deal with each significant factor, the potential for another ''dresser drawer'' hearing aid fitting will be quite high.

REFERENCES

Berkowitz, A., & Hochberg, I. Self-assessment of hearing handicap in the aged. *Archives of Otolaryngology,* 1971, *93*, 25–28.

High, W. S., Fairbanks, G., & Glorig, A. Scale for self-assessment of hearing handicap. *Journal of Speech and Hearing Disorders,* 1964, *29*, 215–230.

Noble, W., & Atherley, G. The hearing measure scale: A questionnaire for the assessment of auditory disability. *Journal of Auditory Research,* 1970, *10*, 229–250.

Rupp, R. R., Higgins, J., & Maurer, J. F. A feasibility scale for predicting hearing aid use (FSPHAU) with older individuals. *Journal of the Academy of Rehabilitative Audiology,* 1977, *10*, 81–104.

REFERENCE NOTES

1. Allen, C., & Rupp, R. R. *Comparative evaluation of a self-assessment hearing handicap scale given to elderly women from low and high socioeconomic groups.* Paper presented at the Convention of the American Speech and Hearing Association. Washington, D.C., 1975.

2. Shotola, R., & Maurer, J. *The development and use of a short screening form for detection of hearing loss in older adults.* Paper presented before the Annual Meeting of the Western Gerontological Society, Tucson, Arizona, 1974.

Roger N. Kasten
William E. Miller

Chapter 23: Modifications of Hearing Aid Evaluation and Fitting Procedures for Elderly Clients

Since the development of the wearable hearing aid, efforts have been made and procedures have been developed for the purpose of comparing the performance of different hearing instruments (Carhart, 1946; Carhart, 1950; Jeffers, 1960; McConnell, Silber, & McDonald, 1960; Zerlin, 1962; Reddell & Calvert, 1966; Ross, 1972; Alpiner, 1975; Hayes & Jerger, 1978). This has been done in order to provide as much assurance as possible that the potential wearer would obtain a hearing aid that would be of substantial benefit to him or her. In some cases, it is not possible to state unequivocally that every recommended instrument was the ultimate of perfection for each individual, but procedures have been developed which take into account many different factors in an effort to approach that goal as nearly as possible. The degree of success in obtaining this goal undoubtedly varies but it is sincerely believed that these procedures avoid selection of an instrument that would be unsuitable for the individual concerned.

In other chapters of this book, it has been pointed out that aging individuals of our society have hearing impairments which present unique problems as a result of their age. These problems are particularly evident when one considers procedures to be used in the selection of hearing aids. There is no question that the same purposes and philosophies apply to the selection of hearing aids for this group as for any other group. But their unique needs, abilities, and limitations demand that the selection and fitting procedures be modified to some extent. The selection procedures used in choosing amplification for older clients must take those special characteristics of aging persons into account.

The large numbers of those who make up this age group may be divided into several different categories, and the selection procedures will need to be modified in different ways to meet the needs of each category. While it is true that we traditionally establish an evaluation procedure that will allow an accurate comparison among performances with a variety of hearing aids, it is also true that we frequently mold the individual to fit the evaluation procedure. With the aging population, however, we find ourselves in a position of most frequently having to mold the evaluation to fit the individual. We cannot talk about a single evaluation procedure, nor can we talk about a single population of aging individuals. In short, it is necessary for the evaluator and fitter of hearing aids, when working with the aging population, to utilize a broad variety of evaluation procedures and tailor these procedures to the specific requirements of each potential hearing aid user.

MODIFICATION ACCORDING TO DIFFERENCES AMONG POPULATIONS

There are several populations included in this age category and the differences among these populations influence the potential use of hearing aids. Likewise, the differences among these populations influence the procedures which can be used for selecting a suitable hearing aid.

Independent

Older individuals in the independent-living group are frequently the easiest to work with and the most successful in terms of hearing aid use. They are still in control of their life styles, and they enter into the process of hearing aid use with their eyes wide open, albeit sometimes reluctantly. It is with this particular group that a high score on the feasibility scale of Rupp, Higgins, and Maurer (1977) is most encouraging. For the factors or prognostic areas that predict hearing aid use, individuals in this population are most frequently amenable to change. These individuals still see a great many varied opportunities available to themselves and frequently are willing to exert themselves to modify behavior and attitude for their own betterment and for the benefit of their spouses or friends.

With this independent-living population, *motivation* is the critical factor. If motivation exists, even to a limited degree, appropriate counseling and sufficient success experiences can serve to bring about change relating to other factors. Sympathetic involvement on the part of a spouse or friend can clearly help to demonstrate the degree of communicative success that can be achieved. Also, sympathetic involvement can soften the impact of the knowledge that certain desirable conditions may remain unattainable due to their inherent difficulty.

To a large degree, potential success with a hearing aid will be tied directly to the extent that the potential hearing aid user can see and experience success in significant and meaningful situations. Successful communication can increase individual adaptability, and the willingness on the part of the ''old dog'' to learn new tricks. Successful communication can bring real insight into personal appraisement and can cause the individual to begin to realize the degree to which rationalization or projection dominated his or her previous communicative endeavors. Success in communication can cause a heightened social awareness and can lead to a genuine desire to expand social horizons and to modify the individual milieu. Finally, success in communication can drastically improve the older individual's mobility by making it apparent that there is still real reason to participate in activities and in events in a variety of locations. All of these changes, with the assistance and encouragement of a spouse or friend, can be demonstrated and documented if the individual possesses the motivation for improvement.

When motivation lags, the audiologists genuinely have their work cut out for them. Motivation is rarely built by applying pressure or through the nagging or ''friendly encouragement'' of spouse or friends. Rather, motivation can be developed through a demonstration of successful communication experiences. If, or when, the individuals learn that they can better themselves, increase their personal enjoyment, and improve their relationships with others, improved motivation will frequently follow. This will require careful structuring of learning situations, which rarely can be completed in one or two brief clinic sessions. The older people must be led to discover for themselves the enrichment of life that can result from improved communication. This discovery will be the key. The spouse or friends must be cautioned to allow the potential hearing aid user to set the pace for his or her communicative growth and must be prepared to reward appropriately individual successes and nondirectively encourage motivational changes.

These are the individuals who determine, to a large degree, their own life style and activity level. They are the ones who can come to the audiology clinic and can be given evaluation procedures that are generally appropriate for any other adult population. However, even within this group, it is sometimes necessary to make slight variations in presentation in order to avoid having the procedures become too difficult, frustrating, or time consuming. It is sometimes necessary to repeat instructions more than once in order to make certain that they are understood, and patience must be exercised in cases where instructions are not followed precisely from the beginning.

Speech Reception Threshold and Speech Discrimination

Test materials designed to investigate speech reception threshold and discrimination ability usually must be presented by live voice rather than recordings in order to vary the rate of presentation and provide adequate time for response. Where there is evidence that the client's attention has wandered or that there is some other distracting factor present, the live voice presentation can be far more personal and successful in obtaining valid results. Also, words of encouragement can be very helpful in maintaining motivation and yielding a more nearly correct measure of the hearing potential.

Speech discrimination test material may need to be modified by presenting shorter lists of words. It also may be necessary to have the individual come back for a greater number of test sessions. If the older person seems to have only a limited vocabulary, it may be necessary to use word lists which have been prepared for children, rather than the usual lists prepared for adults. Also, if this person has extremely poor discrimination ability, it may be necessary to present the material using the alternative mode of auditory and visual stimulation. In a typical audiology suite, the client might be allowed to watch through the observation window in order that he or she might both see and hear the talker. With some minor equipment modification, direct face-to-face discrimination testing can also be accomplished accurately and can be extremely beneficial.

While this procedure does not test the pure auditory discrimination ability, it certainly is a measure of the person's capability of understanding in a normal type of environment. Forcing older people to attempt to understand purely by audition could be quite artificial for their ordinary conversational situation. Utilizing both auditory and visual capabilities is certainly much less frustrating for these individuals than trying to understand by auditory means alone. Also, when hearing aids are evaluated in this way, use of both auditory and visual stimulation provides the examiner with a very practical measure of the individual's ability to comprehend the speech which is presented to him or her. When differences arise among performance with various hearing aids utilizing both vision and hearing, there is just as much reason to make the selection of a particular instrument on the basis of these results as with audition alone.

Use of Competing Signals

Particular care also must be taken in the use of competing signals for the measurement of either unaided or aided speech discrimination performance. Many aging individuals with varying degrees of hearing loss experience rather significant difficulty with speech discrimination even in quiet surroundings. When a competing message is inserted into the listening environment, they very quickly become aware of the fact that their performance in that environment has deteriorated. This fact easily can cause considerable discouragement and can cause aging individuals to reject further attempts for help because of their belief that they are beyond help.

Great care must be taken to explain to these individuals that the insertion of a competing message is going to make the task markedly more difficult. They must realize, before the fact, that the purpose of the competing message is to make the task more difficult, and that this is a function of the test situation and not a function of their performance ability. Also, when we deal with aging individuals who display a maximum speech discrimination performance in quiet of 50 percent or less, the audiologist must question seriously whether any meaningful information can be obtained through routine testing in a competing message environment. It is frequently far more beneficial to introduce a competing message in a more informal rehabilitative environment than in the initial evaluation environment. This allows the aging individual to experience a degree of success in relatively quiet listening situations before the more difficult listening situations are introduced. It also allows the person to become accustomed to the new listening code being presented by the hearing aid, and it allows him to acclimate gradually to the progressive difficulties that he or she will encounter in competing-message environments.

Tolerance

The question of tolerance must be considered as being of vital importance, and extreme care must be taken to avoid selection of a hearing aid with too much gain or too high a saturation sound pressure level. In doing this, one must differentiate between physiological and psychological tolerance. Psychological tolerance might be defined as a level at which the individual objects to the loudness of the sound. This is oftentimes well below the physiological tolerance level but is just as real and just as objectionable as if it were causing physical pain. McCandless and Miller (1972) as well as McCandless (1978) have shown that when the output of a hearing aid becomes great enough to bring about an acoustic reflex, the individual will usually object to the sound as being too loud. Thus, there is reason to believe that the psychological level of tolerance is just as real and just as important as the physiological tolerance. If a hearing aid is to be worn with complete satisfaction, it not only must increase sensitivity for faint sounds, but it also must have a dynamic range that does not go beyond the accepted level of loudness for the individual.

With the aging individual, we must be particularly aware of the influence that a psychological tolerance problem can have in the evaluation procedure. Traditional measurements of tolerance for loud sound call for the individual being evaluated to indicate when sound has become uncomfortably or painfully loud. The older person is also capable of providing this information to the evaluator. Unfortunately, all too often, the aging individual's psychological tolerance level has been exceeded before the physiological tolerance level is reached. These individuals then complain about the hearing aid bringing in too much sound, and they very realistically talk about their inability to live with that kind of sound in a normal environment. They tend to state, "All that sound just drives me up the wall," or "I don't think I could ever get used to that much sound," and they are all too often very accurate in their statements. It is imperative, in regard to aging persons, that we listen carefully to their descriptions of sound quality and modify our evaluation techniques and procedures to take into account their reactions.

Too frequently, we tend to look upon this type of individual as one who really does not want to use or wear a hearing aid. We know that the hearing aid is not amplifying to the level of their physiological tolerance, and yet they continue to complain about the magnitude of sound reaching their ear. Indeed, they are accurately describing a very realistic event, and it is essential that we modify our evaluation to take into account their unique requirements in terms of tolerance ceilings.

Type of Hearing Aid

One factor that must not be ignored is the matter of physical construction of the hearing aid being considered. Individuals are far more likely to accept and wear amplification if it is of a type, size, and appearance with which they feel comfortable. Many older people have very definite ideas as to whether they desire a behind-the-ear, in-the-ear, glasses type, or body-type instrument. It often is advisable to try out several types in order to let the person get experience with more than one style. It then is appropriate to concentrate on the type the person feels he or she would be most willing to wear. However, if arthritis, reduction in the sense of touch, reduction of finger dexterity, or limited ability to control small knobs exists, then it may be necessary to select a general type, or even a specific model, which would be easier for the person to handle.

Although we typically do not associate vanity with the aged when it comes to the use of a hearing aid, we quickly learn that vanity is as important a factor with this population as it is with any other group of individuals. Most aged people ardently reject the concept of a body-type hearing aid with its "ugly cord and big button in the ear." Unfortunately, there is a sizeable number in the elderly group who are physically incapable of manipulating anything smaller than a body-type hearing aid. For these individuals, the evaluator and dispenser of the hearing aid must be extremely adept at counseling and convincing them of their need for good hearing. All too often, aged individuals who are not capable of physically manipulating their own hearing aid will soon learn to reject the instrument. They experience enough dependencies in everyday life that they do not choose to become further dependent upon someone else by having them adjust and insert the hearing aid.

With this in mind, great care must be taken to see that all clients are able to handle and adjust their own instruments. They must be given opportunities during the evaluation procedure to work with a specific hearing aid model and to demonstrate their ability to both use it and adjust it. If they are unable to accomplish these tasks on their own, they must clearly understand that successful hearing aid use will require either a larger instrument or the continual assistance of significant other persons. These facts must be emphasized in order to prevent the individual from later rejecting the instrument as an unsuitable device. Some older individuals will be perfectly willing to rely upon a significant other person, and in this case we can do our best to satisfy their individual desires. Those who are strongly independent in terms of their personal care, however, must be made fully aware of the fact that the hearing aid should be of a size and construction that will allow them to make all necessary manipulations.

In conducting the hearing aid evaluation, it is extremely important to provide the client with clear and precise instructions so that he or she knows exactly what is wanted. Likewise, it is equally important to get as much information as possible from the potential hearing aid user as to his or her preference of a particular make or style of instrument. From a psychological standpoint, it is essential that the hearing impaired older person be convinced that a particular hearing aid is one which will give him or her good satisfaction.

It is extremely important to convince the potential hearing aid user that he or she is not being pushed into purchasing an instrument which is not desired or which will not be personally satisfactory. The audiologist has the responsibility of informing the client that a 30-day trial rental period is not only available but hightly desirable. The client should be urged to take advantage of this period of time to try to evaluate the instrument under normal conditions and then decide whether he or she really wants to make a purchase. Obviously, during the trial rental period, every effort must be made to continue to help the aging individual through this phase of the evaluation procedure. The knowledgeable evaluator and fitter of hearing aids will know those specific listening situations that are of particular difficulty to each individual. These listening situations then can be staged or simulated in order to demonstrate to the aged person the degree of success or difficulty he or she might expect with the new hearing aid. Since the elderly client has a lifetime of knowledge and experience behind him or her, it is genuinely important for the person to have the opportunity to experience aided listening and to make an ultimate decision without undue pressure from the evaluator or dispenser.

During the trial rental period, it is imperative that the potential hearing aid purchaser be provided with counseling to ensure that everyone concerned with the hearing impaired aged person really knows how to help him or her get the most from the hearing aid. This period also provides the maximum opportunity to make any necessary adjustments of the instrument or of his or her own attitude in order to become a truly successful hearing aid user.

Semi-Independent

When we deal with the semi-independent population, we are faced with a different set of circumstances. These individuals frequently have large portions of their life styles dictated by those who control the environment in which they live. Very often, this direction is provided by well-meaning but communicatively naive sons or daughters in whose homes the older people find themselves. All too often, this group of elderly individuals find themselves existing in a relatively comfortable, albeit controlled, environment, and they recognize completely that their only other option is nursing home or care-home placement. As a result, their psychological set and their attitude toward the factors relating to successful hearing aid use is subconsciously dictated to them by the individual or individuals governing their living accomodations.

With this population it is frequently necessary to spend more time with those persons who control the living environment than with the older individuals themselves. If the well-meaning son or daughter is not sold on the value of a hearing aid system, odds are better than even that the older individual will not be able to be sold. If the son or daughter feels that a hearing aid is too expensive to warrant purchase, the likelihood is quite high that the older individual will find no way to afford that purchase. If the son or daughter strongly states that the older person does not seem to have enough problem to warrant hearing aid use, then chances are that the older person will at least verbalize this same statement. If the son or daughter feels that the older person does not have a wide enough range of activities or experiences to benefit from a hearing aid, then the likelihood is quite high that the older person will reflect the same belief and, even worse, may demonstrate it. In spite of the apparent needs of the older individual, decisions regarding amplification and attitudes toward amplification may be shaped or totally formed by others who are not directly experiencing the problem.

This particular situation creates an awkward position for the older hearing impaired individual. He or she may readily recognize the need for the kind of assistance that can be obtained from amplification, but genuinely fear the consequences of a decision that goes contrary to the power structure in his or her environment. Although often not intentional, the older individual in the semi-independent population may become the *recipient* of attitudes and decisions rather than the *originator* of the attitudes and decisions.

In situations such as these, the audiologist and/or hearing aid dispenser must first convince the others in the living environment. A positive outlook on their part will frequently produce a positive, willing, and highly motivated potential hearing aid user. The audiologist must be careful not to give the impression that he or she is relaying pressure to the older hearing impaired individual. We gain little if we win a new hearing aid user but create a miserable and frightened individual in the process. Fortunately, most people who have elderly parents living with them are vitally interested and concerned in the welfare and extended well-being of the older persons. A logical, thoughtful, and in-depth discussion of the fitting and hearing aid orientation activities and the potential benefits to be accrued frequently will provide a major first step toward the acceptance of hearing aid use. If it can be arranged, an opportunity to visit with or observe older individuals who are successful hearing aid users can do much to alleviate the fears or misgivings of the misguided but well-meaning sons or daughters. In short, when working with the semi-independent population, it is critical to deal with the same set of factors or prognostic areas that were discussed earlier but now include in counseling and training those who share the responsibility for the life style of the older individual.

Evaluation Procedures

This group covers a very wide range of capabilities and therefore the hearing aid evaluation and fitting procedures must be varied a great deal to meet the specific needs of the individuals. It must be emphasized that the procedures must be tailored according to their abilities more than their disabilities. It is the responsibility of the person conducting the hearing aid selection to determine what these people are capable of doing and to utilize these abilities to select the amplifier which will be best for their use. This would include investigating the matter of finger dexterity, sense of touch, ability to manipulate the hearing aid controls, desire for communication with others, and ability to socialize with others.

A part of the evaluation procedure would include determination of the interest and involvement of the person or persons responsible for the care of the aging individual. It is important for the audiologist to learn if the relative or friend who is responsible for the care of this person is sincerely interested in his or her welfare. If so, then the relative or friend should be involved in all of the testing and counseling procedures. In this way the relative or friend may be able to provide the type of help that the older person must have in the use of the hearing aid. Obviously, some of the clients in this group would have no need for the help of another, but for many, the successful use of the hearing aid will depend greatly upon such a significant other individual.

The actual testing procedures must be sufficiently flexible to provide quantitative and qualitative information about the assistance provided by the hearing aid. The audiologist must be prepared to use methods which would cover the entire range from the quite formal and objective procedures that are used with independent individuals to the informal and less structured or observational means used with those who are entirely dependent. However, when a method is selected as being appropriate for the particular individual, that procedure should be used for evaluating a number of different hearing aids as objectively and uniformly as possible. In this way, it becomes possible to make a selection of a specific hearing instrument on the basis of performance rather than on the basis of some subjective or biased judgment.

Dependent

The dependent living population frequently requires a totally different approach and demands serious moral judgements on the part of the audiologist or the hearing aid dispenser. Individuals in this population are oftentimes totally controlled and cared for as the result of their physical, emotional, mental, or financial condition. If we view this population objectively in terms of hearing aid use, we are faced with the brutal facts that they frequently have poor motivation, markedly little adaptability, limited insight in terms of personal appraisement, little available money, poor social awareness, and restricted milieu as well as limited mobility and finger dexterity. In addition to the above factors, we must realize that these people oftentimes are cared for by well-meaning and hard-working staff members who know almost nothing about hearing aid use and who are primarily concerned with physical factors relating to the extension of life. Taken as a group, the prospects for successful hearing aid use are limited indeed. This fact has been substantiated in the reports of Grossman (1955), Alpiner (1963), and Gaitz and Warshaw (1964). In particular, Alpiner discusses three general attitudes that appear among those dependent older individuals who chose not to become involved in hearing aid use. They presented a definite denial that a problem was present, displayed a general attitude of hopelessness, and expressed a recognition of the hearing loss but indicated no desire for any type of rehabilitation. It should be emphasized again that this situation is confounded further by the fact that many of the individuals who deal with the dependent older individual know little or nothing about hearing aid use and oftentimes are occupied fully in providing the necessities for meaningful life support.

Successful Hearing Aid Use

For this group, the key to any successful hearing aid use will be the staff members who care for the individual or the volunteers who are present for daily activities. These people must be trained in proper hearing aid use and maintenance and must be made aware of the importance of communication experiences. A statement that we always make when dealing with the staff of care homes is, "A person reacts to people who react." By explaining in detail the methods and procedures they can use to convey information to the hearing impaired older individual, we provide them with extensive knowledge regarding hearing aid use and care. We then encourage them to work with hearing aid users in an attempt to elicit the maximum response from this group of people.

We must realize, however, that there generally is a relatively high turnover of staff in many care-home facilities. As a rule, the work is hard, the hours are long, and the pay is often not commensurate with the work involved. As a result, many individuals stay with a particular job only until they are able to find something else that will provide them with more satisfaction or more money. With this in mind, we must realize that in-service training which deals with hearing aid use and care must be performed on a recurring basis and must include a great deal of demonstration and some rather thorough follow-up evaluations.

Care-home staff must be made aware of the fact that within some states, hearing aids can be provided to needy older individuals under Medicaid and under some restricted insurance coverages. The staff also needs to know the procedures to follow in order to obtain an adequate audiological evaluation. They also must have enough knowledge about hearing aids and the communication process to become familiar with the devices and their workings. They also must develop and promote activities that will require communication by hearing impaired persons. Also, hearing aid users can be coached and prepared by knowledgeable staff members prior to a specific event so that they can experience a degree of success during the actual activity. Dependent hearing aid users need praise and rewards for positive changes in communication, and they continually need to feel that communication is vital and important. Families of dependent older individuals need to be instructed to encourage hearing aid use and communicative interaction using nondirective procedures.

With the dependent group, we must continually remember that a well-fitted hearing aid is not an end unto itself. Successful hearing aid use will result only if there is a need for communication, a desire for personal interaction, and support which includes family and staff encouragement and understanding. Successful hearing aid use will result only when the older individuals can demonstrate to themselves a real benefit from the process.

In working with this group, it will usually be necessary to use much more informal procedures than those appropriate for either the independent or semi-independent groups. However, even with these individuals, who are more limited in their mobility, there will be considerable variability in test procedures from one to another. Here again, it is necessary to investigate thoroughly their capabilities and limitations. Before any real testing procedures are undertaken, it is imperative to determine whether there is a staff member, friend, relative, or some significant other individual who can become knowledgeable and will be available almost constantly to provide help with the placement and operation of the hearing aid. If such a significant other person is not going to be available almost constantly, then the chances for successful use of the hearing aid are very slight. If the hearing impaired elderly adult is unable—physically, mentally or emotionally—to handle a hearing aid and there is no one else available to assist and support him or her, there is probably little need to proceed with the hearing aid evaluation and fitting. If the hearing impaired individual can carry out the responsibilities of operating the hearing aid, this is an ideal situation and the hearing aid selection process should be initiated. If he or she cannot be expected to assume this responsibility, then someone else must be found and trained to take care of these matters for that person. This significant other person must be one who is reliable and available whenever the aging person needs help with the hearing aid.

Clearly, it is never easy for an audiologist to deal with the dependent aged person who is in need of amplification and likely could benefit from such amplification, but who has determined that he or she cannot or will not respond appropriately to this type of hearing assistance. As audiologists, we have traditionally looked upon our role as one devoted to seeking out the most suitable amplification device for individuals and assisting them to obtain this specific amplification system. It is, however, equally important to determine who those individuals might be who are unlikely candidates for use of a hearing aid. When we deal with the person who is incapable of handling his or her own system and who has no one else within his total environment to assist in using the amplifying unit, then we have no choice, as undesirable as it may be, but to recommend against the use of a hearing aid. Clearly, we have the responsibility, along with all others who come into contact with the dependent aged person, to seek out any possible help or assistance for the hearing impaired individual. In this best of all worlds, however, we must recognize that there will be times when our best efforts cannot alter the circumstances, and we will have to acknowledge that the potential hearing aid user cannot respond to hearing aid use.

With the dependent group, we will frequently be dealing with state Departments of Welfare or with well-meaning but physically isolated relatives or friends. It may be possible to demonstrate that an individual might benefit from a hearing aid, and the resources may be available for the purchase of an instrument. However, we must again remember that it is also our responsibility to determine if the dependent individual will be able to use the hearing aid after it is purchased. This decision may frequently be painful and time consuming, but a necessary part of the evaluation process is a determination of the potential for success after the initial fitting.

Evaluation

In order to conduct the preliminary test, a portable audiometer capable of producing pure tones by both air-conduction and bone-conduction tranducers should be utilized. In addition, the instrument should be capable of producing speech test material by means of earphones or small calibrated speakers. It should be possible to present the speech test material not only by means of live voice but also by recording. Recordings provide the opportunity to present test material entirely auditorily and in a very uniform manner from one test to another. However, a live-voice procedure provides opportunities for variation in rate as well as material and easily allows for the necessary combination of auditory and visual presentation. Thus, a live-voice presentation offers flexibility of a type which is most often very necessary with individuals in this type of setting. The actual speech materials may include phonetically balanced word lists, but the examiner may find it necessary to use common phrases or some other type of speech material. Biblical passages or lines from favorite hymns are often appropriate. Tests of speechreading ability, such as those prepared by Jeffers and Barley (1971) or Binnie and Wales (Note 1) are often quite good for use in this type of measurement particularly in regard to visual discrimination. If the hard of hearing individual finds it difficult to understand by hearing alone, frustration can be avoided by use of both vision and hearing in the presentation. Certainly, such speechreading tests are very useful for this type of assessment.

It is often useful to get an estimate of performance utilizing the voices of individuals who normally associate with the older hearing impaired individual. These might include some staff members of the health care facility, friends, or relatives. Since these are the ones who have been conversing with the client and will continue to do so, this is a very practical procedure for obtaining an estimate of his or her communication ability. This also allows an opportunity to utilize very familiar speech-type materials for a gross measurement of discrimination ability. These associated individuals can provide the kinds of questions or statements that are most frequently used in the aged individual's environment. In this manner, the potential hearing aid user is provided with speech test materials that are very realistic and meaningful. They frequently stand a much higher chance of achieving successful recognition when the speech test is administered by a familiar voice utilizing familiar material.

Particular care must be taken when utilizing significant other individuals in the speech testing to ensure that they adhere to reasonable rules of speech testing. Very frequently, these individuals are accustomed to speaking loudly to the dependent aged individual and great care must be taken that they do not continue this practice during the speech test. They must be carefully monitored and supervised, and we must see to it that their messages are of significance and contain real message content. Also, they can frequently provide very meaningful feedback to the potential hearing aid user when successes are achieved and can provide great encouragement for continued success.

Whatever test material or presentation procedure is used, it is necessary to establish a fairly definite method of measuring hearing ability. If possible, it is good to do this in a quiet situation and with a controlled level of background noise. The presentation levels of both the test material and the noise should be appropriately calibrated or measured. Often, however, the nursing home environment includes considerable amounts of background noise that make precise calibration difficult.

As soon as the unaided performance of the individual has been analyzed, the aided test results should be obtained utilizing the same procedures so that both the unaided and aided results can be compared. Before actually starting an evaluation of wearable instruments, it is often helpful to use an auditory training unit to obtain informal estimates of comfortable and uncomfortable levels and also to obtain estimates of aided performance capability.

Part of the testing should be done in a rather informal way by having the staff members, relatives, or friends ask certain questions or make specific statements at various locations within the client's room and record the results for comparison between unaided and aided performance. The test materials must be such that the hearing impaired individual is capable of responding or reacting in an observable manner to such items as words, phrases, hymns, or other types of verbalizations. Although the test procedures that have been described have an element of informality, it is possible to maintain quite good uniformity of presentation and obtain fairly objective results. When this is done, it is possible to compare the results produced by different hearing aids and obtain an unbiased judgment concerning the value of the instrument.

One major deviation from the traditional hearing aid evaluation procedure will very often be necessary when working with dependent aged population. These individuals frequently have a very short attention span and tire quite easily. As a result, it is frequently necessary for the hearing aid evaluation to be carried out in a series of short sequences covering a number of days. Obviously, this will impose a genuine hardship in terms of the amount of time expended for the evaluation of a single individual. It is often most desirable to try to arrange simultaneous evaluations for several individuals within a specific care facility. In this manner, the audiologist can spend a short period of time with each of several individuals on any given day and can return on subsequent days to continue with the evaluative procedure. Any attempt to extend the length of the evaluation beyond the endurance level of the aged individual will only result in frustration, discouragement, and artifactual results.

Extremely Dependent

These are individuals who are truly physically, mentally, or emotionally dependent. In many cases, they will have only very limited ability to communicate, but it may be possible to make their care easier and provide them with some additional contact with the outside world. With individuals of this group, formal testing procedures are often completely impossible and decisions concerning the value of amplification may necessarily be made purely by observation. Before actually attempting the use of a hearing aid, it is necessary to make some type of estimate concerning the degree of hearing impairment. It may be necessary for this test to be conducted with the presentation of various sounds combined with subjective observation of any type of response the individual produces. Predictive acoustic reflex testing should also be accomplished, when possible. Although this may provide only an approximation of the hearing capability, it will give the audiologist some indication as to whether the use of amplification is or is not indicated. Obviously, any type of information concerning the degree of hearing impairment would be most helpful.

As soon as the degree of hearing impairment has been determined, it would be appropriate to evaluate performance with a series of hearing aids while the audiologist carefully observes responses to sound. One might notice whether the individual responds to voice or environmental noises or whether the use of both visual and auditory means are used in making contact with those around him or her. The observer also should watch for any behavioral changes, tolerance reactions, vestibular effects, or aggression toward amplification.

It should be fairly apparent that this type of observational evaluation is not altogether unlike the procedures used with very young infants. With the totally dependent aged individual, however, there is a greater likelihood of receiving interpretable responses. While these individuals may not be able to communicate with us in a conventional manner, they frequently can provide highly observable reactions that often are almost as quantifiable as direct responses to stimuli. Although it is always important to quantify favorable responses to sound, it is equally important to quantify unfavorable responses. We accomplish little if we determine that an individual is capable of responding to sounds and then fit him or her with an amplification system that provides too much sound. We must be particularly aware of facial expressions or eye changes that could indicate an adverse reaction to amplification.

If the person is truly an extremely dependent elderly individual, and we must rely exclusively on observational responses to make a determination of successful hearing aid fitting, it becomes necessary to include in the evaluation process a series of observations with the hearing aid turned at or near the full-on gain setting. This will allow us to determine whether the aid will be objectionable when it is operating near its maximum performance ability. Although we would not consciously anticipate that the aid will be worn in this manner, we must remember that the aid will be placed on the individual and adjusted by a significant other person who may not be knowledgeable in hearing aid use. What might well be an appropriate hearing aid fitting with the volume control turned to some midpoint may well turn out to be a grossly inappropriate fitting if the aid is inadvertently turned near the full-on position. By incorporating this information into the evaluation procedure, we eventually can make a realistic recommendation regarding the appropriate gain setting.

This procedure may appear to lack the true objectivity audiologists generally strive for in evaluating a hearing aid. But, if one can observe and document behavioral changes which result from amplification, there would appear to be reason to recommend use of an instrument based on these results. However, if one can observe no changes between the unaided and aided behavior, one can state that there is no evidence of any improvement, and recommendation of a hearing aid could not be justified, even though evidence of hearing loss suggests that the amplification is needed.

A Final Consideration

One final factor is absolutely essential to consider when dealing with the extremely dependent aged population. By definition, individuals in this group are incapable of caring for themselves and require the constant ministrations of others who care for them. For the hearing aid user within this group, this means that the significant other person must be somewhat knowledgeable and proficient in terms of hearing aid use. He or she must be able to ensure that the hearing aid is working properly, the batteries are appropriate, the earmold is inserted properly, and the aid is set as it should be for the individual. While these do not seem to be overwhelming tasks, they can be major hurdles for a health care facility staff member who has had no experience with hearing aid use.

Since there is a relatively high turnover in nursing home staff, this means that an ongoing program of hearing aid familiarization will be necessary in order to ensure proper hearing aid use for both the dependent and the extremely dependent individuals. It will accomplish little if we provide only a one-time orientation for staff members at the same time that hearing aids are actually evaluated and fitted on elderly individuals. While these staff members may be able to provide adequate care for the hearing impaired individuals, this care will cease if the staff members move on to other occupational settings. The audiologist will need to maintain close contact with the care facility administrators so that they can immediately be available when staff turnover requires a new staff training program so that continuous care can be provided for the hearing aid users.

SUMMARY

The hearing impaired geriatric individual may belong to one of several different populations having any of a wide range of skills and abilities. Because skills and abilities vary so much, it is frequently necessary to modify the procedure for selecting and fitting hearing aids in order to meet amplification needs successfully. However, even while modifying the test procedures to fit individual needs and capabilities, it is possible to carry out relatively objective test procedures which can aid greatly in the selection of a particular hearing aid for an individual.

It matters little which dependency category an aged person may conveniently fit into. The individual presents a unique set of abilities and capabilities, and the audiologist must be fully aware of the major characteristics of the elderly population in order to deal effectively with the individuals within this population. The aged individuals have experienced long and meaningful lives in which they frequently have functioned in a very independent manner. As such, they have formed opinions of their own, and these opinions must be respected. When the aged clients reject amplification and the evaluation of amplification because of their own individual biases, these biases cannot be dismissed casually with the thought of a rapid progress into an evaluation procedure. The elderly individual (and in some cases the significant other person) must be dealt with as mature and knowledgeable individuals who possess unique capabilities and frequently present distinct disabilities. Hearing impairment may be only one of many problems that face the older individual, and we must approach the remediation of the hearing impairment with this fact firmly in mind.

We frequently must modify the length of the hearing aid evaluation, rate of presentation, and type of presentation so that the procedure itself becomes totally meaningful.

In addition, we must take into account the tendency on the part of some elderly individuals toward conservatism and rigidity. The procedures utilized in an evaluation of amplification systems must be conducted in a manner that will instill confidence and a willingness toward adaptation.

The large population of aged individuals poses a unique challenge to all persons involved in the hearing health team. The audiologist must be particularly aware that he or she is not dealing with one large group of homogeneous individuals but rather with several subgroups who have advanced age as a common factor and any level of ability as a distinctive feature.

REFERENCES

Alpiner, J. G. Audiologic problems of the aged. *Geriatrics,* 1963, *18*, 19–26.

Alpiner J. G. Hearing aid selection for adults, in M. Pollack (Ed.), *Amplification for the hearing impaired.* New York: Grune & Stratton, 1975.

Carhart, R. Selection of hearing aids. *Archives of Otolaryngology,* 1946, *44*, 1–18.

Carhart, R. Hearing aid selection by university clinics. *Journal of Speech and Hearing Disorders,* 1950, *15*, 106–113.

Gaitz, C., & Warshaw, M. S. Obstacles encountered in correcting hearing loss in the elderly. *Geriatrics,* 1964, *19*, 83–86.

Grossman, B. Hard of hearing persons in a home for the aged. *Hearing News,* 1955, *23*, 11–12, 17–18, 20.

Hayes, D., & Jerger, J. A new method of hearing aid evaluation. *Journal of the Academy of Rehabilitative Audiology,* 1978, *11*, 57–65.

Jeffers, J. Quality judgement in hearing aid selection. *Journal of Speech and Hearing Disorders,* 1960, *25*, 259–266.

Jeffers, J., & Barley, M. *Speechreading (Lipreading).* Springfield, Il: Charles C Thomas, 1971.

McCandless, G. A. The use of impedance measures in hearing aid evaluation. *Journal of the Academy of Rehabilitative Audiology,* 1978, *11*, 2–9.

McCandless, G. A., & Miller, D. L. Loudness discomfort and hearing aids. *National Hearing Aid Journal,* 1972, *25*, 7, 28, 32.

McConnell, F., Silber, E. F., & McDonald, D. Test–retest consistency of clinical hearing aid tests. *Journal of Speech and Hearing Disorders,* 1960, *25*, 273–280.

Reddell, R. C., & Calvert, D. R. Selecting a hearing aid by interpreting audiological data. *Journal of Auditory Research,* 1966, *6*, 445–452.

Ross, M. Hearing aid evaluation, in J. Katz (Ed.), *Handbook of clinical audiology.* Baltimore: Williams and Wilkins, 1972.

Rupp, R. R., Higgins, J., & Maurer, J. A feasibility scale for predicting hearing aid use (FSPHAU) with older individuals. *Journal of the Academy of Rehabilitative Audiology,* 1977, *10,* 81–104.

Zerlin, S. A new approach to hearing–aid selection. *Journal of Speech and Hearing Research,* 1962, *5*, 370–376.

REFERENCE NOTE

1. Binnie, C. A., & Wales, J. G. *A diagnostic test of speechreading for the geriatric hearing impaired.* Paper presented at the Annual Convention of the American Speech and Hearing Association, San Francisco, 1978.

Section 4: Aural Rehabilitation Procedures for Elderly Adult Clients

Robert M. Traynor

Chapter 24: Hearing Aid Counseling and Orientation for the Elderly

The counseling of hearing impaired clients and their orientation to amplification has long been recognized as an extremely important part of the aural rehabilitation process. This is particularly true among older individuals seeking assistance from amplification: they often possess other concomitant problems which may hinder efficient use of hearing aids. In the past, there have been many theoretical and/or "how-to" pamphlets written regarding client adjustment and orientation to amplification. These pamphlets, however, usually are designed for use by the general population and do not allow for such problems as the reduced manual dexterity often manifested among older persons. The goal, then, of this chapter is to present the audiologist with general techniques for counseling the hearing impaired older person regarding amplification and to present hearing aid orientation procedures for this population.

COUNSELING THE HEARING IMPAIRED ELDERLY INDIVIDUAL FOR AMPLIFICATION

Chermak (Note 1) cautions that the counseling of any age group should include confronting problems and feelings, not simply exchanging information between the two individuals. Such superficial relationships may sometimes be successful among younger adult populations, but the aural rehabilitation process is doomed to failure when conducted in this manner among geriatric clients, particularly when they have come to the audiologist with specific problems. Sanders (1975) has indicated that the counseling of hearing impaired individuals involves two major areas: personal adjustment and informational guidance. These two aspects of the counseling process are closely related since much of the anxiety experienced by the hearing impaired person occasionally arises from the lack of information, or from erroneous information, especially regarding the topic of hearing aids.

Personal adjustment and informational exchanges are greatly facilitated by the participation of a significant other person to assist the older client in developing an understanding of the aural rehabilitation process, specifically the use of amplification. Rupp (1977) indicated that the significant other person acts as a teammate, participant, observer, and interacter throughout the total process. In such a team approach, client and teammate can discuss all aspects of the program, review problems together, and formulate realistic questions to ask the rehabilitational advisors. Rupp further suggested that this significant other person can continue to interact with the hearing aid user after the intensive remedial program has been completed. The team approach to counseling the older person regarding amplification provides for an open confrontation of problems and feelings while presenting needed information about the auditory deficit and possible rehabilitative procedures. Ideally, all counseling and orientation of older individuals should include a friend or relative to serve as the significant other person in an effort to maximize success with amplification.

Discussion of the Hearing Evaluation

For most older clients, particularly those accompanied by a significant other person, the acceptance of a prosthetic device is a positive event. Usually, a simple explanation of the hearing impairment is enough to facilitate trial amplification. The discussion of the evaluation should be put into laymen's terminology so that the older person knows what their hearing impairment is in relation to normal hearing. Further, the client should also realize what the audiologist hopes to accomplish with amplification.

An example of a ''laymen's'' discussion of the hearing evaluation is as follows.

> These graphs represent how you hear. One is for the right ear and one is for the left ear. Across the top of the graphs the pitches of sound are indicated, with low pitches on the left and higher pitches on the right. Loudness is indicated along the side of the graphs; the lower the loudness, the lower the number on the side of the scale. The goal is to determine how loud I have to make each pitch for you to hear it. In today's evaluation you hear the pitches as shown on the graph. [Show the client the audiogram, make sure they are wearing glasses if needed.] Normal hearing is considered to be somewhere between 0 and 25 on this scale. As you can see, your line on the graph is very much below that level. In fact, the speech of a moderately loud conversation is usually about 50 on this scale, and you just begin to hear speech at this level. These scores [demonstrate on the audiogram] suggest that speech must be almost at a normal conversational level for you to just detect that it is present. Additionally, your understanding ability is essentially normal when speech is made loud enough for you.
>
> The type of hearing loss that you have is not surgically correctable and there is no medicine that will cure the problem. We may, however, want to consider a hearing aid. [At this point, the clinician should further discuss hearing aids, their benefits and limitations, and listen to the client's possible prior experiences with amplification.] This is what a hearing aid will, hopefully, do for you. Hearing aids pick up sounds and make them louder so that they are more easily perceived by the person, reducing the frustration of not being able to hear sounds loud enough. Unfortunately, these devices also pick up unwanted sounds such as noise.

This presentation usually generates many questions from the client, which should be appropriately answered at that time.

Although this is the suggested method for discussing amplification, caution should be exercised in either overestimating or underestimating the possible benefits of amplification for the elderly individual. Care must be exercised to present the advantages of amplification without overstating its benefits. Additionally, one must be somewhat enthusiastic about the process in order to entice at least an attempt at utilizing amplified sound.

Getting to Know Your Client

It is necessary to find out about the client and his or her communication deficit. This effort will help you discover the extent of difficulties and, thus, facilitate personal adjustment and/or acceptance of informational guidance. There are many scales and/or questionnaires which may be utilized to gather information about the client that will be helpful for counseling regarding amplification. Most of these formal instruments are either direct descendants of the Social Adequacy Index (Davis, 1948) and/or the Hearing Handicap Scale (High, Fairbanks, & Glorig, 1964). One such instrument is the Denver Scale of Communication Function (Alpiner, Cheverette, Glascoe, Metz & Olsen, 1971). According to Alpiner (Note 2), the Denver Scale of Communication Function originally was intended as a questionnaire evaluating the client's communication self-image before and after rehabilitative intervention. Although the Denver Scale is still utilized for this purpose in many clinics, it also has been suggested as a counseling tool. As a counseling tool, it is used to obtain information needed to assist the clinician in helping the client adjust to amplification. Bate (Note 3) presents the Denver Scale not only to his clients, but to their spouses as well. He allows the client and spouse to take the questionnaire home, fill it out, and return it to the clinic. From the data obtained, the clinician is then informed, first, of specific items and/or comments which suggest areas of counseling need for the hearing impaired person, second, of specific items and/or comments which suggest areas of counseling need for the spouse, and third, of items on which there is considerable disparity between the wife and husband that indicate possible need of resolution. For example, Item number 9 of the Denver Scale is, "I am not a calm person because of my hearing loss." If the hearing impaired person responds "agree," and the spouse responds "disagree," this might suggest that the spouse is not aware of the inner turmoil that the hearing impaired person is experiencing. Utilization of the Denver Scale in this manner can, thus, be expanded upon to include the responses of family members in an effort to understand compounding difficulties which may be experienced by older clients in adjusting to amplification.

Another descendant of the early scales and/or questionnaires that offers some possible value as a counseling tool for use with older clients adjusting to amplification is the Profile Questionnaire for Rating Communicative Performance (Sanders, 1975). The profiles are utilized to identify specific problem areas, including communicative environments. Sanders suggests that the profiles may be designed specifically for each client or for situations in which they find themselves. A scale of this type is ideal for the aging population. For example, the active aging person might well be given the same scale as a younger adult, while the confined elderly person may require the construction of a special scale to determine needs for communication and to assess the possible benefits of amplification. In any event, the Sanders' profiles offer the objectivity of a numerical scoring system and the versatility of individualized construction according to specific client needs.

Ideally, for elderly clients, the audiologist should have the information generated by a Feasibility Scale for Predicting Hearing Aid Use (FSPHAU) (Rupp, Higgins, & Maurer, 1977), which attempts to predict success with hearing aids. The areas probed with this tool are outlined in Table 24-1.

Table 24-1
Patient Information Generated by Feasibility Scale for Predicting Hearing Aid Use

Motivation and mode of referral to professional services
Self assessment of the individual's communication difficulties before amplification
Verbalization on the client's part as to "help" for the communicative difficulties
Magnitude of the hearing loss and understanding difficulties in audiological units before and after amplification
Informal verbalizations during the hearing aid evaluation
Estimate of the patient's general state of adaptability and flexibility
Age of patient
The patient's manual finger and hand dexterity
The patient's visual ability
The patient's financial resources
Presence of a significant other person to assist the client in a rehabilitative program

The Confined Elderly Client

Recently, there has been genuine interest in the evaluation of the rehabilitative potential of confined elderly clients. These tests, too, can provide some real insight into the problems facing the clinician when considering amplification relative to this special population and have a similar ancestry to the other instruments mentioned earlier. The first of these appraisals is the Denver Scale of Communication Function for Senior Citizens Living in Retirement Centers (DSSC) (Zarnoch & Alpiner, 1977) which is discussed in detail in Chapters 7 and 27. The data obtained from the DSSC can provide information not only about the client's counseling needs relative to the hearing impairment and amplification, but also about concomitant problems which may complicate the total aural rehabilitative process.

Building Rapport

Client rapport is extremely important in any rehabilitative endeavor, but it is particularly essential in a client's adjustment to amplification. Proper rapport between client and audiologist allows for greater assurance that specific advice to be offered will be utilized more efficiently. Carkhuff, Pierce, and Cannon (1977) have presented some principles which may assist the audiologist in building desired rapport during counseling sessions with older clients. These principles may be utilized to obtain information about the person through the use of the above scales or in specific client-clinician dialogue during treatment sessions.

The manner in which the audiologist approaches the older client is a manifestation of the professional's interest. The clinician can foster an attentive atmosphere in the session by utilizing the following suggestions:

1. In all discussions with older clients, direct the conversation to the elderly person, not the friend or relative who brought them into the clinic.

2. Make sure the older client understands what is said during the session.
3. The environment should be conducive to good listening. Furniture should be arranged so that there are no desks or barriers between the older person and the audiologist.
4. The clinician should facc the elderly client at a distance of 4 to 5 feet, ideally sitting on the same type of chair. If the person is confined to a wheelchair, the audiologist should be seated on the same level at an appropriate distance.
5. The clinician's posture communicates a readiness to respond to the client's problems. It is best to face the person squarely or, when sitting, with the body inclined slightly forward.
6. Maintaining good visual contact with the client demonstrates that the clinician is offering full and individual attention to the problems being discussed.
7. At times, touching the client in some symbolic way e.g., a pat on the hand or shoulder, but not in a demeaning manner, facilitates an atmosphere of openness and genuine interest.
8. It is a good practice to point out what the client does well before confronting the client's difficulties.

The professional's responses to the problems presented should reflect the feelings being expressed, not impose feelings on the client. This process involves empathy on the part of the audiologist but not sympathy. For example, the older client may express, "I feel left out of conversations." The next task is to discover the situation or situations in which the person feels that they are an outcast. Is the hearing impairment causing these feelings, or is it family/friends simply excluding the person from conversations? This information is derived by asking probing questions as to when, where, how, and why. These questions lead to descriptive statements by the older person such as, "I feel an outcast in some conversations because of my hearing impairment." These answers by the older client provide the audiologist with a basis for understanding the person's problem and their motivation for various behaviors.

The last consideration of Carkhuff et al. (1977) in the building of rapport is termed *personalization*. This process is an effort to help the older client understand where he or she is in relation to where he or she wants to be. Among the hearing impaired older population it means demonstrating to noneffective communicators that they can be effective communicators. This involves discussion of the older client's auditory deficit in laymen's terminology to provide the knowledge necessary to properly understand the hearing loss, its ramifications, and what must be done to facilitate the rehabilitation process. This is accomplished by discussing the person's audiometric thresholds relative to normal hearing as suggested previously. Additionally, the clinician should discuss various difficult communication situations, the usual problems encountered and the advantages and disadvantages of amplification in those situations. For instance, an older person might be counseled as follows.

Clinician: Do you have difficulty communicating with others?

Client: Yes.

Clinician: In what situations?

Client: Well, if someone is close to me I can hear fine but if they are far away, or if its noisy, or if I am among a group of people, I'm lost.

Clinician: Let's consider these problems individually. First, when someone is closer to you, the sound of their voice is more intense, therefore, you should hear and understand what is being said much better. Conversely, when someone is quite a few feet away, some of

> the sound energy is lost before it gets to you. Additionally, some of the critical sounds of speech may be absorbed by the wall, ceilings, furniture, and other environmental objects. Secondly, problems in a noisy environment are usually caused by the noise covering up the low pitched sounds which you hear the best. The pitch of speech sounds which are most important are between 500 and about 4000 Hz on this scale.
> [show client the audiogram, make sure that they have their glasses on if needed.] You hear the low pitched sounds better than the higher pitched sounds . . . .''

In essence, the personalization process involves presenting the hearing impaired older person with the information necessary to understand their auditory deficit. Once the audiologist has the necessary information about the client and rapport has been built, amplification then is suggested.

Suggesting the Use of a Hearing Aid to the Older Client

When suggesting amplification to the older client, the audiologist not only must circumvent physical, social, and psychological limitations, but also must be aware that previous encounters with hearing aids or other amplification devices may have to be overcome. Over the years, the older client may have had either positive or negative experiences with amplification. These experiences may have resulted in preconceived ideas as to the possible benefits of a hearing aid, which in turn affect the client's attitude toward eventual adjustment to the device.

Obviously, positive experiences will enhance a willingness to accept a hearing aid and may include instances where the client knew a spouse, relative, or friend who, when wearing the hearing aid, appeared to function at a normal or near-normal level. The older person who has had such a positive experience may progress into this aspect of the aural rehabilitation program with a very positive attitude. Often these clients are already aware of many of the advantages and limitations of hearing aids and what to expect from them. Additionally, they may ask more sophisticated, challenging questions, which, when discussed with the audiologist, greatly facilitate adjustment to the instrument. On the other hand, some older clients may expect too much from the instrument because of previous experiences or preconceived expectations. This positive attitude may backfire. The client does not understand why this hearing aid does not work as well for him or her as expectations dictated. These individuals usually require in-depth counseling regarding the interaction of their hearing loss, hearing aids, adjustment problems, advantages and limitations of amplified sound, and other specific client needs.

Similarly, previously negative experiences often will contribute to a dissenting attitude toward hearing aids. Such negative attitudes are fostered by bad experiences with family or friends and their amplification devices or the stigma that a hearing aid denotes ''old age.'' For example, the older person may have observed a friend or relative purchase a hearing aid and not be able to hear any better with it than without it; or, he or she might recall a negative remark by an associate about ''false teeth, thinning hair, and now a hearing aid.'' Additionally, other problems relative to the amplification device such as maintenance of a hearing aid, batteries, feedback difficulties, etc., may negate a desire to adjust to amplification. The effect of these negative experiences can be modified by providing information, through the methodologies presented, regarding the possible reasons for the problems others have observed. These questions and subsequent answers should be eliminated as much as possible to reduce the influence of the older client's negative attitudes upon the eventual adjustment to a hearing aid.

The Generation Gap

When presenting the concept of amplification as a viable alternative to the present generation of hearing impaired older persons, we must consider the attitudes toward hearing impairment and hearing aids prevalent in the 1920s. The birth cohorts that are currently 65 to 80 years of age were 7 to 23 years of age in 1925. Generations usually perpetuate the attitudes with which they were reared. In the 1920s, hearing aids were in their infancy, and the hearing impaired were seen as "dumb," or as individuals who possessed reduced intelligence or had become senile. Unfortunately, many older people with hearing loss look upon this deficit as something to hide so that their friends will not think them intellectually deficient. Additionally, the hearing impairment may be seen as another decrement in the aging process. The older person may have reduced ambulation skills, reduced vision, and reduced hearing ability. Therefore, in addition to the normal psychological problems encountered by the adventitiously hearing impaired, the elderly client may look at the hearing aid as a symbol of reduced capacity to function as an independent human being. Often, counseling must include the fact that many of their peers possess some degree of hearing impairment. Further, a discussion of the current types of hearing aids available will, at times, reduce those anxieties. When an older person has unsuccessfully attempted to utilize amplification, they are usually less than anxious to try it again. Whether an earlier trial with amplification was unsuccessful because of poor attitude, health problems, improper fit, poor purchase judgment, or improper counseling and orientation as to its use, the result would be the same—a negative attitude toward a second attempt. These and other issues which are presented by the client during the counseling session must be considered and discussed in simple, nontechnical language.

The client who has not attempted the use of amplification may have misconceptions of what is involved in the process. Many feel that all they must do is go to a store and purchase a hearing aid if they need one. It is the responsibility of the audiologist to instill in the client the need for professional evaluation of auditory function and orientation to the instruments before their purchase. The counseling required in this process usually involves continued discussion of the audiogram in reference to how the client is communicating.

Those with Reduced Needs for Communication

Many older people live alone and communicate very little with others except by telephone, when someone occasionally comes to their door, or by watching television. These individuals may have been relatively reclusive during the active years of their life or, on the other hand, the auditory deficit or other physical problems may have contributed to the client's inactivity. As suggested by Traynor (Note 4), success with amplification appears to be marginal for older people who live alone. Usually they hear well on the telephone since the intensity of the telephone without an amplifier is about 60 dB through the frequencies of 300 to 3000Hz. Most older clients are able to hear this frequency–intensity range rather effectively. Due to utilization of a narrow band of frequencies to present the message, voices on the phone do not sound much different than before the acquisition of the auditory deficit. Telephone amplifiers are, further, quite beneficial for those who do have difficulty. Many older individuals can hear their television set without the aid of amplification if it is turned up loud enough. Further, when people come to their door, they may understand what they are saying very effectively if speaking on a one-to-one basis. Thus, those older clients have reduced communication needs, and it is difficult to justify a $400 to $550 investment in a hearing aid which may only be used twice a year when relatives come to visit. An important role of the audiologist is, however, to assess whether the older client is, by nature, one who does not socialize, or if such seclusion is a result of their hearing impairment. This information is generally available from family and friends.

For the most part, success with hearing aids among this population is due to a real need to communicate. Those who have a reduced need to communicate will present the audiologist with a marginal success rate in the utilization of amplification. It is important to note that many times failure to purchase a hearing aid when there are few communication needs does not indicate a floundering aural rehabilitation program but wise financial management by the client.

ORIENTATION OF THE ELDERLY HEARING AID USER TO AMPLIFICATION

The key to a successful hearing aid orientation program among elderly clients is a detailed explanation of the components and their subcomponents in nontechnical terminology. This approach not only fosters a greater understanding of the instrument, but confirms the fact that the audiologist is someone on whom he or she can depend for assistance. Kasten (1977) suggests that a minimum of 30 minutes should be allowed for the explanation process. Among older clients who possess various psychophysical limitations, however, orientation to the instrument usually will take longer. The actual amount of time is directly related to the person's ability to respond to the instructions and their motivation.

Many of the answers to clients' specific questions depend on whether the audiologist is dispensing hearing aids or if the more traditional referral system is utilized. In either situation, someone must demonstrate the instrument, the manipulation of the controls and power supply, and the idiosyncrasies of amplified sound. This orientation is conducted, ideally, by the audiologist, either as a dispensor/counselor or simply as a counselor as part of a total aural rehabilitation program.

General Knowledge of Amplification

The audiologist should make the older person aware of the major components of the hearing aid and their function. Included in the overall explanation of the instrument is a description of the amplification process, the various devices which control this process, and the manipulation of the instrument.

The following simple diagrams and explanations have been found to facilitate orientation of older clients to amplification.

Microphone

The microphone function is to change sound vibrations into electrical impulses so that they may be amplified (Fig. 24-1).

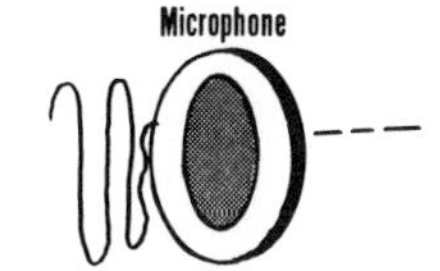

Fig. 24-1. Microphone.

Amplifier

An amplifier, as seen in Figure 24-2, simply magnifies the electrical impulses generated by the hearing aid microphone.

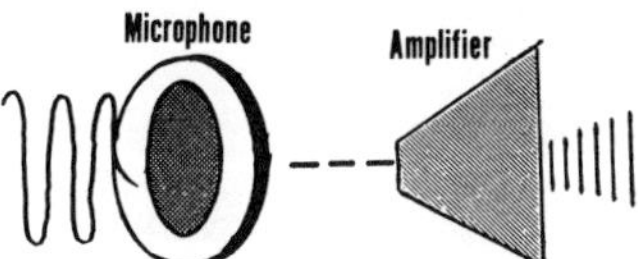

Fig. 24-2. Microphone, electrical impulses, and amplifier.

Receiver

The magnified electrical impulses from the amplifier are changed back into sound vibrations at the receiver (Fig. 24-3).

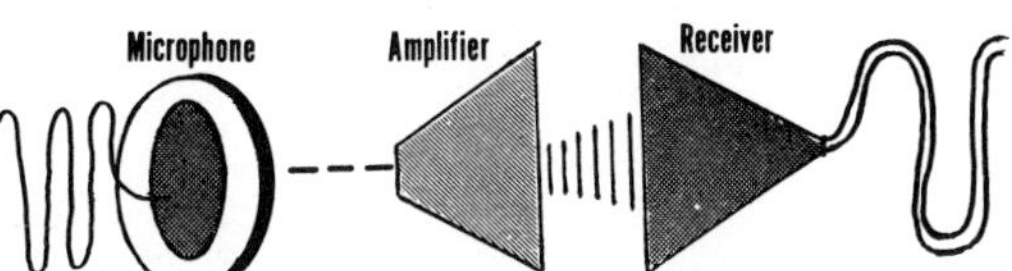

Fig. 24-3. Microphone, electrical impulses, amplifier, magnified electrical impulses, and receiver.

Tubing

The tube attached to the receiver directs the amplified sound vibrations into the earmold (Fig. 24-4).

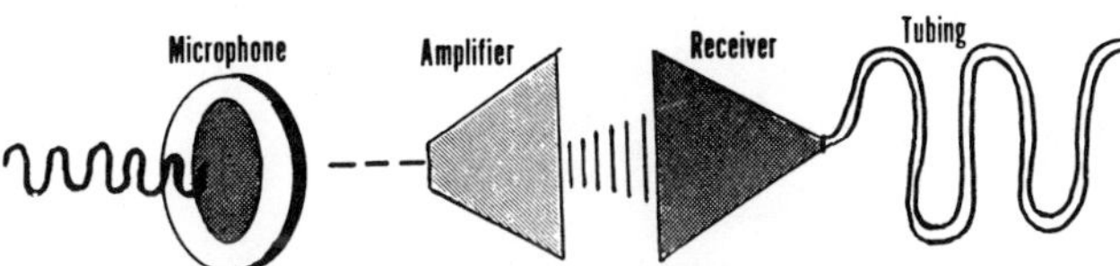

Fig. 24-4. Microphone, electrical impulses, amplifier, magnified electrical impulses, receiver, and tubing.

Earmold

The device which couples the hearing aid to the person's ear is called the earmold (Fig. 24-5). Its purpose is to effectively transmit the magnified sound vibrations from the receiver to the user's ear.

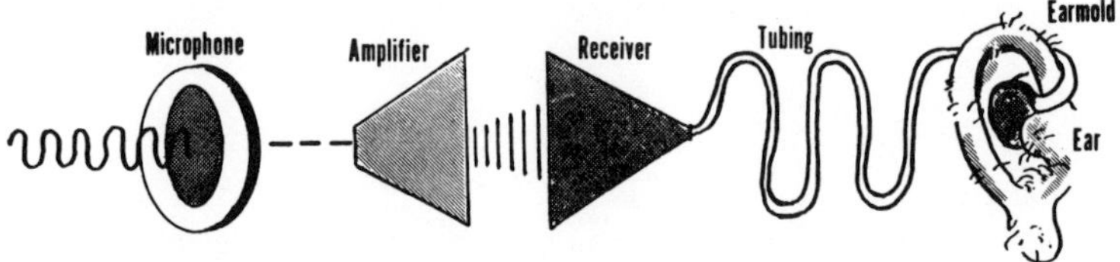

Fig. 24-5. Microphone, electrical impulses, amplifier, magnified electrical impulses, receiver, tubing, and earmold.

Feedback

A byproduct of the amplification process is feedback. This term refers to the escape of the amplified sound into the microphone of the system. This "leak" and reamplification of the signal results in a high pitched squeal of the hearing aid. The most common cause of feedback is an improper fitting earmold. A schematic drawing of this cycle is shown in Figure 24-6.

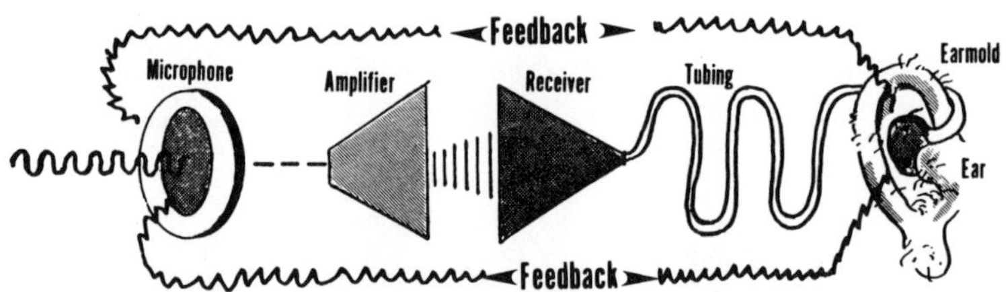

Fig. 24-6. Feedback due to improperly fitting earmold.

Another common cause of feedback is a vented earmold. This type of feedback usually does not occur unless the client puts a hand near the hearing aid and directs the leaking sound into the microphone of the instrument. A vent of this type may be necessary to provide the proper type of amplification (Fig. 24-7). The older hearing aid user should be assured that feedback is undesirable, and that every effort will be made so that feedback does not occur. Many older clients have heard feedback from a friend's or relative's hearing aid and fear that their instrument will also create this difficulty.

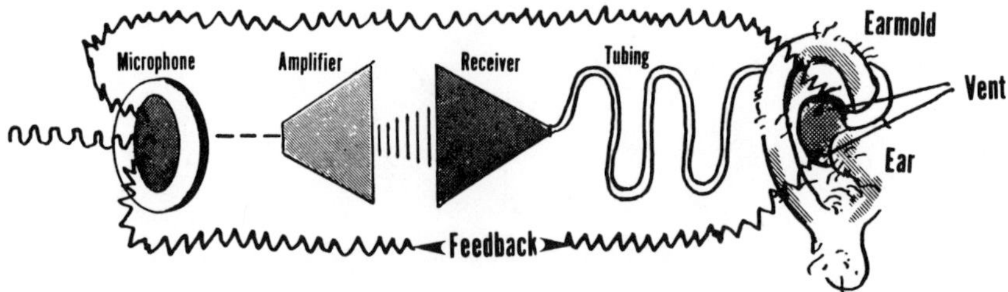

Fig. 24-7. Feedback due to earmold venting.

Batteries

The battery provides power to the instrument; without it, no amplification occurs. Hearing aids utilize different sizes and shapes of batteries. The older client should be instructed regarding the proper battery for the hearing aid he or she uses, proper insertion techniques, battery life, and their cost. Additionally, the hearing aid user should be aware of the recent advances in batteries, such as the air-electrode cells currently available in most sizes. According to Lee (1978), these batteries can provide power to some hearing aids for almost twice the time of regular cells and retain 98 percent of their original capacity after a year of sealed storage. At first observation, the air-electrode batteries appear to be more expensive. However, when the extended life is considered, most types are about the same expense. Thus, the major benefit afforded the consumer by air-electrode batteries is that of changing cells less often. The published battery life of a particular hearing aid is computed utilizing a formula which considers the power drain from the battery at full volume. For example, the published battery life of a given instrument might be 60 hours. If one considers that the normal wearing day of a hearing aid is somewhere between 10 and 16 hours, this instrument would require a new battery about every 4 to 6 days utilizing regular cells or every 8 to 12 days with an air-electrode cell. A common problem encountered by the audiologist who serves elderly clients that utilize hearing aids is that of improper battery insertion. The hearing aid user must know which end of the battery is positive (+) and which end is negative (−). Further, they must know where positive is on the instrument to ensure correct insertion. One method of demonstrating the correct insertion procedure is by instructing the client that the positive side of the battery is flat and the negative side is rounded. Improper insertion of the cell is usually obvious in that the compartment is often difficult to close, and in some cases will damage the case of the instrument.

Telephone Coil

The purpose of a telephone coil is to assist the hearing impaired person in conducting telephone conversation by amplifying the signal in the telephone receiver. The signal is generated by a magnetic coil within the telephone receiver and converted into electrical impulses by the telephone coil located within the hearing aid. These electrical impulses produced by the coil within the hearing aid are then presented to the amplifier so the sounds can be heard. Usually the telephone coil is activated by the input-selector switch. In some instruments it may be necessary to turn the volume slightly higher when listening through the telephone coil. The telephone is shown in Figure 24-8.

Input Selector Switch

If the instrument has a telecoil it also will have a switch that selects between microphone input for environmental sounds and telecoil input for telephone use. The input-selector switch may have many configurations. Some popular ones include

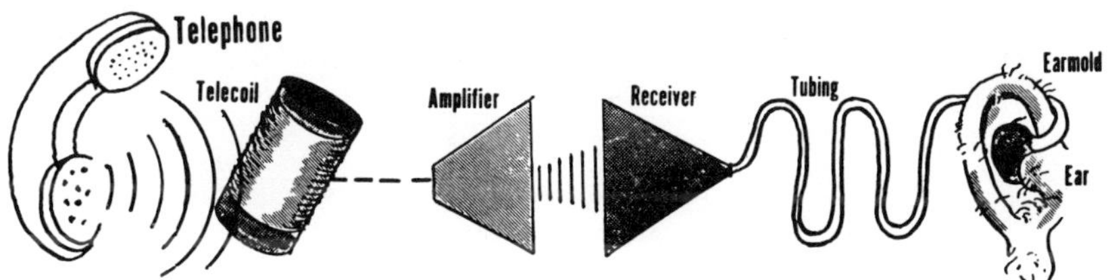

Fig. 24-8. Operation of the instrument utilizing the telephone.

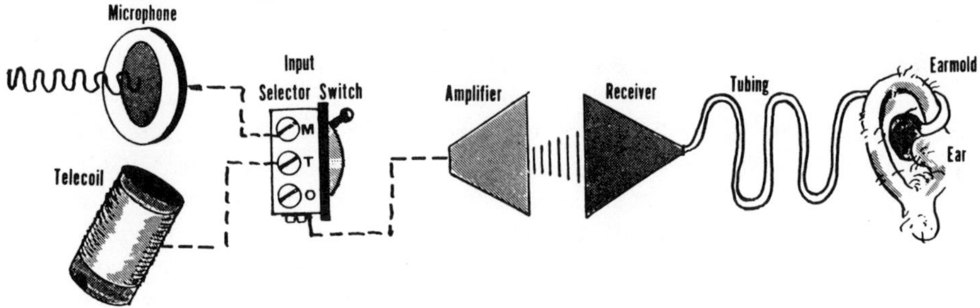

Fig. 24-9. Function of the input-selector switch in the M mode.

1. Two positions—microphone (M) and telephone (T)—with an on–off mechanism that is simply activated by removing or inserting the battery
2. Many body-type aids have a four-position switch—microphone (M), telephone (T), microphone–telephone (M–T) (allows the user to hear on the telephone and environmental sounds simultaneously, often utilized with induction-loop auditory training systems), and off
3. A three-position switch, microphone (M), telephone (T), and off (O)

For example, let's examine the latter arrangement presented in Figures 24-9 and 24-10. The microphone (M) mode is the normal position for most situations. In this mode the hearing aid microphone picks up sound vibrations and converts them into electrical impulses, the amplifier magnifies these electrical impulses, and the receiver turns the magnified electrical impulses back into sound vibrations. When the input selector switch is in the telephone (T) mode, the microphone is no longer in the circuit. The hearing aid is not sensitive to sound vibrations, but responds to the magnetism produced by the telephone receiver. When orienting older clients to their hearing aid, it is important to inform them what is happening to the instrument internally when the switch is manipulated. The client also should realize that if they forget to change the switch back to the M mode after a telephone conversation, the instrument will not pick up environmental sounds, and appear to be inoperative.

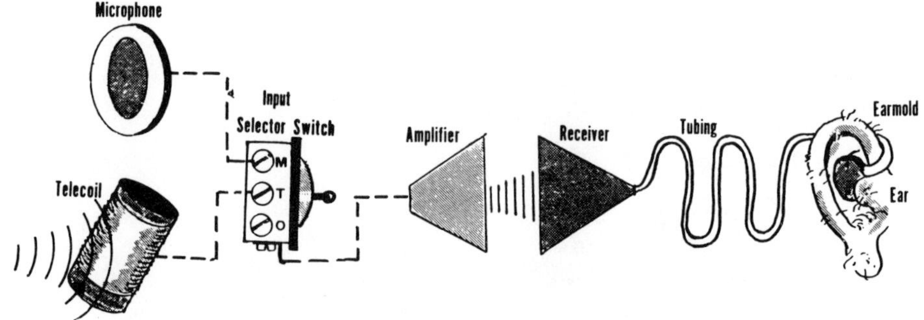

Fig. 24-10. Function of the input-selector switch in the T mode.

Tone Control

Many hearing aids have some type of tone control. Normally such tone controls adjustments modify the response of the instrument to various frequencies of sound input. In most situations, these tone controls are set by the audiologist/dispensor and should not be manipulated by the client. Thus, instructions to the client, in most cases, are that these controls are set for their hearing impairment and should only be manipulated by the audiologist/dispensor.

Ouput Limitation

The older client should be instructed that the hearing aid is equipped with circuitry that will not allow the sound to become intolerably loud for them. In-depth explanations of compression amplification versus peak clipping should be avoided with this population except in rare instances since these concepts are difficult to understand. As in the case of tone controls, the client should be informed that these controls should be set by the audiologist/dispensor and not manipulated by the client.

Volume Control

Obviously, the individual should be aware of how the volume of the instrument is regulated. The older client needs instructions about his or her particular instrument since volume controls vary among hearing aids both in position and direction of manipulation. Additionally, the client should realize that it is desirable to move the volume control according to specific situations since it is common for older clients to feel that the instrument must stay at the same volume at all times, particularly when they have been instructed that several other components are not to be manipulated.

MANIPULATION OF THE HEARING AID BY ELDERLY CLIENTS

Hearing aids can produce numerous problems for the older client particularly when reduced manual dexterity restricts manipulation. For older clients, some types of instruments are easier to use than others. Usually, the less controls and switches to be manipulated by the older person the better they are able to handle the aid.

Probably the easiest of all hearing aids to manipulate is the custom in-the-ear hearing aid. This type of aid is being utilized more among older clients than in prior years. Orientation to this type of instrument includes demonstration of the location of the battery compartment, how the batteries are inserted, and the volume control, with a demonstration of its manipulation, and insertion of the aid into the ear. An approach to manipulating the volume control of the custom in-the-ear hearing aid is to stretch out the forefinger, and place it on the volume control. A twist of the wrist usually moves it. Insertion of the instrument into the ear is best accomplished by instructing the older client to look in the mirror while the clinician inserts it the first few times. The older client then should be allowed to insert it while the audiologist or significant other acts as a "coach." Most older hearing aid users have little difficulty inserting this type of instrument since it is large enough to grasp with little manual dexterity, and the whole instrument fits into the ear canal and concha, requiring no manipulation behind the ear.

Behind-the-ear instruments are usually more difficult to manipulate. Not only does an older person with limited manual dexterity need to place the earmold in their ear, but they must also place the instrument behind the pinna as well. In addition, once the hearing aid is in position, the older user must manipulate the controls of the device behind their ear. This is often a difficult task, particularly for persons with reduced dexterity and tactile sensation, which is frequently found among older clients.

Glasses hearing aids also present their difficulties for use among the older population. Manipulation, however, is not one of the problems, since most glasses aids are controlled reasonably well by new users. In wearing the device, the client simply puts on the glasses and then inserts the earmold. The switches and controls are usually strategically located on the temple portion of the frame for easy movement. When these controls are utilized, the instrument is held firmly in place by the glasses frame rather than moving as is often the situation with behind-the-ear instruments. Some drawbacks to glasses-type instruments for this population include continual difficulties in glasses adjustment, problems inserting batteries, complaints of excess weight of glasses on the nose, and loss of amplification when not wearing glasses.

The body-type instrument is currently the least popular of hearing devices among this population. Although many older clients would actually be better able to operate a body-type aid than some of the other styles, most are willing to ''trade off'' this ease of operation for a better cosmetic effect.

ADJUSTMENT TO AMPLIFICATION

At times, the audiologist will encounter older clients who are able to put the instrument on and leave it throughout the day, subsequent to an initial orientation. These older clients, however, are a minority of the individuals seen for aural rehabilitation treatment. Most clients need to become accustomed to amplification devices gradually. It is often necessary to write out an adjustment plan for the older client. Further, such plans may require custom tailoring for the specific older person involved. These custom plans should be written out for the client so that they can take them home to follow during the ensuing adjustment period. In addition, the client ideally should be scheduled for a series of follow-up sessions to ensure proper adjustment to hearing aid.

The suggested consultations are important to the older individual since these clients need someone to reassure them and answer questions about situations in which they have found themselves during the trial period. These consultations are not required by all older clients adjusting to amplification as some will adjust quickly to the device and others will not. It is obvious to the experienced clinician that when the client is ready to be dispensed the instrument (or referred to a hearing aid dispenser for purchase of the instrument) most questions and problems are rectified.

Training Program

At the time of dispensing, the client should be wearing the instrument on a daily basis at a volume setting which is providing significant benefit. The following program, modified from Downs (Note 5), has been designed by Traynor and Peterson (1973) to meet the needs of some of the older individuals in adjusting to amplification. The client is given the following instructions:

The First Week or Two
For one-half to one hour in the morning, one-half to one hour in the afternoon, and one-half to one hour at night, wear your aid in a quiet room in these situations (start with a low volume setting and gradually increase it to the recommended level).

1. Read aloud to yourself, to learn to adjust to your own voice, as it will sound different to you.
2. Talk with one person at a time, at a distance no greater than six feet. Watch the speaker's face attentively while listening. Ask him to speak in a clear, natural voice—not too fast nor too slow—and *do not* let him shout or "mouth" (exaggerate) lip movements. In the evening, this can consist of a quiet listening hour during which someone can read to you for one-half to one hour. By watching their face all the time, you can put together what you see and what you hear to make speech more meaningful. Watch for the differences on the lips between the /p/, /t/, /s/, /b/, /f/, and /m/ sounds. These are the easiest sounds to see on the lips. Although consciously looking for these sounds, try to obtain the general idea of the conversation.
3. Listen to these sounds:
   a. Radio or recorded music. Try to identify the instruments within the music. Ask one of your family to tune the television so it is comfortable for him at a distance of six feet, and carefully adjust your aid. At first, you may want to sit closer, but gradually move back.
   b. Environmental sounds: Try to identify car or airplane motors, clocks ticking, footsteps, etc., and investigate each sound to determine its origin.

During this time, keep a notebook in which you record your practice. Record notes on the words which were difficult for you to understand. Each night you should give this list to whoever is assisting you so he can make up a sentence with each word that has been difficult for you that particular day. He can then read the sentences to you in a different order while you listen and watch carefully for the visual and auditory clues that will help you to understand these problem words. You should learn to relax during this listening training, as the more tense or nervous you are, the less message you will understand. When this feeling appears, turn off the hearing aid and relax. Later, when you feel refreshed begin your practice listening exercises again. (pp. 1–2)

First Aural Rehabilitation Consultation

This consultation normally is conducted 1 to 2 weeks after the hearing aid evaluation to determine how the client is progressing with amplified sound. It consists of an evaluation of use gain to ascertain the amount of amplification being utilized and how effectively it is being used. Further, a discussion of the client's difficulties is conducted to dispose of misconceptions and facilitate realistic attitudes regarding the possible benefit of the instrument. The clinician and the older client go over the difficulties specifically written in their notebook. For confined clients, the audiologist may need to visit the person at least twice during the first week in order to reinforce the discussions conducted earlier regarding amplification and manipulation of the device. After this session, the client is given the following instructions as an assignment to be completed in the coming 2 weeks and is scheduled for another appointment.

The Next Two Weeks
Increase the time of wearing the aid to one and a half to two hours three times a day. Take care to rest if it tires you or makes you nervous, but wear it as long as you can comfortably tolerate it. Arrange these listening situations in a quiet room:

1. Talk to several people at a time, at a distance of about six feet. Cross-conversation may be difficult at first, as you may have lost the ability to catch the various voices. Pay close attention to each speaker, watching his lips, gestures, and facial expressions as well as listening carefully to him. When that speaker has finished, you can usually tell by the direction of his glance who is speaking next. This will allow you to shift your attention to this next person and eventually you may even be able to follow the "rapid-fire" conversation at bridge or cocktail parties. However, do not attempt these extremely difficult listening situations quite yet!
2. Listen to these things:
   a. News commentators on television or the radio. You should sit close to the loudspeaker at first. Avoiding distortion of sound by setting the volume at a low level, your goal should be comfortable listening at approximately six feet.
   b. Music or singing over television, radio or phonograph. If your loss is greatest in the high pitches, listen especially to string instruments and to soprano singers.
   c. While the vacuum cleaner or refrigerator is on, listen to someone talk. Relax and try to listen to sounds, and not to the motor noise.
3. Continue the listening hour in which someone reads to you quietly.
4. Constantly enlarge the list of words that are hard for you; by now, your notebook should have many pages of these words. Your assistant should be able to think up sentences off hand with these words that are hard for you. Often times others will help you with sentences so you can practice in listening and watching the lips of different people. (p. 3)

Second Aural Rehabilitation Consultation

The second consultation is normally conducted 2 weeks after the first one. At this point, the clinician discusses how the client reacted to the listening situations assigned for the previous 2 weeks, which included listening to news commentators, music or singing, or conversation in the presence of background noise. The second session is also when the audiologist should present some superficial speechreading instruction to assist the older client in utilizing not only the auditory modality but visual clues as well. Usually, the experienced clinician will be able to determine if the instrument will be of significant benefit to the client by the second week and, if so, the device may be dispensed during this session. If adjustment problems which require more experience utilizing the hearing aid still exist, additional consultation sessions may be required before the instrument is dispensed. The following instructions are designed for use by the client, either as practice exercises for use after the instrument has been dispensed or as an assignment for the next visit (often within 2 weeks) for those clients who need extra help.

The Next Few Months
Begin to wear the hearing aid for a longer time so that eventually you will be wearing it all day. By this time you should be able to accomplish this easily at the recommended volume setting. Arrange for these experiences.

1. Turning your volume fairly low, go outside and take a walk. Listen carefully to identify all the sounds you hear—children's voices, dogs barking, horns blowing, etc. Do this every day alone until you are ready to have someone accompany you on your walk and talk to you. Listen for his voice above the street noises.
2. Begin attending public gatherings; start with church services, or lectures. Sit as far front as possible in the middle, so you can watch lips, gestures and facial expressions of the speaker. Experiment with the volume and tone controls to achieve maximum hearing

with maximum comfort. Learn to regulate the volume and tone controls by feel rather than looking at it so you will not need to take your eyes away from the speaker. Later you can go to the movies by following the same procedure. Avoid sitting under a balcony, as the sound will be distorted there. The best seating is in the following locations.
   a. At the movies: 8 to 15 rows from the front, as close to the center as possible.
   b. At church: approximately the fifth row from the front, near the center.
   c. At lectures: four to six rows from the front, near the center.
3. Listen to all types of television or radio programs, music, news commentators, plays, etc. Always listen in a relaxed, attentive manner at a normal distance (approximately 6 feet).
4. Find varied hearing experiences of your own both inside and outside. Continue the listening hour, although by now you should be able to wear your hearing aid most of the time at the recommended volume setting. (pp. 3–4)

PROPER CARE OF HEARING AIDS

The older client should receive some type of a handout describing general cautions about the wearing of the instrument and how to care for it. This reference source assists the client in remembering the discussions and counseling conducted by the audiologist. Among the more important cautions, the client should remember to be certain that the battery is inserted with the + sign at the correct end, remove the batteries from the hearing aid when they are not in use (such as at night; this will conserve battery power and save on monthly operating expenses), and avoid corrosion deposits on the batteries, as they may transfer it into the aid. (Slight corrosion deposits are removed with a pencil eraser, whereas large deposits can be wiped off with a damp cloth.) In addition, it should be emphasized that the client should not attempt to save batteries by lowering the volume, but should wear the aid at its recommended level, and extra batteries should be kept on hand at all times, however, a 1-month supply is usually sufficient. He or she should store extra batteries in an air-tight container *in their original package*. Caution the patient to keep dust out of the microphone, and to avoid exposing the hearing aid to radiation or diathermy (X-rays or excess hot and cold temperatures). The case, receiver, and cords may be cleaned with a damp cloth only, not with alcohol or cleaning fluids as they damage the case. Excessive moisture should be avoided.

For the patient with a body-type hearing aid special reminders to obtain an extra receiver and cord (these are common malfunctions of body aids and will save waiting for a factory order) and to avoid blows to the receiver as it is *very* delicate should be emphasized. Remind your client when pulling the cord out of the hearing aid or the receiver, to grasp the plastic part of the prong connection firmly and pull *gently*; he or she never should jerk at the cord. In addition, the hearing aid wearer should not allow the cords to be pulled, bent, or knotted (if it is necessary to anchor the cord, slip it through a safety pin) and should keep the prongs of the cord clean (if they become corroded, a damp cloth and/or an emery board will clean them very well).

All patients wearing hearing aids should be taught proper care for earmolds. They should learn to wash the earmold daily in a solution of soap and warm water. A pipe cleaner should be used to remove wax and dirt from inside the canal of the mold. Tell them to dry the mold carefully and blow the water out of the canal, but never use alcohol or cleaning fluids to clean the earmold, as these solutions tend to crack the plastic material.

Table 24-2
Simple Trouble-Shooting Techniques for the Older Client

What to do if the hearing aid is inoperative, weak or goes on and off.

Be sure that the aid is at the proper volume.

Ensure that the battery is good, and that it is inserted properly.

Try another battery to see if the aid works better.

Make sure that the battery is clean.

Check the earmold, ensure that it is not clogged with wax.

What to do if your hearing aid squeals when it is in your ear.

Seal the end of the earmold with your finger and turn the volume to the highest setting. If it still squeals, there may be a leak in the hearing aid itself; see your hearing aid dealer.

If the aid does not squeal with your finger plugging it, there is possibly an earmold misfit. Try some vaseline around the canal piece (the part that fits in the ear). If your hearing aid still squeals, a new earmold usually is required.

What to do for scratchy noises or intermittent operation.

Try a spare cord (if a body-type aid).

Move all switches back and forth. This may remove fine particles of dust or lint interfering with proper electrical contacts. Removing and inserting the cord plugs in the receiver, as well as in the hearing aid may also correct the trouble.

SIMPLE TROUBLE-SHOOTING TECHNIQUES

Instruction regarding simple trouble-shooting tends to foster responsibility for the instrument in the client. Table 24-2 shows some simple techniques which can be published for a handout to the older client.

If the client notices any of the conditions, try the trouble-shooting techniques mentioned as they will save money or repairs. However, if these techniques do not correct the problem, emphasize that they should see an *audiologist or hearing aid dispenser*.

REFERENCES

Alpiner, J. D. Evaluation of communication function, in J. Alpiner (Ed.), *Handbook of adult rehabilitative audiology*. Baltimore: Williams and Wilkins, 1978.

Carkhuff, R. R., Pierce, R. M., & Cannon, J. R. *The art of helping III*. Amherst, Massachusetts: Human Resource Development Press, 1977.

Davis, H. The articulation area and the Social Adequacy Index for hearing. *Laryngoscope,* 1948, *58*, 761–778.

High, W. S., Fairbanks, G., & Glorig, A. Scale for self-assessment of hearing handicap. *Journal of Speech and Hearing Disorders,* 1964, *29*, 215–230.

Hull, R., & Traynor, R. *Hearing impairment among aging persons*. Lincoln, Nebraska: Cliffs Speech and Hearing Series, 1977.

Kasten, R. Learning to use the hearing aid, in W. Hodgeson, & P. Skinner (Eds.), *Hearing aid assessment and use in audiologic habilitation*. Baltimore: Williams and Wilkins, 1977.

Lee, R. Space-age zinc-air battery. *Hearing Instruments,* 1978, *29*, 28.

Rupp, R., Higgings, J., & Maurer, J. A feasibility scale for predicting hearing aid use for older people. *Journal of the Academy of Rehabilitative Audiology,* 1977, *10*, 81–104.

Rupp, R. The significant other person: An essential

factor for success with the elderly hearing aid user. *Hearing Aid Journal,* 1977, *30*, 9.

Sanders, D. Hearing aid orientation and counseling, in M. Pollack (Ed.), *Amplification for the hearing impaired.* New York: Grune & Stratton, 1975.

Zarnoch, J. & Alpiner, J. *The Denver Scale of Communication Function for Senior Citizens Living in Retirement Centers*, in J. Alpiner (Ed.), *Handbook of adult rehabilitative audiology*. Baltimore: Williams and Wilkins, 1978.

REFERENCE NOTES

1. Chermak, G. D. *Counseling: An integral component of audiological rehabilitation*. Paper presented at the Annual Convention of the American Speech and Hearing Association, Chicago, 1977.
2. Alpiner, J. D., Cheverette, W., Glascoe, G., Metz, M., & Olsen, G. *The Denver Scale of Communication Function*. Unpublished study, 1971. (University of Denver.)
3. Bate, H. L. *The Denver scale of communication function as a counseling tool*. Paper presented at the Annual Convention of the American Speech and Hearing Association, Chicago, 1977.
4. Traynor, R., & Peterson, K. *Adjusting to your new hearing aid*. Unpublished Clinic Handout, 1973. (Available from ENT Group of Greeley, 2528 16th St., Greeley, Colorado 80631.)
5. Downs, M. *You and your hearing aid*. Unpublished Clinic Handout, 1970. (Available from the University of Colorado Medical Center, Denver.)

Perry G. Thompson

Chapter 25: Techniques for Motivational Counseling with Elderly Clients

Some of the questions that motivational counselors ask their clients are in and of themselves very difficult to pose, much less to answer. Two such questions are, "How often do you feel there is no point in going on living?" and, "As you get older, do you find things becoming better or worse than you thought they would be?" A response to either of these questions requires a good deal of reflection, and the answer can vary depending on how the client feels that day or even at that time of day. But then those are "research" questions, and the question counselors are more likely to ask is simply, "How are you today?" If the answer is not bright and cheery, or at least prompt and politely neutral, one begins to consider possible motivational counseling. Incidentally, phrasing the question as, "How are we today?" is too cute and belittles the client; counselors should come into the room as equals and prepare themselves to listen to an honest answer.

Social systems run on information. A husband who always tells his wife that she looks great and that everything she is doing is fine, no matter what the circumstances are, is not transmitting useful information to her and is setting himself up for a fall. Similarly the professional who asks a question and then becomes irritated upon not hearing the anticipated (proper) answer is also setting him- or herself up for failure.

UNDERSTANDING THE CLIENT

In order to counsel with the elderly we need, first, an understanding of the basic processes of normal aging; sound communication–interaction skills are second; then comes the question of why motivation is necessary. What is it that the counselor intends to motivate the client to do? Motivational counseling may be a philosophy of intervention, or it may be no more than mere techniques or tricks for altering another person's life to suit a standard of appropriateness or propriety.

Intervention is at first a statement of evaluation of the other person, and care must be taken to ensure that the evaluation is not a negative judgment of that person for being too ugly, too short, or too old. Professionally we are aware that to be old is not a necessary moral judgment any more so than to state a person is deaf or blind is a moral statement. We often are drawn, however, into evaluative statements, even against our better professional knowledge. Aging strikes at our adulthood, our sense of competence, and it strikes each of us with some impact. The whiskers, the tapering off of menstruation at menopause, the new gray hairs, and the threats to one's libido create a rising sense of insecurity and questions retaining control of one's life. It is very difficult to avoid evaluative judgments when we couple any of the sensory decrements (dimming of visual acuity or hearing) and our age. How do you respond to a client who comments, "I may be as good as I ever was, but who knows? Worse, who cares?"

Normal aging is a combination of biological and psychological processes and social definitions. Aging is affected by diseases, environment, heredity, and the ravages of one's life-style, all to the accompaniment of a cultural set of attitudes and values. We are, as yet, unable to "cure" aging, but we do feel it proper to repair the ravages of time. Our intervention ranges from cosmetics, hair dyes or hairpieces, and concern for being in fashion to cortisone shots, face lifts, hearing aids, eye glasses, and false teeth. Such simple intervention as the self-administered touching up and smoothing of wrinkles is significant for the motivation it demonstrates.

Most people are normally motivated to present themselves to others as attractively as possible and as complete and in control (or at least competent). If they cannot present themselves well, in keeping with how they feel they ought to be presenting themselves, then they can lose their motivation for a positive presentation of self and either allow or deliberately present a negative self.

People are very dependent on others for the "framework of imagery" (Goffman, 1961) that they use to see and then reflect their sense of self. Much, if not all, human behavior serves to protect this sense of self, however stupid or maladaptive it may appear to others. Counselors need to begin to understand the normalcy and the rationality behind some of the behavior they are about to attempt to change.

This means that counselors must be sensitive to the needs that are being served by their clients' behavior which they label as pathological. For instance, when a counselor corrects a client's hearing loss with an operation or with a hearing aid, he or she probably feels that the intervention has been a success. The client has been counseled—psyched, cajoled, threatened, bribed—into acceptance and utilization (one hopes) of the best available technology. Now the client can function "normally" in society or at least with the family. No longer does he or she have to sit and stew over whether others across the room are talking about him. No longer do people have to repeat every sentence ten times for her to understand the topic of conversation. He even takes his turn in the conversation instead of always dominating it in order to avoid losing control of the topic. Because of all this the counselor expects that the client should be grateful for the intervention and for the medical and mechanical technology that made the new (near) normalcy possible. But the client isn't grateful. He or she may even refuse to wear the damn machine and, worse, is grouchy, irritable, and as yet a far piece from normal. What has gone wrong? The client has been deprived of a retreat that may have been 30 years in the making. The hearing loss that is gradual is also gradually made a part of the personality. Now the client has been robbed of something that at least was a facet of his or her personality and been left very vulnerable to external incursions.

The foremost incursion of course, is noise. Sounds that were long forgotten may be of some renewed interest, but their continuity is annoying and exhausting. In a more important behavioral sense, the communication system, both habitual and deliberate, is immediately altered. The client thinks, "I can no longer choose when, or even whether,

I will hear you. Because I have accepted your prosthesis you can demand that I hear you, understand you, and not be so dependent on you.'' This is a delicate mixture of objective and subjective conditions. It may be the case that such demands are more threatening than is recognized for the client's sense of well-being. It also may be that vanity is rearing its ugly head, since visible prosthetic device is an invitation for others to comment, if they are so bold, and is at least visible evidence of one's infirmities and, hence, a potential threat to a sense of self-worth. A last incursion, too often belittled, is pain. The sound hurts, and the mold hurts, and it feels better not to hurt than to hear.

MOTIVATION

Theories on motivation and aging are essentially specific to a biogenic or psychogenic need as the incentive to some preselected and appropriate behavior, as in memory, appetite, sex drive, or psychomotor activity. Techniques of motivation range from deprivation, aversive stimulation, and drug therapies to sensory exercises and reality orientation. Group processes range from primal scream therapy to music and art therapies.

Something Pleasant

Audiologists interested in counseling older clients are more likely to be working on an individual basis than in group settings. Any technique that works to motivate people to behavior that's desired by their children, their spouses, or their parents is likely also to motivate the older client. This can be something sweet or pleasant, be it either candy or words, or something soft and warm, such as a touch or an expression of concern. Even offering a challenge to be met generally evokes a positive response in people, regardless of their age.

But genuine concern is not to be faked. The sweetness may be cloying and the touch resented as demeaning. Accordingly there are a few rules that counselors should observe in their interactions with elderly clients. As indicated earlier, they should not include themselves in the inquiry into the client's present state of being. If the client is feeling lousy or depressed that day (and there are few people who have not had such feelings), the counselor could offer empathy by saying something like, ''Yes, I've had blue Mondays . . . even blue Tuesdays.'' Counselors also may offer their professional services as an antidote, though that may require that they would have to offer to leave and return at a later time to obtain the client's consent.

Social Space

Counselors should mind their social space. The idea of social distance has to do with the physical proximity between the counselor and the client. The hard-of-hearing and deaf do touch more naturally in order to obtain attention and to pass on conversation. Not all persons are touchers, however, and how one touches can convey very strong messages. A tap on the arm may be read as an imperious gesture, a pat on the head as demeaning (even children hate adults who pat them on the head), a pat or rub too low on the back as too familiar. On the other hand, touching is fun, it is nice, it obviously and directly conveys a sense of warmth and concern. It also says to the client, ''I'm not afraid of catching your wrinkles.'' People do act in many instances as if they believe old age is some sort of contagious disease. Aging is a process of inter-related biosocial events, neither disease nor contagious.

Another aspect of social distance is the evaluational content implied or stated by the manner in which counselors place themselves in relation to their clients. They should not enter the room and move to a sitting position at the clients' feet; they are not dogs, and the clients would certainly think they had lost their marbles. Conversely, counselors should not enter the clients' social space and stand above them as if the clients were the dogs; and in the name of all that is sentient, counselors should not lean over and pat their clients, who then would be perfectly justified in biting their hands. The proper position is one in which the counselor's face is level with the client's and well-lighted, both for good eye contact and ease of communication.

External Snags

The audiologist's desire to fit a hearing aid on a client may next run into some external, or environmental, snags. For one, the clients' wishes may not be the primary reason that professional help and advice have been solicited. Frustrated family or friends may have pushed them into seeing a counselor, with the result that some clients will refuse to admit that they need help. The audiologist's task is then to present in a positive way what a hearing aid will do. Obviously of primary importance is that the ability to hear enables the clients to understand what others are saying. Out of respect for their intelligence, however, audiologists also should counsel clients on what *not* to expect from the hearing aid. The clients' experience should not be undervalued, and the audiologist should solicit information on where and under what conditions clients want the aid to be effective.

Audiologists who succeed in counseling on effective utilization of the hearing aid may then be faced with another client attack on them, and they need to be ready. Nonhearing elderly persons are generally silent and nondemanding, if only because of lack of practice instead of desire. The audiologist is altering the communication patterns of the clients and all those who make contact with clients. Old habits are difficult to change; people still holler at the clients or ignore their comments. In a society that is highly verbal, clients will have missed much of the content of past conversations and so lack information necessary to participate in future conversations. Challenge those persons who will make up the clients' supporting environment to participate in a one-week sound fast (i.e., wear earplugs) and then attempt to re-enter conversations. Both the clients and their support groups may be expecting a restoration of a sensory state that's impossible to achieve.

Self-Worth

If the clients' sense of self-worth is low, then counseling has to help them cope with not only the physical fatigue that accompanies the transition to hearing but also the emotionally devastating question of whether or not it's worth the bother. The essential nature of our society is the social bond of reciprocity. One gives as well as receives. Professionally the audiologist offers the means and techniques of aiding the clients in redressing their social isolation and its attendant problems of social and mental health.

Elderly clients have not survived their allotted three score and ten years of life to be quickly whipped into shape by a pep talk on dignity and worth of Everyman. Their experience has led them to an acceptance, however reluctant, that aging is normal.

Vision, hearing, and memory loss are all "normal." Thus, the clients' rejection of the audiologists' best professional offering should not be read as a rejection of the audiologists. Rather it is more simply that some elderly people are rejecting the notion that you can pour water up hill. Or, if a client defines deafness as "being old," then to accept professional help is also to accept the self as being old, and some clients may not be prepared to make that step. The counselors' intervention here, based on knowledge of the areas in which the clients interact and operate, can offer to maximize their control of those spheres of social space and, hence, of their sense of self.

There exists a range of events and behaviors that need to be met in order to motivate the elderly client successfully. The foremost criterion is that the clients like themselves and the age they are becoming. Contrary to what we believed as adolescents, all growth and sense of future do not cease at age 21!

Retaining Pride and Dignity

A person who finds "old" distasteful will never experience the joy of an exquisite wine or the best cheese nor appreciate the craftsmanship of a 17th century cabinetmaker. He or she also may not acquire the coping skills that can be learned from a generation that has managed to negotiate the transformation from a rural to an urban society, a generation that coped with the social changes involved in moving from the horse and buggy to the moon within a single lifetime.

Counseling and advice (intervention) should be gauged to maximize the clients' independence and their sense of self-worth. Audiologists thus should not be threatened by clients who show a sense of independent judgment not in keeping with their best professional advice. They should understand that intervention may be or may result in a further loss of environmental control than already experienced and be prepared to intervene on their clients' behalf since professional expertise extends their competencies.

Clients' gifts should be accepted. When audiologists offer their vibrant professionalism and concern in addition to their professional billing for services, the clients may find it depressing not to be able to return the vibrancy. They may instead offer stories of their past, morality lessons, or coping skills. It is important that these gifts be accepted as offered, for the clients are saying, "This is from when I was somebody, when I counted." Acceptance of these gifts tells them that they still count. This reciprocity creates a social bond that allows the clients to be dependent on another yet still retain their pride and dignity.

The issue really is the dignity and self-esteem of both client and audiologists. While it is not dignified to be spoken to in baby talk when you are 85 years old, it is not any more dignified to be the person cooing to elderly clients. As stated earlier, it is demeaning to be patted on the head and quite uncomfortable and dizzying to have to look upward to make eye contact. Touching is critical to communication, and, mindful of public mores, touching in appropriate places can convey intimacy in the warmest human sense. The most tragic loss that accompanies aging is often the loss of spouse and friends; the separation from family also can mean the loss of touching. Counselors should remember that as infants born prematurely can die from lack of touching and caressing, so, too, may adults wither, withdraw, and die for lack of touching.

Low Self-Esteem

A major task of motivational counseling is to overcome the clients' feelings of low self-esteem. In addition, counselors may have to deal with and alter the family's concurrence with that feeling. The client needs choices. Offering them will, in itself, bolt some elderly persons out of nonresponsiveness since the elderly are not used to being offered choices, only directions. The choices the counselor offers them are to hear and better understand, to participate in the world around them, and to control again (the hearing aid can be shut off if the preacher is boring).

To Want to

Another task is to encourage the clients to want to: to want to do anything that is contrary to the stereotype of themselves or of ''old people'' that directs their behavior. It is an unfortunate fact of our society that the elderly hold many of the negative stereotypes of aging that their own experience should belie. But there is the chink in this wall of myth and stereotype, and that chink is their own experience. The elderly will estimate that their own condition (i.e., health) is generally better than the ''average'' old person. They can be encouraged to break the mold of what others think they should be like and to be what they want, if they want, if they have already confessed that they are not like others their age.

Labels

Labels are insidious things. We have discovered that our society punishes people who do not conform to our labels and rewards those who do conform to the stereotyped or even deviant role. This is to say, an old person may be receiving more attention, more ''strokes,'' by conforming than by behaving contrary to expectations. Deviance may get a family or friend to say, ''Act your age.'' Of course, no one has yet adequately determined what it means to act one's age. It is a way in which we control others. Children are too young to drive, to court ardently, and to drink and too old to cry about it. The elderly are too old to drive, to court ardently, and to drink and too young to cry about it.

To change the expected dependent behavior, to engage in normal and conventional activities, is to expose the client to some risks. Counseling should explore the myths and suggest how to counter them when confronted. It is possible to sympathize with how much simpler life is or would be if we would only behave as others expect. It is not normal for the young or the middle-aged to stop all activity, learning, loving, and growing, and it is not normal for the elderly either.

HEARING AIDS

It is important to focus on how a hearing aid will help in coping with normal, ordinary social interaction. It is not normal to be always depressed (only in the morning maybe, if you are a night person), and it is not normal to be always anxious. But counselors should avoid the error of Damocles and not constantly sing praises to the happiness and fulfillment of aging, lest the elderly seat them beneath the sword hung by a single thread. The aging process does bring with it some sense of continuous threat to health and to finances. A positive offer is a tool to help cope with the threat, but not a cure.

Effective intervention should not entail any surprises. The most effective motivation is the pulling pressure from family and friends to participate. Counselors need to explain in as much detail as possible and practice in the privacy of clients' environment the clients' hearing aids before hitting the freeway of large gatherings. In preparing elderly clients, counselors arm them with a sense of control and of competence.

And, finally, counselors need to be ready to interpret their clients' efforts as progress and to encourage them to see the signs of aggravation in others as positive signs. They are neither "nonpersons" nor "good patients," but people striving to meet their own needs and goals and continue to lead a meaningful life.

CONCLUSION

Counselors can offer a sense of the future, of goals to be set and achieved, a continuity of adulthood for elderly clients in our society. Then, if clients are depressed that they have given nothing for all that has been done for them, counselors should touch them and tell them that they have offered their strength and knowledge and the courage to have coped with some of the most vexing problems of mankind. They survived, so they need to be thanked for sharing those skills. This is, in a word, motivation.

REFERENCE

Goffman, I. *Asylums*. Garden City, New York: Doubleday-Anchor, 1961, p. 128.

Raymond H. Hull

Chapter 26: Techniques of Aural Rehabilitation Treatment for Elderly Clients

The process of aural rehabilitation for elderly clients is exciting, to say the least. To be involved in the recovery of communication skills which have previously caused the older adult to withdraw from a communicating world is indeed rewarding. Both the client and the audiologist can rejoice in the recovery of those skills. Some elderly clients recover skills that allow him or her to participate on a social basis once again, at least, with a greater degree of efficiency. Others may simply regain the ability to communicate with their family with greater ease. In light of those gains and, perhaps, a step toward a reinstatement of confidence in their own ability to function as independent beings, the client and his or her audiologist have reason to rejoice.

We cannot, under any circumstances, hope to benefit every elderly hearing impaired person. But in attempting to do so, if some are helped who had since submitted to a self-imposed withdrawal from family and friends because of the embarrassment resulting from responding inappropriately to questions they thought they understood, then we can be satisfied that our work is worthwhile.

This chapter will present the components of aural rehabilitation services for the older adult client. The aspects to be discussed are not truly original since professionals in the fields of audiology, psychology, speech/language pathology, and others also use these approaches. Perhaps, however, the manner in which they are organized will be helpful to the reader.

In some ways, the two most difficult clients the audiologist faces are the young adult and the elderly client. Because of the fact that the majority of hearing impaired elderly clients have experienced normal to near-normal auditory function during their younger years, and because they are generally fully aware of the communicative difficulties they face, approaches to aural (re)habilitation must also depend on the client to make us aware of those needs.

Since it is being discovered that the auditory disorder found in older adults is not only peripheral in nature but also involves higher levels of auditory function (Bergman, 1980; Hull, Note 1; and Kasten, 1981), our approaches to aural rehabilitation must accommodate the communication difficulties experienced because of those compounding problems (see Chapter 17). Those seem to include deficits in areas such as (1) auditory/

linguistic closure, (2) the speed of central processing of auditory/linguistic information, and (3) sorting behaviors, that is, sorting meaningful (desired) information (speech) from nondesired, nonmeaningful competing signals (noise). These factors appear to be very similar to those found among children who possess auditorily based language problems, and children with neurologically based learning disabilities. The audiologist is, indeed, facing complex people who possess a complex auditory disorder.

Let us now consider some approaches to the provision of aural rehabilitation services for the older client.

COMPONENTS OF AURAL REHABILITATION TREATMENT FOR ELDERLY CLIENTS

The various physiological and psychological aspects of aging which impact on elderly persons, and in turn those that may affect the services any professional provides them, are presented in Chapter 14. Also, Chapters 19, 20, 21, and 22 present discussions of those aspects of aging which can impact on the provision of audiology services, the measurement of communicative function, and modifications which may be necessary in assessing the elderly client. Many of the effects of the process of aging which can impact on assessment also may effect the manner in which elderly clients can and will respond to remediational procedures. For a review of those important physiological aspects of aging and procedural modifications that may be necessary as a result of the process of aging, the reader will want to review those chapters.

The following are important components of an aural rehabilitation service program for older adult clients that are applicable for either the well older adult in the community or those who are confined to a health care facility.

1. Counseling
2. Hearing aid orientation
3. Adjusting the listening environment
4. Development of positive assertiveness
5. Involvement of family and others

Counseling

As this author talks with his students about aural rehabilitation services for older adult clients, it is emphasized that counseling, for lack of a better term, is one of the most important aspects and is intertwined throughout the process of aural rehabilitation. It is not something that occurs alone and out of context. It is an integral part of everything the audiologist does when working with his or her clients. It is called *talking*. It is called *instilling confidence* in a client who became discouraged when he or she did not do as well as expected on a given communicative task. It is called *listening* to the innermost feelings a client reveals about him- or herself and that person's relationship with an intolerant family or roommate. And, it is called *trust* that must develop between audiologist and client. Counseling is the discussion which develops when the client desires to talk about an incident in which he or she had particular difficulty understanding what another person was saying, and also includes the problem solving which should ensue to unravel the possible reasons for the difficulty.

This aspect of the process of aural rehabilitation is again, for lack of a better term, called counseling. But, whatever it is called, it involves listening, talking, problem solving, facilitating adjustment to a sometimes infuriating disability, and the development of trust between client and audiologist.

When an audiologist comes face to face with a hearing impaired elderly client who says, "I do not desire to be helped. I am old and I do not know how much longer I will live," the attitude of that elderly person certainly will impact in a negative manner on how much potential progress that person will make. This is particularly true if that person has isolated him- or herself from the outside world as a result of that attitude and resigned him- or herself to not seek help because of advanced age.

The Audiologist as Counselor

If there are no other significant contraindicating factors which would hinder responsiveness to aural rehabilitation services, the audiologist is in a position to intervene in a counseling role. It is possible that this person has said what was said because he or she has been told by others that "you are too old." A well-meaning physician may have said, "You know you're no spring chicken any more." Or, a child may have said unthinkingly, "Mom, you know you can't care for yourself as well as you used to, so we should start thinking about moving you to a nursing home," not realizing that the older adult is convinced that placement in a nursing home will be terminal. Such statements, perhaps said in a well-meaning way, are understandably defeating to the elderly adult. They further may cause the person to develop doubts regarding his or her survival. Death must be imminent. One of my clients, a female of 89 years, told me that when her 50-year-old daughter told her that they should sell her house and she should then move into an efficiency apartment, she was so hurt and angry that she could not think of anything to say. She felt convinced that if her mature daughter felt that she could not care for her house, then she must be doing a worse job than she thought. I asked her what she would have said if her daughter would have suggested that to her when she was 45 years old and her daughter was 15. She said she would have told her to mind her own business. But, she said, when you are 85 years old, perhaps it is not worth it to fight back.

If the medical records of an individual indicate satisfactory health, and there appears to be nothing that would contraindicate the provision of aural rehabilitative services, then the self-defeating attitude of the potential client may be the only thing that stands between the provision of services and reasonable progress in aural rehabilitation. Although an older person's realistic view of becoming older may be a healthy one, long-term mourning because of age and the possibility of death is not. The audiologist can be a positive catalyst in helping adjustment to aging, particularly for those who are barred from social interaction as a result of their auditory deficit.

Feelings to which the Audiologist Must Respond

Phrases exemplifying attitudes typical of many older hearing impaired adults were recorded by this author during initial aural rehabilitation interviews with six elderly clients. The feelings which prompted these revealing statements are those that can and do stifle the desire for aural rehabilitative services or the progress that they may be capable of. They are, further, those which the audiologist must respond to. It should be noted that the ability to communicate with others improved to some degree among all of these persons and none dwelled upon these topics as frequently after improved communication skills were evident. The following are those statements, out of context, recorded by this author:

> ''I feel that I'm on trial . . . incompetent.''
>
> ''My son is right behind me. He comes down to see me as often as he can, but he has a lot of business to handle there. . . . I don't see him very often anymore.''
>
> ''I can't hear and my eyes bother me. Surgery won't help my ears or my eyes. I'm too old.''
>
> ''My arthritis bothers me . . . all over, especially with the weather. I used to walk a lot. I can't hear now . . . I'm too old.''
>
> ''I fear being alone—being melancholy—with no future to look forward to. I need to find some way to be useful . . . I can stand a lot. I'm still sturdy.''
>
> ''I would like, more than anything, to be able to get out, to socialize, but I can't hear very well. I would like to go to church, but the children don't come on Sundays and there is no one to take me.''

One statement stands out from all of the rest. It is a statement by a physically strong and mentally alert 82-year-old hearing impaired man who is torn between giving up or submitting to the opportunity to improve his ability to function communicatively through aural rehabilitation treatment. It is as follows. ''I'd like to put a younger person on my shoulders to ride intellectually and hear for me, and to go on from there. I suppose I need to learn to rely on myself . . . relationships with people are important, but I've lived my life. . . .''

The statements above are representative of those heard by audiologists who are faced with the opportunity to provide a significant rehabilitative service to older adults. These people are, in many ways, crying out to be recognized not simply as an old person, but as adults who have grown older, who have something to offer, and who do not want to be left alone, only to die. Their resolution to ''not be a bother'' and their resignation to ''being old'' is in some cases the most logical choice in their minds for lack of alternatives. The audiologist, in those instances when one of the reasons for such negative reactions is an inability to cope in a communicating world due to an auditory deficit, can be the catalyst in developing a desire for rehabilitative services and self-improvement.

The audiologist must not be afraid to work with clients in a close but professional manner. He or she must not be hesitant to intervene in a counseling role but must be cognizant of those instances when a client's state and emotional problems are beyond the scope of the audiologist's knowledge. For those persons, it is the responsibility of the audiologist to refer the individual to other appropriate professionals. Above all, the elderly client must be confident in the audiologist who is providing the aural rehabilitation service. The client must realize that the audiologist understands the communicative impact of presbycusis through his or her experience in working with other elderly clients. The elderly client must know that the audiologist feels that he or she can, indeed, be helped to communicate more efficiently through aural rehabilitative services, and that feeling has justification on the basis of evaluation, not sympathy. A feeling of justified trust is the true key to motivational counseling.

> Listen—talk—empathize—listen—encourage where appropriate—remember the status and age of the client—provide support—counsel—listen—ask questions—expect answers—listen—provide guidance. Add an appropriate amount of inspiration and we may have the key to successful motivational counseling (Hull, 1977).

Counseling as a part of the aural rehabilitation process is presented later in this chapter under "The Process." The psychosocial implications of aging are presented in Chapters 18, 24, and 25.

Hearing Aid Orientation as a Part of the Aural Rehabilitation Treatment Process

Information in Chapter 24 deals with hearing aid orientation procedures for the elderly. As stated in that chapter, the process of adjustment to the use of a hearing aid and orientation to its efficient use can be facilitated with greater ease for some elderly clients than others; this depends upon prior exposure to and knowledge of the use of hearing aids and factors of memory, manual dexterity, and others. The process of adjustment to a hearing aid and orientation to its use can be logically carried over into daily or weekly aural rehabilitation treatment sessions, as can the trial use of various hearing aids as part of the hearing aid evaluation.

Through carry-over of orientation to hearing aid usage into the aural rehabilitation treatment program, slight adjustments to the hearing aid can, for example, be made pursuant to communicative problems encountered during treatment sessions. Questions can be answered regarding its use, and discussions regarding certain difficult listening environments can be entertained that may benefit not only that individual client, but others, for example, in a group session. More experienced hearing aid users can be an important catalyst in the new user's successful adjustment to amplification. Further, experimental adjustments in hearing aid gain and frequency response can be made in accordance with the activities in various treatment sessions.

Carry-over of the hearing aid orientation process into aural rehabilitation treatment sessions can be as important as the orientation process itself, and is a logical extension. The consistency of client contact itself is a valuable asset in facilitating adjustment to amplification. In group treatment sessions, the catharsis and camaraderie which arises as various clients describe their own difficulties experienced during the initial adjustment period is a healthy environment for efficient adjustment to hearing aid use. Procedures for hearing aid orientation that are applicable for the older adult are well outlined by Downs (Note 2), and modified by Traynor and Peterson (Note 3). Hearing aid orientation for the confined elderly has been prepared by Smith and Fay (1977).

Adjusting/Manipulating the Listening Environment

As will be observed in "The Process" section of this chapter, elderly clients are initially asked to set priorities in favor of those communication situations in which they desire to function more efficiently. After this is completed, they are asked to choose one or two in which they *most* desire to learn to function more efficiently. They are, of course, requested to be reasonable in their selections. In this way, the aural rehabilitation treatment program can be designed to meet their specific communication needs. In those instances where a client's auditory difficulties are so severe that group sessions are not practical or cannot be tolerated by the client, individual treatment is scheduled. The goal, however, is to integrate that client into a group situation as soon as is possible, if at all possible. Another situation in which it is desirable that individual treatment be instituted is in the case of a client whose priority communication environment is so unique as to warrant individual work. A situation in point is a client who was provided services individually by this writer. His most difficult communication environment, as a semi-retired physician from a small town, was his examination room. His treatment sessions, therefore, centered around physical/environmental adjustments in that specific room. His priority communication environment did not warrant exposure in group sessions. He, further, did not desire that his difficulty be exposed to the group at that time. He had little difficulty in other more social environments.

Group Sessions

Group sessions center around discussions of the clients' chosen and priority communication environments. Priority environments most frequently center around the church (understanding the minister or Sunday school teacher, or at church committee meetings), other social environments in which groups of people meet, understanding what females or children are saying, and understanding what people are saying in other environmentally distracting environments, such as on the street corner, in a restaurant, or at the theater. The inevitable commonality of their choices allow for group sessions that are beneficial for everyone, since the majority of clients can enter into each discussion as it relates to him or her.

A problem environment is brought before the group. The client (or clients) who presented that communication problem is asked to describe it in detail by giving examples of instances when it has occurred and the physical environment of each. As the physical environment is described, the audiologist diagrams it on the blackboard as accurately as possible from the client's description. It is generally necessary for the audiologist to ask for guidance as the diagramming is completed. After the client's problems in that environment are adequately described, and the room or other physical environment is drawn on the blackboard by the audiologist (including windows, doors, partitions, furniture, and so on), the remainder of the group is asked to give suggestions, as they see it, regarding how this client may have adjusted to that communication environment by manipulating it, making physical adjustments, or manipulating the speaker as to the cause, in their opinion, of the client's difficulty functioning in that environment.

As those suggestions are made, the audiologist lists suggestions and makes the suggested adjustments on the blackboard diagram, e.g., moving the client's chair into a better situation for listening, changing position away from a window, moving closer to a public address system speaker, asking the person being conversed with to move closer, walking out into a hallway where it is quieter, and so on.

The group participation in this treatment activity can be extremely motivating. As the client joins the group discussion by explaining the difficult environment more fully, and as questions or assumptions are made, ways in which he or she may have been able to manipulate the listening environment or those within it to his or her benefit become more clear. Others in the group also benefit because most may have or may find themselves in a similar environment.

Creating Positive Assertiveness

A trait that appears to become more typical as people grow older is to be less assertive, or more passive. This is particularly true of older adults who have been placed in a nursing home (health care facility) or who have been pressured to move from their home to a retirement complex. Some may act stubborn, but those responses are generally out of self-defense, because they may not have heard or understood what the nurse or other personnel was going to do or what was expected of them. In all too many instances, older persons in health care facilities simply are not told what is going to be done to them. Rather than continuing to react against the health care facility personnel and, thus, being listed as "uncooperative," they generally become more passive.

Whether an elderly person is residing in a health care facility or in the community, it regretably becomes more usual for dramatic and sometimes unpleasant things to occur in that person's life. In light of the unexpected occurrences that are prompted by people doing things *to* elderly persons rather than *for* them, it becomes easier to remain passive and wait rather than to become assertive. To refuse to do something a son or daughter wants you to do, or to become assertive and say "no," may result in the use of force to make you do it anyway. "Dad is getting stubborn in his old age," may be the label placed on that elderly person. Many elderly persons feel powerless because of a lack of independence. It is difficult to respond to a rapidly changing world when one does not possess the finances, transportation, physical mobility, quickness of analytical thought, or strength to manipulate one's environment. When dependence is related to a small social security check, one will strive to please a son or daughter whose only gesture of good will may be to drive him or her to town once a week for 1 hour to shop for food. Otherwise, he or she simply may be left at home. Further, it may be deemed better to remain passive rather than even positively aggressive when it is feared that the son or daughter may be planning to suggest selling the house and moving him or her to a retirement center. It is a normal human response for people to feel more vulnerable when their finances are such that, for example, they must wear 15-year-old clothes because they can afford no others. An elderly adult may, further, remain too proud to purchase others from the Salvation Army store. Elderly persons also tend to feel more vulnerable when they are confined within a two-block radius of their house because arthritis restricts walking and the bus to downtown stops four blocks away from the grocery store. And, if they did ride downtown on the bus, there may be nothing to do there. Church may be a person's only independence, but his or her ride may be coming less frequently.

To remain passive, in many elderly persons' minds, is survival. "If I become a bother" as one elderly woman put it, "my family may put me away. I don't want to be a bother. It is too dangerous. So, I sit here in my house and remain quiet." For a hearing impaired elderly person, "out of sight, out of mind" may have become the only choice for lack of alternatives.

Examples of Passive Behavior

One of this author's clients, an 80-year-old male, was asked to chair a committee in his church because of his knowledge of religion. He was flattered to be asked to accept that position, but then shortly resigned since he could not understand what his committee members were saying. When I asked him why he did not ask the members to speak up, he said that he did once. He, further, stated that it worked for a short time, but then they returned to their old speaking habits. When I asked him why he did not again ask them to speak up, he said that he did not want to be a bother to them. When I asked him why he did not change the room arrangements so he could place himself in a more advantageous position for communication, he said that the room had been in that same arrangement for years, and he did not want to disrupt it. Those attitudes can defeat an otherwise productive person.

Another example which illustrates the feelings of many hearing impaired elderly persons is one that involved a 72-year-old female client who had just returned from a lecture on South East Asia that she had been looking forward to attending for some time. She explained that the lecturer, a woman who had a rather soft voice, began talking and then walked away from the public address system microphone and sat down in front of the podium with the statement, ''I'm sure that you can all hear me without the microphone.''

The client said that she hardly understood a word the speaker said throughout the entire evening, but she was too embarrassed to leave the auditorium. When I asked her why she did not say ''Please use the microphone,'' when the speaker moved away from it, her reply was that she just could not bring herself to do it. She desperately wanted to, but was too embarrassed. ''Besides,'' she said, ''maybe I was the only person there who couldn't hear her.'' When I asked her whether she was important enough to warrant that speaker's consideration, this client's response was simply, I hope so.'' I said, ''Don't you think that the microphone was put there for a purpose? A public address system generally helps everyone to hear more comfortably. If you would have said something, I am sure that others in the audience would have been pleased that she had returned to the podium and used the microphone.'' Her reply was that she had not thought of that. ''But still,'' she said, ''I didn't want to make a nuisance of myself. I'm just an old woman who can't hear very well.''

That prevailing attitude among older adult clients is one that must be combatted, or at least altered, if these persons are to learn to cope and function more efficiently in the world outside and in their homes.

In many instances it can be done, at least to some degree. In light of the fact that apparently some people are not willing to accommodate hearing impaired elderly persons or, perhaps are not aware of what accommodations can be made to facilitate communication, elderly persons themselves must be taught ways to become assertive enough to manipulate their communication environment and those with whom they desire to communicate.

One way in which this can be done is, again, by asking individual clients to describe communication situations they have found themselves in during the past week or month. The situation described above, in which the 72-year-old woman found herself, is a good example of the problems that are brought to the treatment sessions. Suggestions by group members are brought forth after questions by the group and the audiologist are satisfied. When group members courageously state what *they* would have done in that situation, e.g., to have told the woman speaker that, ''I would appreciate it if you would use the microphone,'' in front of the entire audience, they are asked if they really would have done it. If they hold fast to their commitment, they are asked to do it at the next lecture they attend when the speaker hesitates to use the microphone. Occasionally, a group member returns after such an experience and triumphantly proclaims that, ''I did it!'' On occasion, another member of the aural rehabilitation treatment group may have been in attendance at that meeting and confirms that that individual did a very nice job in changing a poor listening situation to a more pleasant one. Also, others at the meeting may have thanked our client for asking the speaker to use the microphone by saying, ''We just did not have the courage to speak up like that!'' The triumph is great, and does much toward encouraging the other clients to also become more positively assertive.

Other difficult situations brought before the groups may include family dinners, going to a noisy restaurant, talking to timid grandchildren, talking to one's attorney with other members of the family in attendance, following more than one request in a sequence, and many others. The bywords in these treatment sessions are, "If those with whom we desire to or must communicate cannot seem to be accommodating, then we must assert ourselves by showing them how they can best communicate with us! Suggestions or adjustments must be made without hesitation. To do otherwise is to place ourselves back where we started." These are powerful treatment sessions and act to instill confidence, which may not have existed for some time in clients.

Involvement of Family and Others

The client's family and significant others in the client's life are critical elements for a successful aural rehabilitation treatment program. This is particularly true if, for example, the client's spouse is willing to become involved in the aural rehabilitation process. This includes attending the individual or group treatment sessions and participating in follow-up assignments.

A significant other's involvement in the aural rehabilitation treatment sessions provides that person with a better understanding of the difficulties and frustrations with which the friend, spouse, or family member undergoing treatment is faced, particularly if they can attend the first sessions when discussions of presbycusis and difficult communication situations are emphasized. It, further, aids the client's significant other to understand the commonality of communication difficulties when other clients discuss similar problems. That involvement prompts a realization that the communication difficulties that have arisen because of the auditory deficit are not limited only to their spouse, family member, or friend, but are found in others as well. That enhances understanding hopefully will be passed on to others who are close to that client.

This author frequently requests that those who attend the treatment sessions with individual clients be fit with noise suppressing ear plugs and participate in various activities during the sessions. Some of the same frustrations revealed by the clients are often felt by them during that brief period of time. It is explained to them, however, that ear plugs do not replicate the discrimination problems being encountered by the person with whom they are attending the sessions, but simply demonstrate a moderate loss of auditory acuity. Still, their use enhances a feeling of empathy for the frustrations the hearing impaired person must feel.

One important by-product of encouraging the involvement of a significant other in the aural rehabilitation treatment program is that carry-over of the treatment process into the everyday life of the client is greatly enhanced. If, for example, the elderly client asserts him- or herself before the remainder of the family by suggesting certain adjustments regarding seating arrangements for Thanksgiving dinner so that he or she can become involved in the conversation more efficiently, the significant other can reinforce and strengthen that positive assertive step. It is, further, not as much fun to go to a restaurant or the movie by oneself. The significant other can not only strengthen and encourage carry-over, but also make some potentially apprehensive situations more enjoyable. It helps to have someone there to back you up when the going gets rough.

One of the most discouraging aspects of the provision of any rehabilitative service to elderly clients is the lack of family involvement. In many instances, if a spouse has passed away, the family may live quite a distance from the client. Children may visit only once a year if the distance is great, and that may be for only a few days around a principal holiday. Even if grown children live in the same community, their desire for involvement with their parent on a social basis may be lacking, let alone a desire to become an important part of their mother's or father's rehabilitation program. The excuse is generally, "We just don't have time." In this remarkably advanced society, it is sad that we lose sight of the needs of our family. But, it seems to be the case, and alternative means for carry-over support for elderly clients must, in many cases, be sought.

As stated earlier, the client's spouse can be the most effective significant other, if the spouse is emotionally supportive of his or her husband or wife. If the spouse is not willing or capable of aiding in the support or carry-over process, then a friend is appropriate and can be a most effective partner in the aural rehabilitation process. In fact, at times it is common for people to discuss inner feelings with supportive friends prior to bringing them before a spouse or other family members. In any event, a close friend can be a very significant other. A case in point is that of a 70-year-old male client who was provided aural rehabilitation services by this author. He had been a widower for 4 years. On the first day of his group aural rehabilitation program he brought a female companion. Both were avid fishermen and were almost inseparable. They both enjoyed attending social gatherings together, but my client was experiencing great difficulty hearing and, in particular, understanding what was being said in such environments. His female companion was willing to explain what was being said, but was becoming discouraged at the consistency with which she had to function in the capacity of interpreter. In this instance, she attended all treatment sessions with the client; she wearing her ear plugs and he his hearing aid. A great deal of warmth and understanding developed between them, and as his ability to function communicatively increased so did her willingness to aid in the treatment process through carry-over. The assignments, which included experimentation at social gatherings, were carried out in an excellent manner. Problem situations which were to be discussed during treatment sessions became less, and likewise his dependence upon his female companion for communication support.

The support and carry-over by this significant other was instrumental in this client's achievements in learning to use his residual hearing, to use supplemental visual clues, and to manipulate his most difficult listening environments. Without such support and assistance, the audiologist may have great difficulty facilitating such improvements. In the end, he or she may never be able to aid the client in making such significant and positive strides as will the significant other.

THE PROCESS

As previously discussed, the aural rehabilitation program for the older adult includes

1. Knowledge of the client's desires and needs for communication through setting priorities
2. On-going motivational counseling as an integral part of the process of aural rehabilitation
3. Carry-over of hearing aid orientation, at least for those who are felt to benefit from amplification
4. Learning how to manipulate one's environment to enhance communication
5. Learning to become positively assertive
6. Throughout all of the above, learning to use one's residual hearing and supplemental visual cues to enhance comprehension of verbal messages

To put all of the above together into a meaningful aural rehabilitation treatment program for the older adult is not really difficult. As a matter of fact, the process becomes quite logical once a number of older clients have critiqued your approach in relation to its meaningfulness and benefit to them.

The following is an example of an approach to aural rehabilitation treatment for the elderly adult client, utilizing and intermingling the six areas listed above. There are subtleties involved in clinician–client interaction which can make or break an effective treatment program. Those subtleties are difficult to discuss, but in any event, the process is herewith displayed. This process has been found effective for use with both the confined and community-based elderly.

The On-Going Aural Rehabilitation Program

Some structure in the treatment process is desired by the majority of elderly clients. But, on the other hand, overly structured sessions can be counter productive. For example, it is not uncommon for audiologists who utilize traditional speechreading approaches which emphasize a progression from phoneme analysis to syllables, words, phrases, sentences, and stories (which, for example, stress several like-phonemes), to begin to realize in a fairly short period of time that the clients who seemed motivated initially are attending speechreading sessions with less regularity. Soon they may cease attending all together. Excuses generally range from, "My family is coming to visit and I will be spending time with them," to "We have several church suppers coming up, and I have to help with them." It is embarrassing to see them downtown later with apparently nothing to do. They may, further, call to tell your secretary that they really do not feel the need to come to "class" anymore, even though the audiologist knows that they have made little or no progress in treatment.

Those clients are telling us something that we *should* receive loudly and clearly. That is, if they felt that aural rehabilitation services were benefitting them they probably still would be attending, since when they began they evidently were motivated. If the aural rehabilitation treatment program was geared to their specific needs, they would probably be taking advantage of the audiologist's expert services. But, for those reasons, and because the audiologist perhaps began the first session from a book of strict unalterable approaches to speechreading, the clients were not interested in receiving those services anymore. A few faithful clients may continue to attend, but probably will leave the final session as able or unable to communicate with others as he or she was in the beginning. The audiologist may wonder why these otherwise apparently alert older persons have not improved, even though they may say, "I enjoyed your class," and pat him or her on the shoulder. Further, why does this audiologist have to coerce clients in health care facilities to attend aural rehabilitation treatment sessions, or have to depend on a gracious activity director to bring them from their rooms to attend sessions that should be helping them cope in the everyday world more efficiently? Again, it may be because the audiologist has lost sight of the fact that the treatment must be designed with the needs of the clients in mind. Other treatment procedures used by speech/language pathologists, occupational therapists, physical therapists, and others, are based on a treatment plan which is designed around the *assessed needs* of the client. Why are some audiologists, then, still opening their "lipreading" lesson book and beginning at page one to provide services to clients who have varied and individual communication deficits and needs? Those speechreading books too often are used as hymnals, and the session begins with the audiologist saying, "And for the next session we will turn to page 15." That is not treatment.

Individualizing Your Approach

How does one develop a meaningful approach to aural rehabilitation treatment for the elderly client? Hardick (1977) described basic characteristics of a successful aural rehabilitation program for older adults. They are well defined, and provide comprehensive guidance for those who intend to provide services for older clients. Those characteristics are as follows:

1. The program must be client centered
2. The program must revolve around amplification and/or modifying the client's communication environment
3. All programs consist of group therapy with some individualized help when necessary
4. The group must contain normally hearing friends or relatives of the hearing impaired person
5. Aural rehabilitation programs are short-term
6. The program is consumer oriented
7. Promotion of a better realization by colleagues and other professionals of the existence of aural rehabilitation programs and their potential benefits
8. Make use of "successful graduates" as resource people in group activities whenever possible (pp. 60–62)

These characteristics are extremely important for consideration prior to the initiation of aural rehabilitation programs for the older adult. They go far beyond the more traditional "lipreading" procedures that continue to be utilized by some. Even though Hardick (1977) and others recommended group treatment for the elderly, some will require individual sessions. As has been noted by this author and others including Miller (Note 4), there is a tendency among some to hesitate to participate or refuse to participate in individual treatment unless they, themselves, have requested it.

Other more current client-centered approaches to aural rehabilitation include that by McCarthy and Alpiner (1978), discussed in detail within Chapter 6 of this text, Alpiner (1963), Miller and Ort (1965), Colton and O'Neill (1976), McCarthy and Alpiner (1978), discussed in detail within Chapter 6 of this text, and others. The aspect stressed throughout those is the fact the older adult clients possess needs that are specific to them, and each client's aural rehabilitation program must be centered on his or her needs and priorities.

If the ingredients presented on the previous pages are combined properly, a possible sequence of services emerges. An example of such a sequence includes the following.

An Awareness of Reasons for Auditory Dysfunction

Facilitating an awareness of the reason for the auditory communication difficulties through an understanding of the process of aging and its effect on the auditory mechanism is an important part of the aural rehabilitation process. Included is a discussion of the processing of auditory/linguistic information and the effect of aging on the speed of that important component in communication, particularly in noisy or otherwise distracting environments. The level of terminology is determined by the individual or group in question. The audiologist is cautioned *never* to speak down to clients. It is important to use the correct technical terminology, but immediately explain it at the level of the persons involved. Always remember that you are speaking to adults, no matter what their educational level. They deserve to be treated as such.

Charts are used in this discussion, perhaps along with 35-mm slide presentations on the ear. If individuals in the group are severely hard of hearing, projected slides should be used only if enough light can be left on in the room to facilitate the use of visual clues. Charts, diagrams, slides, and blackboard drawings are used for that discussion, and presentations on the aging ear, hearing aids and their uses, benefits and limitations, environmental factors that affect communication, poor speakers versus good speakers and their make-up, and a general discussion of the aging process are included.

The basis for this first session (or sessions) is to facilitate a basis for the remainder of the treatment program, to develop a better understanding among the clients of what has occurred to them, and to assure them that in all probability they can improve, at least to some degree. Most persons come away from that session or those sessions, with a better understanding and greater acceptance of what is occurring to them and a desire to participate in the aural rehabilitation treatment program. It cannot be emphasized enough that a significant other in each client's life should attend these sessions. Whether it be a spouse or a family member such as a child, or a friend, they will gain much greater insight into the auditory/communication problems with which that person is attempting to cope.

Priority Communicative Needs

The second step in the aural rehabilitation treatment program is, as stated earlier, to ask each client to list those difficulties in communication which affect them most. They may include specific communication environments, such as a meeting room, church, certain restaurant, table arrangement at their child's home, and so on. They also may list certain individuals who they have difficulty understanding. They are to list those difficulties on paper even if someone else must write for them.

The next step is for those clients to set priorities in those situations or persons on the same sheet of paper, from most important to least important. And, if they had their choice, in which of those would they most like to improve. They are asked, of course, to be realistic in their final choices. For some, the choice is a simple one. For others, it is more difficult. It is important to note, however, that if gains are made in one category, there is the probability that they will observe improvement in others.

They are asked to discuss their choices, present a situation in which they experienced difficulty, and explain what prompted them to make those choices. Particularly in a group situation, it is interesting to note the general consistency of priority areas which emerge. The clients generally feel a sense of comaraderie develop out of this discussion. For the first time, many of them realize that they are not the only ones who experience difficulty in those environments.

In many instances, clients put part of the blame for their auditory/communicative difficulties on others who possess poor speech habits. That is acknowledged and discussed. The discussion centers around the fact that there are, indeed, many poor speakers in this world, and a demonstration of some of their habits which interfere with efficient communication is appropriate. Immediate identification is generally evident among the clients. Even though there are many poor speakers, we must develop ways to cope in those communication environments. The encouraging acknowledgement that they can, in many instances, manipulate those difficult situations in such a way as to at least be able to function more efficiently in them, and the fact that they will be working on those devices, ends that discussion.

The above items generally do not consume more than a 1 or 2 full-hour session. The discussions of priority difficulties and circumstances that interfere with efficient communication should not be curtailed, however, because the airing of frustrations and concerns will greatly facilitate future progress. For many, this may be the first time those concerns have been discussed. To prematurely conclude such a discussion simply on the basis of a rigid schedule can stifle the airing of emotions and adjustment that may have otherwise been made.

On Becoming Assertive

Weekly assignments for each client are made and include noting a communication situation in which they had particular difficulty and, in the end, interfered with communication. As discussed earlier, they are to write them down and diagram the physical environment if necessary (or simply be able to recall it as accurately as possible). In any event, they are to bring the specifics of the situation to the next treatment session for presentation and discussion. Each client (or in the case of individual treatment, the client) presents his or her difficult situation, if one has been noted. It is imperative that the client who was involved in the situation be the one who presents it and not the significant other who may be present with the client.

After thorough presentation, with diagrams if necessary, the situation is discussed by the group (or in the event of individual treatment, by the client, the audiologist, and the significant other who is present, if he or she was involved). Suggestions regarding possible ways the client might have manipulated the communication environment to his or her best advantage, including the physical environment or the speaker, are made by the group under the guidance of the audiologist, and are accepted as viable or discarded. As stated by this author previously (Hull, 1980), insights into ways of manipulating the communication environment to their best advantage, along with methods of coping with and adjusting to frustrating situations are, in turn, developed among clients under the guidance of the audiologist. This form of self- and group-analysis is an extremely important part of the aural rehabilitation program. Clients, then, are helped to develop their own insights into methods of adjusting to situations where communication is difficult. If, for some reason, they find that it is impossible for them to make the necessary adjustments, perhaps they can, in a positive—supportive—assertive manner, ease the difficulty they are experiencing by requesting that others make certain adjustments. Perhaps they could request that the physical environment be adjusted so that they can function more efficiently in it.

It becomes difficult for some older clients to develop even mildly assertive behavior. They do not want to be noticed as a ''demanding'' older person. Many do feel rather vulnerable; perhaps feeling that the people who invited them to a party did so more out of a feeling of obligation than desire. They may feel that if they request that others in attendance change positions by moving to a more quiet place to talk, or request that someone change the position of their chair so that they are in a better position to talk, then, perhaps, the people who invited them will feel that it is more trouble than it is worth to invite them again. In light of such fears, it becomes quite logical to avoid that possibility by simply remaining quiet, and maintaining the fear that if asked a question, he or she might become embarrassed once again by answering inappropriately. In light of those occasional fears that are brought forth by clients, discussion should center around them as they arise.

Examples of those discussions may include one that was initiated by one of this author's clients who was being seen on a group basis. The woman in question was discussing a situation involving another woman with whom she had morning coffee on almost a daily basis for a number of years. The client's complaint was that her friend was an incessant gum chewer, and her manner of chewing gum almost negated ongoing conversation since chewing continued as she talked, thus, interferring with precise articulation. Her friend interpreted the client's inability to understand what she was saying to be the result of the hearing impairment, not her imprecise manner of speaking which resulted from her enthusiastic gum chewing, compounded by the client's hearing loss. This apparent interpretation of the situation infuriated my client. But, she continued the morning coffee time because there were few other women her age in that geographic area, and besides, they had been friends since childhood.

This woman's major concern was how to tell her friend that her manner of speaking and gum chewing had, for several years, interfered with her ability to understand what she was saying and, in the end, made what might have been a pleasant conversation, an almost intolerable one. She was particularly afraid to say anything because of the embarrassment her friend might feel since the situation had been going on for so long, and nothing had been said. "Almost like," as the client said, "being associated with a person for a long time and never knowing her name. As the days pass, you become increasingly embarrassed about asking her name, particularly when she knows yours." The suggestions that came from the group varied from an enthusiastic "Tell her that if she wants to talk to you, to take her gum out of her mouth," to a timid, "If you value your friendship, maybe it is best to say nothing and simply tolerate the situation." The latter suggestion was immediately discarded. The ultimate conclusion was to simply tell the truth. It was the consensus of the group that they would respect their own friend more if he or she would say something like, "You know, we've been friends for a long time. You realize, as I do, that I have some difficulty hearing what people say to me. I have particular difficulty with men who wear mustaches or beards, people who do not move their lips enough, or people who talk with their hand near their mouth, since I depend upon seeing the face of persons with whom I am talking. You know, I have difficulty understanding what you say sometimes, and I think that I may have discovered why. I know that you like to chew gum a great deal, and like me, it helps my mouth not to become so dry. I do think, however, that because you—probably not realizing it—chew your gum while we are talking, it doesn't allow me to see your lips move properly, and besides, you aren't able to talk as plainly when you chew it so hard. I just bet that if you don't chew gum while we are having our coffee, I will be able to understand you better and we'll have a nicer time talking. do you want to give it a try?" *Positive-assertiveness* are the key words in this instance. For that client, the strategy she and the remainder of the group determined as most effective, did prove to be successful. And, she maintained the friendship.

Other Topics

Other topics for discussion and development of strategies may include weekly socials at private homes where the furniture arrangements interfere with efficient communication. Some, as experienced through this author's work with older clients, involved the table arrangement at one client's son's home where they usually had Thanksgiving dinner; the television set at a male client's friend's home; the seating arrangement and acoustics at a church meeting room, and others. Even though the discussions and thought-provoking suggestions generally aid the individual whose situation is being discussed, they also provide insights for the remainder of the group on how they, too, can manipulate their communication environment.

These assertiveness discussions can be extremely stimulating for the clients involved and for their significant other in attendance. Clients have told this author that those sessions are probably the most valuable for them, particularly because we are working and sharing on behalf of their problems in communication. As clients identify with other client's difficult communication situations and relate to solutions as they see them, insights into solutions for their own difficult situations emerge and are strengthened. A reawakening of self-confidence is evidenced when clients return to state that the solution as contrived during the last session did not work as planned, but with a few adjustments developed by him- or herself, it did! Most older clients, no matter how hearing impaired or how distraught because of his or her inability to communicate, can benefit from these assertiveness sessions. The topics of self-worth and, ''I'm important too,'' which become a part of the discussions are an extremely important part of the total aural rehabilitation program.

The Use of Residual Hearing with Supplemental Visual Clues

Even though the use of visual clues and every possible bit of residual hearing individual clients can muster is discussed and practiced throughout all aspects of the aural rehabilitation program, some sessions should emphasize those aspects of communication. Again, it is not suggested that strict approaches to speechreading/auditory training be stressed. Rather, the fact that the majority of older clients possess normal to near-normal language function should be capitalized on to encourage the use of innovative and useful approaches toward an increased efficiency in the use of a very natural compliment in communication, that is, the compliment of vision to audition.

The premise on which these sessions are instituted is that speech (including the phonemic patterns of words in the English language, the use of gestures, inflectional clues, and the English language itself) is generally quite redundant, although, understandably, there are differences among individual's speech patterns, use of gestures, words, etc. A further premise is that the average listener has been taking advantage of the redundancies inherent in American English speech and language patterns to aid in verbal comprehension for the majority of his or her life. When hearing declines with age—as does the precision and speed of the processing of phonemic verbal/linguistic elements of speech—it becomes more difficult to comprehend (understand) what others are saying. This is particularly true in environmentally distracting or otherwise difficult listening situations. The purpose of these sessions, therefore, is to remind clients of what they have been doing for years at an almost subliminal level; that is, using important parts of auditory/verbal messages, when heard, and supplementing what was not heard with visual clues. By visual clues, this author means the face of the speaker, including lip, tongue and mandibular movements, gestures, facial expression, shoulder movements, and so on used to ''fill in the gaps'' between what was heard, what was not heard, and what was observed visually.

A further purpose of these sessions is to discuss the redundancies of the phonemic and linguistic aspects of spoken American English, and to encourage clients to take advantage of them when they are communicating with others. This aspect of the aural rehabilitation treatment program is called, for lack of a better descriptive title, ''A Linguistic Approach to the Teaching of Speechreading'' described by this author (Hull, 1976). It depends on essentially normal language function among clients. Further, a great deal of time is spent using the blackboard. If, however, a client is visually impaired, these sessions help to enhance auditory closure. The term ''closure'' is the byword during these sessions, as the reader soon will realize.

Linguistic Closure

As the reader will observe below, clients are asked to determine the correct information within sentences from the least number of words provided. The clients are asked to imagine that the word, or words, given on the blackboard are those that were heard. The blanks provided between words are imagined as those not heard or not heard well. Clients are, first of all, asked to tell the audiologist what the sentence is about (out of context), when perhaps, only one word is provided out of a total of seven, with six blanks indicating that those words were not heard. Clients are encouraged to venture guesses as to what the sentence might be. Let us say, for example, that the word presented is ''street'' located as the last word in the sentence. The clients are asked to let their minds wander. ''Take a guess.'' As clients accept that encouragement and begin to guess, the fear of being wrong appears to decrease. Many are genuinely surprised, in fact, to find that their ''educated'' guesses are often extremely close, if not correct. Guesses in this instance may, for example, range from ''the man was walking down the street'', to ''a giraffe was seen running up the street.'' They are, however, encouraged to be rational in their decisions. The question may appropriately be asked, ''How many times have you heard someone say, 'A giraffe was running up the street?' '' Think more realistically about the possibilities. The word, ''street'' as the last word in a sentence tells you what? It tells you, generally, that *something* is happening. If the word came as the second word in a sentence, maybe after the word ''the,'' I may have been describing the street, such as, ''the street was very bumpy.'' But, since it is located at the end of the sentence, we know that something is probably happening either on or to the street. Now, let's set the stage. Let us say that your neighbor's child, Billy, has run away. You and other people from around the neighborhood are searching for him. Suddenly, someone runs to you and says something about, ''______ ______ ______ ______ ______ _____ _____street!'' You observed that the speaker had obviously been running, and was pointing up the street as he was talking. Now, what do you imagine the speaker was telling you?'' Since the audiologist has now set the stage for the clients, their guesses will probably be quite close to what he or she had intended.

The audiologist's next step is to say, ''Now I am going to allow you to fill in the gaps by observing my face and gestures as I take the place of the excited neighbor who is talking to you.'' The audiologist then presents the sentence in a slightly audible manner and with full visible face and gestures. If clients are not able to ''make closure,'' then another word is added at the blackboard, and the clients are allowed to try again. An example of the sequence of presentation, if additional words are required, is presented below.

1. ______ ______ ______ ______ ______ ______ street!
2. ______ ______ is ______ ______ ______ street!

3. ______ ______ is ______ down ______ street!
4. ______ ______ is running down ______ street!
5. The ______ is running down ______ street!
6. The ______ is running down the street!
7. The boy is running down the street!

Each time an additional word is given, the entire sentence also is presented to the client(s) by the audiologist as described above. As clients become aware of what the message is, the audiologist continues by discussing, first, the importance of the position of each word within the sentence that was required before they were able to determine its content, second, their linguistic value in terms of the probability of determining the meaning of the sentence, third, the importance of the environmental clues which were available to them, and fourth the supplemental use of visual clues.

An important element which is involved in any of these sessions is the audiologist's enthusiasm over the fact that, perhaps, the clients needed only to ''hear'' one or two words out of a sentence to make closure and grasp the meaning of the sentence. It is encouraging for older clients to be made aware of the fact that with their knowledge of the English language and their successful use of visual and auditory clues, they were able to determine what the message was.

On more difficult sentences and more complex contrived situations, clients may require more ''heard'' words to be provided via the blackboard. Nevertheless, they are being reminded that with a relatively small amount of visual, auditory, and environmental information, they are generally able to determine at least the thought of what is being said.

Linguistic, Content, and Environmental Redundancies

Linguistic redundancy. The American English language is redundant in its formal usage in regard to the position of various parts of speech. In other words, the position of principal words such as nouns, pronouns, and direct objects are generally constant, as are function words, descripters such as adjectives and adverbs, and action words such as verbs. Some dialects within the United States do, however, deviate from those standard rules. During these sessions, although the technical names of the parts of speech are not stressed at all, the importance of those words which fall within various positions in verbal messages are discussed as they relate to deriving the meaning of those messages.

This aspect of treatment capitalizes on the fact that most older hearing impaired clients will possess at least near-normal language function. It stresses the fact that as people listen to others, they zero in on words within conversations that permit them to at least derive the thought of what is being said so that the conversation can be followed. In some distracting environments, less of the message may actually be heard, but most persons can still maintain the gist of what is being said. It is normal in those circumstances, if a word was missed, to ask the speaker to repeat it, because it appeared to be an important one in regard to the content of the statement. The point that is stressed to the clients here is that the reason the listener was able to determine that the word was an important one for permitting him or her to continue to follow the conversation was an almost innate knowledge of the structure of the American English language which has progressively expanded since early childhood.

The treatment sessions which stress this important aspect of efficient listening revolve around bringing that functional language capability to a more conscious level.

Occasionally, clients have become so despondent over an inability to communicate with others that such otherwise natural compensatory skills become repressed.

Content and environmental redundancies. These discussions stress the fact that, as we observe human behavior, it is discovered that not only do the same people generally say similar things on similar occasions, but they also say them in similar places. In other words, in a given environment, depending on who the person is with whom one will be speaking, what the listener knows about him or her, and if the listener is aware of those influences, the general content of some conversations can be predicted with reasonable accuracy.

Clients are asked to describe the environments they frequent. In all probability they will be those which were set as priorities earlier. They are also asked to describe those persons who are generally there, including their speaking habits, their facial characteristics, and their known interests. During these treatment sessions, the clients also are asked to write down the more frequent topics of conversations that are observed among those whom they have described. These not only include frequent topics, but also words and phrases which those people may use habitually. They are asked to keep those lists and add to them as they remember additional items or as they find out more about the person after speaking with him or her. Clients also are asked to begin new lists as they meet new people. The more one knows and remembers about a person, the more communication is enhanced.

An awareness of the predictability, or redundancy, of people and what they will say within known environments is sometimes surprising to hearing impaired older adults. If it is surprising, it is generally because they had not really thought about it prior to that time. If nurtured, however, this awareness can facilitate increased efficiency in communication.

Reducing Auditory or Visual Confusions

Other activities which, by necessity, are important for adults may include information on why certain confusions of words occur in conversations. This particularly concerns older adults because word confusions may be occurring with some frequency. These discussions not only include information on the fact that the nature of the majority of auditory disorders which older adults face enhance the probability of auditory confusions, but also that the nature of certain sound and visual elements within many words enhance the probability of confusions because they may either sound like or look like other words. When words are confused with others, the meaning of a sentence or conversation may appear to be different than what was intended.

An example of an activity which can bring about an awareness of how these confusions can occur centers around typed lists of sentences, or sentences written on the blackboard. It is generally best to use those sentences which contain visually and/or auditorily confusing words within mock conversations to more accurately exemplify the difficulties clients may experience in their real worlds. In this instance, the first sentence on the clients' list may be presented by the audiologist within a short "conversation." The conversation is presented with voice, but as close to the clients' auditory thresholds as possible. Full-face and gestures are used. When the sentence within the "conversation" is presented, the clients are asked to determine if the sentence the audiologist said was "the same as" or "different" from the one on their list. If they determine that there was a word or words that were different than observed in the sentence on their list, then they are asked to explain why they felt that there were differences. Further, if they felt that the sentence presented by the audiologist was the same as the one on their sheet or on the blackboard, they also are asked to explain why.

If, in the context of the short conversation the clients determine what word or words in that sentence "threw them off course" in terms of following the conversation, they not only are asked to analyze those confusing words, but attempt to determine why they were confusing. They also are asked, in light of what they derived from the remainder of the conversation, to determine the words or the thought that the sentence should have contained so that it would make sense. When that analysis is completed, the clients again are asked to listen to and observe the conversation and the possibly confusing sentence to determine if it then appears to be what they thought it should have been within the context of the intended message. If the word or words within the sentence still do not appear to be what they should have been to complete the thought of the conversation, then they again are asked to attempt to determine what the confusion was. An example of the type of brief conversation and stimulus sentence used in this exercise is as follows.

1. Stimulus sentence: She bought a new coat.
2. Stimulus conversation: "Alice came over yesterday to see me, and had some news to share. She said that she now has a new friend who is soft, black and white and weighs about 1 pound. Well, she bought a new *coat*. She has named him 'Mike.' "

In the above stimulus conversation, the possible visual confusion occurs with the word *coat,* which was given to the clients within the stimulus sentence they were expecting as per their list. Again, if clients, in this instance, determine that the word in the sentence they were expectiong did not make sense within the context of the conversation, they are asked to explain why that word seemed to be misplaced, and what the word should have been. Further, the visual and auditory similarities and differences between the word they were expecting and the one they saw and heard are discussed.

These exercises should progress toward truly homophenous and homophonous words within sentences. The mental gymnastics required during these sessions allows for practice in making on-the-spot decisions regarding misunderstood messages by determining *why* a sentence within a conversation was visually and/or auditorily confusing, or otherwise did not make sense. The process generally involves

1. Analyzing the information derived from the previous portions of the conversation
2. Determining that a confusing word has been received which may change the content of what is being said
3. Sifting mentally through other words which look and/or sound like one that would make more sense in light of the previous portions of the conversations
4. Simultaneously projecting what that word "should have been" from the continuing conversation

Communicating Under Adverse Conditions

One of the most frequent priority communication problems that older adult clients view as their most difficult is communication in noisy environments including, for example, social events and meetings. Many clients' primary complaint, after finding themselves in an adverse listening environment, is that the noise and the resulting difficulties they experience in attempting to sort out the primary message from the chatter of other voices makes them tense and nervous. They describe the nervousness as, perhaps, the greatest detriment to their ability to successfully manage a conversation in those environments. They tell this author that as they begin to experience difficulty within the noisy communicative environment, they begin to detect feelings of nervousness. The nervousness, as they describe it, results in a further deterioration of their ability to cope in that environment, and thus also their ability to sort the primary message from the noise. For many, the only alternative that appears to be available is to excuse themselves from the situation by ceasing the conversation. By submitting to that less-than-satisfactory option, however, they generally feel some embarrassment. Unless they are quite resilient, many will simply avoid those situations in which they consistently fail. Since those include social events, meetings, the theater, church, and other desirable environments, the decision to avoid them can be quite self-defeating. Nervousness in that sense and as they describe it may not lessen since they are concerned over their inability to function communicatively in those environments and are torn between making another attempt at coping or giving up all together.

In regard to the above communication problem, treatment sessions are not only designed to aid clients in the development of skills for communicating in those distracting environments but also to develop coping behaviors. The terms ''desensitization,'' ''reciprocal inhibition,'' and others may be appropriate to use here, but ''coping behaviors'' will stand as the most meaningful for this discussion. Within this framework, clients again choose as priorities those environments in which they have most difficulty and/or those within which they most desire to function more efficiently. Those situations are recreated within the treatment room as accurately as possible around individual clients' description of their chosen difficult environments. It is stressed that in the treatment environment no one can fail but can feel free to discuss their concerns or frustrations as they arise. Use of the language-based speechreading instruction previously discussed further, is emphasized during these sessions. Those areas which are stressed in the discussions during these noise exercises, but not in order of importance, are outlined in Table 26-1.

These sessions are used as the culminating treatment experience. Clients are asked to take everything that they have gained from the previous sessions and put them to use here. Some may never learn to cope in environmentally distracting situations. Others develop such self confidence that they feel more comfortable in the most adverse environments. One aspect of coping is stressed. That is that few persons, whether they possess normally functioning auditory mechanisms or are hearing impaired, can tolerate every noise environment. They must learn to recognize their limits in attempting to develop coping behavior.

As each client's difficult communication environment is recreated by the audiologist and other members of the treatment group, taped noise that is the same as or similar to the environment the client(s) described is introduced into the room. It is best to utilize a stereophonic tape system to more accurately recreate the noise environment. The noise is introduced gradually at the beginning of those sessions and increased as tolerance and coping behavior likewise increase, until the noise is presented at such a level as to become difficult to tolerate. If clients wear hearing aids, they also are asked to experiment with them as they participate in the mock noisy communication environments.

The clients are told that the situation during treatment is going to be made more difficult in regard to noise levels and/or visual distractions than they will probably ex-

Table 26-1
Responses Stressed during Auditory Treatment Sessions

- Relaxation under stressful conditions.
- Confidence that clients can, indeed, piece together the thought of the verbal message, even though not all of it was heard.
- Remembering that because of their normal language function and their knowledge of the predictability of American English, they can determine what is being said if supplemental visual clues are used, along with as much auditory information as is possible under the environmental circumstance.
- Knowledge that other people in the same environment may also be having difficulty understanding what others are saying, and they also may or may not be coping successfully with the stress.
- Freedom to manipulate the communication environment as much as possible by, for example, asking the person with whom they are speaking to move with them to a slightly quieter corner where they can talk with greater ease, move their chair to a more advantageous position so the speaker can be seen and/or heard more clearly, or other positive steps to enhance communication.
- Remembering that if difficulty in that communication environment seems to be increasing and feelings of concern or nervousness begin to become evident, they should feel free to interrupt the conversation and talk about the noise or the activity around them that seems to be causing the difficulties in understanding what the person with whom they are speaking is saying. The other person will probably agree with that observation, and in talking about it, feelings of stress may be reduced and communication enhanced.
- Remembering that the amount of noise used in treatment sessions was probably greater than will be experienced in most other environments. If success was noted in their treatment sessions, then similar success may be carried over into other stressful environments.

perience in the "real world." Clients inevitably desire such an approach since they would rather practice in such difficult situations in the friendly environment of the treatment room than among less tolerant people.

A discussion of noise per se and its natural effect on speech perception is also introduced before the actual re-creations begin. An awareness of different types of noise, their general acoustical characteristics, their emotional impact, and other factors give clients a better understanding of the "situation" as they see it. When one begins to gain an understanding of feared elements, the fear generally subsides.

Almost without fail, some persons begin to become nervous and frustrated during the noise sessions. The susceptability of certain clients to an intolerance for noise can be observed by the alert audiologist, even when low levels of noise are introduced.

In an instance where the group (or individuals) begin to become obviously frustrated, the audiologist, rather than ceasing the activity immediately, terminates it momentarily at a logical point and begins to discuss general feelings about the noise rather than attempting to pinpoint individual personal feelings about it. The audiologist might appropriately say, "Noise makes me feel nervous. How about you? Sometimes during these sessions I want to turn it off. When I'm in a situation where I can't turn it off, it even makes me angry sometimes. Is that a little like the feelings you have when you find yourself in a situation like that?" Generally the response will be affirmative, and clients will agree that those feelings are real for them also.

The "time-out" periods are used to talk about those feelings. When feelings of frustration and even anger are expressed freely by them, the reality that those feelings are not uncommon among others occasionally brings relief to clients who, perhaps, thought that they were among only a few older adults who had such difficult times. These persons are, thus, learning to cope with their feelings and realizing that they are normal reactions to adverse and frustrating communication environments.

Discussing those feelings freely, without fear of negative response or reprisal from others, is an important part of the aural rehabilitation process. As frustrations and anger are expressed regarding their difficulties tolerating and communicating in a noisy world—and occasionally at the whole process of growing older—the way opens for the aural rehabilitation program to move forward toward the development of coping behaviors and techniques for manipulating their communication environments as positive, assertive attributes. As one of this author's clients has so aptly stated, "In a noisy world of generally poor speakers, we usually have to fend for ourselves. But, we are looking to you to teach us how, and to give us the inspiration to use what we learn."

THE USE OF COMPRESSED SPEECH IN AURAL REHABILITATION TREATMENT

When one speaks of auditory training, we generally expect to hear about bringing sounds of various types to a higher level of awareness, including environmental and speech, teaching the congenitally deaf about sounds in his or her environment, speech and language therapy for the hearing impaired, and others. Another approach to auditory training has also been found to be an effective tool in training the hearing impaired to make more efficient use of their residual hearing. It involves the use of time-compressed speech. This technique has been used at the University of Northern Colorado Aural (Re)Habilitation Clinic by this author for the past three years. Data regarding improvements in speech discrimination among various ages of hearing impaired clients are presently being logged for release to the public.

The basis for the use of compressed speech as a method of auditory training has its roots in the use of another form of time compression that has been used successfully for a number of years—speed reading and the use of the tachistoscope in assessing and training for speed of visual closure.

Listening skill requires speed in making auditory closure involving the levels of both the brain stem and brain, i.e., taking the bits and pieces of phonemic/linguistic information derived from a conversation, lecture, or sermon, sorting them and making closure. The premise was that if the central visual system can be taught to make closure more rapidly through speed-reading instruction, perhaps the same principle could be used in teaching the central auditory system to accept and utilize progressively less phonemic/linguistic information and still make closure at usable comprehension levels.

The procedure appears to be successful in strengthening skills in speech discrimination, particularly among adventitiously hearing impaired adults from younger to older. Some older adults have, however, not been able to tolerate the pressure of attending to speech compression for even short periods of time. After 6 to 10 weeks of instruction at ever increasing levels of compression, speech discrimination scores have revealed improvements of up to 48 percent for monosyllabic words and up to 42 percent for paragraph comprehension among older hearing impaired adults. The words and paragraphs are also presented in signal to noise ratios ranging from +20 dB to +10 dB.

These results are encouraging and will perhaps eventually confirm an approach to auditory training for the adventitiously hearing impaired adult that will merit further consideration for use.

CONCLUSION

It is important for older adult clients to be given the opportunity to make decisions regarding areas of communication in which they desire to improve. Even though many may feel discouraged, not only because of the embarrassing difficulties they experience in their attempts at understanding what others are saying but also because of the whole process of aging that they are experiencing, they generally are totally cognizant of those communication situations which cause them the most difficulty. They, as adults who probably possessed normal hearing and were once vital social beings (whose case history may reveal nothing except the fact that they have become older), deserve to participate in the decisions regarding their treatment program. These persons, above all, are adults, and deserve to be treated as such. Guidance in the decision-making process must be provided by the audiologist. However, allowance for prescription of certain aspects of treatment by individual clients must be made simply because *they* feel that they are important for enhancement of their ability to function in their own communicating world.

REFERENCES

Alpiner, J. G. Audiological problems of the aged. *Geriatrics,* 1963, *18*, 19–26.

Bergman, M. *Aging and the perception of speech*. Baltimore: University Park Press, 1980.

Colton, J., & O'Neill, J. A cooperative outreach program for the elderly. 1976, *Journal of the Academy of Rehabilitative Audiology,* 1976, *9*, 38–41.

Hardick, E. J. Aural rehabilitation programs for the aged can be successful. *Journal of the Academy of Rehabilitative Audiology,* 1977, *10*, 51–66.

Hull, R. H. A linguistic approach to the teaching of speechreading: theoretical and practical concepts. *Journal of the Academy of Rehabilitative Audiology,* 1976, *9*, 14–19.

Hull, R. H. Aural rehabilitation of aging persons: Problems and strategies for their solution, in L. Bradford (Ed.), *Audiology: an audio journal for continuing education*. New York: Grune and Stratton, 1977.

Hull, R. H. Aural rehabilitation for the elderly, in R. L. Schow & M. A. Nerbonne (Eds.), *Introduction to aural rehabilitation,* Baltimore: University Park Press, 1980, pp. 311–348.

Kasten, R. N. The impact of aging on auditory perception, in R. H. Hull (Ed.), *The communicatively disordered elderly*. New York: Thieme-Stratton, Inc. 1981.

McCarthy, P. A., & Alpiner, J. G. The remediation process, in J. G. Alpiner (Ed.), *Handbook of adult rehabilitative audiology*. Baltimore: Williams and Wilkins, 1978, pp. 88–120.

Miller, M. & Ort, R. Hearing problems in a home for the aged. *Acta Oto-laryngologica,* 1965, *59*, 33–44.

Smith, C. R., & Fay, T. H. A program of auditory rehabilitation for aged persons in a chronic disease hospital. *Journal of the American Speech and Hearing Association,* 1977, *19*, 417–420.

REFERENCE NOTES

1. Hull, R. H. *Aural rehabilitation treatment for the older adult: A new look at an old subject*. Paper presented at the Aspen Symposium on Aging, Colorado, July, 1980.
2. Downs, M. P. *You and your hearing aid*. Unpublished manual, University of Colorado Medical Center, Denver, 1970.
3. Traynor, R. M., & Peterson, K. E. *Adjusting to your new hearing aid*. Unpublished manual, University of Northern Colorado, Greeley, 1972.
4. Miller, W. E. *An investigation of the effectiveness of aural rehabilitation for nursing home residents*. Paper presented at the Convention of the American Speech and Hearing Association, Houston, 1976.

Raymond H. Hull

Chapter 27: Evaluation of Communication Function and Successes in Aural Rehabilitation of Elderly Clients

One of the most discouraging aspects of the provision of aural rehabilitation services on behalf of the adult, and particularly the elderly client, has been the frustrations in attempting to assess the impact of those sevices on their communication behaviors. Perhaps the most discouraging have been those instances in which persons from other professions, or within our own, who have doubts as to the worth of aural rehabilitation services have asked us to show them *how much* improvement a given client has made or have asked a pointed question such as, "How do you know that the elderly clients with whom you are working have improved enough to warrant payment for your aural rehabilitation services?" It's simpler to note the speech and language progress of a congenitally hearing impaired child than to pinpoint the social gains of an adventitiously hearing impaired 68-year-old adult.

THE FACTORS OF AGE AND ASSESSMENT

The complexities involved in presbycusis, and aging in general, compound the difficulties one faces in attempting to evaluate communication ability and the potential for and/or progress in regaining such skills among elderly clients. There are several factors which must appropriately be considered prior to developing a procedure for assessing communication skills or in the use of any of the presently available methods in relation to older clients.

An apparent reduction of the central auditory system's ability to transmit a complex acoustic signal with the speed and accuracy it once may have possessed. This appears to be an important overriding factor in the speech perception difficulties noted among persons who possess presbycusis. When compounded with a peripherally located high-frequency hearing loss, the elderly client can become quite depressed and/or angry as a result of frustrating difficulties experienced when attempting to understand what another person is saying and at difficult test materials. The speed of administration of any test or assessment procedure must take into consideration the above neurological factor frequently seen in presbycusis. This aspect is discussed in Chapter 21.

The elderly person's emotional response to his or her auditorily based communication difficulties. Occasionally positive change in a client's emotional response to his or her auditory difficulties will reflect itself in enhanced communication abilities.

The clients' most frequented communication environments. Audiologists must realize that not all persons frequent active social environments, but rather they may be content to remain at home with a family member or a friend. Their requirements in regard to aural rehabilitation services are, thus, based upon that environment, and the assessment of communication abilities and subsequent determination of improvements or lack of them resulting from aural rehabilitation services must be capable of reflecting such differences among elderly clients.

The communication priorities of the client. Linked to the previous factor, but important to discuss further, is the establishment of priorities by the client relative to his or her communication needs. In Chapter 26 this author discussed prioritization as an important part of the provision of aural rehabilitation services for elderly clients. If the priority communication needs of each client are the basis upon which treatment services are developed and provided, then any evaluation of progress must also be based on them. Only then can progress or lack of it be determined.

Aside from established client needs or desires for communication as a basis for services and subsequent evaluation, is the *importance of determining those which are realistic for individual elderly clients*. If, for example, a profoundly hearing impaired bedridden client has established as a priority the ability to communicate with absolute precision at social gatherings, that goal may not be realistic for that person. If the goal is held at that level, treatment may be doomed to failure and the evaluation would reflect little or no improvement. However, a realistic goal of increased skill in social communication within his or her confined environment may be reached, and pre- and post-evaluation may reveal those gains. This is not to say, however, that goals should be set so low that improvement in communication skills is inevitable. The point stressed here is that goals for individual clients should not be set so high that failure is inevitable. The insightful audiologist will be aware of communicative heights to be attempted. The most important criteria for goals, again, are the communication needs of individual clients. As stated in Chapter 26, they, too, must be considered in the establishment of treatment goals to be eventually evaluated. We find that most older adults are realistic in their expectations and their knowledge of their limitations. It is tragic to observe audiologists who have established the same aural rehabilitation goals for all clients or, perhaps, had established no real individual goals at all at the time that speechreading services for a group of older clients were begun.

ATTEMPTS AT ASSESSMENT

Elements to Be Assessed

Research designed to investigate factors that influence the ability of hearing impaired persons to communicate has historically included such areas as the visibility of phonemes of speech, intelligence versus lipreading ability, factors of memory, synthetic abilities among good and poor lipreaders, and others. Those and other studies have led to the ultimate conclusion that the person's language level is one of the most important factors that influence compensation for a hearing loss (Lowell, 1969). This not only includes vocabulary level, but also the client's ability to efficiently use the level of language that he or she possesses. This involves the rules of language and the ability to make closure when not all of the linguistic information is available within a given moment of communication. This also inevitably involves factors in the speed of processing linguistic information from moment to moment.

The mental gymnastics that are involved when a hearing impaired person is required to take the threads of phonemic and linguistic information obtained through an impaired receptive auditory system and combine them with what is received visually (if the speaker is visible), and derive information from what is being said is mind boggling, to say the least. To measure that ability appears to be equally difficult, especially when we are dealing with complex adult or elderly clients who differ greatly in relation to

1. Their response to their hearing impairment
2. Their communication environments
3. Their response to noise and other distractions
4. Those with whom they communicate
5. Other multiple factors

These important aspects are, in one way or another, addressed in the scales of communicative function. In terms of evaluating changes in social/communication behavior, the use of such scales may be leading us in the right direction.

In view of the complex nature of the requirements for efficient communication which may be compounded by a hearing impairment and advanced age, the remainder of this chapter will concentrate on sorting through the factors involved in assessment of progress in communicative function and among elderly hearing impaired clients who are involved in aural rehabilitation treatment. Even though there is evident diversity among philosophies relative to assessment of speechreading, general communication abilities, and other factors involved in communication by the hearing impaired, common denominators appear to be emerging. Those common denominators will be presented as the focal point during the remainder of this chapter in relation to procedures which appear to have promise in noting progress in communicative function among elderly hearing impaired clients.

A HISTORICAL PERSPECTIVE

Filmed Tests

Studies of filmed tests of lipreading ability have generally demonstrated that hearing impaired persons perform at least similar to persons with normal hearing. Further, they have generally shown that adult clients perform as well or as poorly after completion of a speechreading treatment program as when they began. Most importantly, it has been demonstrated that it is difficult to separate the quality or efficiency of the aural rehabilitation treatment procedures from invalid tests of lipreading.

Morkovin Life Situation Films

Early filmed tests include those which were introduced in the 1940s as an attempt to both evaluate and teach lipreading. Mason (1943) developed a series of 30 silent films for purposes of lipreading instruction. Morkovin (Note 1) introduced the Morkovin Life

Situations films. These films depicted various "real life" situations for lipreading therapy that advocated a theme approach. They were also utilized as an approach to assessing lipreading skills. The films were made with sound and, for example, depicted a girl and her mother buying shoes at the shoe store, youngsters receiving dancing lessons, and Monty Montana (the roping and cowboy movie star) demonstrating rope tricks for children. The films were generally interesting, but difficult to use either for instruction or for assessment. They, further, became quickly dated due to the actors' clothing and other aspects. In the majority of instances, they were certainly not suitable for work with adults.

Utley Test

The first actual filmed test of lipreading was developed by Utley (1946). It has also received the majority of attention by researchers. This silent film was developed from the most frequently used words in Thorndike's *First Word Dictionary*. It is not known whether the use of those words hindered the validity of her test or not, since those words contained in that dictionary are the most frequently written words, not the most frequently spoken.

The test contained three parts. Part 1 utilized words, and Part 2 contained sentences. Both Parts 1 and 2 were filmed in black and white. Part 3 was a five-part story test filmed in color. Utley investigated the reliability of the forms of the tests and found that in Parts 1 and 2, the internal reliability of each portion was high enough to be significant. Those parts were presented to 761 deaf and hard-of-hearing subjects for purposes of standardization.

The validity of the Utley test has been investigated on numerous occasions. DiCarlo and Kataja (1951), for example, found that the test was probably, although not necessarily, reliable. Even though they found a 0.77 correlation level between the Utley test and the Morkovin "Family Dinner" film, they questioned the validity of the test. They felt, due to the method of filming and its length and speed of presentation, that the test primarily assessed persistence and frustration tolerance of the viewers.

O'Neill and Stephens (1959) studied the Mason, the Utley, and the Morkovin films. They did not find a significant correlation between the responses of viewers of the Utley and Morkovin films, but did find a correlation between the Mason films and Parts 1 and 2 of the Utley film test and the Morkovin films. They concluded that the lack of correlation between the Utley Tests and the Morkovin films was probably because the Morkovin films were originally constructed as a series of lessons and not as an assessment tool.

Simmons (1959) concluded that the Utley and Mason films seem to measure something related to lipreading ability. But the "something" was thought to be only a part of the general ability of hearing impaired persons to communicate in face-to-face situations.

Pestone (1962) determined that no filmed tests met all the criteria that are needed in a test. She felt that a filmed test should utilize presentation of material by two speakers—one male and one female. Further, she advocated that the films should be in color to make them more realistic, two equivalent forms should be developed to facilitate measurements, and the test should have a wide range of difficulty and be easy to score. Pestone used this philosophy to develop a filmed test which utilized sentences, evenly divided between statements and questions. She found the test to be reliable, but it has not been heard of again to any great extent.

Table 27-1
Criticism of Filmed or Videotaped Tests

The distractions caused by the tester on the film holding up a card with the number of the test item.
The stolid appearance of the presenter.
The usual presentation mode of showing the speaker from the shoulders upward.
The erratic rate of presentation of stimulus materials.
The dated clothing and hair styles which may prove distracting to the client.

Reprinted with permission from Alpiner, J. G. *Handbook of adult rehabilitative audiology.* Baltimore: Williams and Wilkins, 1978, p. 36.

John Tracy Test of Lipreading

Donnelly and Marshall (1967) developed a filmed multiple-choice test of lipreading using the John Tracy Clinic Test of Lipreading (Note 2). The test was filmed in color and with sound. Hearing impaired college-age students were utilized as subjects in a study to assess its reliability. The subjects controlled the intensity of the sound. Multiple choice answers were based on (1) the correct answer, (2) the most frequently incorrect response of persons tested previously, and (3) the second most frequently missed. They found the test to be highly reliable.

Even though filmed tests of lipreading have consistently shown at least some level of reliability on test–retest and between tests, their validity has continually been questioned. Perhaps Lashley (1961) has stated it best by saying, "It is possible that validity of lipreading tests will not be established until an understanding of what factors involved in lipreading are agreed upon" (p. 182). Alpiner (1978) has, further, listed criticisms of filmed or videotaped tests (see Table 27-1).

Other Earlier Attempts at Assessment

Other attempts at measuring speechreading or lipreading abilities included interview procedures for determination of hearing impaired persons' communicative function. These have included the use of panels of judges (Simmons, 1959) who were to determine individual clients' lipreading ability and to note progress or lack of it. The basis upon which Simmons attempted the use of judges rather than previous standard tests of lipreading was the lack of quantitative measures of lipreading ability. She felt that this was the major problem in attempting to establish a relationship between lipreading ability and other physical or psychological factors.

Interview Methods

Simmons (1959) used five judges who were qualified therapists of hard-of-hearing adults to attempt to determine the reliability of an interview method for assessing lipreading abilities. Subjects included 12 men and 12 women. All were hard of hearing, with a mean pure-tone average of 33.8 dB and mean speech discrimination scores of 58.7 percent. The rating scale devised was based upon three simple categories of "good, average, and poor" lipreading abilities. Each classification had its own set of criteria for determining the level of skill. The judges engaged in "everyday" conversation with the subjects, keeping their voices at an intensity level that was below the threshold of each subject. Comparison of the judges' decision as to lipreading ability of individual clients yielded a relationship of 0.92, indicating a high positive correlation.

If such correlations can be maintained, perhaps such interview techniques could be used with success. Close monitoring of the intensity level of the judge's voice below, at, or above clients' thresholds could yield important pre- and post-treatment information about their ability to utilize visual and supplemental auditory clues in everyday speech. The most difficult aspect when dealing with such methods, however, is the scoring procedure. It is suggested that further investigation of such approaches be made relative to their possible routine use with older adults.

Multiple Choice Tests

Other procedures, such as that developed by Hutton (1959), included the use of multiple choice tests. Hutton's procedure, for example, utilized two simultaneous word presentations in visual-only, auditory-only, and auditory–visual modes. The subjects were asked to choose the correct word from a multiple choice answer sheet of eight words.

Further, Black, O'Reilly, and Peck (1963) developed a self-administered multiple choice procedure which was presented on silent film. The filmed stimulus items were used for training in lipreading. The projector speed could be slowed. Subjects were first tested using the normal speed of projection. The film was then slowed 15 percent and subjects were tested again. The subjects, after reviewing their scores, were permitted to adjust the speed of the projector until they could achieve a score of 100 percent. Results revealed that even with that brief period of practice, subjects improved in their ability to lipread even when viewing a different speaker. Although this procedure was basically self-administered training in lipreading, the assessment procedure was unique.

Assessment through Bisensory Modalities

The current consensus of opinion is that assessment of the ability of hearing impaired persons to understand speech should involve the combined use of vision and audition. Innumerable studies confirm the reciprocal compliment of vision and audition (Binnie, 1973; Binnie, Montgomery, & Jackson, 1974; Duffy, 1967; Erber, 1971; Erber, 1972a and 1972b; Erber, 1975; Ewersten, Neilsen, & Neilsen, 1970; Hutton, Curry & Armstrong, 1959; Miller & Nicely, 1955; Neely, 1956; O'Neill, 1954; Prall, 1957; Sumby & Pollack, 1954; Van Uden, 1960; and Note 3). Their results, as do the results of numbers of other studies, continually confirm the benefits of bisensory modalities for speech reception. No matter how restricted the auditory component, the compliment continues to exist. If an individual client's ability to recognize the visimes of speech or to discriminate auditorily is to be assessed, then those sensory modalities must be isolated. If assessment of the ability to communicate is held as a priority, however, then both vision and audition should be combined.

Use of Live-Voice Tests

The criticisms of filmed or videotaped tests of lipreading cited earlier by Alpiner (1978) are valid ones. Further, people do not communicate with others via film or videotape in the course of everyday conversations. Therefore, the use of live voice for the presentation of assessment materials to determine skill in the reception of speech among hearing impaired clients is preferred by this author.

For live-voice testing, the use of sentences is preferred over single words. Sentences as stimulus items most closely approximate the types of stimuli found in the conversations experienced by hearing impaired clients. Sentences also lend themselves to greater ease of scoring. Even though paragraphs most closely resemble the conversations which people listen to in the everyday world, they are more difficult to score, and other compounding factors such as auditory and visual memory may impact on the results. For a more accurate determination of skill in auditory–visual reception of speech, sentences continue to be beneficial.

Sentence materials which lend themselves well to assessment of speechreading skills include the Central Institute for the Deaf (CID) Everyday Speech Sentences (Davis & Silverman, 1970), the Denver Scale Quick Test (Alpiner, 1978), and the University of Northern Colorado (UNC) Sentence Test of Speechreading Ability (Note 3).

The CID Everyday Speech Sentences include ten lists of ten sentences each. The sentences vary in length and are common to most adults. (See the appendix to the text for the CID lists of sentences, Lists A through J.)

The Denver Scale Quick Test is made up of 20 simple sentences, 8 questions, and 12 declarative statements. Although no information is available regarding consistency of sentence ease or difficulty or consistency of phonemic visability, the list lends itself well to assess client abilities in the identification of sentence material. It is suggested by Alpiner (1978) that the test be administered under the visual-only condition, although it can be used with an auditory–visual mode. Each stimulus item has a value of 5 percent, and scoring is based only on identifying the thought of the sentence rather than on verbatim repetition. (See the Denver Scale Quick Test in the appendix.)

The UNC Sentence Test of Speechreading is based on a study by Hull and Alpiner (1976) in which they investigated linguistic factors in speechreading. Three lists of 36 sentences each were developed based on a sentence length of eight words, which was found by Taaffe and Wong (Note 2) to be as visually intelligible as shorter sentences. Since shorter sentences are limited in content and complexity, it was felt that longer sentences would provide a greater opportunity for comparisons between conditions and allow for greater experimental manipulation. Further, the sentences were developed according to specific requirements (see Table 27-2).

Scoring is based on the thought or idea of the sentence. Each sentence is valued at 1 point, and it is suggested that the lists be presented live voice, at a just-audible level for the client (See the appendix section for the UNC Sentences.)

Presentation of Sentence Material

The presentation of the assessment materials can be made in the same room as the client at a distance of approximately 5 to 6 feet, with the voice of the tester just audible to the client. The determination of audibility can be made by asking the client to close his or her eyes and, with tester reading words or sentences, by judging when the tester's voice is audible, but the stimulus items are not understood. Any level of desired voice presentation can be determined in that fashion.

Another method of live-voice presentation that has been found to be useful is through the use of a sound-treated audiometric suite where a window separates the tester from the client. If lighting can be adjusted so that the face and shoulders of the tester are easily observable, the free-field speech system of the audiometer can be used for presentation

Table 27-2
Guidelines to Development of Sentences for UNC Sentence Test

An equal number of interrogative and declarative sentences (forty-five each).
All sentences contained an equal number of words (eight).
All words within each sentence were taken from the Jones and Wepman (1966) list of 1,000 most commonly spoken words.
Parts of speech within each sentence were varied as much as possible in terms of position so identifying cues could not be obtained from word position.
Percentage of words among parts of speech was based on norms established by Templin (1957) regarding the structure of the English language.
No common phrases such as "good morning," "in the U.S.," or "how are you" were used in the sentences developed.
No contractions that might be confusing in terms of completing written answers were included.
No bisyllabic proper nouns were included that might be confusing.
No highly visible words that could influence the visual intelligibility of sentences were included (Fisher, 1968).

of the auditory portion. Further, the just-audible level, or other intensity levels, of voice presentation can be more easily established, and the intensity levels varied. The most difficult aspect in the use of an audiometric sound-treated suite is the visability of the tester, particularly through the two to four panels of glass between most prefabricated enclosures.

SCALES OF COMMUNICATIVE FUNCTION

One viable approach to assessing the handicap of hearing impairment on elderly clients' ability to function within their everyday worlds as well as changes that occur as the result of aural rehabilitation treatment, are rating scales of communicative function. This approach is particularly recommended for use with older adult clients.

Hearing Handicap Scale

A number of such scales which are designed to assess the impact of hearing impairment on an adult's ability to function communicatively have been developed over the past decade and a half. One forerunner of the current scales is the Hearing Handicap Scale (HHS) developed by High, Fairbanks, and Glorig (1964). Both forms of this scale are presented in the appendix section. As can be seen, the scale concentrates on questions related to communication per se; that is, the impact of hearing impairment on communication in various environments. It does not delve into other aspects related to hearing, such as the social or psychological impact of hearing impairment (Giolas, 1970; Sanders, 1975), which appears to be one of its weaknesses. Responses for this Scale include the options of (1) almost always, (2) usually, (3) sometimes, (4) rarely, and (5) almost never.

Even though the above scale is somewhat limited by probing only into various communication settings (including the impact of distance on communication, etc.) those questions do lend themselves well for interviews with elderly hearing impaired clients. Their subjective judgments relative to their ability to function communicatively within typical environments provides important treatment data. Since there are two forms for the Scale which are similar in terms of the area of communication queried, the Scale can be used on a pre- and postassessment basis to determine if clients' opinions of their ability to communicate in various similar environments have changed to the positive or the negative. Further, the pretreatment administration can, as with other scales, be used to guide the emphasis of treatment and the procedures. The fact that the psychosocial impact of hearing impairment is not included in the scale is, as stated before, a drawback to its possible usefulness. It does, however, provide some very specific information on the client's attitudes regarding their ability to function in common communication environments.

The Denver Scale of Communication Function

The Denver Scale of Communication Function (Alpiner, Chevrette, Glascoe, Metz, & Olsen, 1978) is an attitude scale which provides hearing impaired adults the opportunity to make subjective judgments relative to the impact of their hearing impairment on, for example, relationships with family, their ability to communicate with others, image of self, and the impact of the hearing impairment on the social and/or vocational aspects of life. (This scale is presented in the appendix section of this text.)

It is suggested by Alpiner (1978) that the scale be administered prior to initiating aural rehabilitation treatment so that the client responses will not be influenced by discussions that take place there. Client's respond to 25 statements on a seven-level semantic differential continuum, from 1 (agree) to 7 (disagree). The scale contains four categories: family, self, social–vocational, and general communication experience. Alpiner (1978) recommends a time limit of 15 minutes for administration of the scale.

Client responses are recorded on the Denver Scale Profile form (Alpiner, et al., 1971). The abscissa numbers represent the statements on the scale, and the ordinate points represent the clients' responses to each statement, ranging from agree to disagree. The responses are plotted along the abscissa, and lines are drawn from response to response. The profile is studied by the client and audiologist in relation to the communication problems which need attention. That information is then used to design individual clients' aural rehabilitation treatment program.

One aspect of the Scale has been confusing to some clients, and their ratings are probably affected. That is the fact that the middle point on the semantic differential, that is exactly between 1 (agree) and 7 (disagree), is meant to be marked if the statement on the scale is, to an individual client, "irrelevant or unassociated" with his or her communication situation. Some clients, perhaps not understanding the instructions, have placed marks in that position believing that their response would then mean that it is somewhere between agree and disagree, perhaps as a "maybe." Alpiner (1978) has stated that that aspect will be altered on future revisions of the scale.

Even though this scale is not designed specifically with the older adult in mind, it is applicable and useful for pinpointing areas of communication which concern individual clients. These are important in planning the treatment program. The majority of the Denver Scale is applicable for the well noninstitutionalized older adult. Zarnoch and Alpiner (Note 4) have developed a modified version of the Denver Scale which is designed for the older adult who is confined to a health care facility (nursing home). This scale will be presented later in this discussion.

Test of Actual Performance

A brief scale to assess the communication habits of hearing impaired persons has been developed by Koniditsiotis (1971). (The test is shown in the appendix section.) The purpose of the design of the test was to study the extent of relationship between the amount of hearing loss as determined by pure-tone and speech audiometry and the actual disability experienced by the person who possessed the hearing loss. The test contains seven items that are scored in terms of 1 (poor), 2 (adequate), 3 (good), or 4 (excellent). Little correlation between the test judgments and actual hearing impairment has been found. The least correlation was found when comparing the test judgments and client scores for speech discrimination.

The strongest limitation to the test is the fact that the test judgments are made by the clinicians who work with the clients and not the clients themselves.

The Hearing Measurement Scale

Noble and Atherley (1970) devised the Hearing Measurement Scale (HMS), which was designed to probe the handicap of hearing impairment. Even though the purpose of their scale is to assess handicap of hearing loss acquired as the result of industrial noise, all of the questions lend themselves well for use with other persons including the elderly. (This scale is shown in the appendix.)

The Scale is divided into seven Sections.

Section 1: Speech Hearing
Section 2: Acuity for Non-Speech Sound
Section 3: Localization
Section 4: Reaction to Handicap
Section 5: Speech Distortion
Section 6: Tinnitus
Section 7: Personal Opinion of Hearing Loss

The HMS contains a valuable assortment of questions that not only aid in the determination of the client's opinions of the extent of his or her hearing impairment, but also those aspects which interfere most and their reactions to the handicap. A set of instructions accompany the assessment forms. Noble and Atherley (1970) stress that the scale cannot be administered without reading the instruction manual.*

Profile Questionnaire for Rating Communicative Performance

A Profile Questionnaire for Communicative Performance has been developed by Sanders (1975). Two aspects of the profile—Communicative Performance in a Home Environment and Communicative Performance in a Social Environment—are quite ap-

*The manual and the scale can be obtained from Dr. W. Noble, Department of Psychology, University of New England, Armidale, N.S.W., 2351, Australia.

plicable for older adults. A third profile, which may or may not be applicable for use with older adults, is the questionnaire entitled Performance in an Occupational Environment. The former two profiles are suitable for the noninstitutionalized older client. For older adult clients in a health care facility environment, responses to the profile relating to the home environment would need to be interpreted as being their typical environment. (The profiles on social and home environments are presented in the appendix section of this text.)

These profiles and the Hearing Handicap Scale (High, Fairbanks, & Glorig, 1964) discussed earlier, differ from the Denver Scale since they probe into specific communication environments, rather than client's attitudes regarding their ability to communicate. All, however, provide valuable pre- and post-treatment information for assessment of progress or lack of it.

The scales, or profiles, discussed above by High, Fairbanks, and Glorig (1964), Alpiner et al. (1971), Noble and Atherley (1970), and Sanders (1976) can appropriately be used with noninstitutionalized older adult clients. In some instances they can be utilized with regard to older clients who are more confined at home or in a health care facility, but usually in those instances where they are otherwise alert social persons.

Scales for Older Adult Clients

The Denver Scale Revised

The Denver Scale of Communication Function for Senior Citizens Living in Retirement Centers is the result of a modification of the Denver Scale of Communication Function, and was developed by Zarnoch and Alpiner (Note 4). (This scale can be seen in the appendix of this text.)

The content of the questions has been designed to be suitable for confined elderly clients. Further, rather than the scale being self-administered as in the original Denver Scale (Alpiner et al., 1971, and Alpiner, 1978), the questions are presented to the clients, who then respond verbally. This provides control for variables such as client inability to respond to written tests, fatigue, and others. The Scale for Senior Citizens is based on seven major questions regarding their feelings about themselves and their communication abilities. Each question is followed by Probe Effect questions which delve more extensively into the principal question. Probe Effect questions range in number from two to five depending on the principal question. To determine the relevance of the principal question and the Probe Effect questions, Exploration Effect questions are also asked.

Each of the seven major questions, including the Probe Effect and Exploration Effect questions, are categorized according to family, emotional, other persons, general communication, self-concept, group situations, or rehabilitation theme. Responses are based on yes or no answers, and scores are indicated by a plus or a minus. Scoring is identical in relation to the principal questions, the Probe Effects, and Exploration Effects.

As stated earlier, the Denver Scale for Senior Citizens appears very useful for interviewing the confined elderly person on a pre- and post-treatment basis. The only drawback observed by this author is the scoring procedure. A semantic differential format which allows for degrees of yes-to-no responses is generally more desirable for any age of client. Otherwise, the scale provides valuable information for the developement of aural rehabilitation treatment programs and evaluation of progress based on the attitudes of the client about him- or herself.

ASSESSMENT BASED ON COMMUNICATIVE PRIORITIES

This procedure, developed by Hull (1978), lends itself well for both the nonconfined and confined older adult. Since those highest priority, but realistic, communication environments should be stressed in planning aural rehabilitation treatment for the older adult, assessment of successes, or lack of them should also be based on them.

Prior to the initiation of treatment, clients are asked to rank the difficulty they experience in a variety of communication environments on a form which can be seen in the appendix. The ratings of difficulty range from 1 (no problem) through 2 (only in specific instances) to 3 (definite problem). A section for ''Other'' is included on the form in anticipation that an environment which was not included originally may be felt to be important to an individual client. After they have rated those 13 communication environments, they are asked to choose those which are most important to them. When that task is completed, they are then requested to rank them in terms of their priority, from highest to lowest. The priorities, if realistic for individual clients, are used as the basis for the design of their treatment program and evaluation of successes or lack of them.

At the conclusion of a specified number of treatment sessions, clients are again asked to complete the identical form and rank the communication environments in terms of the difficulty that they experience within them. The client and the audiologist then review both the pre- and post-test ratings, particularly noting those communication environments considered high priority by the client. Success, or lack of it, is based only on changes in client attitudes relative to the priority environments. It is interesting to note, however, that on occasion, if positive progress is noted on one priority item, there appears to be a progression of attitude change regarding other ''near'' environments as they are ranked according to their difficulty. For example, if participation in church group meetings was rated as the highest priority communication environment by an individual client, but other near environments such as other formal meetings, at the dinner table, and at parties or other social events were also ranked as being a definite problem but not high priority, the client's rating in those other environments also may begin to change toward positive.

In any event, evaluation of progress or lack of it based on clients' priority communication environments, whether they be related to people or places, appears to have merit. Further, clients' feel a sense of confidence in audiologists who hold their priorities as pre-eminent in aural rehabilitation treatment.

HEARING PERFORMANCE INVENTORY

This comprehenseive assessment tool has been developed by Giolas, Owens, Lamb and Schubert (1979). It probes six areas that can either impact upon communication or involves communication. Those areas are (1) understanding the speech of various talkers, (2) intensity, or the person's awareness of social and nonsocial sounds in his or her environment, (3) response to auditory failure (4) social, or the person's ability to converse in groups of two or more persons in social environments, (5) personal, or the person's feelings about his or her hearing impairment in relation to its personal impact, and (6) occupational.

This inventory can be used effectively with older adults. All categories—except, in most instances, the one entitled "occupational"—will be used for both the elderly who are well and confined. Due to its length, selected categories may be desired for use in regard to establishing priorities for aural rehabilitation treatment and for assessment.

SUMMARY OF ATTEMPTS AT EVALUATING COMMUNICATIVE FUNCTION

By whatever method used to determine whether a hearing impaired person can perceive speech or the symbols of speech, communicative function is being evaluated. Those methods may include determining if he or she can visually recognize phonemes, words, or sentences; use his or her residual hearing to recognize units of speech; utilize both vision and hearing to recognize them; or use various factors of language to determine the meaning of statements. What matters is the emphasis that is placed on the interpretation of the results of the evaluation.

Phoneme Identification

If lipreading ability for phonemes per se is intended to be measured, then a visible mouth, mandible, and neck may be all that is necessary to determine if the hearing impaired person can identify the various vowels, consonants, and dipthongs as they are viewed on film, on slides, or in ink-drawn pictures. If the score that is derived is presented as that person's score for the recognition of phonemes of American English in isolation, then it would be described accurately. If the score was described as a measure of communicative ability, however, then it would be misrepresented, as would that client's probable ability to communicate. The emphasis would have been inappropriately placed, although a high score may indicate that the person has less difficulty recognizing phonemes of speech, which is, indeed, a part of communication. The score does not, however, tell us how well that person may be able to recognize those same phonemes within continuous discourse, which is the near totality of verbal communication with other human beings.

Word Identification

Tests of lipreading ability which include filmed, videotaped, or live visual-only presentations of single words out of context as test items do not provide information on a hearing impaired person's ability to recognize words within continuous discourse, nor his or her ability to communicate in various social or business environments. However, the scores are, indeed, still used by some to predict abilities in social communication, even though they may only provide information regarding the person's visual recognition of those words. Such tests, presented in an auditory-only format, would provide information on the accuracy with which that person's peripheral auditory mechanism can receive and transmit the acoustic/phonemic elements of those words. This procedure can, however, provide important bits of diagnostic information regarding auditory and visual speech discrimination. If the mode of presentation included both the auditory and visual portions of the stimulus items, then information would be obtained regarding that person's ability to utilize the additive compliment of visual clues on audition and vice versa.

Although the components discussed above can provide important information regarding a given hearing impaired individual's ability to utilize audition and vision in the recognition of phoneme and word elements, they do not provide clues as to that person's ability to communicate in his or her most frequented environments, nor in those other situations where the person must function communicatively.

Sentences and Paragraphs

The use of sentences and paragraphs as stimulus items for assessment of a person's ability to communicate in spite of hearing impairment have been recommended (Hirsch, 1952) but, again, the use of sentences still leaves us without important information regarding the client's ability to contend in his or her communication environments. Assessment of a person's ability to receive and interpret at least the thought of sentences does, however, provide us with information on that person's ability to receive and synthesize content while using visual and auditory modalities. The use of paragraphs in analyzing a person's ability to use visual and auditory clues is generally compounded by such factors as memory and attentiveness, although those are also important in most communication environments. Difficulties in administration of such test batteries, standardization of the tests, and client variables such as the elderly person's emotional response to his or her hearing impairment and the testing environment, compounded by problems in scoring, make the use of paragraphs relatively inefficient as measures for determination of improvements in communicative ability, particularly among older clients.

Vision versus Audition

The visual-only mode of presentation of test batteries generally is not satisfactory. There are very few older adults who do not possess at least some usable hearing no matter how severe their discrimination problem. Any formal assessment and treatment procedure should include the use of both audition and vision. Since clients also will seldom find themselves in situations where they will not be using hearing and vision, any assessment of the ability to receive and interpret verbal information should emphasize the advantage of the bisensory mode of presentation. Among elderly persons who possess severe visual disorders, assessment and treatment will obviously involve the use of residual hearing as the primary sensory modality.

Communication Scales and Profiles

Scales of communicative function—including those which stress attitudes of hearing impaired people and those concentrating on situations or communication environments—seem to be taking us in the right direction. This is particularly true when attempting to assess the communicative behaviors and needs of the elderly client. The majority of the scales and profiles appear to be based on the important fact that the audiologist is dealing with adult clients, and in this instance, older adult clients who have communication needs and priorities which are unique to them. Even though many persons may benefit from enhanced visual and/or auditory skills and awareness, they also desire that the efforts involved have meaning for them, and that the treatment have relevance to their specific communication needs.

Assessment and treatment based on the feelings, attitudes, and priority communication environments of elderly clients will surely enhance a reality of maturity in the services provided by audiologists. These procedures have brought us a long way from the days of the filmed tests of lipreading.

Validity

The scales of communication function face similar questions in regard to validity as have tests of lipreading and other procedures. Test–retest reliability among the various scales and profiles has been generally found to be acceptable. A major question that is inevitably asked, however, is do we know that clients are answering the questions or responding to the statements honestly? In that regard, the reliability of the client is in question. Hopefully, a wise audiologist will be able to, in the majority of cases, "see through" the client who appears to be attempting to fool the audiologist or, perhaps more regretably, fool him- or herself. Occasionally, there are clients who provide answers he or she feels that the provider of services *wants* to hear. Clients do not like to see audiologists fail, either. It is up to the audiologist to assure clients that their answers or responses are to be honest ones. How else can real progress, or lack of it, be noted? And, how can adjustments in the treatment program be made, if they are needed?

The question of validity is indeed, for lack of a better phrase, a valid one. However, Alpiner (1978) responded to that question well when he stated that, "Their (the scales or profiles) successful use depends on the audiologists' judgment, not on tests of validity" (p. 32).

SUMMARY

To recommend an approach to assessment, not only of the handicap that elderly adult clients are experiencing as a result of an auditorily related disorder, but also gains or lack of them as a result of aural rehabilitation treatment, is difficult. The audiologist, however, must be responsible for determining those aspects of communicative function to be assessed, treated, and again, assessed as to the value of the treatment procedures used.

A comprehensive approach to assessment is recommended. This includes:

1. Observing the results of the case history relative to the possible causes of the auditory deficit, its duration, and the current social and environmental status of the elderly client.
2. Utilizing the audiometric results, particularly the type, degree, and configuration of the hearing loss, and very importantly the results of speech discrimination assessment.
3. The results of a hearing aid evaluation and the possible benefits of amplification.
4. Assessment of the clients' ability to utilize visual clues with minimal auditory clues. This assessment may include: (1) monosyllabic words, (2) sentences, and (3) everyday conversation. Sentence lists recommended are the Denver Quick Test of Lipreading, the CID Everyday Sentences, or the UNC Sentence Test of Speechreading.
5. Assessment of the impact of the hearing impairment by the use of one of the scales of communication function. Those recommended are: (1) the Denver Scale of Communication Function, (2) the Denver Scale of Communication Function for Senior

Citizens, (3) the Profile Questionnaires (Home and Social), or (4) the Communicative Priorities Assessment.

6. Plans for aural rehabilitation treatment and post-treatment assessment should only be based upon the clients' communicative needs and priorities. Only then will the audiologist be adding validity to his or her treatment goals. "Cookbook" approaches usually do nothing more than consume valuable time.

REFERENCES

Alpiner, J. G., Chevrette, W., Glascoe, G., Metz, M., & Olsen, B. The Denver Scale of Communication Function, in J. G. Alpiner (Ed.), *Adult rehabilitative audiology*. Baltimore: Williams and Wilkins, 1978, pp. 36, 53–56.

Alpiner, J. G. *Handbook of adult rehabilitative audiology*. Baltimore: Williams and Wilkins, 1978, p. 36.

Binnie, C. A. Bi-sensory articulation functions for normal hearing and sensorineural hearing loss patients. *Journal of the Academy of Rehabilitative Audiology*, 1973, *6*, 43–53.

Binnie, C. A., Montgomery, A. A., & Jackson, P. L. Auditory and visual contributions to the perception of selected English consonants. *Journal of Speech and Hearing Research*, 1974, *17*, 619–630.

Black, J. W., O'Reilly, P. P., & Peck, L. Self-administered training in lipreading. *Journal of Speech and Hearing Disorders*, 1963, *28*, 183–186.

Davis, H., & Silverman, S. R. *Hearing and Deafness*. New York: Holt, Rinehart and Winston, 1970.

DiCarlo, L. M., & Kataja, R. An analysis of the Utley Lipreading Test. *Journal of Speech and Hearing Disorders*, 1951, *16*, 226–240.

Donnelly, K. G., & Marshall, W. J. A. Development of a multiple-choice test of lipreading. *Journal of Speech and Hearing Research*, 1967, *10*, 565–569.

Duffy, J. K. Audio-visual speech audiometry and a new audio and audio-visual speech perception index. *Maico Audiological Series*, 1967, *5*, 9.

Erber, N. P. Auditory and audiovisual reception of words in low-frequency noise by children with normal hearing and by children with impaired hearing. *Journal of Speech and Hearing Research*, 1971, *14*, 496–512.

Erber, N. P. Speech-envelope cues as an acoustic aid to lipreading for profoundly deaf children. *Journal of the Acoustical Society of America*, 1972a *51*, 1224–1227.

Erber, N. P. Auditory, visual, and auditory-visual recognition of consonants by children with normal and impaired hearing. *Journal of Speech and Hearing Research*, 1972b, *15*, 413–422.

Erber, N. P. Auditory-visual perception of speech. *Journal of Speech and Hearing Disorders*, 1975, *40*, 481–492.

Ewertsen, H. W., Birk Nielsen, H., & Scott Neilsen, S. Audiovisual speech perception. *Acta Oto-laryngologica (Supplement)*, 1970, *263*, 229–230.

Fisher, C. Confusions among visually perceived consonants. *Journal of Speech and Hearing Research*, 1968, *11*, 796–804.

Giolas, T. G. The measurement of hearing handicap: A point of view. *Maico Audiological Library Series*, 1970, *8*, 6.

Giolas, T. G., Owens, E., Lamb, S. H., & Schubert, E. E. Hearing performance inventory. *Journal of Speech and Hearing Disorders*, 1979, *44*, 169–195.

High, W. S., Fairbanks, G., & Glorig, A. Scale for self-assessment of hearing handicap. *Journal of Speech and Hearing Disorders*, 1964, *29*, 215–230.

Hirsh, I. J. *The measurement of hearing*. New York: McGraw-Hill, 1952, p. 131.

Hull, R. H., & Alpiner, J. G. The effect of syntatic word variations on the predictability of sentence content in speechreading. *Journal of the Academy of Rehabilitative Audiology*, 1976, *9*, 42–56.

Hull, R. H. Aural rehabilitation of aging persons: Problems and strategies for their solution, in L. Bradford (Ed.), *Audiology—An Audio Journal for Continuing Education*. New York: Grune and Stratton, 1978.

Hutton, C. Combining auditory and visual stimuli in aural rehabilitation. *Volta Review*, 1959, *6*, 316–319.

Hutton, C., Curry, E. T., & Armstrong, M. B. Semi-diagnostic test materials for aural rehabilitation. *Journal of Speech and Hearing Disorders*, 1959, *24*, 318–329.

Jones, L. V. & Wepman, J. M. *A Spoken Word Count*. Chicago: Language Research Associates, 1966.

Koniditsiotis, C. Y. The use of hearing tests to provide information about the extent to which an individual's hearing loss handicaps him. *Maico Audiological Series,* 1971, *9,* 10.

Lowell, E. L. Rehabilitation of auditory disorders, in *Human communication and its disorders—An overview* (Monograph No. 10). Bethesda, Md.: National Advisory Neurological Diseases and Stroke Council, National Institutes of Health, 1969.

Mason, M. K. A cinematic technique for testing visual speech comprehension. *Journal of Speech Disorders,* 1943, *8,* 271–278.

Miller, G. A., & Nicely, P. E. An analysis of perceptual confusions among some English consonants. *Journal of Acoustical Society of America,* 1955, *27,* 338–352.

Morkovin, B. S. *Life-situation speechreading through the cooperation of senses (movie),* Los Angeles: University of Southern California. 1948.

Neely, K. K. Effect of visual factors on the intelligibility of speech. *Journal of the Acoustical Society of America,* 1956, *28,* 1275–1277.

Noble, W. G., & Atherley, G. R. C. The hearing measure scale: A questionnaire for the assessment of auditory disability. *Journal of Audiology Research,* 1970, *10,* 229–250.

O'Neill, J. J. Contributions of the visual components of oral symbols to speech comprehension. *Journal of Speech and Hearing Disorders,* 1954, *19,* 429–439.

O'Neill, J. J., & Stephens, M. C. Relationships among three filmed lipreading tests. *Journal of Speech and Hearing Research,* 1959, *2,* 61–65.

Pestove, M. J. Selection of items for a speechreading test by means of scalogram analysis. *Journal of Speech and Hearing Disorders,* 1962, *27,* 71–75.

Prall, J. Lipreading and hearing aids combine for better comprehension. *Volta Review,* 1957, *59,* 64–65.

Sanders, D. A. Hearing aid orientation and counseling, in M. C. Pollack (Ed.), *Amplification for the hearing impaired.* New York: Grune and Stratton, 1975.

Simmons, A. A. Factors related to lipreading. *Journal of Speech and Hearing Research,* 1959, *2,* 340–352.

Sumby, W. H., & Pollack, I. Visual contributions to speech intelligibility in noise. *Journal of Acoustical Society of America,* 1954, *26,* 212–215.

Templin, M. C. *Certain Language Skills in Children.* Minneapolis: University of Minnesota Press, 1957.

Utley, J. Factors involved in the teaching and testing of lipreading ability through the use of motion pictures. *Volta Review,* 1946, *38,* 657–659.

Van Uden, A. A sound-perceptive method, in A. W. G. Ewing (Ed.), *The modern educational treatment of deafness,* Washington, D.C.: Volta Bureau, 1960, pp. 3–19.

REFERENCE NOTES

1. Morkovin, B. S. *Life-situation speechreading through the cooperation of senses* (movie). Los Angeles: University of Southern California. 1948.
2. Taaffe, G., & Wong, W. Study of variables in lipreading stimulus material. *John Tracy Clinic Research Papers III.* Los Angeles: The John Tracy Clinic, 1957.
3. Hull, R. H. *Sentence test of speechreading.* Paper presented at the 1971 Convention of the American Speech and Hearing Association, Houston, November 20–23, 1971.
4. Zarnoch, J. M., & Alpiner, J. G. 1977. *The Denver Scale of Communication Function for Senior Citizens Living in Retirement Centers.* Unpublished study, University of Denver, 1977.

A. Implications and Supportive Procedures for the Confined and/or Multiply Handicapped Hearing Impaired Elderly

Raymond H. Hull

Chapter 28: Programs in the Health Care Facility

Even though only approximately five percent of all persons over age 65 years reside in various levels of health care facilities, that percentage still represents almost 1.5 million persons. According to Atchley (1972), over 14 percent of persons age 85 or over are institutionalized. Of those who are institutionalized, most are in nursing homes or other personal-care facilities. Further, according to Chafee (1967), approximately 92 percent of those persons residing in health care facilities possess hearing impairment of sufficient degree to interfere with communication.

Although a vast majority of those persons will, for all practical purposes, remain confined for the remainder of their lives due to chronic illness and other physical or mental problems, some can benefit from aural rehabilitation services from the audiologist. They, too, deserve the opportunity for enhanced communicative skills in spite of impaired hearing and to experience the heightened social and personal communication which may result. Further, with effective inservice education for health care facility personnel relative to hearing impairment, the use of hearing aids, and communication with the hearing impaired, coordinated with educational programming for elderly persons and their families, the daily lives of elderly persons within the confines of the health care facility can be enhanced.

HEALTH CARE FACILITIES

Before this discussion of services for confined older persons proceeds, a description of what is meant by the ''health care facility'' is appropriate. The term means different things to different people.

Health care facility is a currently accepted term denoting any facility that provides long- or short-term residential care for older adults who require medical or other health services other than that provided by hospitals. The facilities may provide intensive care services, including 24-hour-a-day nursing care for posthospitalized stroke patients, or simply a place to live where there is nursing or other health care near by.

Outpatient Residential Facilities

These may include apartment or condominium living for ambulatory older persons. The apartments or condominiums, in this instance, are a part of a health care facility, perhaps in a separate wing or simply on the same grounds. Health care is usually a button push away. Those older persons who reside in the outpatient or residential facility may have been ill enough at some recent time to desire the proximity of those services. These facilities most nearly resemble retirement communities. The only difference, again, is that they may be a part of a health care facility complex.

Short-Term Care

Many health care facilities possess an intensive care or a skilled nursing wing or may be an intensive-care or skilled nursing facility. These are generally considered short-term care facilities. A stroke patient, for example, when known to be recovering, but still too ill to return to his or her own home due to the need for rather constant monitoring and nursing care, may be dismissed from the hospital and taken to the intensive-care facility. The stay may be only a few days or may last for several weeks. These facilities play an important role, not only for recuperative purposes, but also as an alternative to higher-cost extended hospital stays. For stroke patients and others who may require other services, rehabilitation personnel—such as occupational therapists, audiologists, speech/language pathologists, and others—are generally available, perhaps at least on a contractual basis.

When placed in short-term facility, it is expected that the patient will be released within a fairly short period of time. The most desirable destination is the patient's home. Unfortunately, however, for some older adults, the destination is to an intermediate or long-term care facility, for lack of other alternatives.

Intermediate and Long-Term Care Facilities

The most frequently observed facilities for older adults are these, most often called nursing homes. They represent facilities where older adults reside who may or may not require nursing or other health care. Although the primary reason for placement is generally some health or psychologically related problem, recent studies have shown that some persons who reside in intermediate or long-term care facilities do not possess health or mental problems. Intermediate care facilities all too frequently become long-term in nature. Other reasons for placement in these health care facilities may be no place else to live, a spouse has passed away and the elderly survivor fears living alone, or—and the most devastating to older persons—the elderly person's family "feels that it is best." As one older woman told this author, "I thought my daughter was out looking for an apartment for me, and I ended up here."

These facilities offer a room (usually with a roommate), balanced meals, some social and recreational activities, and a nursing staff. Larger health care facilities may have a social services director, an activity director and rehabilitative services such as occupational therapy and physical therapy. Some facilities are Medicare and/or Medicaid approved, but for those programs to provide payment for services and residence, a medically related problem must be the reason for placement in the facility. Further, some health care facilities do not desire to be approved by either program due to the relatively low rate of reimbursement for care of the resident.

THE RESIDENTS OF HEALTH CARE FACILITIES

Those older adults who are placed in skilled or intensive-care wings of health care facilities or in skilled nursing care facilities are there because of specific health or mentally related reasons. They may have been transferred from a hospital to the skilled nursing facility because they are still too weak or unable to care for themselves at home, but well enough to be released from the hospital. It is anticipated that the facility and the 24-hour-per-day nursing care which is available will, in that respect, be the ''halfway house'' for the patient between hospitalization and home. In some instances, however, due to lack of sufficient recovery, some older patients must be transferred to an extended-care facility because they are not able to care for themselves sufficiently to live at home and, further, there may not be others available at home to aid the person. Therefore, the adult is placed in a longer-term health care facility so that the necessary services for daily needs are available.

In all too many instances the elderly person views this placement as terminal. And, for many persons, it is true. It is, however, a fear that can interfere with the elderly person's desire for rehabilitative or health services. The audiologist and other health care professionals must be aware of that as well as other responses and feelings that can have a negative impact on their desire for supportive services.

Reasons for Placement

What are the reasons for placement in extended care facilities? Since placement for any reason can result in a lessening of desire for self-maintenance and/or improvement, the audiologist should be aware of them. According to Atchley (1972), the major factor in placement in health care facilities (nursing homes or other residences) appears to be their state of mental or physical health, their previous residential setting, or the family system. Older people in nursing and other health care facilities tend not to have a spouse or children who live nearby, although many have living children. Indications are that many older people would be able to avoid institutionalization if they had relatives to help care for them, and if they possessed adequate finances. Breakdown in the support system appears to be the primary cause for placement in nursing or other forms of residential facilities. Others include loss of residence due to urban renewal projects, a child who has urged them to sell a house (that according to the child is just too much for the elderly family member), or other reasons.

The placement of an elderly person in a health care facility does not generally occur rapidly. A series of events usually take place prior to placement. Those events may include serious illness. They may include attempts at residence with relatives who, in the end, find the older person to be too much of an emotional or financial burden. For whatever reason, placement in a health care facility (nursing home) was felt to be a necessity, and the factors leading to that decision frequently may effect the morale of the elderly person and his or her family.

In view of the fact that the majority of older adults view residence in a nursing home as a last resort and, in all probability, terminal placement, its impact on the older person can have a number of negative implications, which the audiologist or other health professionals who may attempt to provide diagnostic and rehabilitative services must be cognizant of. Those include:

1. Depression
2. Loneliness
3. A growing lack of desire to receive rehabilitative services when they may be indicated
4. The shock and stress associated with the move from a residence where the person may have lived for many years to the nursing home
5. A lessening of self-image due to the routine of the nursing home
6. Gradual dependency upon persons who, for all practical purposes, are strangers
7. A lessening of awareness of occurrences in the outside world due to the isolating effect of the nursing home
8. Personality changes resulting from isolation and/or certain medications
9. A loss of independence
10. A loss of personal control including who his or her roommate will be, time for sleeping and eating, and other aspects of life
11. The depressing influence of illness
12. The dehumanization of people which can occur in more institutionalized nursing homes
13. A lack of personal stimulation, which occurs from a loss of close interpersonal communication
14. A reduction of sensory capabilities which come with age, including sense of smell, touch, sight, and hearing

These effects, and many others not mentioned, are difficult ones to overcome. The audiologist who expects the hearing impaired elderly resident of a nursing home to readily accept his or her services to assess and restore communicative function to his or her maximum potential without hesitation is, in most instances, being naive. When depressed communicative function due to presbycusis is only one of many distressing aspects of the elderly person's present life state, should he or she be forced to make a choice as to which is most important? No, a choice should not be forced. However, when an inability to communicate with other people, watch television, or participate in other enjoyable activities may be one of the reasons for increasing depression and decreased feelings of self-worth, then it is reasonable that the service offered by the audiologist should be presented to residents as being very important. When so much else is taken away, an enhanced ability to communicate with other people can encourage increased personal, emotional, and physical function and a desire for survival.

ESTABLISHING AURAL REHABILITATION PROGRAMS IN HEALTH CARE FACILITIES

The population of hearing-handicapped persons who reside in various levels of health care facilities were, for many years, either ignored or avoided because it was felt that they possessed little rehabilitative potential. Others believed that they were experiencing so many other problems that it was probably best to leave them alone. Further, many audiology services on behalf of elderly clients have been provided as parts of practicum experiences by graduate students in audiology training programs. In the greatest majority of instances, however, those students did not possess the insights into aging and aging persons to provide effective aural rehabilitation services. Rather, they may have begun with "lesson number one" in a book of speechreading lessons and proceeded to provide "speechreading instruction" that had little or no meaning for the clients involved. The majority of clients, then, had to be "rounded-up" before each weekly session, and the gradually disillusioned graduate student clinician wondered why so many would not leave their room to come to "class." This experience is discouraging to say the least. The clinician may have felt that the book of speechreading lessons must contain *something* that would benefit the older clients or else it would not have been written. More importantly, the clients were told that the aural rehabilitation program may help them to learn to communicate more efficiently with others in spite of impaired hearing, only to realize later that it did not.

It is no wonder, then, that so few audiologists graduating from training programs have had a desire to initiate audiology service programs in health care facilities. The fact is that many of those graduate students may not have had a positive practicum experience in that setting. They also may not have had a positive instructor model who provided concrete information and personal examples on how to provide meaningful services to elderly clients. Further, many professionals who could have served handicapped older adults did not take the time to *listen* to their potential clients, to find out what their functional needs and desires were. That information is probably the most critical for developing a viable rehabilitation program for elderly clients.

It must be made clear that residents of health care facilities are individuals who have specific goals and needs. Among the 92 percent of health care facility residents who possess some degree of hearing impairment, the sense of need and urgency for interpersonal communication is as great as for other human beings. After all, is verbal communication not one of the traits that identify us as humans? The isolation which occurs as the result of impaired hearing can be even more devastating to persons who are already isolated due to their confinement to a nursing home. Their sense of urgency to break through the barriers to communication caused by an inability to hear and understand what others are saying may be much greater than evidenced by their statements or emotions. They, further, may have suppressed a desire to accept those services since they may feel that perhaps nothing will help at this late stage of their life.

In chapter 26, suggested procedures for aural rehabilitation services for the older adult client were presented. If geared toward the specific needs and priorities of the client, those services will benefit many of them. Prior to their initiation, however, the clients must be encouraged to develop the courage and desire to at least "give it a try." If the desire is awakened or reawakened, it is then the responsibility of the audiologist to demonstrate to the client that his or her communication needs and priorities are of prime importance in the treatment program. And that, within reason, improvements can be made if they also accept responsibility as adults to participate in the treatment program.

Above and beyond the service aspect is the important fact that the audiologist must remember that he or she is working with adults—no matter what the age or temperament—adults who, beyond their desire or control have become older. And, with age, an increasing inability to efficiently hear and understand what others are saying has added to the isolation and depression they may be experiencing after being taken from their home and placed in, what may be to them, their terminal environment—a health care facility.

If the audiologist offers the time, energy, and commitment to learn about the process of aging and listen to what his or her clients are saying relative to their needs, desires, and concerns, then viable aural rehabilitation treatment programs can be developed.

Another important aspect of this facinating work must be acknowledged. That is, the audiologist must be realistic in her or his efforts on behalf of elderly persons. There are some, no matter how much we would like to effectively serve all persons, who, because of physical or mental problems, do not have the potential to benefit from aural rehabilitation services. The audiologist must be aware of who these persons are and provide services to those who can benefit from them, no matter to what slight degree. It must also be remembered that even a hearing impaired, terminally ill, bedridden person's last weeks or months may be brightened by a health care facility nursing staff who has learned from the audiologists' inservices how to communicate more efficiently with hearing impaired persons. That is in itself a tremendously significant service.

Determination of the Need for Services

As is described in Chapter 32, a marketing survey lays the ground work for establishing service programs. In most health care facilities, however, it can be assumed that there are at least a number of persons who reside there who are hearing impaired and can benefit from some aspect of an assessment and aural rehabilitation program. As stated earlier, effective inservice education can enhance communication between health care facility personnel and hearing impaired residents and, thus, ease one reason for frayed nerves on both parts. Suggestions for alterations in the furniture arrangement in a lounge area to enhance communication can be of great service in a health care facility where residents may have previously avoided the area where the greatest amount of activity and communication was to have taken place. Effective hearing aid orientation programs can provide the impetus for previously inefficient users of hearing aids to benefit from them in their daily activities. An effective assessment program can identify hearing impaired persons who may have been thought to be noncommunicating or confused for other more debilitating reasons. Further, well-designed aural rehabilitation treatment programs can provide for enhanced skill in the use of residual hearing and supplemental visual clues for those who can benefit from that service.

For others, the aural rehabilitation program may consist of discussions of their most difficult communication environments and suggestions for manipulation of the physical environment or those persons with whom they have difficulty communicating. These programs, if geared toward clients' specific communication needs, can be extremely beneficial for confined elderly residents, and some persons can generally benefit from the services discussed above.

Surveying for Hearing Impairment

The determination of the need for any of the services discussed above must begin with a survey of the residents of the health care facilitty and, in specific terms, a demonstration of the results of the survey to the health care facility administration. Those include the director, the head of nursing, the activity director, and the social services director. It is suggested that all residents who can respond to a threshold evaluation be included in that survey.

A typical screening for hearing has generally not been found to be a satisfactory method for use in a health care facility since such large numbers fail. The most efficient procedure has been described by Traynor (Note 1) and includes establishment of pure-tone thresholds and the use of impedance audiometry to confirm the type of loss or the presence or absence of middle pathology. Even if a quiet environment for assessment can be found, the use of impedance audiometry is important because of the probability of even low noise levels interfering with bone conduction testing.

For those who are found to possess hearing impairment, assessment of speech discrimination ability with and without visual clues provides relevant information for discussion of individual client's handicap and need for aural rehabilitation services. Speech discrimination, in the absence of a sound-treated room and audiometer with speech capabilities, can be assessed with relative accuracy by live voice, with the audiologist seated approximately 5 to 6 feet from the client. Monosyllabic words, sentences, and brief conversation with and without visual clues and with and/or without the use of amplification, administered at a comfortable listening level for the client, is a reasonable mode of administration, but only in the hands of a skilled audiologist.

Results of the survey then are presented to the administration of the health care facility and, if that facility is a part of a corporate body, a representative of the corporation. If the administration is convinced that an aural rehabilitation program is desired, the program format is outlined. It is stressed here that the initial screening/threshold survey be conducted only after the administration has contracted for the assessment program, and the avenue for reimbursement of that service has been established. In discussing the assessment program and reimbursement, it should be emphasized that Medicare and, in most states, Medicaid cover diagnostic evaluations, including special assessment procedures, in accordance with charges which are reasonable and typical in that geographic area. The testing must be justified on an individual basis. Routine testing will not be reimbursed. Audiologists who are certified or eligible for certification as audiologists by the American Speech-Language-Hearing Association, or licensed by states where licensure laws exist, are eligible to become Medicare approved providers of audiology services by award of a Medicare provider number (Hull, 1978). If the audiologist has been awarded a provider number, he or she can bill for services directly. If the health care facility is Medicare approved, its own accounting office can bill for the service. In whatever manner, then, an agreement for reimbursement for the audiological survey should, in all instances, be arranged prior to the survey. Chapters 31 and 32 provide a thorough explanation of the contracting and reimbursement process and laws involved. The survey alone will provide important information for the health care facility staff. Residents who may have previously been described as confused and/or disoriented may be found to possess a severe enough auditory impairment to account for at least a portion of that behavior. Modifications in patterns of communication by health care facility staff alone may result in positive behavior change on the part of those residents. The modifications in communication strategies can, for example, result from an effective staff inservice program. An antagonistic elderly man, previously described as stubborn, inattentive, withdrawn, and antisocial, may begin to interact more with his environment. Others may demonstrate positive personality change as the result of a properly fitted hearing aid and, again, through modifications of speaking habits by health care facility staff as the result of an effective inservice program.

With information on the incidence, severity, and communicative impact of hearing loss within that health care facility available for discussion with the administration—including the possible positive impact of a viable aural rehabilitation on the residents, the health care facility staff, and the programs within the facility—a full assessment and aural rehabilitation program can be outlined and initiated. Those remaining components are treated as follows. It should be remembered that all effective aural rehabilitation programs begin with a knowledgeable assessment.

Inservice and Involvement of Health Care Facility Personnel

Inservice training for health care facility administration and staff not only supports the assessment and aural rehabilitation treatment program, but also provides carry-over of the treatment aspects into the daily life of the clients. Inservice provides administration and staff with insights into: (1) the cause and effects of presbycusis on residents' ability for communication, (2) the resulting psychosocial impact, (3) the structure of the aural rehabilitation program, (4) hearing aids—what they can and cannot do, (5) trouble-shooting procedures for hearing aid malfunction, and (6) methods for more efficient communication with hearing impaired residents. Included during inservices are discussions of individual residents who are involved as clients in the program. Those discussions include the hearing impairment those clients possess, its impact on their communicative function, their progress (or lack of it) as a result of the aural rehabilitation treatment program, and the development of plans for follow-through and carry-over of those clients' programs into their daily life within the health care facility. The health care facility staff, including the director of nurses, activity director, physical therapist, occupational therapist, and other personnel including the cooks and janitors, can all be vital forces in the carry-over process.

The techniques offered through inservice for more efficient communication with hearing impaired elderly persons can impact positively on the lives of both the staff and the elderly residents. It is generally found, to everyone's relief, that some of the emotional encounters resulting from futile attempts at communication between hearing impaired residents and staff members are sometimes soothed after the techniques for communication that the staff learned during inservice and that the elderly clients are learning during their treatment sessions are utilized.

Topics for inservice training should include

The structure of the auditory mechanism and theories as to the cause of presbycusis.

The manifestations of presbycusis and its impact on the elderly person's ability to function communicatively is another important point. This discussion includes presentations of audiometric configurations and examples of what the client who possesses presbycusis might hear, compared with a normally hearing person.

Hearing aids, their uses and mis-uses, are discussed relative to what hearing aids are, what they sound like, what they can do, and what they cannot do. The reasons why some persons cannot benefit from hearing aids are also presented, along with the necessity for a thorough hearing aid evaluation by a hearing professional. Instruction on the use of hearing aids, placing the earmold properly in the ear, the switches (including the use of the gain control), the battery, the care of ear molds, and others are presented, in turn, to alleviate some of the difficulties some elderly residents have due to manual dexterity or memory problems. The staff of health care facilities can, further, aid the carry-over of hearing aid orientation for recently fitted residents if they are familiar with the component parts and their use.

Hearing aid trouble-shooting procedures also are stressed. Those include:

1. Knowledge of the causes of acoustic feedback
2. Battery longevity and placement
3. Checking for broken receiver cords
4. Procedures for cleaning ear molds
5. Correct use of the telephone switch, and others

The nurse aide, for example, can reduce the stresses involved in adjusting to a hearing aid by possessing the knowledge required to conduct a quick check on an aid that a frustrated elderly resident feels is not working. A simple adjustment of battery placement, or reminding the resident that the earmold needs cleaning can eliminate non-use of an otherwise beneficial hearing aid. Since these adjustments and reminders may be necessary at times when the audiologist is not present in the health care facility, this aspect of inservice is extremely important.

The components of an aural rehabilitation program are discussed so that administration and staff are aware of the intricacies involved not only in the assessment of auditory function, but also in the treatment sessions per se. These insights, and a resulting staff who is knowledgeable of the role of the audiologist, permits an enhanced working relationship between audiologist and staff. A program that flows more smoothly generally results.

The role of the staff in carry-over is also discussed. This includes the fact that the staff can be the vital catalyst in providing an enhanced climate for communication in the health care facility.

Methods for effective communication with hearing impaired elderly persons is a critical part of inservice training. The stresses that grow out of frustrated attempts at communication, both on the part of residents and staff, can stifle an otherwise pleasant living environment. The suggestions provided the staff include the Thirteen Commandments for Communicating with Hearing Impaired Older Adults (Hull, 1980). (See the appendix following this chapter.)

PROVISION OF AURAL REHABILITATION TREATMENT SERVICES IN THE HEALTH CARE FACILITY

The specific strategies for providing aural rehabilitation treatment services on behalf of older adult clients in the health care facility remain essentially the same as those outlined by this author in Chapter 26. They are procedures which lend themselves well for any level of client. There are, however, some considerations that one must be aware of when providing aural rehabilitation services for confined elderly clients, including:

1. Motivation of clients
2. The environment of the health care facility
3. The health-state of individual clients
4. Family involvement
5. Compounding visual problems
6. The impact of death on both the client and audiologist and its inevitability

Motivation

Some audiologists prefer not to attempt to provide aural rehabilitation services to elderly persons who reside in health care facilities. Their reasoning is based on the lack of motivation of so many potential clients to receive these services. As we observe these clients, many of them have good reason for their lack of motivation. We can, however, blame ourselves as audiologists in some instances for not being able to provide motivation. Alpiner (Note 2) has described a number of reasons for lack of motivation among many elderly persons, presented in Chapter 16 of this book. Lack of available finances, the death of a spouse or friends, lack of efficient modes of transportation, children living a great distance away, and physical problems which may restrict mobility are among those which impact on the older adult.

As we view the elderly resident of health care facilities, we observe other more dramatic effects which impact on their motivation to receive rehabilitation services. According to Atchley (1972), the most depressing aspect of placement in a health care facility (nursing home) is the move from a home where the person may have lived for many years to a strange, and to that person, a probable terminal residence. The events leading to placement in the health care facility were in all probability equally depressing, including, perhaps, the loss of a home due to rezoning laws or lack of finances, severe enough illness to require constant nursing care, or slowly decreasing health simply because of advancing age. And, if the elderly resident has read the statistics on the longevity of residents of nursing homes, he or she will know that the probability of survival after the first month of placement is only about 73 percent. Further, only about 20 percent ever leave health care facilities except for burial (Moss & Halamandaris, 1977).

The well elderly in the community do not experience that reason for depression, nor are they experiencing that single dramatic change in their lives. The fear of the necessity for that change can, however, result in motivation to work toward preventing it.

Motivation of potential clients who have been placed within a health care facility to receive aural rehabilitation services can, indeed, be a problem, particularly when positive results may be slow to emerge. Audiologists must also be realistic in their attempts at motivating clients. Some hearing impaired residents of health care facilities do not possess real potential for rehabilitation. Their state of physical or mental health may contraindicate their participation and the benefits they otherwise may have derived. For audiologists who attempt to motivate and provide services for *all* persons, the results may be disappointing. Inservices to provide staff with insights into more efficient communication with those residents may be sufficient, at least for the present, and would relieve some of the depression those residents were experiencing.

For those who can benefit from aural rehabilitation services, however, efforts toward motivation should be made. If for no other reason than to enhance communication abilities with family and friends in that confined environment, to be able to enjoy watching television once again, or to participate more efficiently in social activities within the health care facility, motivation toward receiving aural rehabilitation services should be given a high priority. It must be kept in mind, however, as was discussed in Chapter 16, the aural rehabilitation treatment program must be developed around those clients' priority communication needs, and no others.

Once an elderly client is motivated to receive aural rehabilitation services, working lesson by lesson through an activity manual on speechreading can be deadly, and motivation can be quickly lost. The audiologist has, then, lost the trust of the clients. ''She said that aural rehabilitation treatment would help, and that learning to communicate in spite of hearing impairment would be a priority, and all we did was try to figure out what the sounds, words, and sentences were from a book she was giving our lessons from. Is that aural rehabilitation?'' That is a common complaint by previously motivated clients who desired to be helped. But, the audiologist did not help. Thompson, in Chapter 15 of this text, presents an excellent discussion on motivtional counseling for elderly persons.

The Environment

Discovering an area within the facility where aural rehabilitation services can be provided in a pleasant and the least restrictive environment for clients is also frequently a problem. Most health care facilities do, however, possess an area that is at least a pleasant place to be. That area may be an activity room, a lounge that is not the main lounge or lobby area, a staff dining room, or other sections of the health care facility which are not considered by the residents as ones where, for example, people go when they are ''not well.'' Places to avoid include the infirmary and the chapel. The chapel has special meaning for many persons, and it is not a place where therapy is held. Further, the infirmary is usually thought of as a place to avoid, and it is not a place where one goes voluntarily once or twice a week for self-improvement. This is particularly true among older adults.

The only available space where frequent disturbances will not be observed may be in relatively undesirable space such as the laundry room or the rear portion of the cafeteria. In that instance, modifications will be necessary. This is not always greeted with enthusiasm by health care facility administrators, particularly when many are faced with tight budgets. Such modifications for improvement of the therapy environment, however, may be necessary for the aural rehabilitation program to be effective to any degree.

Some remodeling of an otherwise drab room can be done relatively inexpensively. Some wallpaper, a moveable partition, some paint, and carpeting can do wonders for the environment. There are few health care facilities that do not possess at least a small amount of money for such improvements. If the audiologist has some talent for painting and minor carpentry, then labor costs may be reduced. Even some of the health care facility residents may enjoy chipping in on the labor. A retired carpenter or painter may find it a joy to lend an experienced hand. Women who have had experience making throw rugs may enjoy reawakening that skill for the good of the ''audiology room.'' If the health care facility agrees to hire professionals to do the remodeling work, then such innovations may not be necessary.

Within the University of Northern Colorado Aural Rehabilitation Program for the Aging, rennovations for the installation of sound-treated rooms and audiometers, including carpentry, electrical work, painting, and others were funded by the health care facilities involved. When one health care facility was being constructed, the corporate owner's plans included a sound-treated room as part of the initial construction in support of their aural rehabilitation program. The room was, further, to double as a staff lounge. That aspect, for obvious reasons, was not a satisfactory arrangement, and the staff later found other quarters for coffee and conversation.

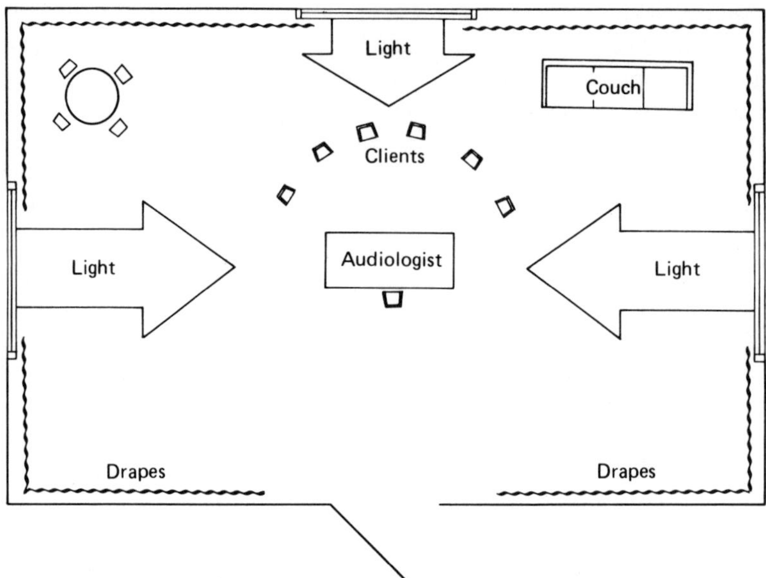

Fig. 28-1. Desirable room arrangement for aural rehabilitation services for older adults.

Another health care facility remodeled a large linen closet, one provided a large vacant resident room, another provided remodeled space in what originally was an alcove area off of a hallway, while yet another built new walls for a new room for the audiology services. Interest level in the program varies from facility to facility, but the general commitment remains the same. Figure 28-1 illustrates a desirable room arrangement for the provision of aural rehabilitation services, including counseling, hearing aid orientation, and speechreading/auditory training.

The Health-State of Clients

As stated earlier, the audiologist must be realistic regarding the elderly client's potential to respond to aural rehabilitation services. A terminally ill resident of a skilled nursing wing of a health care facility may possess impaired hearing, but not be able to respond to a diagnostic evaluation. It is not reasonable to ask that person to participate in a complex aural rehabilitation program. A knowledgeable staff, however, as the result of effective inservice, may ease some of the frustrations the resident may be experiencing due to an inability to understand what they are saying. If the state of health of some individuals was the catalyst for placement in the health care facility, but those persons can, indeed, benefit from audiology services, additional considerations will be necessary.

For example, accomodations for persons who are confined to a wheelchair are mandatory. Ramps into sound-treated testing booths, tables used in therapy which conform to the height of wheelchairs, and doors which permit maneuvering in and out of the rooms are necessary. Other considerations for elderly residents of health care facilities are as follows.

Attention Span

Many elderly persons cannot tolerate long periods of concentrated effort on any task. Audiometric evaluations where attention to an almost inaudible pure-tone is required, or aural rehabilitation sessions which have as their purpose instruction on more efficient means for communication can become intolerable for some elderly persons, even when the program is specifically designed around their needs. This is equally frustrating to some audiologists who have difficulty understanding the reason for the low attention/tolerance span. The problem does exist, however, and must be accounted for.

Audiological evaluations may be required to be broken up into two, even three shorter periods, particularly if a hearing aid evaluation is included. Speechreading/auditory training sessions should not extend for more than 45 minutes. If clients appear to be less tolerant on a specific day, short breaks during which time something else is talked about will be necessary. An alert audiologist will realize when those "stretch breaks" are required.

Other Modifications for an Effective Aural Rehabilitation Program

The following additional considerations previously described by this author (1977) are also important.

Number of clients. The number of clients that facilitate optimal group interaction ranges from six to eight, the aural rehabilitation groups should not exceed this number. If at all possible, it is necessary to control admittance to specific groups to assure that hearing levels among participants are as equal as possible. It can become frustrating for the group members, the audiologist, and the client if one client has extreme difficulty communicating, and thus great difficulty participating in the group. The audiologist, out of necessity, will tend to spend most of the group time attempting to facilitate that person's participation. The latter does not enhance positive and facilitory group interaction. As the clients progress in their communicative skill, the development of advanced classes may be warranted, depending upon the needs of the clients.

Individual versus group treatment. The more severely impaired individual will require individual aural rehabilitation treatment. If the person progresses to the point that group involvement is possible, then he or she should be referred to that treatment setting. Some audiologists prefer to begin all clients' treatment on an individual basis so as to attend to any immediate needs they may have.

Physical environment—acoustics and lighting. Consideration of the acoustic environment of the aural rehabilitation treatment facility is critical. At least initially, the environment should be a quiet one, free of undue reverberation, and with adequate lighting. Fluorescent lighting is not suggested for use with elderly clients. Both the hue of the light and the "flicker" can cause visual difficulties. Indirect and incandescent lighting is suggested, but glare from hard tables, floors, walls, and ceilings is to be avoided at all costs. Aging results in a thickening of the lens of the eye and a narrowing of the pupil aperture. Further, the muscles of the eye do not function as well so that accommodation of light changes is not as efficient. Woodruff (1975) stated that it takes more light energy to have the same effect on the older eye as the younger eye. In other words, the older eye is less responsive to light, and cannot compensate for changes in light as quickly as it could when it was younger. It behooves the audiologist, therefore, to avoid moving from light to shadows as he or she is involved in aural rehabilitation treatment sessions.

The suggested acoustic environment is one that consists of carpeted floors, textured walls or walls that are carpeted one-third to one-half up from the floors, spackled acoustic tile ceilings or spackled dry wall, and chairs that at least have a padded seat and back. From this initial design, the audiologist can modify it to suit his or her own acoustic desires relative to aural rehabilitative tasks engaged in.

A little reverberation gives sound ''life;'' too much causes distortion of speech. A study by Bergman, Blumenfeld, Cascardo, Dash, Levitt, and Margulies (1976) determined that unfavorable acoustics (reverberated speech) contributed most to difficulties in speech discrimination among older hearing impaired persons.

The time of day for treatment. The process involved in aural rehabilitation treatment is fatiguing for both the client and the audiologist. In providing those services, particularly on behalf of the older adult clients, the factors of fatigue and alertness must be kept in mind. That includes remembering that most people function better at certain times of the day, and that attention span and periods of maximum alertness are different as one becomes older.

In working with the older adult, the period immediately following lunch and anytime in the evening will provide the least benefit for the client. The inefficiency of those times will be seen most dramatically among the confined or less active older person.

The time periods that will be most advantageous for the client and the audiologist are those toward the middle of the morning and perhaps one to two hours after lunch. The audiologist should be alert to the behaviors of his or her clients and change times as needed. It is generally best to ask the client to suggest the time of day when he or she feels best. However, we must also be reminded that the audiologist has a schedule to meet during daily working hours.

The length of aural rehabilitation sessions must also be considered. This author has found that most alert–active older adults can work for at least one hour, as long as periodic breaks are taken that include brief chats about things other than the treatment session. Many older clients will not be able to tolerate strenuous sessions for longer than 30 minutes. The alert audiologist will be able to judge the tolerance levels of his or her clients.

The Family

Although the role of the family or other significant others in the aural rehabilitation process is discussed throughout this text, it is a critically important aspect to be presented as per the elderly resident who is confined to the health care facility. The discouraging component of this discussion, however, is the fact that many family members of these persons either do not wish to become involved or live such a great distance away that they cannot be involved in any consistent manner. The former reason, it is sad to say, is generally the most frequent. It is disheartening, not only on the part of the audiologist, but more so on the part of the elderly client, to observe a family member who agreed to come to the health care facility to become involved in the aural rehabilitation process, to gradually dissolve the commitment. If such a possiblitiy exists, it is generally better to not ask the family member to participate at all. A genuine commitment is necessary before such participation is initiated, mostly for the mental health of the elderly resident. The anguish felt by elderly persons, who eventually realize that their child or other family member apparently did not possess a geniune desire to become involved, is heartbreaking.

If family involvement is possible, however, the enhanced awareness among them regarding the potential for communication by their elderly family member can enhance family bonds. The importance of this involvement cannot be stressed enough.

Compounding Problems of Vision

As discussed in Chapter 30, the multiple handicaps of vision and hearing impairment are very real among elderly persons. The majority of these persons who may possess significant visual problems are generally found within health care facilities. This is particularly true if they have not been able to remain mobile and self-sufficient in their own homes. These clients have told this author that the isolation they feel is deadly, and some would prefer death when both audition and vision become nonfunctional.

For those persons who possess rehabilitative potential, the aural rehabilitation process revolves around work toward enhancement of auditory function; basically auditory training, since visual clues may be of little advantage. The audiologist's efforts must be combined with those of a vision specialist who can work to aid the person in becoming more mobile, including furniture arrangements in his or her room, use of cosmetics, and self-help skills. That team effort, along with the help of the activity director can supplant the terrible isolation which may otherwise face the elderly resident. The audiologist can play a vital role in providing input to those person's rehabilitation programs.

The Impact of Death

The possibility of death and/or its inevitable presence not only impacts on potential clients desire for services in health care facilities, but also on the person who can potentially serve those elderly persons in a rehabilitative role. Many elderly persons, as stated earlier, feel that placement in the health care facility—particularly after the many events which may have led to such placement—is terminal. That feeling is generally supported by the all too frequent visits at the health care facility by the ambulance or hearse, which usually are visible to the residents. They wonder if they are next, especially when a person who may have become a friend in the health care facility was one who was recently "taken away."

Death and the fear of death certainly takes its toll among those who may otherwise benefit from the services of any professional who offers rehabilitation services. A common response by elderly residents when the benefits they may derive from aural rehabilitative services are described to them is, "Why should I work to become better when I may die at any time? What is the use?" On the other hand, many audiologists do not desire to become professionally involved with persons who they may grow to care for and respect; persons who may not be there tomorrow for the next session. How is this barrier on both parties part dissolved?

A Positive Approach

Helping elderly people accept the inevitability of death is not the responsibility of the audiologist. However, the manner in which the audiologist approaches the provision of services can change opinions of older clients regarding their potential to benefit from them. To learn to communicate more efficiently, to be able to interact with family and friends with greater ease can give more meaning to life and increased satisfaction as a result of those interactions. That, in and of itself, can add greatly to an individual's life, particularly for a confined individual.

It is a part of human nature to fight back against adversity. For many confined elderly persons the inability to hear and participate in social or personal conversation is a great adversity. A hearing aid may have been tried as an attempt for a ''quick cure.'' When it may have been found not to help as well as it was hoped that it might, some persons may give up the fight, particularly when they are facing other adverse elements including declining health, decreased mobility, and loneliness.

The audiologist who approaches confined elderly clients with an attitude of positive anticipation regarding assessment and aural rehabilitation services will do much to override a client's possible preoccupation with thoughts of impending death. This is especially true when the services are centered around those client's communication priorities. Further, with many confined elderly persons' resignation to an apparent attitude that people within the health care facility will continue to do things *to* them, without a great deal of explanation, rather than *for* them, an audiologist who presents him- or herself as one who wishes to provide a beneficial service to that adult may observe a change in attitude regarding their potential to be helped.

Elderly Clients as Adults

Probably the most important word in the previous statement is ''adult.'' Elderly persons who are confined and who may be quite lonely and fearful that death surely must be imminent are all too often treated not as adults, but as something other than that state which they have attained. Negative responses to food they may not desire to eat, vaccinations or medication which are administered without consideration for human dignity, and roommates they do not desire to have are often considered to be child-like. Staff too frequently respond as parent figures by either scolding or responding in condescending tones as though speaking to a child. The hurt and the disappointment felt by elderly persons in response to those actions may not be expressed for fear of reprisal. Some elderly persons resign themselves to the treatment as inevitable and continue to live with the emotional pain.

Nurses, nurses aides, activity directors, social workers, physicians, speech pathologists and audiologists, and others who serve elderly persons may be guilty of those responses to elderly persons. The thoughts of elderly persons who have confided in this author illustrate their feelings toward ''well-meaning'' persons who work for them. ''Do they feel sorry for me? If so, they should really feel sorry for themselves. I feel sorry for them because they don't seem to know how to care without making me feel bad about their caring.'' As one confined elderly client stated, ''I dread being here. Nurses come into my room and hurt me with the shots they give, and don't tell me why they are giving them to me. Why don't they bother to tell me—to talk to me? When they do talk to me, they sound like they're talking to a child—as though they know I'm going to die tomorrow and don't want to tell me.'' Another client aptly spoke of her feelings about life and herself when she stated, ''I know I'm not pretty any more. When I look in the mirror, I look like death. I know that it will come soon. I'm lonely, I'm hungry for love; and I know that people do not like to look at me. It is time to die.''

It is unquestionably important to remember that these persons and others who are crying out for considerate attention are adults, and they must be treated as such. They are adults who have become older, may have wrinkled skin, may possess health problems that frighten them, and, for various reasons, may feel very vulnerable and alone. For obvious reasons they know that death is more probable than when they were younger—a depressing thought to anyone. They however, adults, and deserve that status. They are, further, dying, as is every human, tree, and insect from the day birth occurs. Most persons, however, do not dwell on that inevitable fact until death appears to be nearer than before. Suddenly an awareness that life may end tomorrow; that this may be the last day of living results in a sense of urgency, of fear, of a resolution to either fight back or give up. In the majority of instances, however, the latter is the most frequently observed. Life's precious moments are not precious anymore. This usually occurs out of default rather than choice, however, when a reason to fight back and to improve one's life state would have been the most desirable alternative.

It is interesting to note that most elderly adults have accepted the fact that death is inevitable and have developed a rather healthy attitude toward it. The depression and mourning generally occur when they find that there is nothing left to live for. For those elderly who feel that the isolation they are experiencing as a result of depressed hearing is the dawning of the end, and audiologist can provide the catalyst for renewed hope that they can, indeed, fight back.

Why Bother with Me?

A common expression heard by most helping professionals when their services are offered to elderly persons is ''Why bother with me? I am old and may die any day. You should give your time and help to children.'' This author's response to those and similar statements is, ''Don't deprive yourself of all the good that is in store for you during this time.''

Statements about Dying

If statements about dying are made, they should not be ignored. The ignored statement may reconvince the elderly person that death may be more probable than they wanted to think about. And, those reconfirmed thoughts can be defeating. Also, do not laugh them off with a shrug of the shoulders and an off-the-cuff jest about, ''You don't have to worry about that.'' Those statements by elderly persons are only made because the concern is real, and they have been thinking about it. The response that they desire to hear contains (1) a realization that the concern is real, and (2) the fact that you still desire to serve them. The statement, occasionally resembling a ''joke'' on their part, is sometimes a test of the person who has offered his or her services. The test involves their concern that perhaps your interest in serving them is not genuine, and they are thereby giving you a way out. As stated so many times by elderly persons, either overtly or covertly, ''I am afraid that I may be a burden to you.'' If that feeling is at any time evident on the face or the words of those serving those persons, they will avoid the service and the person providing them.

A healthy attitude toward the inevitability of death, an acceptance of the fact that these persons, too, deserve the best services of the audiologist for the years, months, weeks, or days of life that remain for them, must be developed by any audiologist who serves elderly clients. The elderly clients we serve must be considered fortunate, for they have experienced more years of life than many others. The audiologist can learn much from these people if he or she takes advantage of that invaluable opportunity.

CONCLUSION

This chapter has presented some important considerations for the provision of services on behalf of persons who reside in health care facilities. It is stressed, however, that as with other clients, these persons' communication priorities must be addressed. Even though they are residing within the confines of the health care facility, they are still individuals and, most importantly, they are individual adults with unique goals and concerns. The audiologist and other professionals who serve these people must be constantly aware of that fact. The clients must be fully aware that they are involved in treatment, not simply another activity within the ''home.'' They must be aware of the reasons for the communication problems that they are experiencing, the steps that will be taken to help them, and the strategies involved. Only then will the services and the audiologist be accepted.

REFERENCES

Atchley, R. C. *The social forces in later life*. Belmont, California: Wadsworth, 1972, p. 123.

Bergman, M., Blumenfeld, V., Cascardo, D., Dash, B., Levitt, H., & Margulies, M. Age-related decrement in hearing for speech. *Journal of Gerontology,* 1976, *31*, 533–538.

Chafee, C. Rehabilitation needs of nursing home patients: A report of a survey. *Rehabilitation Literature,* 1967, *18*, 377–389.

Hull, R. H. *Hearing Impairment Among Aging Persons*. Lincoln, Nebraska: Cliffs Notes, Inc., 1977.

Hull, R. H. The thirteen commendments for talking to the hearing impaired older person. *Journal of the American Speech and Hearing Association,* 1980, *22*, 427.

Moss, F. E., & Halamandaris, F. E. *Too old, too sick, too bad: Nursing homes in America*. Germantown, Md: Aspen Systems, 1977.

Woodruff, D. S. A physiological perspective of the psychology of aging, in D. S. Woodruff & J. E. Birren (Eds.), *Aging: scientific perspectives and social issues*. New York: D. Van Nostrand, 1975, pp. 179–198.

REFERENCE NOTES

1. Traynor, R. M. *A method of audiological assessment for the non-ambulatory geriatric patient*. Unpublished dissertation, University of Northern Colorado, Greeley, 1976.
2. Alpiner, J. G. *The feasibility of rehabilitating the elderly hearing impaired*. Presented at Workshops on Geriatric Aural Rehabilitation, University of Northern Colorado, Greeley, September 14, 1973.

APPENDIX: THE THIRTEEN COMMANDMENTS FOR COMMUNICATING WITH HEARING IMPAIRED OLDER ADULTS

- Speak at a slightly greater than normal intensity.
- Speak at your normal rate, but not too rapidly.
- Do not speak to the elderly person at a greater distance than 6 feet but no less than 3 feet.
- Concentrate light on the speaker's face for greater visibility of lip movements, facial expression, and gestures.
- Do not speak to the elderly person unless you are visible to him or her, e.g., not from another room while he or she is reading the newspaper or watching TV.
- Do not force the elderly person to listen to you when there is a great deal of environmental noise. That type of environment can be difficult for a younger, normally hearing person. It can, on the other hand, be defeating for the hearing impaired elderly.
- Never, under any circumstances, speak directly into the person's ear. Not only cannot the person make use of visual clues, but the speaker may be causing an already distorting auditory system to further distort the speech signal. In other words, clarity may be depressed as loudness is increased.
- If the elderly person does not appear to understand what is being said, rephrase the statement rather than simply repeating the misunderstood words. An otherwise frustrating situation can be avoided in that way.
- Do not overarticulate. Overarticulation not only distorts the sounds of speech, but also the speaker's face, thus making the use of visual clues more difficult.
- Arrange the room (living room or meeting room) where communication will take place so that no speaker or listener is more than 6 feet apart, and all are completely visible. Using this direct approach, communication for all parties involved will be enhanced.
- Include the elderly person in all discussions about him or her. Hearing impaired persons sometimes feel quite vulnerable. This approach will aid to alleviate some of those feelings.
- In meetings or any group activity where there is a speaker presenting information (church meetings, civic organizations, etc.) make it mandatory that the speaker(s) use the public address system. One of the most frequent complaints among elderly persons is that they may enjoy attending meetings of various kinds, but all too often the speaker, for whatever reason, tries to avoid using a microphone. Many elderly persons do not desire to assert themselves by asking a speaker who has just said, "I am sure that you can all hear me if I do not use the microphone," to *please* use it. Most persons begin to avoid public or organizational meetings if they cannot hear what the speaker is saying. This point cannot be stressed enough.
- Above all, treat elderly persons as adults. They, of anyone, deserve that respect.

Reproduced with permission from Hull, R. H. The thirteen commandments for talking to the hearing impaired older person. *Journal of the American Speech and Hearing Association,* 1980, *22*, 42.

Jacqueline Heppler

Chapter 29: The Nurse in the Aural Rehabilitation Process

The nurse can play a vital role in support of the audiologists' services on behalf of the elderly. It is, therefore, felt to be important that audiologists be aware of the various avenues of nursing care to, in turn, more knowledgeably utilize her or his services. With the proliferation of new roles for health care workers, the newly awakened collective social conscience, and the growing numbers of people over age 65 years, it is time (actually past time) to explore nursing roles in the care of elderly persons with communication handicaps.

This chapter will discuss the roles of nurses and ancillary health care workers in various settings. The focus will be on health care, not sickness care. Thus, the emphasis will not be on nursing care in the acute care setting, hospitals and physician's offices, but rather on the potential for nursing intervention primarily through patient education and counseling in long-term care settings.*

It is noteworthy that in some states there is little or no differential in state reimbursement for Medicaid patients in skilled nursing facilities versus intermediate care facilities. Hence, one can expect that staffing patterns, both in levels of nursing personnel and in actual numbers of personnel in long-term facilities, may often preclude the rehabilitative care that is needed by the patients. It is stressed here that members of the nursing profession must take an active role both in health care planning and in legislative action on health matters through involvement in the political process. Nursing professionals, along with other health professionals, can help effect changes in reimbursement levels so that qualified personnel can be present in sufficient numbers so that they may intervene in a therapeutic role with patients, rather than on a custodial basis such as so often is found in long-term care facilities. The nurse and ancillary health care workers can find personal satisfaction and professional pride in helping restore the elderly impaired patient to his or her maximum level of functioning.

*Long-term care settings are defined in their broadest sense. home, adult day care, well oldster clinics, residential living units (hopefully staffed with a nurse on an ongoing basis), and finally, nursing homes encompassing different levels of care.

THE GERONTOLOGICAL NURSE PRACTITIONER

The role of a new health care worker, the gerontological nurse practitioner, should be discussed in some depth for the edification of physicians, audiologists, and other professionals who view the nurse in an expanded role of support for preventative and restorative services on behalf of the elderly, including the hearing impaired elderly.

This nursing speciality prepares registered nurses to help the patient who is experiencing the normal processes of aging, in a variety of settings. The coping mechanisms of the individual, the concomitant pathological diseases present, the availability of social supports, the health history and physical status, and the treatment regime are considered by the nurse practitioner as part of the data base that this nurse must integrate into the plan of nursing care. Heppler (1976) speaks both to the preparation and potential for practice by the gerontological nurse practitioner.

The gerontological nurse practitioner functions as a team member of the health-care team; as an independent, accountable health care professional, as a patient–client advocate, and in a collaborative role with the patient's physician. In addition, and perhaps most importantly, the nurse practitioner involves both client and his or her family in a goal-directed plan of care. The literature of chronic disease management abounds with studies citing lack of patient compliance with therapeutic regimes. It is critical to realize that unless the client–patient is made a true partner in his or her plan of care, the dresser-drawer syndrome, originally used to describe failure to utilize birth control measures, could aptly describe improper utilization of hearing aids and other prosthetic devices.

The following broad areas of expanded nurse practice, as noted in the Department of health, Education and Welfare's (DHEW) 1971 report, entitled, "Extending the Scope of Nursing Practice," delineates the capabilities of this new health care worker in long-term care. They are as follows.

1. Assessing physical status of patients at a more sophisticated level than is now common in nursing practice
2. Securing and maintaining a health history
3. Within protocols mutually agreed upon by medical and nursing staff, make adjustments in medications, initiate requests for certain laboratory tests and interpret them, make judgments about the use of accepted pharmaceutical agents as standard treatments in diagnosed conditions, assume primary responsibility for determining possible alternatives for care settings (institution or home), and initiating referral
4. Conducting nurse clinics for continuing care of patients
5. Conducting community clinics for case finding and screening for health problems
6. Assessing community needs in long-term care and participating in development of resources to meet them
7. Assuming continuing responsibiliy for acquainting patients and families with implications of health status, treatment, and prognosis
8. Assuming responsibility for the environment of the care setting as it affects the quality and effectiveness of care (pp. 11–12)

The following definition of health care, again found in the DHEW 1971 report, clearly speaks both to the totality of health care and its interdisciplinary nature.

> Health care in its entirety, from the point of view of providers and consumers alike, is the sum total of care rendered by all disciplines. It comprises more than diagnosis, treatment, and rehabilitation associated with acute and chronic illness; it includes health education,

health maintenance, prevention, and early case finding. As such, health care is not the province of any one profession, nor does it lend itself to delivery through a rigid professional hierarchy. (p. 3)

Nursing practice itself may be compartmentalized under three headings: (1) primary care, (2) acute care, and (3) long-term care. These categories, while broad, are not mutually exclusive but rather speak to the changing needs of patients and clients and the changing settings in which health care is offered.

The term primary care needs clairification since the definition is the crux of the nurse practitioner's practice. As noted by Booth (1972), two important facets of most definitions of primary care are (1) first contact with the health care system and (2) assurance of continuing contact. Primary care givers are concerned with patient education, prevention, and long-term management of chronic diseases in a continuous, coordinated manner. All of the above elements are important when caring for the hearing impaired elderly, and/or elderly persons who possess any chronic disability.

THE NURSE AND THE HEARING IMPAIRED ELDERLY CLIENT

What are the clues of hearing deficits that the nurse and the ancillary workers should be aware of on first contact with the elderly person? What must these workers remember when caring for the auditorially disabled over time? What are the multifaceted roles of the nurse as a member of a health care team when that team may vary widely both as to the kinds of professionals involved and the time spent by the various members in direct contact with the patient? The nursing role and responsibilities, therefore, may expand services on behalf of the hearing impaired elderly in the absence or presence of other health care workers in the various settings. Moreover, in Barney's (Note 1) insightful speech, the registered nurse was noted as the professional most frequently present in long-term care institutions. The physician's presence in the nursing home was so limited that the amount of time spent could not be noted in that published survey.

Hopefully, with the trend toward the inclusion of gerontological content in basic curricula for both physicians and nurses and the advent of geriatric medicine as a specialty, the care of the elderly across various health settings will improve. Certainly, the success of programs in aural rehabilitation of the elderly do much to sensitize the health care workers of all levels both to the need for intervention and the potential for restoring functional abilities in communication in the hearing impaired elderly. In that regard, the nurse can be a strong ally in the continuity and carry-over of aural rehabilitation programs, not only in health care facilities, but in other settings as well.

Ways in which the Nurse Can Facilitate Communication with Hearing Impaired Aging Persons

Since the etiology of presbycusis has been well covered elsewhere in this text along with the various procedures involved in aural rehabilitation, the remainder of this chapter will focus on suggestions on how nursing personnel can not only enhance communication between them and the hearing impaired elderly in various health settings, but also aid in the carry-over of aural rehabilitation programs. The suggestions by Hull and Traynor

(1977) can, for example, help to ease the frustrations of the nursing staff and, more importantly, the patient in their daily attempts at communication.

Given that nursing personnel within any given long-term care facility tend to follow a revolving pattern, it is submitted that the following suggestions for efficient communication with hearing impaired elderly be an integral part of the orientation process for new staff members. These are discussed below.

Give the Patient Time

The nursing staff in their continuing contact with the elderly, can allow the elderly person *time;* time to respond to requests, time to reminisce, time to give the pearls of wisdom about his or her needs and life in general. The technique and value of reminiscing as a methodology for group therapy with the aged is skillfully covered by Ebersole (1976). The reader is referred to that author for an in-depth coverage of this important treatment modality.

Stimulate the Patient

Nursing staff, housekeeping personnel, and families of the institutionalized elderly resident should be sensitive to the lack of sensory stimuli found in some nursing homes. The use of calendars, clocks, bright colors, and appropriate lighting for the tasks at hand must be considered. The older adult in an institution may be surrounded by people yet still be living in relative sensory isolation. It is well known that sensory deprivation may lead to delusions of persecution and hallucinations in the elderly. The overuse of many sedative–hypnotic medications, along with the decrease in sensory cues that occur with darkness, may lead to confusion, falls, and fractures. At the very least, cognitive functioning during the day is impaired by oversedation at bedtime.

The Nurse and the Hearing Aid

Nursing staff should reinforce proper care of hearing aids if, indeed, one has been prescribed. They should seek help from audiologists to expand their own knowledge as to both the potential and limitations of hearing aids.

The above communication suggestions should also be internalized by public health nurses who may be communicating with the hearing impaired elderly in less than optimal settings. Well-oldster clinics are held in various community settings such as church basements, trailer park community rooms, senior citizen centers, and other locations which are not equipped with soundproofing or often even the rudiments of privacy. Thus, the all-important patient teaching that is a prime benefit for the well elderly who seek monitoring of their health status through regular attendance at these low-cost or free clinics may not be internalized by the client. Inservice training by audiologists relative to the communicative effects of hearing impairment on the elderly and suggestions for efficient communication in a variety of settings should be viewed as essential for those nurses who work with the ambulatory elderly on a preventative health basis.

Inservice and Plans for Care

It is the responsibility of the director of nurses or the in-service staff development nurse of all long-term care facilities and public health agencies to orient staff to techniques of reality orientation, remotivation, and resocialization. In addition, the audiologist who is providing aural rehabilitation services to the patients should also provide in-service to the nursing staff so that continuity of care is ensured. Further, the director of nurses should relinquish the majority of the administrative functions and reallocate priorities toward improved patient care. If this were the case, the paper work resulting from the plentitude of federal and state rules and regulations would be done properly by nursing home administrators and clerks. The registered nurse should be free to plan for care which is based on nursing knowledge and knowledge of the individual patient. Further, the registered nurse would accept the responsibility for evaluating the nursing intervention on a continuous basis. If this reordering of priorities were done, perhaps the well-known "transfer trauma" from home to health care facility would be lessened. The elderly population and their offspring might then view nursing homes in the proper perspective in the continuum of care. The often verbalized dread and despair associated with nursing home placement might, over time, be overcome.

Other Nurses' Roles with the Hearing Impaired Elderly

It is recognized that only 4.5 to 6 percent of the elderly are to be found in long-term care institutions, accounting for approximately 1.5 million persons. It is distressing, however, to find that of the 978,649 active registered nurses in the United States, only 79,649 are found in nursing homes (National Survey and Inventory of Registered Nurses, Note 2). Therefore, we must recognize that other nurses are depended on to frequently interact with the elderly in homes, doctors' offices, clinics, and community settings other than long-term care facilities. The nurse practitioner in the physician's office, for example, has an obligation to follow the techniques of successful communication with the hearing impaired elderly to reinforce the physician's instructions. In addition, the review of medications with elderly patients, both initial and ongoing, is a task that is best performed by the nurse in a quiet, unhurried atmosphere.

DRUG REGIMENS

Elderly people frequently have difficulty comprehending a complex drug regimen. Virtually all elderly people who, for example, have six different medications to take during any given day make some kind of error either in timing or dosage. Given sensory deficits, child-proof bottles which frustrate arthritic hands, complex drug regimens, and subtle differences between prescription and over-the-counter medications drug therapy remains problematic for health care systems and for the elderly persons themselves both in terms of drug abuse and misuse. Kayne (1976) cites the following estimations which speak to the magnitude of the drug therapy problem in relation to the elderly.

1. While the elderly constitute roughly 10 percent of the population, they account for approximately 25 percent of the drugs used.
2. Three to five percent of all hospital admissions of elderly persons are a consequence of adverse drug reactions.
3. Of all hospitalized elderly patients, 10 to 30 percent have a drug reaction during their stay in the acute care setting.
4. One-seventh of all days in the hospital are devoted to the care of drug reactions, at the cost annually of approximately three billion dollars (p. 439).

Further indication of the need for efficient communication between the nurse and the hearing impaired elderly is that it is becoming common place for the aged patient to continue to take a medication long after a rational need for the drug has disappeared. Conversely, the elderly may discontinue essential medications if symptoms have disappeared. Further, antihypertensives and cardiovascular drugs tend to be taken in response to symptoms rather than as prescribed. Kayne (1976) describes a study of ambulatory patients that demonstrated that patients over the age of 65 had the lowest comprehension level of the prescribed medications (Boyd, 1974). Therefore, the time spent by the professional nurse in reviewing the medication regimen and in devising methods to enhance compliance should be considered as vital in the planning of client–patient flow in any busy clinic.

It goes without saying that the hearing impaired elderly person is at extremely high risk for making medication errors. Therefore, the nurse must be creative and patient in teaching those patients. The nurse must not only consider the physiological changes of normal aging, but also the presence of multiple chronic disease states and possible sensory deficits. The need for complex drug regimens for the elderly potentiates the possibility of drug interactions and reactions. In addition, the nurse should be aware of the following behaviors: (1) doctor-shopping resulting in several different prescriptions for the same condition, (2) stockpiling of out-dated medications, and (3) the propensity of well-meaning friends, neighbors, and family to give the elderly some "of what worked for me."

SUMMARY

The nurse can be a vital force in helping the hearing impaired elderly person toward efficient communication, particularly in what otherwise could be life-frightening situations. The nurse, as a member of a health-care team, should accept the responsibility of educating staff, families, and patients, in concert with the physician and other professionals, in the potential for aural rehabilitation regardless of age.

All nurses can make meaningful contributions to the hearing impaired elderly in the various settings where health care encompasses the totality of human needs. In addition, the gerontological nurse practitioner has the responsibility to develop written nursing management protocols to be used in the care of the hearing impaired elderly that encompass assessment, maintenance, referrals to other professionals such as audiologists and otologists, patient education, and expected outcomes. The nurse can continue to add life and not just years for the elderly, and can be a powerful force in the support and carry-over of the audiologist's efforts.

REFERENCES

Booth, R. Z. Primary care: The role of the nurse. Baltimore: *The University of Maryland, Baltimore Ambulatory Services Newsletter,* 1972, *June 15,* 1–6.

Boyd, J. R. Drug defaulting, II: Analysis of noncompliance patterns. *American Journal of Hospital Pharmacy*, 1974, *31*, 485–491.

Ebersole, P. P. Reminiscing and group psychotherapy with the aged, in I. M. Burnside (Ed.), *Nursing and the aged*. New York: McGraw-Hill, 1976.

Extending the scope of nursing practice. A report of the secretary's committee to study extended roles for nurses, Washington, D.C.: Department of Health, Education, and Welfare, November, 1971.

Heppler, J. M. Gerontological nurse practitioner: change agents in the health care delivery systems for the aged. *Journal of Gerontological Nursing,* 1976, *8*, 38–40.

Hull, R. H., & Traynor, R. M. The hearing impaired aged patient: The structure of aural rehabilitation programs and the role of the nurse in the rehabilitation process. *Nursing Care,* 1977, *June,* 14–15, p. 32.

Kayne, R. C. Drugs and the aged, in I. M. Burnside (Ed.), *Nursing and the aged.* New York: McGraw-Hill, 1976, pp. 436–451.

REFERENCE NOTES

1. Barney, J. *Community presence as a key to quality of life in nursing homes.* Paper presented at the 100th Annual Meeting of the American Public Health Association, Atlantic City, 1972.
2. National Survey and Inventory of Registered Nurses, American Nurses Association, 1977.

Milledge Murphey
Jane E. Myers

Chapter 30: Visual and Multiple Impairments in Older Persons

Most elderly persons are affected by visual impairment or blindness to some extent. These impairments create a variety of adjustment problems and activity limitations. When coupled with other physiological losses normally associated with the aging process, multiple and compounding complications occur (Perlman, 1977). In this chapter, the visual decrements experienced by older persons are explored and the effects of these losses discussed. Emphasis is given to the causes and impacts of visual changes in terms of the behavioral limitations they impose on the elderly. Also considered are strategies for helping persons so afflicted to cope with the multihandicapping conditions often present in persons beyond 65 years of age. Interestingly, the presently available literature covers each sensoriperceptual loss of aging separately, and in no instance is information regarding multihandicapped aged persons reported (Wolanin & Phillips, 1981).

DEMOGRAPHY

Kohn (1980) states that one half of the 500,000 legally blind persons in the United States are over 60 years of age. According to Kohn, legal blindness is defined as "central visual acuity of 20/200 or less in the better eye after correction, or visual acuity of more than 20/200 if there is a field defect in which the widest diameter in the visual field subtends an angle distance no greater than 20 degrees" (p. 230). While blindness is a significant problem for the elderly, defective vision is a major area of loss with 85 percent of those persons 75 to 79 having visual acuity of less than 20/40 (Hess & Markson, 1980). A 50-year-old person needs twice as much light to see as well as a youth of 20, and an 80-year-old needs three times as much light (Manney, 1975).

Defective vision among persons 12 to 17 years of age is found in only 22 percent of the population (defective vision is defined as less than 20/40 without correction). This proportion actually decreases until age 45, at which point the proportion of persons having defective vision again increases. Although defective vision is the norm in old age (90 percent of those over 65 years wear corrective lenses), serious visual defects are less common, affecting 7 percent of those 65 to 74 and 16 percent of those 75 years of age and older. The incidence of blindness and other serious visual difficulties increases with age and the incidence of blindness is twice as high among nonwhites as whites. The rate of absolute blindness is three times as high among nonwhites (Hess & Markson, 1980).

VISUAL CHANGES IN OLD AGE

Among the normal visual changes with age is decreased lens transparency. Yellowing of the lens results in decreased ability to discriminate all colors in the spectrum, particularly shades of blue or purple (Saxon, 1978). Other visual changes include decreased acuity, improved accommodation to distant objects, decreased near vision accommodation, reduced adaptation to light or dark, and reduced color vision (pastels less readily discriminated, color blindness worse). Also common are decreased flicker adaptation, decreased peripheral vision, decreased pupillary response (smaller pupil), and decrease in interocular fluid reabsorption (making glaucoma more likely). Additionally, less tearing is present in the eyes of older persons. The combined effect of these changes in vision creates a reduction in mobility and increases in the probability of an accident or injury for the elderly individual (Malasanos, Barbanskas, Moss, & Stoltenberg-Allen, 1981).

EYE DISEASES IN OLDER PERSONS

Stryker (1977) estimate that about 80 percent of all blind persons lose their sight in adulthood and that 40 percent of all blindness is caused by cataracts, glaucoma, and diabetes. These diseases are, in most instances, developed in late adulthood or old age and can be successfully medically treated in most cases. The leading cause of blindness in olders persons is cataracts (Kart, Metress, & Metress, 1978). This condition, the yellowing and ultimate opacity of the lens, is common to some degree in most persons who live to extreme age. It is correctable through surgical removal of the affected lens and prescription of contact lenses or glasses (Villaverde & MacMillan, 1980). Glaucoma, on the other hand, is irreversible. However, blindness usually can be prevented by early detection and medical treatment (Stryker, 1977). While not the most common visual problem of older persons, it is the most serious, and all persons over 40 years of age should have regular tonometry examinations (available from ophthamologists) to ensure that this virtually symptomless disease is detected early. The increased interocular pressure present in glaucoma can result in irreparable damage to the optic nerve, and can cause early loss of peripheral vision. Glaucoma will result in total blindness if undetected. Treatment for this condition includes surgical intervention and/or drug therapy to reduce interocular pressure by diminishing the aqueous humor (fluid) production within the eye.

Diabetes and hypertension, when present in older persons, may cause and exacerbate the condition known as senile macular degeneration, which is relatively common among older persons. Early signs of this disease usually appear in persons in their fifties and include inability to discriminate fine print and loss of central vision. Control of diabetes and hypertension with drug therapy and magnifying lenses usually ameliorates the symptoms of this condition, as peripheral vision remains unaffected. These and other less common visual conditions, alone or when combined with other losses experienced as one ages, can lead to a psychophysiological complex of problems which defy all except the most tenacious approaches to rehabilitation (Hogstel, 1981).

CASE STUDIES

In order to more accurately consider the feelings, thoughts, frustrations, and plight of the multihandicapped older person, several case studies will be considered. The impact of the visual difficulty coupled with hearing loss, economic loss, mobility limitations, inability to communicate effectively, and other limitations may produce depression, despair, hostility, and exacerbation of the isolation many elderly persons experience (Rossman, 1979). The goals of improved quality of life and increased feelings of self-worth among multihandicapped elderly can become realistically attainable through careful study of individual personal losses. Persons who are not totally blind and deaf, but very nearly so, often find themselves in a grey area of life with few, if any possible solutions to their problems.

Case I

The first case is that of a 92-year-old widowed housewife, living alone in rural central Mississippi. Her two primary handicaps include gradual onset, nonspecific macular degeneration resulting in light perception only, and presbycusis with resulting near total deafness. Her initial limitations were loss of her driver's license and substantial oral communication difficulty. Later, she was unable to crochet or play her organ and could not correspond with her friends due to her loss of ability to read and write legibly. In her mid-eighties, she could no longer attend church, nor could she cook, wash clothes, or accomplish her basic personal hygiene needs. At this point she expressed frustration, saying, ''What can I do? What can be done for me? I feel worthless and I'm ready to die.''

Her almost total blindness and deafness left her experiencing only fragments of what was occurring in her environment, and she often expressed the desire to become totally blind and deaf so she would not be aware of *any* of the occurrences around her. The effect of the cumulative losses was that she was unable to cope with the fragments of perception which she experienced. She said, ''Life as I experience it is stifling.'' A housekeeper was employed for her during the evenings to clean the house, cook, and serve as a companion. As she continued to live in the home she had occupied when sighted, she was able to maintain a realtively high degree of mobility. Illumination was increased throughout the home; contrasting colors in red, yellow and orange were used to color code certain areas (doors, medication containers, steps, telephone, etc.) so that she could more easily distinguish them. All persons with whom she came in contact were advised to speak slowly, to repeat if necessary, to speak in a lower pitch, to give basic information first, and to touch while speaking.

These efforts enabled her to function in her home but did not address her isolation, deprivation, anxiety, and feelings of worthlessness. She experienced the disinterest of her physician and often had hypocondriacal reactions which further reduced the physician's patience with her. She accelerated her attempts to converse with the family and friends, resulting in heightened anxiety among all who came in contact with her.

The first and only (to date) non-drug-related therapy which partially improved her feelings of self-worth and mood elevation was her introduction to swimming at the age of 91. She found that exercise in the buoyant medium gave her an uplift in both her physical feelings and mental outlook. She enjoyed the exercise, kept count of her lap progress, and seemed to feel better. She left the house for her daily swim, enjoyed ''getting out'' without endangering herself, falling, or other possible negative outcome. Further, she did not require communication for success in this activity, visual acuity was not a requirement, and a full-time support person to pursue her new, healthful activity was not necessary. Presently, at age 93, she continues to swim and has a reasonably positive outlook for the future. Family members are supportive and provide transportation for her daily swim, as the benefits in terms of her mood elevation are apparent to all (Note 1).

Case 2

Another case of interest concerns an 81-year-old male with no relatives, living in a long-term care facility in Florida. He is a diabetic amputee, has tunnel vision secondary to glaucoma, and has severe bilateral hearing impairment. He had little interest in activity of any kind. He could not read, was immobile, and was considered senile by institutional staff. He was docile and appeared confused by his environment and routine of the facility. He received meals regularly and was fed by an aide, was escorted to the bathroom on a regular basis, and received occasional visitors, but did not respond to any of these activities in a positive or interested manner. He said he ''worried about others because he couldn't see or hear them'' and, therefore, ''did not know how they were.''

Intervention for him came when a graduate student in gerontological counseling began visiting him and attempting to relieve the anxiety and confusion he was experiencing. This occurred at the same time that a unique elementary school program called ''Adopted Grandparents'' began to have children visit the facility twice each week, resulting in his ''adoption'' by a child (Whitley, 1976). The student/counselor and the ''adopted grandchild,'' over an extended period of time, were able to isolate certain vocal levels and words that the elderly man could hear and understand. Further, since the client would talk and was lucid mentally, it was discovered that he felt trapped inside ''his physical prison.'' As he began talking about himself, his life, and the limitations his physical decrements imposed upon him, he became more alert, talkative, and responsive. He responded to the touch and affection of the child and looked forward to her visits each week. His mood improved, he began feeding himself, and he was less passive. Communication between the student/counselor, the child, and himself had been virtually one way, but through talking things out with these concerned and interested others, he had become better able to function within his institutional life setting. He is currently a resident of the same institution and does not have any reasonable prospect of living in a noninstitutional setting. He is no longer confused and anxious, and he maintains a positive attitude concerning his life and its meaning. He often talks of the feelings of being needed as the adopted grandparent of the child and how much that has meant to him.

Case 3

The third case study involves a 76-year-old woman living in the home of a daughter. At 61, she began to experience mild confusion, and following the death of her husband, she became increasingly unable to accomplish personal care tasks in her own home. When she developed cataracts, her daughter became distressed and invited her to move to Florida from her native Michigan. Following surgery for the cataracts at age 66, it was discovered that she was unable to hear female voices. She was examined and found to possess hearing impairment bilaterally, which was not amenable to medical treatment. Her confusion continued to exacerbate, and when she was 70, she was diagnosed as having irreversible chronic brain syndrome. The daughter was unwilling to place her in a nursing home as she was often very loud, physically active, and had a tendency to wander if not attended constantly. She did not have control of bowel or bladder function and, as a result became an embarrassment to the family. Ultimately, when she was age 74, her daughter's marriage ended in divorce, resulting in she and her daughter relocating to a small apartment, leaving the husband and children in the home.

The resolution of this case study is the least satisfactory of the three cases presented since, currently, she is 76 years old and still living with the daughter (they now reside in a mobile home). She is now frail and continues to be loud, very active, and have no control of body functions. The daughter spends virtually all of her time caring for her, and they subsist on the mother's Social Security income and a small allotment from the former husband of the daughter.

The three case studies described above are illustrative of typical developments involving multiple handicaps including vision, hearing, and a variety of decrements in psychoneural responses in older persons. The outcomes in each case depended to a considerable extent on the chance availability of special services or on interested persons with commitment or family ties. They were more or less successful (in terms of improved quality of life for the older persons) depending on the severity, number, and type of disability(s) which were experienced.

CURRENT DEVELOPMENTS

One of the major difficulties in treating geriatric visual impairment is the lack of knowledge among the elderly concerning the diseases that occur most frequently in old age. Additionally, there are many misconceptions among older persons regarding prognosis, treatment, and limitations imposed by these conditions. Recently, an ophthalmologist at Fitzsimmons Army Hospital in Denver, Colorado, developed, with the author, a listing of rehabilitative concerns experienced by physicians when dealing with older patients who have cataracts, glaucoma, macular degeneration, and other eye diseases. Among the major issues of concern expressed by the medical practitioners are:

1. Lack of knowledge of the general public concerning visual conditions in old age
2. Fear and anxiety of older persons regarding eye diseases
3. Lack of knowledge of the probability of occurrence and/or prognosis for older persons who have cataracts (it is believed that the above concerns are due primarily to lack of knowledge of modern treatment/preventive measures and to "old wives' tales" concerning blindness and age.)
4. Physician concern over how to most appropriately inform an elderly patient of the presence of eye disease in order to reduce anxiety, fear, stress, and other psychological trauma due to the diagnosis
5. Physician desire for training in techniques or for counseling staff to use these techniques when dealing with severely visually impaired older persons
6. Physician desire for information on how best to work with family members of the severely impaired older family member
7. Physician interest in developing positive approaches to working with elderly, visually impaired, institutionalized patients, with a goal of improvement of quality of life for those persons

These issues are areas in which further research is indicated in order that the physician–patient link may become a more positive experience for both. The result of such improvements should enhance the ability of older persons to effectively deal with multihandicapping conditions. Further, physicians may become more willing to accept the limited successes possible when treating frail impaired elderly persons.

The availability of innovative programs and concerned persons has increased during the past decade (Gelfand & Olsen, 1980). Much of this new concern and interest in gerontology and geriatrics has developed as a result of the implementation of programs funded by the Administration on Aging (Cohen, 1979). The United States National Institutes of Health, National Institute on Aging, and Veterans' Administration have funded expanded programs of geriatric research in recent years (Butler, 1979). In reviewing materials reporting results of many of these studies, it was found that none dealt with the multihandicapped older person in terms of intervention techniques or methods for ameliorating their probems (U.S. Department of Health, Education, and Welfare, 1980). Further, it has been reported that physicians in practice are most often familiar with those elderly patients who are preoccupied with their bodily functions, giving rise to a negative stereotype for the aged among many of the physicians who treat them. For these and other reasons, it appears that medical research and medical practitioners have not yet developed a universal interest in and/or compassion for multihandicapped aged persons or their problems.

Today the White House Conference on Aging, which has been conducted once each decade since 1961, remains the major force in considering the multihandicapped elderly. Mini White House conferences on vision, hearing, and a variety of other infirmities associated with the aging process are conducted and the proceedings published and distributed. These serve as guides for further research, training, and workshops conducted at or by centers for gerontological studies across the country. Further, institutional, hospital, and medical literature reflect new and promising technologies which may be of value in rehabilitating the multihandicapped elderly.

In long-term care and institutional settings, research is being directed toward increasing the quality of care and enhancing the life experience of severely impaired older persons. One such study was recently funded by the U.S. Home Health Care Financing Administration and deals with appropriate staffing in nursing homes nation-wide. The outcomes will include recommendations for provision of more adequate counseling and mental health intervention for severely impaired residents of these facilities.

The VA programs dealt with a population of more than 2.97 million persons over 65 years of age in 1980. This population of VA eligibles will continue to increase until it reaches a ceiling of 8.05 million in 1995 (USVA, 1980). The VA has reported cataract surgical repair as the most frequently occurring surgical procedure performed for discharged patients over 65 years of age. The VA is currently accomplishing a large volume of corrective medical care on behalf of eligible veterans, and is developing significant programs designed to rehabilitate the multihandicapped elderly.

Programs for the "well elderly" have been developed primarily subsequent to the passage of the 1965 Older Americans Act. These community-based programs include a variety of health screening components conducted at sites including senior centers, congregate meal sites, senior day care facilities, Foster Grandparent program sites, and in a number of other contexts. A recent development in community-based aging programming is the Community Care for the Elderly concept in which funding is provided for the establishment of comprehensive service sites for the elderly on a seven-day-per-week, 24-hour-per-day basis. These programs are typically funded in existing long-term care facility settings and provide total care to community elderly on an immediate, short-term basis. Current demonstration projects of this concept are being funded and evaluated in Florida. Preliminary evaluation of the existing programs appear positive (Collins, 1980).

PRESENT AND FUTURE NEEDS

With the rapid expansion of programs and services for the aged during the past two decades has come an awareness of the paucity of trained persons presently employed or available to develop and implement new and innovative programming for them. In a recent interview, former Administration on Aging Commissioner Robert C. Benedict stated that National Aging and Rehabilitation officials had begun initial efforts toward joint planning of services for handicapped elderly (Note 2). It appears that if these two agencies can work together in an effort to increase function, improve quality of life, and aid the multihandicapped elderly in coping with the progressive and cumulative losses they face, a more positive image of the potential among the aged population may be forthcoming.

Among possible new approaches to effectively assisting the multihandicapped elderly are the establishment of regional and local comprehensive geriatric opthalmology/audiology/internal medicine centers. Such centers can be joint funded by the Administration on Aging, the Rehabilitation Services Administration, and other sources, and can include staff with gerontology and rehabilitation experience, education, and training. Further, a holistic health care model can be implemented in these centers which does not consider the ''time left to live'' constraint which has been traditionally used to avoid providing positive services to the severely handicapped elderly. Research, treatment, and therapy can be conducted at these centers simultaneously, thus avoiding the duplicative administrative costs presently encountered in the separately sponsored RSA clinics and university medical center research and treatment efforts.

The sheltered workshop concept has been successfully developed by RSA for the retarded, delinquent youth, the severely physically handicapped, and the mentally ill for more than 30 years; however, such programs for multihandicapped elderly persons have not yet been developed. It appears that in order to gain such attention and concomitant funding for sheltered workshop establishment, a national effort must be mounted on behalf of this special category of disabled persons. It is suggested that existing long-term care facilities are plausible locations for demonstration projects for the severely handicapped elderly. With special funding, selected long-term care facilities can implement programs which include additional staffing of counselors, social workers, recreational therapists, physical therapists, physicians and nurses with specialization in rehabilitation medicine, and other personnel committed to gerontology/geriatrics. Special and innovative approaches to mobility training, communication problem solution, and a variety of other areas of concern can be explored within such settings and with such staffing. These demonstration programs, when conducted nationally, can provide the base data for developing new and more positive approaches to dealing with the psychophysiological losses that occur with advanced age. Initial research inquiries in areas such as gerontological counseling, hydrotherapy, touch, cohort relations, family sociology, and numerous other high-risk concerns can be undertaken in the proposed sheltered workshop environments (US House of Representatives, 1980).

In order to realize the benefits of new and innovative gerontological programs, facilities, and personnel, continued and expanded funding is mandatory. At the time of this writing, funding in all social program areas is being reduced nationally. There is, however, a positive perspective in regard to aging funding; among social programs so affected, aging has received significant cuts only in the areas of research, training, and discretionary grant funding (US Senate, 1980). Other social service agencies have experienced recent cuts in direct service budgeting with resulting program reductions. If the present funding trend continues, aging funding, because it is tied to a large and increasing segment of the population, will fare well relative to other special population programs. The cuts in research, training, and discretionary funding do, however, exist now, and contingency planning must be developed to prevent loss of existing educational programs, ongoing longitudinal research efforts, and viable model projects which have made positive impacts on specific problems of the aged.

A suggested solution to this dilemma is attracting private trust and foundation resources in support of educational, training, and research efforts in rehabilitative gerontology. A major factor in the success or failure of such efforts will be the ability of present aging related organizations and professionals in the field to disseminate the demographic projections concerning the aged to the public, and in turn, the private funding sector. If basic gerontological training for the families of older persons can be initiated including, and beginning with, all elementary school children, the cost/benefit ratio of money presently being spent on long-term care can be significantly impacted. Further, quality of life for both young and old can be dramatically improved far beyond the conditions we now experience.

An additional major issue when contemplating future needs is that of provision of increased educational and training opportunities for gerontologists, physicians, nurses, and all service provider staff in aging programs. Few universities or colleges are presently providing this training, and with the previously discussed funding cuts, this small number may be reduced. In-service training for persons presently working in gerontological settings who have not had the opportunity to receive specialized training in gerontology is one of the most pressing and significant current needs. This need has been partially addressed in the past through grant funding (Title IV-A of the Older Americans Act), however the future of in-service gerontological education is now in jeopardy due to the previously discussed funding cuts. Research data indicates that few persons presently working with the elderly have had any formal or in-service training in gerontology (Note 3).

SUMMARY

The emerging awareness of and concern for the multihandicapped older person is a relatively new social concern, and one which cannot be ameliorated by provision of medical services alone. A much broader and more personal solution to the decrements of age appears to be an approach of choice. dissemination of information concerning aging, disability, and death, in the elementary schools nation-wide may well be one of the key elements in developing a social ability for long-term successful aging in our culture. Public interest and acceptance through education and public information programs can expedite and enhance these efforts. Funding, from both public and private sources, coupled with intergovernmental agency cooperation will further stimulate problem solution for impaired elderly persons. Finally, realistic self-acceptance and adjustment among the aged themselves can become a major positive factor. Personality integration in old age facilitated by trained gerontological counselors can become a catalyst for successful aging for all. The continued development and proliferation of innovative local programs (such as the Adopted Grandparent program), which enhance the positive aspects of the process of aging for multihandicapped individuals can further impact the isolation and helplessness now experienced by many of these persons.

We have witnessed a spontaneous shift against "ageism" during the past two or three decades. This movement has included government, scientific bodies, consumer groups, the general public, and the aged themselves. As sources of funding begin to dry up in many public funding sectors, a greater commitment on the part of educators and older persons is needed to ensure a continued expansion of the trend toward lifelong learning (Reinhardt & Quinn, 1979).

Social psychologist Anselm Strauss states that: "the chief business of a chronically ill person is not to stay alive or to keep his symptoms under control, but to live as normally as possible despite his symptoms and his disease" (Manney, 1975). Many older people fail at the task of living as *normally as possible*. Many merely succumb to the limitations of multiple chronic illness because they lack the judgment or the assistance to make necessary adjustments in life style. Without adequate personal and social resources, the multihandicapped older person may sink into miserable and crushing isolation, either self-imposed or imposed by the circumstances of the social situation of which he or she is an integral part. To manage the inevitable losses, older persons must solve social as well as medical problems. These solutions will be developed through the interaction of the aged with family, friends, and trained professionals who all accept the belief contained in the following quote from Saxon (1978)

> Growing old is really not so bad when you consider the alternative. If we live, we grow old, so we may as well do it as gracefully as possible. But we have to work at it. When the print gets smaller, the steps get higher, and the sounds get softer, we have to make adjustments that may not come easily. If we learn to cooperate with the inevitable, life can be a joy to the very end. (p. 177)

REFERENCES

Butler, R. N. Geriatrics and internal medicine. *Annals of Internal Medicine*, 1979, *91*, 903–908.

Collins, L. The many faces of aging, in *Proceedings of the 1980 Florida Governors' Conference on Aging*. Tallahassee, Florida: Florida Council on Aging, 1980.

Gelford, D. E., & Olsen, J. K. *The aging network: Programs and services*. New York: Springer, 1980.

Hess, B. B., & Markson, E. W. *Aging and old age*. New York: Macmillan, 1980.

Hogstel, M. O. *Nursing care of the older adult*. New York: John Wiley & Sons, 1981.

Kohn, J. A new look at the aging blind, in C. W. Hoehne (Ed.), *Opthalmological considerations in the rehabilitation of the blind*. Illinois: Thomas, 1980.

Kart, C. S., Metress, E. S., & Metress, J. F. *Aging and health: Biological and social perspectives*. Menlo Park, California: Addison-Wesley, 1978.

Malasanos, L., Barbanskas, V., Moss, M., & Stoltenberg-Allen, K. *Health assessment*. St. Louis: C. V. Mosby Co., 1981.

Manney, J. D. *Aging in American society: An examination of concepts and issues*. Ann Arbor, Michigan: University of Michigan Press, 1975.

Perlman, L. G. (Ed.), *Rehabilitation of the elderly blind person: A shared responsibility*. Washington, D.C.: National Rehabilitation Association, 1977.

Reinhardt, A. M., & Quinn, M. D. *Current practice in gerontological nursing*. St. Louis: C. V. Mosby Co., 1979.

Rossman, I. (Ed.), *Clinical geriatrics*. Philadelphia: Lippincott, 1979.

Saxon, S. V., & Etten, M. J. *Physical change and*

aging: A guide for the helping professions. New York: Tiresias Press, 1978.

Stryker, R. *Rehabilitative aspects of acute and chronic nursing care*. Philadelphia: Saunders, 1977.

United States Department of Health, Education and Welfare, Public Health Service, National Institute on Aging, *Recent developments in clinical and research geriatric medicine: The N.I.A. role*. Washington, D.C.: U.S. Government Printing Office, 1980.

U.S. House of Representatives, House Select Committee on Aging, Hearing: Families, *Aging and changing*. Washington, D.C.: U.S. Government Printing Office, 1980.

United States Senate Special committee on Aging, Information Paper, *The proposed fiscal 1981 budget: What it means for older Americans*. Washington, D. C.: U.S. Government Printing Office, 1980.

United States Veterans' Administration, *The aging veteran: Present and future medical needs*. Washington, D.C.: Veterans' Administration Central Office, 1980.

Villaverde, M. M., & MacMillan, D. W. *Ailments of aging: from symptom to treatment*. New York: Van Nostrand Reinhold, 1980.

Whitley, E. *From time to time: A record of young childrens' relationships with the aged*. Gainesville, Florida: College of Education Research Monograph No. 17, University of Florida, 1976.

Wolanin, M. O., & Phillips, L. R. F. *Confusion: Prevention and care*. St Louis: Mosby, 1981.

REFERENCE NOTES

1. Murphey, M. *Case study of the multi-handicapped elderly*. Unpublished manuscript, University of Northern Colorado, Greeley, 1980.
2. Benedict, R. *Personal communication*, 1981.
3. Murphey, M. *Counseling services for older persons as perceived and provided by selected Florida aging program administrators and direct service personnel*. Unpublished doctoral dissertation, University of Michigan, Ann Arbor, 1979.

Section 5: The Future of Services for the Hearing Impaired Elderly Adult and Their Implementation

Robert M. McLauchlin

Chapter 31: Legislation and Regulation Affecting the Aging Hearing Impaired Adult

The purpose of this chapter is to briefly review some of the principal laws and regulations affecting older Americans who have hearing impairment. Legislation and regulations are governmental decisions which afford rights to or restrict rights of individuals. Legislation is statutory law developed by a body of elected representatives, whereas regulation is a rule developed by a governmental agency with authority for rulemaking granted to it by a legislative body. However, a regulation has the same effect on individuals as a law. There are many types of law, such as criminal and civil law, but this chapter will confine itself to legislative law.

TERMINOLOGY

It is useful to understand the process and terminology unique to legislation. For example, Congress passed the Older Americans Act of 1965, which was labled Public Law 89-73. These numbers mean that this law was the 73rd act of the 89th Congress signed into law by the President. Initially, proposed law is introduced into the Senate and House of Representatives as a bill. If agreement is reached between the Senate and House versions of the bill, Congress votes on whether to adopt the bill as an act. If the bill is enacted, the Presidennt either signs the act into law or exercises his veto power. Once signed, the law is eventually recorded in the *United States Code* (USC) in sections under an appropriate title. Public Law 89-73 is recorded under Title 42 beginning with section 3001, thus designated as 42 USC 3001, et seg. The law also can be found intact published in the *US Statutes at Large*.

Similarly, there is a unique process and terminology related to regulations. Governmental agencies with authority to develop regulations must publish proposed regulations in the *Federal Register,* seek public comments, review and consider comments, and eventually publish the final rule in the *Federal Register* with the effective date of implementation. This Register is a daily publication of the US Government Printing Office. A pertinent regulation impacting on the rights of hearing impaired aging Americans is the regulation on ''Professional and Patient Labeling and Conditions for Sale of

Hearing Aid Devices,'' adopted by the US Food and Drug Administration (1977). In the proposed form (1976), the regulation might be cited as 41 FR 16756–16763, meaning it was published in volume 41 of the *Federal Register* on pages 16756 through 16763. In the same way, the final rule could be cited as 42 FR 9286–9296. To locate the permanent record of this 1977 regulation, one might be confronted with the designation ''21 CFR 801.'' This code indicates the rule can be located in Part 801 under Title 21 in the *Code of Federal Regulations*.

LEGISLATIVE AND REGULATIVE EFFORTS

Numerous influences can be cited for increased legislative and regulative efforts on behalf of older hearing impaired Americans. These influences might include:

1. The education of congressional members and their staffs by special interest groups such as the American Speech-Language-Hearing Association and National Council of Senior Citizens
2. An enlarged proportion of American citizens 65 years of age and older
3. An increased activism and sophistication among older Americans
4. A predominance of middle-aged and older Americans in major positions of influence in Congress and governmental agencies
5. An enhanced public awareness about the extent of hearing impairment among the aging and its detrimental impact on social interaction and quality of life
6. An expanded professional and scientific base of knowledge about hearing impairment among the aging

To illustrate the impact of such influences, this author recalls hearing testimony presented by Arthur S. Flemming (1976), former Secretary of the Department of Health, Education and Welfare (DHEW), and, at the time of this testimony, Commissioner of the Administration on Aging. At a Federal Trade Commission (FTC) hearing on a proposed trade regulation rule for the hearing aid industry he stated:

> Hearing impairment often inhibits opportunities for socialization of older persons, many of whom are already underinvolved in the main stream of life. Hearing impairments and/or improperly fitted hearing aids can lead to alienation from family, neighbors, friends, employers, and employees. Many older persons with hearing impairments withdraw from family and society, and thus increase their isolation. (p. 610)

He further remarked,

> Withdrawal from life leads to rapid mental, physical, and, I believe, spiritual deterioration. This is why we put the emphasis that we do on opening up opportunities for continued involvement. When noninvolvement takes place, it is serious as far as the older person is concerned, but it is likewise very serious as far as our society is concerned, because we are denying the older person the opportunity of making the unique contributions to the life of our day growing out of their experiences and their training . . . . (p. 625–626)

Commissioner Flemming was testifying in support of the proposed FTC trade regulation rule. Clearly, the impact of hearing impairment on the quality of life for aging Americans was understood at the highest level of the Administration on Aging: and this understanding was playing an important part in influencing the rulemaking process in another governmental agency, namely the FTC.

PERTINENT LAWS AND REGULATIONS

The collective impact of federal laws and regulations on hearing impaired older Americans is substantial. Several of these more important laws and regulations are reviewed in the remainder of this chapter.

Medicare

Medicare is a federally operated health insurance program for people 65 years and older as well as for severely disabled persons under 65 years of age. This program was enacted in 1965 as an amendment (PL 89–97) to the 1935 Social Security Act, becoming Title XVIII. The legislation pertaining to the Medicare program can be found under Title 42 in the US Code and in the US Statutes at Large. The Health Care Financing Administration, in the Department of Health and Human Services, oversees this program which has two major parts: hospital insurance (Part A) and medical insurance (Part B). Medicare hospital insurance is for helping qualified persons defray costs associated with hospitalization and posthospital care provided in a skilled nursing facility or provided in the home by a home health agency. Persons qualify for the hospital insurance if they have made contributions to Social Security and have reached the age of 65, or are under 65 and severely disabled.

Medicare medical insurance is for helping to defray costs of services rendered by physicians in any setting and those provided immediately following hospitalization by other health care personnel in skilled nursing facilities or through home health agencies. Any person who qualifies for Medicare hospitalization insurance can obtain this medical insurance by paying a monthly premium.

Patients are responsible for paying deductibles and copayments established under these insurance programs. Thus, the programs do not provide full coverage. Moreover, the consecutive days of certain services or numbers of visits are limited under both programs. Exact values of these payments and limitations on amount of services will not be mentioned in this chapter because they frequently change, but current details are available at any local Social Security office.

Audiological assessment and rehabilitative services can be covered under Medicare hospital or medical insurance, except when assessment is for the sole purpose of determining the need for or the appropriate type of hearing aid. Covered audiological services, rather, must be requested by a physician. Otological evaluations as well as medical and surgical treatment rendered by physicians are covered under Part B. Unfortunately, hearing aids and related services specifically are excluded as Medicare benefits. During 1975, the American Speech-Language-Hearing Association worked with members of Congress who introduced legislation in both the Senate (S 1784) and House of Representatives (HR 7971) to cover the cost of hearing aid evaluations and partial cost of hearing aids. These bills, however, were never reported out of the Senate and House committees.

Medicaid

Medicaid is the Medical Assistance Program also enacted as part of PL 89–97 as Title XIX of the Social Security Act (1965). Similarly to Medicare, the legislation on Medicaid may be found in Title 42 of the US Code and in the US Statutes at Large. Under this program, the Federal government provides matching grants to help states offer medical and rehabilitative services to financially needy persons, regardless of age. Many elderly persons on fixed and reduced incomes can qualify for Medicaid benefits. The Health Care Financing Administration, in the Department of Health and Human Services, manages the Federal aspects of the Medicaid program. Participating states are required to provide certain Medicaid services within Federal guidelines, while other services merely are recommended and optional. Medicare deductibles and copayments can be covered by Medicaid. Most audiology and speech–language pathology services presently fall into this optional category. Thus, the type and extent of these services varies substantially from state to state. States can choose to provide hearing aids to persons who qualify for Medicaid.

Federal Rules and Regulations for Intermediate Care Facility Services under the Medical Assistance Program state that speech pathology and audiology services shall include ". . . (1) screening and evaluation of residents with respect to speech and hearing functions, (2) comprehensive audiological assessment of residents, as indicated by screening results, . . . and the assessment of the use of visual cues, (3) assessment of use of amplification, (4) provision for procurement, maintenance, and replacement of hearing aids, as specified by a qualified audiologist. . . ." [42 CFR 442.496 (C) (b) (G) (1) (4), 1980] Additional audiology and speech pathology services are detailed in subsection 442.496 and subsequent subsections of this regulation. Depending on the state, further information about any particular state Medicaid program can be obtained at a local welfare, social services, human services, or social security office.

Supplemental Security Income

Supplemental Security Income (SSI) is a Federal income maintenance program designed to augment Social Security benefits for the aged, blind, and disabled. It was enacted into law as Title XVI of the Social Security Act in 1972 (PL 92–603) and became effective on January 1, 1974. The legislation may be found in 42 USC 1381. Eligibility for SSI is based on monthly income and financial resources. It also is related to eligibility for Medicaid because states have the option of using the SSI definitions of aged, blind, and disabled, as well as the SSI payment to assign eligibility for Medicaid. States, on the other hand, can establish more stringent eligibility requirements. Therefore, aging persons who receive SSI payments are not automatically considered needy and thus eligible for Medicaid. They need to inquire about their state's Medicaid requirements for eligibility. Irrespective of eligibility requirements, for those who qualify, this supplemental income could allow older hearing impaired persons to purchase needed audiological rehabilitative services and hearing aids.

Labeling and Conditions for Sale of Hearing Aids

The US Food and Drug Administration (FDA, 1977), with authority granted to it by Congress, promulgated a regulation to require professional and patient labeling and restrict the conditions for sale of hearing aid devices. With respect to labeling, first, each aid must be marked with the make, model, year of manufacture, and serial number, and second, electroacoustical data must be measured and reported in a uniform manner and accompany each aid. Third, used or rebuilt aids must be labeled as such, and fourth, all labeling information must be submitted by manufacturers to FDA for review. Lastly, a

"User Instructional Brochure" prepared by the manufacturer or distributor must be given to each prospective hearing aid user by the hearing aid dispenser (a copy of any brochure can be requested in writing by a hearing aid professional, user, or prospective user). Moreover, the prospective user must be given an opportunity to read the brochure before he or she can be sold an aid. This brochure is to contain at least 13 different types of information about such things as use, maintenance, care, and limitations. This information is reviewed in greater detail in Chapter 5.

The conditions for selling hearing aids are restricted because the FDA regulation precludes a hearing aid dispenser from selling a hearing aid to any person unless he or she has acquired an otological examination within the preceding 6 months. To verify the examination, the prospective user must present the dispenser with a statement signed by a licensed physician indicating the patient's hearing impairment has been medically evaluated, and the patient may be considered a candidate for hearing aid use. Persons 18 years of age and older may waive the medical evaluation by signing an FDA prepared statement, but dispensers cannot actively encourage the prospective hearing aid purchaser to waive the evaluation.

In this author's opinion, the labeling aspect of this regulation is a formidable improvement in services to hearing impaired Americans of all ages. The FDA had the authority to restrict the sale of hearing aids due to problems related to hearing aid effectiveness. However, this agency chose not to require an audiological evaluation to determine the necessity and effectiveness of wearable amplification, even though a waiver was proposed similar to the one adopted for the physician's evaluation. Requiring evaluations by audiologists would have reduced greatly an estimated 20 to 40 percent of hearing aid sales, many to elderly persons, that were inappropriate or unnecessary under the existing hearing aid delivery system (ASHA, 1976). A more detailed review of the entire FDA regulation is provided by McLauchlin (1979). FDA (1980) recently ruled that state laws may not require a mandatory audiological assessment for adults except as a condition of payment for third-party funds.

Federal Trade Commission Regulations

Under authority delegated by Congress to the Federal Trade Commission (FTC), this agency has promulgated at least one regulation and may finalize a second very important one that will affect all hearing impaired Americans. Presently, a person has a legal right to cancel a door-to-door sale of a hearing aid or any product by midnight of the third business day following the sale [16 CFR 429] (FTC, 1973). If a proposed FTC Trade Regulation Rule for the Hearing Aid Industry (1975) is finalized:

1. Hearing aid buyers will have a right to cancel the sale or rental of a hearing aid within 30 days following receipt of the instrument for any reason and be refunded most of the purchase price.
2. Hearing aid advertisements will have to follow prescribed forms of disclosure.
3. Hearing aid sellers will have to obtain prior written consent from prospective buyers before going to their home or place of business for the express purpose of selling hearing aids.
4. Hearing aid sellers will be prevented from representing themselves as physicians or audiologists unless they are such practitioners and from representing hearing aids as being or accomplishing something that is impossible or untrue.

McLauchlin (1979) provides a more detailed discussion of the proposed federal regulation elsewhere. Twelve weeks of hearings were held on this proposed regulation during the spring and summer of 1976. The reports of the FTC Presiding Officer (1977) and legal staff (1978) provide an extensive and excellent review of the proposed rule and public comments. These reports also contain recommendations for a final rule. Both reports make frequent references to the aging hearing aid consumer. This proposed regulation has not been finalized as of late 1981.

Older Americans Act

Congress passed the Older Americans Act of 1965, PL 89–73, [42, USC, 3001 et seg.] to improve the quality of life for aging Americans. The act authorized grants to states for community planning and services as well as for training, research and development, and model projects. Additionally, this legislation created the Administration on Aging to serve as the focal point for implementing the programs of the Older Americans Act. This governmental agency is located in the Office of Human Developmental Services under the Department of Health and Human Services. Programs authorized under the initial act and subsequent amendments are providing funds to train and retrain specialists in gerontology including those persons interested in hearing rehabilitation and health, conduct research into hearing problems associated with aging, develop public information about hearing impairment among the aging, and establish model projects. Most notable are the 1975 amendments to the Older Americans Act (PL 94–135).

Again, the Commissioner of the Administration on Aging, Arthur S. Flemming in 1976, emphasized, as he testified before the FTC hearing alluded to earlier in this chapter:

> It is clear under the law [Older Americans Act of 1965, as amended] that audiological testing, education about the purchase and use of hearing aids, and council for the hearing impaired can be supported under the Older Americans Act. In passing the 1975 amendments to the Older Americans Act, Congress placed special emphasis on the utilization of funds for this particular purpose.
>
> The Administration on Aging, as the body responsible for administering The Older Americans Act, is committed to doing everything we can by exercising leadership and by utilizing our authority and resources to assist older persons in obtaining the best hearing health care available through The Older Americans Act comprehensive and coordinated service programs (p. 612–613).

Additionally, the language of a House report (1975) clarifies the Congressional intent by declaring that the House Committee on Education and Labor ''believes the Administration on Aging should support, under section 308(a), the development or operation of (1) model projects designed to inform hearing impaired elderly citizens of the need for and availability of appropriate professional evaluation, diagnosis, and aural rehabilitation, and (2) model projects designed to expand or improve the delivery of aural rehabilitation services to the hearing impaired elderly'' (p. 17).

Closed Captions for Television

The Federal Communications Commission (1976) approved a regulation to restrict Line 21, an unused portion of the television screen, for ''closed captions.'' The term ''closed'' indicates a decoding device on the television receiver is necessary to view the captions. Hopefully, the broadcasting companies will televise captioned programs to attract the over 14 million hearing impaired Americans, of which approximately half are 65 years of age and older. By the end of 1980, the National Captioning Institute was captioning 30 hours of programing each week (Ball, 1980).

Tax Deductions

Hearing impaired persons of all ages are able, under Internal Revenue Law, to claim deductions for the cost of medical and rehabilitative hearing services, transportation to and from such services, as well as hearing aids and other technological sensory aids. The deaf can even obtain tax information by calling a toll-free television–phone or teletypewriter number.

OTHER FEDERAL AGENCIES SERVING THE AGING

Several governmental agencies other than those already mentioned have been created by legislation, to assist aging persons. The Division of Long-Term Care, in the Public Health Service under the Department of Health and Human Services, sponsors programs to foster additional and improved quality of personnel who can provide health services to the aging and others with chronic health conditions. This agency, for example, sponsored a workshop on February 25–26, 1975, to determine ways of educating the community and providers of long-term care services about how to meet the hearing rehabilitation needs of this population. Raymond Hull, Robert Trainer, and Jerome Alpiner were contracted by this agency to conduct the Workshop.

There are two institutes within the National Institutes of Health (NIH) concerned with hearing disorders in the aging. Those are the National Institute of Neurological and Communicative Disorders and Stroke (NINCDS) and the National Institute of Aging (NIA). NIH is also part of the Public Health Service under the Department of Health and Human Services. NINCDS conducts and funds research in many areas of communicative disorders, including hearing impairment associated with aging. NIA is a newer institute established by the Aging Research Act of 1974 (PL 93–296). Because of overlapping authority with respect to aging, a research proposal on hearing problems in the aging submitted to NIH might be forwarded to one or both of these institutes.

With respect to prevention, the Occupational Noise Exposure and Hearing Conservation Amendment, promulgated by the US Department of Labor (1981), provides the foundation for preventing—or at least reducing substantially—one of the major causes of hearing impairment among aging Americans.

Finally, the Veterans Administration provides hearing rehabilitation services and, in some instances, can provide hearing aids to older veterans even when the hearing impairment is not service connected. Otological evaluations also are provided to aging veterans.

SUMMARY

In this chapter, some of the processes and terminology of legislation and regulation were reviewed. Moreover, six influences contributing to increased legislation and regulation for aging hearing impaired Americans were mentioned. The primary focus of this chapter, however, was to provide a synopsis of federal legislation and regulation impacting on this population of hearing handicapped older citizens. Hopefully the reader has gained a better appreciation of the enormity of federal legislation and regulation affecting aging hearing impaired Americans and a better understanding of how to locate and review pertinent federal laws and regulations.

REFERENCES

American Speech-Language-Hearing Association. *Comment by Frederick T. Spahr and Robert M. McLauchlin in the matter of proposed professional and patient labeling requirements and conditions of sale for hearing aid devices*. Food and Drug Administration, Docket No. 76N-0019, 1976.

Ball, J. E. D. Reaching millions of viewers through closed captioning, *Public Telecommunications Review,* November/December, 30–38, 1980.

Federal Trade Commission. *Cooling-off period for door-to-door sales. Code of Federal Regulations,* 16, 429, 1973.

Federal Communications Commission. *Regulation to reserve line 21 of the vertical blanking interval of the television broadcast signal for captioning for the deaf.* Part 73, Subpart E, 1976.

Federal Trade Commission. Proposed trade regulation rule for the hearing aid industry. *Federal Register*. 40:26646–26653, April, 1975.

Federal Trade Commission. *Report of the Presiding Officer on proposed trade regulation rule for the hearing aid industry*. 16 CFR 400, 1977.

Federal Trade Commission. *Hearing aid industry staff report with appendices A and B*. 16 CFR 440, 1978.

Flemming, Arthur S. Federal Trade Commission hearing on proposed trade regulation rule for the hearing aid industry. *Public Record*. 215–44: 606–634, April, 1976.

McLauchlin, R. The impact of laws and regulations on services for the hearing impaired, in L. J. Bradford & W. G. Hardy (Eds.), *Hearing and hearing impairment*. New York: Grune & Stratton, 1979.

Medicaid Act of 1965, U.S.C. 42, 7, 1976.

Medical assistance program: Intermediate care facility services. *Code of Federal Regulations, 42*:442–496 (c) (b) (G), October, 1980.

Medicare Act of 1965, U.S.C. 42, 7, 1976.

Older Americans Act (P.L. 89-73) of 1965, U.S.C. 42, 35 Sec. 3001, et seg., 1976.

Older Americans amendments of 1975. *House of Representatives Committee on Education and Labor,* Report No. 94-67, 17, 1975.

Supplemental Security Income Act of 1972, U.S.C. 42, 7, XVI, 1976.

US Department of Labor. Occupational noise exposure: Hearing conservation amendment. *Federal Register*. 46: 4078–4179, January 16, 1981.

US Food and Drug Administration. Hearing aid devices: Proposed professional and patient labeling and conditions for sale. *Federal Register*. 41: 16756–16763, 1976.

US Food and Drug Administration. Hearing aid devices: Professional and patient labeling and conditions for sale. *Federal Register*. 42: 9286–9296, or Code of Federal Regulation, 21, Part 801, 1977.

US Food and Drug Administration. Medical devices: Applications for exemption from federal preemption of state and local hearing aid requirements. *Federal Register*. 45: 67325–67338, 1980.

Sondra LV. Gerhardt
Raymond H. Hull

Chapter 32: The Development of Programs for the Communicatively Handicapped Elderly: General Business Considerations

The portion of the population defined by the term "geriatric" is growing in numbers. Along with this growth is an increased recognition of the needs of this group and of our specific professional responsibility to them. This chapter deals with certain business considerations important to independent clinical audiological services on behalf of elderly clients.

PROGRAM CONCEPTION

Prior to spending money on equipment or office rent, a great deal of time must be devoted to determining precisely what services an audiologist seeks to provide. Premature incorporation and premature sales account for over a third of the difficulties encountered by new businesses (White, 1977). It takes many months to fully investigate all aspects of a proposal before committing to opening a clinic.

Assume that as a practicing audiologist, a decision is made to eventually initiate a private practice, to provide services for hearing impaired elderly clients within a chosen geographical area, and the audiological services will be provided under contract arrangements with area hospitals and nursing centers. Careful definition of the program makes the market survey and subsequent analysis easier in that it restricts and identifies areas of investigation and targets anticipated results.

After having defined the service to be provided, one needs to evaluate his or her own ability to deliver that service. There are certain characteristics helpful to a person in business that are neither sought by nor taught in a training program. One way of evaluating yourself would be to complete a business philosophy–personal attitude inventory such as the one developed by Myers (1968).

There are numerous books written on starting a business (Hicks, 1971), financial and management principles (Park & Chapin-Park, 1978), pricing practices (Hanan, Cribbin, & Donis, 1978), forming corporations without legal assistance (Nicholas, 1977), and financing a business (Loffel, 1977). These and many other sources will help teach necessary business language and principles. In this way, business practices can be determined prior to meeting with a lawyer or accountant. Spend a few hours with this individual asking questions, and leave with a smaller bill. Write a sample contract and have a lawyer review it if necessary. Have an accountant set up bookkeeping procedures and then leave until tax time. Be a prudent buyer; only buy what is absolutely required.

PROGRAM RESEARCH

Several separate investigations are necessary prior to commitment to opening a business. Payor status and patronage motivation and preference are of major concern. In order to conduct a market survey for analysis, it is necessary to understand certain health care payment programs.

Third-Party Payors

In any sales situation, there is a first party and a second party; typically the person who is providing and the person who is receiving, respectively. In health care, a third party has entered the picture. This is the person or agency paying for the service or product. With the elderly, this is increasingly a state or federal program. However, it might also be an insurance company or an executor of an estate. In each of these instances, the patient's need for the service is neither the final nor only determining factor as to whether the bill will be paid.

Banks and Executors

Simply because there is a bank or executor of an estate paying the bills for the patient, do not assume that they will automatically pay any bill presented. They have the legal authority and moral obligation to determine what is in the best interest of their client or ward. If they do not understand the value of hearing tests and hearing aids, the bill will not get a favorable response. Depending on how many of the targeted population are under the responsibility of this type of third-party payor, it may be advantageous to introduce yourself and your services as a separate action to sending a bill for services rendered. Prior knowledge on their part could smooth the path at a later date.

Insurance

Insurance policies will require some investigation. There are two types of policies, group and individual. The individual policies will not reimburse for audiological services. By rewording the bill, however, it is possible to convince the company to pay for diagnostics and treatment. It may be a requirement of the policy that a physician be on the premises or that testing be done on an inpatient hospital basis. Do not believe, for example, that every Blue Cross policy has identical coverage. There are over 300 Blue Cross offices in the United States and each is independently incorporated and operated.

Group policies have buyers representing a collection of people, usually an employee group. The buyer's responsibility is to negotiate a rate for coverage with an insurance company for the provision of certain predetermined services and products. These services and products will be provided in the event of need as defined and agreed upon by both parties.

Group policies may refer directly to audiological services in the policy. It may again be necessary to bill for services under another title. The insurance industry at the present time does not, as a general rule, cover hearing aids or evaluations, although it appears some unions have negotiated this coverage.

Medicaid and Medicare

There is generally more confusion regarding Medicaid and Medicare than just about anything operated by the government. Medicaid is a program supported jointly by the state and federal government and operated by the state. It is a health care coverage program for welfare recipients of any age. Whether Medicaid covers audiological services in any specific state will depend not on federal requirements, but on the state. Audiological services, including hearing aids, are not a portion of the requirements as stipulated by the federal government. The state has its choice. Most choose not to provide these services. However, whatever the ruling, it must be obtained from the state—and in writing.

Medicare is a program supported solely by the federal government and is operated by the federal government and its chosen agents. It is a health care insurance program for individuals 65 years of age or older who have paid social security taxes, their dependents, and those tax-paying individuals with disabling conditions of 2 years duration no matter what their age. The criteria automatically eliminate government employees, military personnel, railroad workers, self-employed persons, and a few other categories.

Medicare will reimburse the lesser of costs or charges to recognized providers in those cases where a recognized beneficiary needs recognized services as the result of an accident or illness requiring an inpatient hospital stay of at least 3 days duration. Everything is recognized and spelled out in volumes of tightly printed rules, regulations, stipulations, and exceptions.

Because someone provides health care does not mean they are a Medicare-recognized provider of care. In order to be a recognized provider, the organization must enter into an agreement with the government to provide services to these patients. The agreement stipulates that the provider will abide by certain rules and regulations in the provision of services in return for an agreed-upon rate. Recognized providers include hospitals, skilled nursing facilities, home health agencies, physicians' clinics, and rehabilitation agencies providing either outpatient physical therapy or speech pathology services.

A recognized beneficiary meets those conditions of age, disablement or dependency, and tax status, and has notified the local Social Security office that he or she wishes to participate in the program; a procedure similar to voter registration.

Recognized audiological services are limited in terms of reimbursement. Under Medicare Part A, reimbursement is allowed for therapeutic treatment of Medicare beneficiaries hospitalized as the result of an accident or illness and whose diagnosis or treatment is required as the result of that accident or illness. This means that Medicare does not recognize developmental problems, e.g., presbycusis, under Part A. If a beneficiary goes to a hospital with a hip fracture and has a hearing loss, one should be prepared to prove the hip fracture caused the hearing loss or send the bill somewhere other than to Medicare. At the present time, the Medicare program does not cover hearing aids or evaluations, even if required by an accident or illness. Diagnostic services on an outpatient basis by an audiologist who has been awarded a Medicare provider number are reimbursed under Medicare Part B when the audiological assessment was administered to aid in the determination of the existance or cause of a hearing loss.

One last caution regarding Medicare, Medicaid, or insurance. Not all providers of care have the same coverage allowances. So, the coverage allowed in a hospital as an inpatient may not be the same as allowed in a clinical setting. Investigation of the situation will be necessary.

PLANNING AND CONDUCTING A MARKET SURVEY

Since improper market testing accounts for problems in 73 percent of new businesses (White, 1977), one of the most serious undertakings in program research is the market survey. It would be financial suicide to open a practice where there are no potential clients. It would also be foolish to underestimate the size and needs of the targeted population, as one would get a reputation for not being able to meet business demand. A weak business design can be helped and tightened by a good market survey and its analysis.

What if it is determined that 2,000 clients can be handled comfortably in 1 year's time, and it is then discovered that there are only 2,000 people in that area with hearing losses? If they were all encouraged to come to you, you would effectively work yourself out of a job in 1 year, and it would not be wise to sign a long-term lease. Let the market survey tell you if this is so.

Assuming the program has been defined and the geographical area targeted, the next thing to do is to obtain the statistics on the chosen population within that area. This material is available from many sources, chiefly the United States Bureau of the Census. Other sources are the local Chamber of Commerce, local health-planning commissions, and the Department of Public Health. A common library source is Rand McNally's Commercial Atlas and Marketing Guide, which is frequently updated.

Statistical Information

Third-party payors will probably become the major source of revenue and, therefore, are very important to the program proposal. This is particularly true since the target is the elderly. There is a decreasing tendency for the elderly to pay for their own health care services. It will be necessary to determine to what extent the elderly in the area pay their own bills and to what extent their bills are covered by other payors.

It is necessary to verify the actual statistics for the chosen area, however the figures available from the American Hospital Association (Kessler, Ashby, & Wilson, 1978) may provide a general guide. From these, approximately 44 percent of the clinic patients pay their own bills, but only 12 percent of the hospital inpatients do so. The clinic should have about 13 percent Welfare and Medicaid recipients while the hospital will have 31 percent in outpatients.

There are two more significant reasons for knowing payor status; billing and collections. First, if 31 percent of the outpatients at the hospital are on public aid, then public aid's coverage criteria for services are of programming importance. It will be necessary to know what they can be billed for, how to bill, and what amount can be collected. On this last issue, what if they only pay 80 percent of the billing fee and the expected percentage was 100 percent?

Statistics and opinions regarding payor status should be checked with colleagues from occupational therapy, physical therapy, and speech pathology. Also, ask hospital social workers and discharge planners. Determine if the Department of Public Health has a survey on payor status for that particular community.

There are other things to watch for in gathering statistical information. Since patients with chronic diseases appear to have a higher-than-average incidence of hearing loss (Carter & Webber, 1966), then the potential caseload will probably be higher from the nursing center than from the hospital, based on concentration of patients with chronic illnesses. Also, since there is a higher incidence of hearing loss among the age group over 75 years (Carter & Webber, 1966), then again the nursing center population will provide more potential clients than the hospital. This means that the delivery system will have to be carefully designed to the nursing centers since the greatest number of patients will come from that group.

Another statistic important to your ultimate program concept and design is the poverty status of the elderly in the area. Nation-wide statistics indicate that of those elderly without families, 31 percent are below the poverty level (Kessler et al., 1978). Those with families fare better in that only 11 percent are below the poverty level (Kessler et al., 1978). This may mean that a significant portion of the potential clients will not have the means to pay for the services offered. It is probably best not to have a clinic policy allowing free services. Instead, bill for the service, and account it to a nonbillable or bad debt. This way your private pay patients and Medicare cannot request similar consideration, i.e., free treatments, and the bad debt account will assist at tax and audit time. This is obviously an area to discuss with an accountant and with the Medicare auditor.

EVALUATING A MARKET SURVEY

Statistics can be misleading. For instance, evidence may indicate there are 100,000 elderly living in a geographical area. If 10 percent have hearing losses, then 10,000 potential clients reside within this vicinity. The clinic proposal determined that eight patients could be seen per day. This number multiplied by an average 21-day working month equals 168 patients per month and 1916 patients per year. This number (1916) is below the 10,000 potential clients anticipated, and this is a good factor for success. However, the naive entrepreneur may take one further step and doom him- or herself to financial failure. At this point, it is estimated that an average billing per patient would be $30. This dollar amount times the 1916 clients per year equals $57,480, which sounds so good that a lease for office space in the most expensive building in town is signed immediately and $100,000 in audiological equipment is purchased. Bankruptcy will probably occur within 2 years or ulcers will result from worrying over the possibility. What was done wrong? Three things; first, it was assumed that the eight patients would visit the clinic each and every day from the start to the finish of the year. Second, it was not taken into account how many patients would pay full fees, reduced fees, or none at all. Third, consideration about whether the 1916 patients would either seek or desire the services was neglected.

In order to complete this task correctly, start with the number of patients guaranteed to be in the test suite on day one and at 3-, 6-, 9-, and 12-month intervals. Then, based on the research statistics, estimate how many of these patients will pay for their own services at your billed fee, how many will bring in reduced reimbursement due to a third-party payor, and how many will not pay the bill at all. Then determine an estimated monthly income for the first month and at 3-, 6-, 9-, and 12-month intervals. Take this figure and balance it against the estimated personal and business expenses. Finally, consider the current tendency of potential clients to seek what the audiologist has to offer. This should give an indication whether this is the best business and location for business.

Establishing Contracts with Other Agencies

It soon becomes obvious to any audiologist, whether in clinical or private practice, that it is not always possible to have the clients come to the test suite. Often they are inpatients of another facility and unable to leave the premises, such as Medicare Part A beneficiaries. So, the audiologist has to go to the client, which requires him or her to be inventive and creative in on-site testing. It also requires a contract with the facility regarding provision of services to their patients.

There are various types of contracts which are negotiable with a facility. One of these is the fee-for-service contract. In this type, the audiologist is paid for specified services according to a specified reimbursement schedule stipulated in the contract. There are different ways to establish the reimbursement schedule. The audiologist could be paid for every hour spent on facility premises regardless of activities or functions performed. Or, the hourly payment could be limited to only direct patient contact, which protects the facility against payment to the audiologist for time spent drinking coffee. For protection of the audiologist, direct client contact should be defined to include patient care conferences and report writing. Other contracts are established on a fee for a specific service no matter how long it takes to complete the service; so much is paid for an air-bone test and so much for a hearing aid evaluation.

A separate type of arrangement from the fee-for-service contract is referred to as a percentage or commission arrangement. In this type of contract, the facility would reimburse the outside contractor—the audiologist—a specified percentage of either the billed or collected amount. It is important that both parties agree to which amount would be used and include this in the contract. For instance, if the facility receives 80 percent of the bill, does the audiologist receive a percentage of the 80 percent or the 100 percent billed? This must be included, in writing, in order to avoid later unhappiness. Without written verification of the agreement, the facility could at a later date choose to reimburse at a reduced rate in those instances where reduced reimbursement is received. Or the facility could determine that they are not responsible for reimbursing the audiologist for bad debts or nonreimbursed services. This is particularly important where the client population is comprised of patients with third-party payor status. If the payor reimburses, not on the bill submitted but on a payment schedule devised by another means (such as percentile, salary equivalents, or all inclusive rates), the audiologist must take particular care in establishing a contract equitable to both parties.

Percentage arrangements are often easier to negotiate with health facilities because they are accustomed to the language. It is also much easier for the bookkeeper to take a percentage of the total monthly billing than to figure an hour-by-hour or service-by-service accounting. Finally, there is some peace of mind for the facility by working with tangible billing slips. However, it is to your advantage to avoid such wording in a contract while using percentage wording during contract negotiations with the administrator. For instance, the rate established by the facility to charge for the service is $40. The fee you want is $30 for this service, which is 75 percent of the facility's charge. In speaking with the administrator, use the 75 percent figure, but write the $30 figure into the contract. Be careful to use both figures during conversations so the administrator does not suspect a change in the agreement.

Many times, the facility prefers that the audiologist handle all billing for accounts. Investigate what this might mean to one's own business. Can reimbursement be given for what is done other than in the confines of the clinic? Will the facility provide supporting documentation necessary for billing third-party payors? Even if this arrangement is negotiated by the facility and the audiologist, the agreement must be put in writing. The facility must give written permission to treat their patients and to review the medical and financial records. If the audiologist agrees to handle their own billing, it is not professional to bill the patient and expect him or her to get reimbursed from his or her insurance company or Medicare. At this point, the audiologist would be contributing to a denial of the patient's rights, as most third-party payors will not accept bills for services directly from patients.

Arrangements to Avoid

There are several things to avoid when entering into a contract with a facility, one of them being investigating the reputation and competency of the facility. Other situations to avoid include an agreement which is essentially a "don't call us, we'll call you" contract. This facility is probably only planning on using your credentials and good will to satisfy an inspection or to advertise a total rehabilitation program without actually providing total care. This contract is also called a "paper compliance" contract. In other words, it is only sought for the printed implications of a program. Once the paper is in existence, the chances of being asked to demonstrate actual performance are slim.

Avoid entering into or maintaining a contract with a facility where questionable practices exist. For instance, when a facility requests the names and license numbers of other staff in the clinic or proof of costs for equipment purchased for the clinic, they may be interested in this information for billing or auditing purposes. If the facility presents blank billing forms to be signed, start walking and take your credentials. No matter how innocent the explanation or forthright the intentions, it can only lead to possible abuse. It may, in truth, be that the bookkeeper is only present on days when the audiologist is not and needs to get the billing out on a timely basis. Either make an extra visit on the day the bookkeeper is there or make some other arrangements. Never sign a blank billing form.

The facility may try to deduct third-party denials from the payment. This may or may not be reasonable depending on whether the denial was the audiologist's fault. For example, a certain insurance policy covers hearing evaluations if perscribed by a physician and necessary as part of the treatment resulting from an accident or illness. A patient is treated for a situation caused by a developmental process, e.g., presbycusis. The insurance company is going to deny the payment to the facility for the claim and rightly so. Also rightly so, the payment should be denied since the audiologist knowingly did not play by the rules. If this patient was to be treated for this type of complaint, it should have been clearly understood prior to treatment who would get the bill.

However, if the denial was due to the facility's actions, the audiologist should not suffer. Instances of this latter type are those in which the bookkeeper does not bill in a timely manner. Or, perhaps the nursing department documented conflicting information, such as the admission assessment stating the patient's hearing is good. Although it is obvious nursing is not qualified to make such an evaluation, their statement in the nursing log may cause denial of reimbursement. This is not the audiologist's fault, and he or she should not be penalized.

The most potentially dangerous situations derive from the language used in the financial arrangement. Avoid statements, either verbal or written, such as "I have an arrangement with the facility in which I give them 20 percent of the fee for their overhead and profit." That statement means that there is a "kickback" arrangement with the facility, which is not true. For one thing, the fee is the facility's fee not the audiologist's. One can't give the facility something that belongs to them. Instead, they are paying you a portion of their fee as reimbursement for services provided. The only true instance in which a "kickback" could occur is when the billing is done independent from the facility and the audiologist pays the facility a fee for the "right" to treat their patients. Never enter into this type of agreement. It is not illegal to rent space or equipment from the facility. However, the rate must be reasonable and not inflated to cover other purposes.

REFERENCES

Carter, H. W., & Webber, I. L. *The aged and chronic disease: Research in a local health department* (Monograph Series No. 9). Jacksonville: Florida State Board of Health, 1966.

Hanan, M., Cribbin, J., & Donis, J. *Systems selling strategies*. New York: Amacom, 1978.

Hicks, T. G. *How to start your own business on a shoestring and make up to $100,000 a year*. West Nyack, New Jersey: Parker Publishing Company, 1971.

Kessler, M. S., Ashby, S., & Wilson, K. *Comparative statistics on health facilities and population*. Chicago: American Hospital Association, 1978.

Loffel, E. W. *Financing your business*. New York: David McKay Company, 1977.

Myers, D. B. Starting a business. In B. Greisman (Ed.), *J.K. Lasser's business management handbook* (ed. 3) New York: McGraw-Hill, 1968.

Nicholas, T. *How to form your own corporation without a lawyer for under $50.00*. Wilmington, Delaware: Enterprise Publishing Company, 1977.

Park, W. R., & Chapin-Park, S. *How to succeed in your own business*. New York: John Wiley and Sons, 1978.

White, R. M., Jr. *The entrepreneur's manual*. Radnor, Pennsylvania: Chilton Book Company, 1977.

Robert M. Traynor

Chapter 33: Vestibular Rehabilitation: The Role of the Audiologist

Although this text is primarily concerned with the rehabilitation of hearing impaired elderly individuals, the audiologist may also encounter older clients who demonstrate dysequilibritory difficulties which may be either associated with or separate from a hearing disorder. In recent years, many audiologists have been involved in the assessment and subsequent interpretation of diagnostic vestibular evaluations as well as diagnostic hearing evaluations. Just as the older person with hearing impairment is treated by aural rehabilitation techniques, clients with nonmedically or nonsurgically treatable dysequilibritory disease should receive vestibular rehabilitation. Although the audiologist has not traditionally been involved in this area, it appears to be an emerging role for these professionals. This chapter will assume that the reader has a working knowledge of the anatomy, physiology, and terminology of the vestibular mechanism. This assumption will facilitate the discussion of dysequilibritory disease among the elderly and suggestions for rehabilitative treatment.

THE NATURE OF DYSEQUILIBRITORY DISEASE AMONG THE ELDERLY

According to Sheldon (1960) and Droller and Pemberton (1953), over one half of the elderly population demonstrates a significant amount of dysequilibrium. More recently, Steele and Crowe (1970) have indicated that 75 percent of women over 85 years of age experience symptoms of dizziness. It is logical that this should hold true for men as well, except that most men expire before age 80. The loss of equilibrium among elderly individuals has been termed by Krompotic-Nemanic (1969) as "presbystatis." Factors that influence dysequilibritory difficulties are extremely complex since these disorders may affect any of three systems and/or their nerve pathways. These systems are the proprioceptive, ocular, and vestibular mechanisms.

Proprioception

Proprioception, as presented by Teitelbaum (1967), is the sensory system which provides input regarding the discrimination of the position of arms and legs in space and the perception of their movement without looking at them. Rubin and Norris (1974) indicate that the proprioceptive mechanism may represent the greatest problem of all the associated systems relative to presbystasis. This is most observable when noting older people who, perhaps by necessity, reveal a significantly different gait than their younger counterparts.

Ocular Disorders

Ocular difficulties may also be a significant part of presbystasis. According to Vaughn and Asbury (1974), the lens substance of the eye is soft and pliable at birth and easily altered in shape to facilitate near and far vision by the action of the ciliary muscles. Throughout life there is a gradual hardening of this lens substance, beginning with its nucleus, so that it gradually becomes more resistant to changes in shape. By his or her mid forties the average person with normal vision may have difficulty focusing on near objects and reading fine print. These are early symptoms of presbyopia or "old sight" usually manifested by the blurring of objects when doing close work, visual discomfort, or fatigue. Further, as people become older, pupil diameter diminishes, thus increasing the older person's requirements for light to facilitate adequate vision. Additionally, Gordon (1971) indicated that among the aging there are three common disorders which may also affect the ocular modality. These disorders are (1) macular disease, affecting about 45 percent, (2) cataracts, about 35 percent, and (3) glaucoma, about 5 percent.

RESEARCH ON THE AGING VESTIBULAR SYSTEM

Although research on the aging vestibular mechanism is somewhat limited, there is important information available. For example, through anatomical research, Rosenhall (1974) indicated that among patients 75 to 95 years of age there are 21 percent fewer macular hair cells within the utricle and 40 percent fewer hair cells within the crista ampullaris. Further, Bergstrom (1973) found 37 percent fewer fibers in the vestibular nerve among a group of elderly temporal bone specimens as compared to younger specimens. These studies seem to provide some support for Weiss's (1959) observation of a decrease in the incidence, magnitude, and duration of nystagmus induced by caloric irrigation among older individuals. Additionally, Schuknect (1974) has also outlined some possible causes of dysequilibritory disorders due to the aging process, the first of which is cupololithiasis.

Cupololithiasis appears to be manifested by severe vertiginous episodes of short duration precipitated by head movement and characterized by a difficulty in walking. This type of dysequilibritory disease is thought to be caused by a substance called lipofusin. This inorganic residue is a waste product from the atrophy of the superior and posterior semicircular canals. This material, lodged within the cupula, is acted upon by gravity with each step, thus causing sporatic firing of the hair cells within the crista ampullaris.

The second possible cause of dysequilibritory disorders due to the aging process is ampullary dysequilibrium. Ampullary dysequilibrium is manifested by angular near movement, such as extending the head or turning it quickly to the right or left. This particular disorder is similar to cupololithiasis except that it affects other areas of the system, such as the utricle and lateral semicircular canals. As with its counterpart, ampullary dysequilibrium is caused by gravitational forces acting upon cupula lipofusin granules and the crista ampullaris.

Macular dysequilibrium, the third possible cause, is manifested by changing head position relative to the direction of gravity after such a position has been maintained for some time, as in getting out of bed. This problem is thought to be caused by degenerative changes in the utricle and saccule, particularly within the otolithic membranes. Johnsson (1971) examined the differences among the temporal bones of a group of individuals from 30 to 60 years of age. The study revealed reduced otoconium populations in the utricle and saccule among temporal bones 60 years of age, while younger individuals possessed normal otoconia populations.

Vestibular ataxia is Schuknect's final possible cause, and it is characterized by a constant sensation of dysequilibrium during ambulation. Often these individuals walk from side to side in an effort to avoid dysequilibritory attacks. These problems are thought to be associated with lesions in the descending vestibular tracts.

Although these disorders have been suggested as possible causes of dysequilibritory problems among the elderly, the functional interaction of the proprioceptive, ocular, and vestibular systems must be considered. Additionally, McCabe (1973) indicates that there are many other body systems that can produce balance problems, including, among others, the cardiovascular system, the cardiopulmonary system, the metabolic system, and the hormonal system. The problem of dysequilibritory disease among any population is one which may involve any of these systems at once, and, therefore, suggests an extremely complex etiology.

THE EFFECT OF DYSEQUILIBRITORY DISEASE ON OLDER INDIVIDUALS

Lindsay (1967) suggested that large percentages of individuals over age 55 years demonstrate a persistent, non-life-threatening paroxysmal nystagmus. Smith (1976) suggested that such vertiginous symptoms may induce alarm, confusion, bewilderment, and utter hopelessness into the person's life.

It is an alarming, often debilitating experience to suddenly become dizzy for no apparent reason or to awaken from a sound sleep with these symptoms. Older people often think they are dying and express this openly to their physician or audiologist. Younger adults are often distressed about the vocational limitations of dysequilibritory problems. For example, the bread winner who cannot work due to those symptoms is understandably concerned. Or, an older person who finds that his or her activities are significantly reduced may feel even more confined. Many older clients have seen their friends and relatives get dizzy, fall down, break their hip, go to the hospital, and never return. Jonkees (1975) indicated that people with dysequilibritory problems tend not to go out, notice weight increases, smoke and drink more, and live under the strain of psychological disturbance brought about by their ailment. It appears that the more devastating the symptoms, the greater the person's sedentary tendencies.

Confusion often results when the persons refer themselves for medical treatment.

This self-referral is usually to a general or family practitioner. This may result in an otology referral with subsequent counseling, or it may not. Many times the person is still vague as to the possible causes of their deficit even after medical consultation. Often this is a result of the amount of time the physician has available to spend counseling each patient regarding such deficits. Problems in obtaining professional assistance may generate feelings of hopelessness in the patient.

VESTIBULAR REHABILITATION

Vestibular rehabilitation is usually only conducted by the audiologist upon the direct referral from an otolaryngologist, and may be conducted in conjunction with the services of a physical therapist. The role of the audiologist generally is in four major areas of treatment. These include:

1. Complete subjective and objective audiovestibular evaluation
2. Counseling regarding the anatomical and physiological aspects of the particular dysequilibritory disorder
3. Labyrinthine exercise treatment to promote compensation or habilitation to the problem
4. Dysequilibrium induction to promote the patient's adjustment to noncompensatable dysequilibritory symptoms

Audiovestibular Evaluation

Any investigation of dysequilibritory disease logically involves the evaluation of both the hearing and balance mechanisms. The subjective evaluation of the system is usually conducted utilizing a "dizziness questionnaire" such as the one that follows. This form, developed by Peterson and Peterson (Note 1), is typical of those utilized to subjectively assess balance problems among all ages of patients. The subjective evaluation is extremely important since it provides the audiologist not only with information regarding diagnostic matters, but also allows patients to verbalize how they are reacting and coping with this deficit. Busis (1973) suggests that the dizziness questionnaire should consist of four major areas of inquiry.

Definition of Symptoms

Patients usually present the symptom of "dizziness" which can mean anything from true vertigo to lightheadedness. Therefore, the goal of the first portion of the questionnaire is to clarify the exact symptom to determine the patient's specific difficulties. The types of questions which are appropriate are listed in Table 33-1 (Note 1).

Associated Symptoms Suggestive of Neurological Disease

Since the vestibular nuclei comprise the largest nuclear mass in the brainstem, vertebral basilar insufficiency (common to the elderly population) frequently causes dysequilibrium. In localizing the patient's difficulty to the brainstem, however, there are usually other disturbances present as well, such as visual problems or numbness of face and extremities. These concerns are all investigated by the second portion of the questionnaire, as presented in Table 33-2.

Table 33-1
Portion of the Dizziness Questionnaire Relating to the Definition of Symptoms

When you are dizzy do you experience any of the following sensations? Please read the entire list first. Then circle Yes or No to describe your feelings most accurately.

Yes	No	Lightheadedness	
Yes	No	Swimming sensation in the head	
Yes	No	Blacking out	
Yes	No	Loss of consciousness	
Yes	No	Tendency to fall:	To the right?
Yes	No		To the left?
Yes	No		Forward?
Yes	No		Backward
Yes	No	Sensation of being thrown toward ceiling or floor	
Yes	No	Objects spinning or turning around you	
Yes	No	Sensation that you are turning or spinning inside, with outside objects remaining stationary	
Yes	No	Loss of balance when walking:	Veering to the right?
			Veering to the left?
Yes	No	Headache	
Yes	No	Nausea or vomiting	
Yes	No	Pressure in the head	

Reproduced with permission from Peterson, K. E. & Peterson, J. H. *Dizziness questionnaire*. Unpublished clinical form utilized at ENT Group of Greeley, Colorado, 1977.

Table 33-2
Portion of the Dizziness Questionnaire Investigating Associated Symptoms that May Be Suggestive of Neurological Disease.

Have you experienced any of the following symptoms? Please circle Yes or No and circle if Constant or if in Episodes.

Yes	No	Double vision	Constant	In episodes
Yes	No	Numbness of face or extremities	Constant	In episodes
Yes	No	Blurred vision or blindness	Constant	In episodes
Yes	No	Weakness in arms or legs	Constant	In episodes
Yes	No	Clumsiness in arms or legs	Constant	In episodes
Yes	No	Confusion or loss of consciousness	Constant	In episodes
Yes	No	Difficulty with speech	Constant	In episodes
Yes	No	Difficulty with swallowing	Constant	In episodes

Reproduced with permission from Peterson, K. E. & Peterson, J. H. *Dizziness questionnaire*. Unpublished clinical form utilized at ENT Group of Greeley, Colorado, 1977.

Characteristics and Etiology of the Symptoms

The time of onset and the duration of the vertigo are very important. Dizziness that began many years before and has been constant probably represents functional disease. On the other hand, dizziness beginning months before may be indicative of early serious disease, such as an acoustic neuroma. Episodic vertigo that is severe, lasting several hours, with complete freedom from symptoms between episodes, is more suggestive of peripheral labyrinthine disorders. Vertigo that is produced by a change of position is also more suggestive of a peripheral disorder. Additionally, Busis (1973) continued, it is also important to take time to discuss the patient's lifestyle with him or her as anxieties and pressures at home or at work may account for exaggeration or precipitation of the attacks. This portion of the subjective evaluation often suggests the possible effectiveness of rehabilitative techniques that will be utilized with the patient. Those questions are presented in Table 33-3.

Associated Auditory Symptoms

An obvious hearing loss suggests a primary ear disorder. Careful consideration of the responses to the auditory portion of the dizziness questionnaire are necessary. Particular concerns are tinnitus, hearing loss (progressive, nonprogressive, speech discrimination difficulties, etc), diplausis, paracusis, and fullness in the ear. Suggested questions are presented in Table 33-4.

Objective evaluations of the ear would include a standard audiometrical evaluation, site of lesion battery, possibly a central auditory battery, and electronystagmography.

In essence, the subjective–objective assessment of the audiovestibular mechanism may suggest that the patient may be treated medically. It may also indicate that attenuation of the symptoms may occur spontaneously, while simultaneously requiring other rehabilitative intervention by the audiologist.

COUNSELING THE DYSEQUILIBRITORY PERSON

Hecker (Note 2) has noted that when patients are counseled about dysequilibrium, their adjustment to the problem is greatly enhanced. Counseling the dysequilibritory patient is as important as counseling the hearing impaired person since they possess a disorder which they may or may not understand (Traynor, McHugh, & Goertzen, 1977). It is proposed that the audiologist counsel the person about the dysequilibritory problem utilizing colorful charts and models. These discussions usually involve a general presentation of the anatomy and physiology of the auditory and vestibular mechanisms. This is followed by a discussion of the patient's particular disorder and its effect upon the anatomy and/or physiology of the mechanism and upon themselves. It is imperative, particularly for the elderly, that this counseling be conducted in layman's terminology so that the information is effectively assimilated by the person.

LABYRINTHINE EXERCISES

The concept of labyrinthine exercises is not a new one, in fact, one might suggest that it began some 35 years ago when Cawthorne (1946) and Cooksey (1946) first discussed them. Although the Cawthorne–Cooksey labyrinthine exercises have demon-

Table 33-3
Portion of Dizziness Questionnaire Relating to the Determination of Characteristics and Etiology of the Disorder

Please circle Yes or No and fill in the blank spaces

Yes	No	My dizziness is: Constant?
Yes	No	In attacks?
		When did dizziness first occur? ______
		If in attacks: How often? ______
		How long do they last? ______
		Do you have any warning that the attack is about to start? ______
Yes	No	Are you completely free of dizziness between attacks?
Yes	No	Does change of position make you dizzy?
Yes	No	Do you have trouble walking in the dark?
Yes	No	When you are dizzy, must you support yourself when standing?
Yes	No	Do you know of any possible cause of your dizziness? If so, what? ______
Yes	No	Do you know of anything that will: Stop your dizziness or make it better?
Yes	No	Make your dizziness worse?
Yes	No	Precipitate an attack?
Yes	No	Were you exposed to any irritating fumes, paints, etc., at the onset of dizziness?
Yes	No	Do you have any allergies?
Yes	No	Did you ever injure your head?
Yes	No	Were you unconscious?
Yes	No	Do you take any medications regularly? If so, what? ______
Yes	No	Do you use tobacco in any form? If so, how much? ______

Reproduced with permission from Peterson, K. E. & Peterson, J. H. *Dizziness questionnaire*. Unpublished clinical form utilized at ENT Group of Greeley, Colorado, 1977.

strated some success in the past, McCabe (1970) indicated that little has been said to support them as a practical tool in the armamentarium of the otolaryngologist. Sparse support has been observed, further, as to their physiological basis in medicine. Subsequently, for lack of other alternatives, a compensation phenomenon has been advocated by a number of investigators (Hecker, Haug, & Herndon, 1974; Herndon, Herndon, Horowitz, & Lynes, 1975; Traynor et al., 1977). This phenomenon is characterized by an attenuation of the dysequilibritory symptoms through physiological compensation. McCabe (Note 3) indicates that when input from some part of the inner ear is lost, the brain compensates by virtue of building up the equivalent of that lost impulse in the

Table 33-4
Portion of the Dizziness Questionnaire which Evaluates Possible Associated Auditory Symptoms

Do you have any of the following symptoms? Circle Yes or No and circle the ear involved.

Yes	No	Difficulty in hearing?	Both ears	Right	Left
Yes	No	Noise in your ears? Describe the noise. ______	Both ears	Right	Left
Yes	No	Does noise change with dizziness? If so, how? ______			
Yes	No	Fullness or stuffiness in your ears?	Both ears	Right	Left
Yes	No	Does this change when you are dizzy?			
Yes	No	Pain in your ears?	Both ears	Right	Left
Yes	No	Discharge from your ears?	Both ears	Right	Left

Reproduced with permission from Peterson, K. E. & Peterson, J. H. *Dizziness questionnaire*. Unpublished clinical form utilized at ENT Group of Greeley, Colorado, 1977.

vestibular nuclei. McCabe (Note 3) further suggested that it is the ''spell'' or the dysequilibrium itself that is the adequating stimulus to the rebuilding of this spontaneous vestibular nuclear activity.

The Cawthorne–Cooksey program as described by Hecker et al. (1974) in Table 33-5 is presented to illustrate examples of exercises which have proven to be valuable in vestibular rehabilitation.

Although compenstion is a fairly common occurrence among adults and young people, it appears to be less common among individuals over 60 years of age. Goertzen and Jacobson (Note 4) found that while utilizing labyrinthine exercise, elderly patients did not compensate as easily or as rapidly as their younger counterparts. Similarly, Black (1975) indicated that the amount of vestibular compensation is critically determined by the patient's age. That is, the older the patient, the poorer the prognosis, and the less-active central processes which were designed to suppress or increase the input from each end-organ are not as well coordinated. Thus, the audiologist should not expect compensation for the dysequilibritory disorder among older individuals to occur rapidly, or even be reduced significantly. Indeed, the symptoms may not attenuate at all, but at least the patient will have been given all possible opportunities to compensate physiologically and psychologically to the problem.

DYSEQUILIBRIUM INDUCTION

Labyrinthine exercises are most commonly utilized for positional disorders, such as those often encountered by older clients. Even though such compensation may never occur in response to the exercises, habituation might be achieved. Batin (1974) defines habituation as a process by which normal individuals adapt to new and complex stimuli, e.g., a child learning to ride a bicycle.

Simmons and Goode (1972) have utilized caloric irrigation to facilitate habituation to dysequilibritory symptoms. This technique, referred to as Diliberate Dizziness Therapy

Table 33-5
Cawthorne—Cooksey Labyrinthine Exercise Program

Aims of Exercise

- To loosen up the muscles of the neck and shoulders in order to overcome the protective muscular spasm and tendency to move "in one piece"
- To train movement of the eyes, independent of the head
- To practice balancing in everyday situations with special attention to developing the use of the eyes and the subcutaneous and kinesthetic senses
- To practice head movements that cause giddiness, and thus gradually overcome the disability
- To become accustomed to moving about naturally in daylight and in the dark
- Generally, to encourage the restoration of self-confidence and easy spontaneous movement

All exercises are started in exaggerated slow time and gradually progress to more rapid time. The rate of progression from the bed to sitting and then to standing exercises depends upon the vertigo of each individual case. It has been found that group exercises encourage a more steady rate of progress.

- *In bed-supine* (only if patient cannot sit up, otherwise in sitting position without arm rest)

  A. Head immobile, eye movements: at first slow, then quick

  1. Up and down
  2. Side-to-side
  3. Repeat (1) and (2), focusing on finger
  4. Focusing on finger, moving about 3 feet to 2 inches away from face and back

  B. Head mobile: head movements at first slow, then quick; later with eyes closed

  1. Bending forward and backward
  2. Turn from side to side

- *Sitting position without arm rests*—Repeat as in A and B of previous section

  C. Shrug shoulders and rotate

  D. Bend forward and pick up objects from the ground

  E. Rotate head and shoulders slowly, then fast—Rotate head with eye open, then closed

  F. Rotate head, shoulders, and trunk with eyes open, then closed

- *Standing*—Repeat as in A, B, then E

  G. Change from a sit to stand position, with eyes open, and then shut

  H. Throw ball from hand to hand (above eye level)

  I. Throw ball from hand to hand under knees

  J. Change from sitting to standing and turn around in between

  K. Repeat F

(continued)

Table 33-5 (continued)

- *Walking*

  L. Walk across room with eyes open, then closed

  M. Walk up and down slope with eyes open, then closed

  N. Do any games involving stooping or stretching and aiming, such as bowling, shuffleboard, etc.

  O. Stand on one foot with eyes open, then closed

  P. Walk with one foot in front of the other with eyes open, then closed

Reproduced with permission from Hecker, H. C., Haug, C. O., Herndon, J. Treatment of the vertiginous patient using Cawthorne's vestibular exercises. *Laryngoscope,* 1974, *84,* 2067–2068.

(DDT), involves the use of self-induced, irregular-repetitive, cool-water calorics to create ''artificial'' vertigo. These treatments have been utilized mostly among Meniere's disease patients to attenuate the frequency and intensity of the dysequilibritory symptoms. DDT is, however, a rather devastating procedure for the patient and, therefore, has not gained general acceptance as a rehabilitative procedure.

Although similar, Dysequilibrium Induction is not usually as disturbing to the client as the DDT of Simmons and Goode (1972). Rather than caloric irrigations, the clinician works with the patients to put them into a situation which aggravates their symptoms. Once the symptoms begin, the clinician assists the patient in ambulation, falling safely, and other essential tasks. Clients generally accept this procedure more readily as being therapeutic in nature.

The process of dysequilibrium induction may be utilized as part of a program in labyrinthine exercise or singularly to facilitate habituation to the symptoms of dysequilibrium. It further demonstrates to patients their abilities and limitations during their dysequilibritory attacks, thus fostering psychological adjustment to the problem.

REFERENCES

Batin, R. *Vestibulography*. Springfield, Illinois: Charles C Thomas, 1974.

Bergstrom, B. Morphology of the vestibular nerve: Analysis of the calibers of the mylinated vestibular nerve fibers in man at various ages. *Acta Oto-Laryngologica,* 1973, *76,* 31–338.

Black, O. Vestibular causes of vertigo. *Geriatrics,* 1975; *30,* 123–132.

Busis, S. N. Diagnostic evaluation of the patient with vertigo. *Otolaryngologic Clinics of North America,* 1973, *6,* 3–23.

Cooksey, F. S. Rehabilitation in vestibulator injuries. *Proceedings of the Royal Society of Medicine,* 1946, *39,* 273.

Cawthorne, T. Vestibular injuries. *Proceedings of the Royal Society of Medicine,* 1946, *39,* 270.

Droller, H., & Pemberton, J. Vertigo in a random sample of elderly people living in their homes. *Journal of Laryngology,* 1953, *67,* 689–694.

Gordon, D. M. Eye problems of the aged, in A. B. Chinn (Ed.), *Working with older people,* Washington, D.C.: U.S. Government Printing Office, 1971, pp. 28–37.

Hecker, H. C., Haug, C. O., & Herndon, J. Treatment of the vertiginous patient using Cawthorne's vestibular exercises. *Laryngoscope,* 1974, *84,* 2065–2074.

Herndon, J., Herndon, O., Horowitz, M., & Lynes, T. Benign paroxysmal positional vertigo. *Annals of Otology, Rhinology and Laryngology,* 1975, *84,* 218–222.

Krompotic–Nemanic, J. Presbycusis, presbystasis, and

presbyosimia as consequences of the analogus biological process. *Acta Oto-Laryngologica,* 1969, *67,* 217–223.

Jonkees, L. B. W. Vertigo: research, diagnosis, therapy. *Journal of Vertigo,* 1975, *1,* 1–7.

Johnsson, L. Degenerative changes and anomalies of the vestibular system in man. *Laryngoscope,* 1971, *81,* 1682.

Lindsay, J. R. Paroxysmal postural vertigo and vestibular neuronitis. *Archives of Otolaryngology,* 1967, *85,* 544–547.

McCabe, B. F. Labyrinthine exercises in the treatment of diseases characterized by vertigo: Their physiologic basis and methodology. *Laryngoscope,* 1970, *80,* 1429–1433.

McCabe, B. F. Vestibular physiology: Its clinical application in understanding the dizzy patient, in M. Paparella & D. Shumrick (Eds.), *Otolaryngology.* Philadelphia: W.B. Saunders, 1973, vol. 1.

Rosenhall, U. Degenerative pattern in the aging human vestibular neuroepithelia. *Acta Oto-Laryngologica,* 1974, *76,* 208–220.

Rubin, W., & Norris, C. *Electronystagmography—what is ENG?* Springfield, Illinois: Charles C Thomas, 1974.

Schuknect, H. F. *Pathology of the ear.* Cambridge, Mass.: Harvard University Press, 1974.

Sheldon, J. Natural history of falls in old age. *British Medical Journal,* 1974, *2,* 1680–1690.

Simmons, F. B., & Goode, R. L. Deliberate dizziness therapy (DDT). *Archives of Oto-rhino-laryngology,* 1972, *95,* 221–224.

Smith, B. H. Reflections on vertigo. *Journal of Vertigo,* 1976, *2,* 1–11.

Steele, H. C., & Crowe, C. B. *How to deal with the aging and the elderly.* Huntsville, Alabama: Strode Publishing Company, 1970.

Teitelbaum, P. *Physiological psychology.* Englewood Cliffs, New Jersey: Prentice-Hall, 1967.

Traynor, R. M., McHugh, E., & Goertzen, D. Vestibular rehabilitation techniques for geriatric clients. *Journal of the Academy of Rehabilitative Audiology,* 1977, *10,* 19–24.

Vaughn, D., & Asbury, T. *General ophthalmology.* Los Altos, California: Lange Medical Publications, 1974.

Weiss, A. Sensory functions, in J. Birren (Ed.) *Handbook of aging and the individual.* Chicago: University of Chicago Press, 1959.

REFERENCE NOTES

1. Peterson, K. E., & Peterson, J. H. *Dizziness questionnaire.* Unpublished form utilized at ENT Group of Greeley, Colorado, 1977.
2. Hecker, H. C. *Labyrinthine function and possible rehabilitation of the spatially disoriented patient.* Unpublished Master's thesis, University of Utah, Salt Lake City, 1969.
3. McCabe, B. F. *Current concepts in the treatment of vertigo.* Presented at a symposium, San Francisco, California, December 3, 1973.
4. Goertzen, D., & Jacobsen, E. Unpublished data, Swedish Hospital, Denver Colorado, 1975.

Raymond H. Hull

Chapter 34: The Future of Aural Rehabilitation Service Programs for the Aging

WHERE HAVE WE BEEN?

The field of aural rehabilitation has come a long way during the past decade, particularly in regard to the establishment of services for elderly clients. In the past, the primary locale for service delivery for those clients was in or through university clinics, and aural rehabilitation services were provided principally by practicum students in audiology (Alpiner, 1978). It appeared that services to elderly clients were provided somewhat out of default if younger clients were not readily available so that students could acquire the clinical practicum hours in aural rehabilitation required for their certification as audiologists.

It appears that one of the primary reasons why a majority of aural rehabilitation services for elderly clients has been provided in university clinics rather than by professionals in hospital and outpatient and private clinics has been due to the fact that reimbursement for those services has been difficult, if not impossible, to obtain. Many elderly clients do not possess the financial resources to pay for them. Likewise, there are few philanthropic organizations that support programs for the handicapped elderly. The majority have concentrated their efforts on children and young adults. The majority of insurances do not reimburse for aural rehabilitation services, although most, including Medicare, do reimburse for the audiological evaluation. As stated in Chapter 32, Medicare does reimburse for aural rehabilitation services, but there are stringent requirements attached. In the meantime, it is evident that more professionals are becoming interested and committed to serving the hearing impaired older adult.

Another note of progress toward greater services on behalf of the hearing impaired older adult is in the area of training. More graduate training programs in audiology are developing course work that specifically relates to strategies for assessment and treatment of auditory disorders among elderly persons. Much of the course work and areas of concentration are still in an early stage, but they are growing rapidly among college and university training programs.

THE LARGEST POPULATION

It is estimated that 95.5 percent of the hearing impaired in the United States are over 17 years of age, as reported by the National Advisory Neurological Diseases and Stroke Council (1970). Within that percentage, the prevalence of hearing impairment becomes ten times greater in the fifth, sixth, seventh, and eighth decades of life. When one considers, then, that the largest population of hearing impaired persons fall within the range of age 60 and beyond, it is astonishing to note that aural rehabilitation treatment programs specializing in the older adult are only now beginning to evolve. Prior to this time, children with a hearing impairment have received the highest priority in regard to early identification and therapy services. They do deserve our very best efforts. Those children must be given every advantage to maximize their communicative, educational, professional and social potential. However, even though children and young adults deserve the audiologist's best professional services, so do the millions of elderly persons who possess hearing impairment.

WHAT DOES THE FUTURE HOLD?

It is encouraging to observe the numbers of professionals who are showing an interest and desire to provide aural rehabilitation services on behalf of these elderly clients. From reviewing the some 250 letters and telephone calls that this author has received over the past 2 years on that subject, the future looks bright. Further, the growing numbers of graduate students who are applying to training programs with the express purpose of learning how to provide audiology services on behalf of elderly clients causes this author the view of the future as being even brighter. Some students are seeking training programs where they can even acquire a second major in gerontology or related studies in aging. That interest among students was not as apparent even 5 years ago, and it appears to be growing.

TRAINING PROGRAM

As mentioned previously, there appears to be a growing interest among students of audiology to learn to provide assessment and aural rehabilitation services on behalf of older adult clients. What, however, do training programs have to offer those students?

Survey of Training Programs

In 1977, through a Federal grant, the Area of Audiology of the University of Northern Colorado was funded to expand that program's efforts on behalf of the hearing impaired elderly. The thrust of the project was to establish the University of Northern Colorado audiology program as a model training center in the area of aging and to develop training materials on aural rehabilitation for the elderly for national dissemination. As a part of that project, a national survey was conducted to determine the extent to which other graduate training programs in audiology were developing and teaching courses which concentrated on the provision of services for the aging and/or offering practicum experiences with that age of client (Note 1).

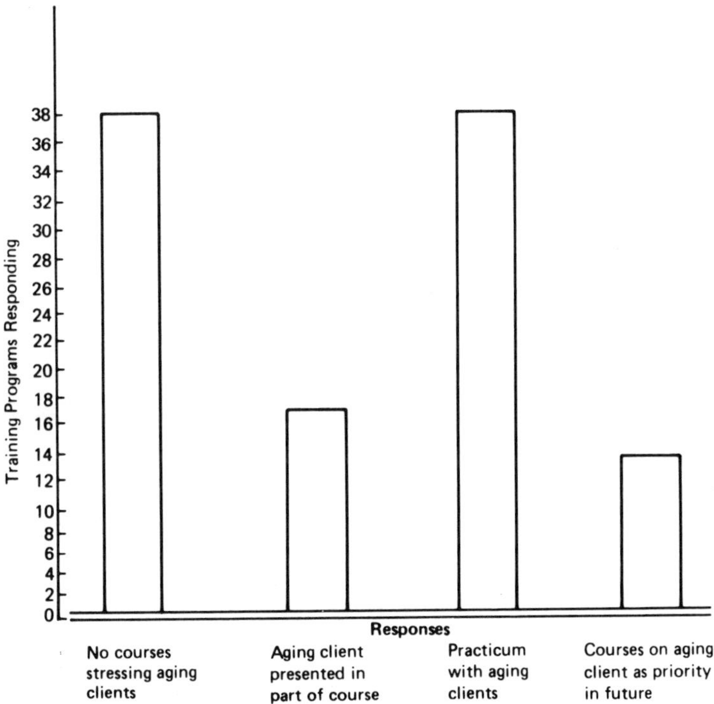

Fig. 34-1. Results of survey of training institutions, 1977.

The results were disheartening to say the least. The results (as illustrated in Fig. 34-1) revealed that out of the 38 programs responding, no programs offered a course which concentrated on the assessment procedures or strategies for aural rehabilitation for aging hearing impaired clients. Further, 17 programs offered course information in that area only as a portion of a general course in aural rehabilitation. The majority stated that the area of the aging client was offered in perhaps as few as one or two class periods. Two programs indicated that they encourage their students to take a course in aging from a department of gerontology or public health. The discouraging aspect of the results of this survey was that all of the programs that responded required their audiology students to participate in practicum experiences with elderly hearing impaired clients. In other words, all programs that responded to the survey required their students to participate in providing services to elderly clients when those students had received little or no academic training relative to the special considerations and techniques required for service provision on behalf of those clients. This, of course, would be unheard of relative to courses and practicum experiences with hearing impaired children. This was a sad state of affairs. The situation was changing toward the positive, however. For example, of the 38 training programs responding, 14 stated that coursework in the area of the elderly client is held as their priority within the next 2 to 3 years. Six had applied for federal monies to expand that area of their training program. Whether that priority became a reality is yet to be seen. In any event, the desire appears to be even stronger today, and increased training efforts among university programs are evident.

Other areas of professional training are also becoming aware of the need for specific academic and practical experiences as they relate to services for the older adult. Those include occupational therapy, physical therapy, nutrition, nursing, psychology, and others. In terms of working on a team approach in providing services for the elderly, the emphasis placed in this area by those areas will certainly strengthen the training and services by the audiologist.

It is interesting to consider that the dearth of professionals within many areas of allied health who have concentrated on the elderly client and gained knowledge in the area may be the principal catalyst in the corresponding lack of courses and training programs concentrating in that area. As more professionals and students strive to become knowledgeable in the area of aging, then coursework and subsequent services will undoubtedly expand, probably toward the past and current levels of concentration that we have experienced in the area of the young child.

Public Awareness

As the general population of the US gradually becomes older, so are attitudes changing relative to aging persons. The 1976 population figures perhaps bear out one reason for this attitude change. For example, the US Office of Human Development Services (1978) presented data which indicate that of the 214,659,300 persons in the US, 32,244,900, or 1.0 out of every 8.5 persons are over age 60 years. Further, their survey figures show that 22,934,400, or 1.0 out of every 9.0 persons, are over age 65 years. It is estimated that by 1980, 1.0 out of every 8.7 persons will be age 65 years or over, and 1.0 out of 8.3 will be age 60 years and older. That does not account for an anticipated undercount of 2 percent that generally occurs with such national surveys (Report of the Office of Human Services, AOA [Administration on Aging], DHEW, 1978).

As the numbers of persons over age 60 continue to grow and if the number of births remain stable, as the result of significant medical advances, the ratio of older persons to those who are younger will continue to be reduced.

Employ the Media

The media has a significant impact on attitudes and attitude change. A reduction in the numbers of very young models and actors for television commercials, for example, is becoming evident. The principal buying power for cosmetics, clothing, and other such expensive luxuries currently lies within the realm of those who are within their middle to late twenties. According to the US Bureau of Census (1974) by 1990, the most frequently occurring population of people will be within the age range of 35 to 44. And, from decade to decade the mode age will continue upward. As Cutler and Harootyan (1975) have stated, the baby boom of the 1950s will mean a gerontology boom of the years 2010 to 2020. The outcome of this is that as positive medical advances continue to save and prolong lives, persons who 30 years ago may have, for example, not recovered from an accident or severe illness, now remain alive. They may, however, possess disabilities that may or may not respond to rehabilitative treatment. In other words, the general public has been made very aware that our average life span is continually increasing, but little note is made of the fact that more persons are surviving who are disabled. Likewise, little notice is made regarding the rehabilitative services that these people require.

How is the public made aware of these requirements for services on behalf of the growing numbers of elderly persons? Undoubtedly the best way is for audiologists, for example, to notify their local media (newspapers, radio, and television stations) of the things that they are doing within the realm of their professional services. Whether we realize it or not, the public is interested in knowing about the good that is being done on behalf of an otherwise isolated hearing impaired elderly client. They, further, are interested in the fact that the aural rehabilitation services being provided for those persons possess a concrete structure and that persons who have been concerned over their potential to participate in society as a result of hearing impairment are learning to communicate more efficiently once again.

Speak Up

Professionals in communication disorders have long been silent about the good that they do. It is no wonder that bumper stickers are observed which state, ''What Is An Audiologist?'' In surveys among the general public, great numbers of them are, indeed, not aware of what audiologists or speech–language pathologists are, let alone what they do. We are certainly not embarrassed to be professionals in these fields, but perhaps have been hesitant to reveal to the world that our services impact heavily on persons who possess a communication handicap. We do not save lives in the strict sense of bringing a patient with a failing heart back to life as a physician might, but we do provide services which bring a failing emotional, psychological, or social life back to as normal a state as possible. An inability to communicate with other human beings due to a disorder of hearing can cause emotional death in an elderly person that is, according to many of this author's clients, as agonizing or perhaps even more agonizing than dying a physical death.

To restore life to the living is as exciting and challenging as restoring life to the dying. Further, successes in research, not only in regard to new assessment techniques, but also the development of new treatment procedures, are important. Newspaper stories on the types of services that audiologists provide and the techniques and equipment used are newsworthy. And, the public would like to hear about them. The audiologist, however, has generally failed to notify the press that those stories are available. Perhaps he or she did not feel that it would match up to the life that was saved by a paramedic or the attorney who saved his or client from the gallows. The audiologist must realize that his or her successes are equally significant, and the world should be made aware of them.

If public awareness is to increase, and with it a heightening of public knowledge regarding the professionals who are involved in providing these significant and exciting services, the audiologist must shed some of his or her humility and write and talk about them to those persons whose job it is to let the public know. And, generally speaking, when the general public is aware of the significance of such services, positive pressure can be brought to enhance other aspects of their provision, including increased reimbursement and other funding.

Administrative Models

Few administrative models for the establishment and maintenance of aural rehabilitation programs exist at the present time. As stated by Gerhardt (Note 2) and Hull (1978), the primary reason for this situation has been the lack of reimbursement and other funding for such programs. One model does exist at the present time, and can be utilized to demonstrate programs for the hearing impaired elderly.

This program was initially described by Hull and Traynor (1975) as the Community-Wide Program in Geriatric Aural Rehabilitation, and was primarily developed as an outgrowth of the University of Northern Colorado (UNC) Graduate Training Program in Audiology. As in most aural rehabilitation service programs for elderly adults, the majority of services were provided by graduate students under faculty supervision. The unique aspect was that the services were provided under contract with various health care facilities (nursing homes) in that community. So, as a service provider, this remained one of the few aural rehabilitation programs for the elderly where reimbursement for the services had been obtained. The old administrative structure of the program is illustrated in Figure 34-2. The graduate students, under supervision, were still the principle providers of services. So, as an administrative model, an important ingredient was missing; that was the provision of services by certified professionals and substantial enough reimbursement to pay for their services. An efficient administrative model should, however, also provide room for an ongoing training component.

The latest administrative model for the UNC Program is presented in Figure 34-3. There are three major additions, and one subtraction. The three additions are (1) increased reimbursement, not only through modified contracts with the individual health care facilities, but also through direct billing for audiological assessment to Medicare and Medicaid fiscal intermediaries by an accounting secretary, (2) monies provided through the county's Council on Aging, and (3) the employment of a certified audiologist to provide services on a full-time basis as the result of the increase in reimbursement for services both on behalf of clients from within the health care facilities but also the well-elderly person from the community. The employment of the audiologist has, thus, released two audiologist faculty members of this training program to be able to provide services on a demonstration basis for student observation, and to supervise other ancillary supportive services which graduate students can aid in providing as a part of their practicum experience with the adult and aging client.

In other words, both professional services which are reimbursed through the services per se and professional training have reached a healthy balance, and this program no longer must depend upon graduate students as the primary providers of services, although they do participate. Through contracts for services and third-party reimbursement, aural rehabilitation service programs can, indeed, be self-supporting.

REIMBURSEMENT FOR AURAL REHABILITATION SERVICES

Chapters 31 and 32 cover, in some detail, federal laws regarding reimbursement for audiology services. It is important, however, to discuss strategies for total reimbursement of service programs for the elderly. This information is difficult to discuss, and the information is always tentative. The following, however, is where reimbursement stands at the present time.

As discussed by Hull (1979), at the present time federal health insurance, or Medicare, does not reimburse for any aural rehabilitative services except under Part A when the hearing impairment was the direct result of the accident or illness that necessitated the client's hospitalization. That service, at least currently, can only be reimbursed when provided by an American Speech and Hearing Association (ASHA) certified speech pathologist, or one who is licensed by that state, eligible for ASHA certification, or under a certified person's supervision. Audiometric evaluations, however, are reimbursable to the audiologist usually on an 80 percent basis, first, if the audiologist is ASHA

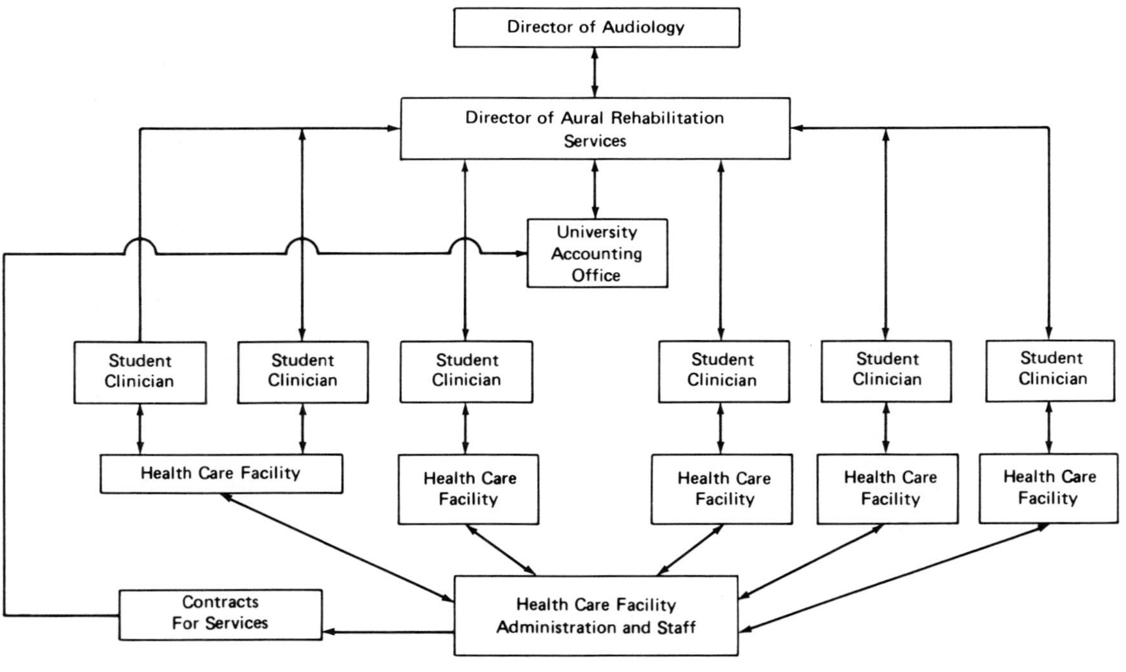

Fig. 34-2. Earlier program emphasizing training through services.

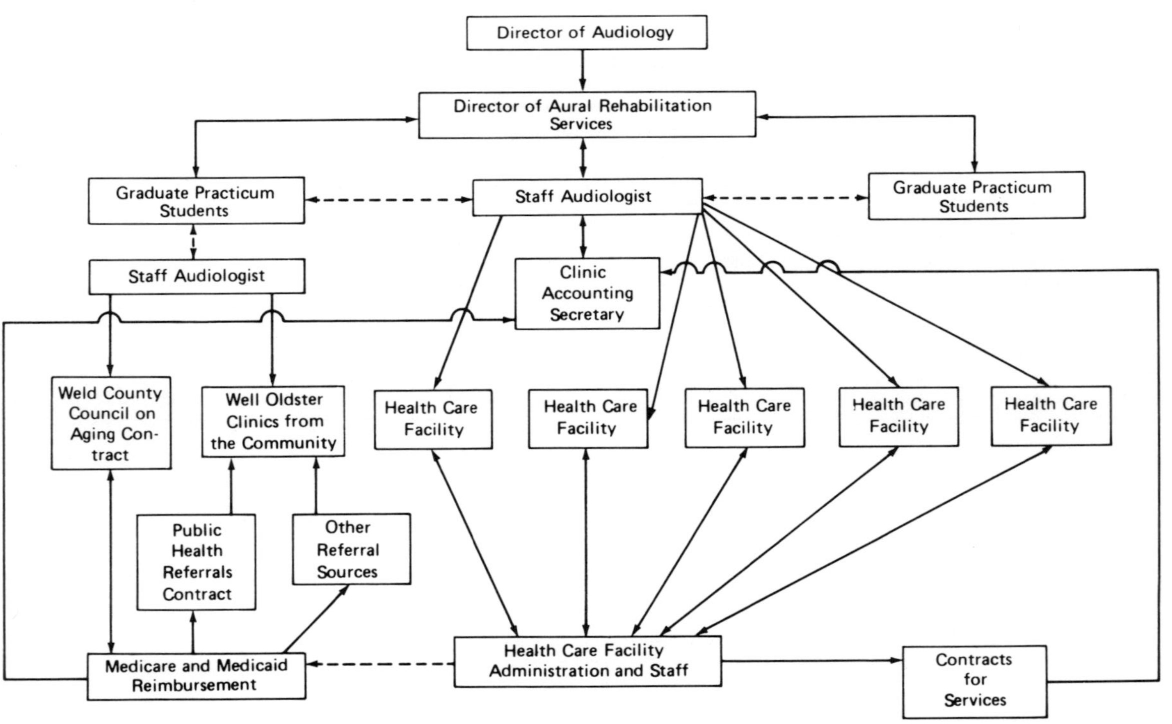

Fig. 34-3. Expanded program of service and training.

certified, licensed by that state, or is eligible for ASHA certification. Reimbursement also can occur when the amount charged by the audiologist is reasonable, proper, and customary as compared with other such services provided locally, and when it is conducted as a part of an examination of the cause of a hearing impairment and/or to determine whether or not the hearing impairment is medically treatable. Lastly, reimbursement takes place if the audiologist has been awarded a Medicare provider number. If the audiologist has not requested and/or been awarded a provider number through Medicare or a Medicare fiscal intermediary, audiometric assessment will only be reimbursed if it is conducted under the supervision of a physician or an audiologist who possesses a provider number. Hearing aid evaluations for the purpose of prescribing and fitting a hearing aid are not reimbursable at the present time.

The allowable charge for services under the Medicare Program depends on the type and extent of services described on the claim form. The benefit approved in this case is based on the information reported on the Medicare form and is in accordance with the maximum allowable charge for the type of services described. It cannot be stressed enough that the description of services provided must be clearly stated. Terms familiar to the audiologist, but not to the claims reviewer at the Fiscal Intermediary's office, can, and usually do, result in reimbursement that is lower than it would have been or listing of the service as a "non-allowable charge." For example, rather than using the term "hearing test," the term "hearing evaluation" or "audiometric evaluation" should be used. Rather than using terms such as "special test battery" to refer to tests for site of lesion, precise descriptive terms such as "acoustic impedance testing" or "assessment for site of auditory lesion: short increment sensitive index and assessment for tone decay," are more appropriate. Under "Nature of Illness or Injury Requiring Services," terms such as "mixed severe to profound sloping sensorineural loss, right ear, and moderate sensorineural hearing loss sloping into the higher frequencies, left ear" should be used rather than "moderate hearing loss, right and left ears," or "sensorineural hearing loss, bilaterally." The more descriptive the terminology, a greater the probability for reimbursement. The terminology to be used always should be worked out with personnel from the disbursement and claims review division of the Fiscal Intermediary. Since there is always the possibility for change-over in staff within that office, however, as descriptive a terminology as possible should always be used so that new personnel will have fewer questions.

Charges

In accordance with Health Care Financing Administration regulations, the maximum allowable charge for a specific service is based on the charge most frequently submitted by the individual supplier or physician for that specific service. This must be taken into consideration when the supplier is contemplating an increase in price for various services. This charge is compared to the charge for that same service which has been most frequently submitted by all other suppliers or physicians in the same specialty in that state. The Medicare Program is authorized to allow benefit equal to the *lower* of the two charges. In addition, an economic index is applied to all charges, which limits the percentage of increase in benefits from year to year. Each fiscal year, the benefits allowed for every service provided are re-evaluated using this comparison. If a supplier of services was not in practice prior to October 1, 1977 (had not provided services under a Medicare Provider Number), allowable charges are based on that 50th percentile—Area of Specialty.

Review Determination

If a supplier of services is not satisfied with a determination of reimbursement rate or has asked for a review determination of his/her reimbursement rate and is still not satisfied, the supplier may request, in writing, within 6 months of the date of the notice, a hearing before a hearing officer if the amount in controversy (the amount of benefits in question) is $100.00 or more. To meet the $100.00 limitation, the supplier may combine other of their claims that have been through the review or reopening process within 6 months of the date of the hearing request. This request must be sent either to the Office of Professional Relations Division of your Fiscal Intermediary, or to any Social Security Office.

To avoid difficulties in obtaining third-party reimbursement for assessment services and to ensure that the audiologist's procedures are correct, it is again stressed that a meeting with the person who is responsible for disbursement and claims review for his or her Medicare Fiscal Intermediary should be held to discuss the use of forms, terminology, coverage versus noncoverage, billing procedures, and so on. Such a meeting will resolve many potential problems which could, otherwise, occur. Ignorance of the law is not an acceptable excuse in the eyes of any state or federal court.

The information and procedures for reimbursement through federal health insurance is such a complex topic that a brief presentation as this could be misunderstood by some. This author would be most happy to talk with any of the readers to help unravel some of those complexities. It is again urged that persons interested in becoming a provider through the Medicare Program should meet with persons in the office of their Fiscal Intermediary to review procedures and forms. Sometimes the audiologist must make the personnel of the Fiscal Intermediary aware that audiology services are reimburseable.

THE FUTURE OF FEDERAL REIMBURSEMENT

Recommendations by the US House of Representatives Select Committee on Aging, Sub-Committee on Health and Long-Term Care (1976a), have been made concerning Medicare coverage for hearing aids which could eventually impact on the audiologist who dispenses hearing aids. Even though the report was published in 1976, the Sub-Committee is still actively working toward congressional acceptance of its recommendations for inclusion in the laws governing provisions under Medicare (Bracknell, Note 3).

As Representative Claude Pepper has stated, "The elderly of this nation are entitled to the best health care that is available in the United States. As the House Report demonstrates, in the area of Medical appliances, they are not getting it" (p. v):

The Sub-Committee (1976a) states, "Over one half of all persons 65 years of age and over suffer from impaired hearing . . ." (p. 19), so they do have a good estimate of the incidence at hand. One disturbing statement in their report, however, relates, "for millions of elderly Americans, the solution to these problems . . .," e.g., the seriousness of the hearing impairment, ". . . is the use of a suitable hearing aid" (p. 19). The use of a suitable hearing aid as a part of a total aural rehabilitation program for those who require amplification to cope with their communication deficit is not mentioned in their report, and must be stressed in future reports which may include implementation of services for the aging. The Staff Director of this House Sub-Committee asked this author to comment on the statements in the report, and I did stress the need for statements to include aural rehabilitation as a part of a total service to the hearing impaired elderly which may or may not include the use of a hearing aid (a hearing aid is not always the solution).

The Sub-Committee Report stresses abuses in the dispensing of hearing aids, particularly the selling of unnecessary hearing aids to the elderly for inflated prices. They do, further, include costatements by representatives of ASHA, such as the need for rejection of the waiver of medical examination prior to purchase of a hearing aid, particularly for those persons over age 65 years, and the inadequacy of most "hearing aid dealer" study courses in preparing the salesperson to make objective judgments and recommendations necessary for viable and ethical rehabilitation of hearing impaired persons.

In regard to their recommended provision of reimbursement for hearing aids, the House Sub-Committee's suggested restrictions and safeguards appear to be well founded. These include the "freedom of choice" concept, the necessity for examination by a hearing specialist for the elderly client prior to being fit with a hearing aid, the barring of certain "dispensing" practices such as door-to-door sales, and the encouragement of continuing education and training programs for audiologists and physicians in order to improve the quality of services to the hearing impaired elderly. The major weakness in the recommendations in the report is that no specification was made as to who would be allowed to dispense hearing aids. The major emphasis in regard to safeguards appeared to be in the area of the costs of hearing aids, which is of course important but certainly not the only consideration. They, further, state that the audiologist or hearing aid dealer can teach the hearing impaired to best use the hearing aid, perhaps inadvertently suggesting that the typical hearing aid dealer is equally qualified to work with the hearing impaired person. They do state, however, that the hearing impaired elderly can "receive further training in lipreading and other skills that will improve hearing comprehension at a hearing clinic." They fail to specify what a "hearing clinic" is or who should provide the service.

In conclusion, relative to the US House of Representative's 1976 recommendations (1976b) for reimbursement for hearing aids through Medicare provisions, they appear to be cognizant of the necessity for stringent safeguards, but the audiologist in the provision of a total aural rehabilitation service, of which the hearing aid may be a part, is not stressed. That appears to be a major weakness in their recommendation. If Congressman Abner Mikva's (HR-9413) bill which was submitted in 1977 is eventually passed as written, the provision of aural rehabilitation services by the audiologist would be greatly enhanced. The bill would add aural rehabilitation to the services now covered by Medicare. The American Council of Otolaryngologists has criticized the bill, stating that it would remove physician control over audiological services stipulated under Medicare.

ASHA is working with the Social Security Administration and Congress to encourage passage of legislation to include comprehensive aural rehabilitation services by audiologists as a reimbursable service under Medicare. This author is encouraged enough to feel that such legislation will be passed.

OTHER SOURCES FOR REIMBURSEMENT

Medicare and, in those states where reimbursement is permitted, Medicaid, are not the only sources for the financial reimbursement of audiology services for elderly clients. Hull (1977), in discussing alternatives for obtaining reimbursement for aural rehabilitation services, presented another important avenue. That was the contracting for services directly with health care facilities for those clients who are confined to that environment, and contracts with other agencies for well-older clients who reside in the community.

For example, if the health care facilities under consideration are a part of a corporate body which owns or provides fiscal management for them, negotiations for contracts must eventually end there. However, as stated in Chapter 31, the administration of individual health care facilities must first be convinced of the need for the audiologist's services. If discussions of the financial reimbursement for those services does reach the negotiation stage, there are two viable alternatives.

Contracts with Health Care Facilities

One option generally places health care facility administrators more at ease, particularly when they may be attempting to maintain their facilities on a very tight budget. This is an arrangement whereby the audiologist, as a Medicare (Medicaid) provider, bills Medicare (Medicaid) directly for diagnostic services. This, then, will provide a portion of the salary reimbursement for the audiologist. The remaining services which include (1) aural rehabilitation treatment for those clients who require those services, (2) in-service for health care facility staff, (3) consultation on efficient communication within the health care facilities, (4) hearing aid orientation programs for individual clients, and (5) other such services are reimbursed on the basis of a negotiated contract either on a per-client basis or on a flat-fee schedule determined by the number of residents within each facility and the number of hours of services required. If the audiologist is working among several health care facilities, the financial burden for these services not covered under Medicare or Medicaid are shared.

A second option which is not generally as acceptable since it places the burden of requests for Medicare or Medicaid reimbursement on the shoulders of the health care facilities, is the alternative of the audiologist negotiating a straight fee-for-services contract with each health care facility. If the audiologist, again, is working on an itinerant basis among several health care facilities, contracts for provision of *all* services, including diagnostic services, are negotiated. The health care facilities, if they are Medicare and/or Medicaid approved, bill directly for reimbursement of the certified audiologists' diagnostic services, and the remainder of the aural rehabilitation services, including in-service and others, are reimbursed to the audiologist under the contracts for services.

Most health care facility directors or corporate heads are not as enthusiastic about this arrangement. They generally hesitate to become involved in contracts in which they are not assured of at least partial coverage of the costs, although some are willing, particularly if they are convinced of the benefits of the audiologist's services to their residents. This type of contract is generally based on a per-client basis, based on the number of clients to be seen. Again, a sharing of the costs between the health care facilities involved lessens the financial burdens.

Contracts with Other Agencies

For the many potential clients who do not reside in health care facilities, there are a number of alternatives for reimbursement for diagnostic and aural rehabilitation services for the audiologist who is either involved in private practice or working in another form of clinic environment. They are as follows.

If the audiologist is a Medicare (Medicaid) provider, direct reimbursement for diagnostic services (excluding evaluation for the purpose of fitting and dispensing hearing aids) is available for those clients who qualify as Medicare (Medicaid) recipients. Reimbursement, as stated earlier, is made in accordance with charges that are reasonable and typical within that geographic area. If the audiologist dispenses hearing aids, the client stands the cost, including the cost of other aural rehabilitation services.

For clients who are financially able to pay for aural rehabilitation services, charges can be made directly to them, perhaps on a sliding scale. Charges are generally based on a per-session fee schedule. Fees may be established for counseling, hearing aid dispensing, hearing aid orientation, speechreading/auditory training, and others as deemed appropriate. The fee schedule for aural rehabilitation services may differentiate between individual and group treatment.

With fee schedules remaining as presented above, contracts with service agencies can provide reimbursement for services for those persons who do not possess the available finances to pay for them. Those agencies include local county health departments which are funded through state departments of health, county area agencies on aging which are funded by federal regional offices on aging, and other such agencies. They are generally willing to expand health-related services for the elderly if they are convinced that the service is to the definite benefit of their clients.

The most desirable contracts through those agencies, in their eyes, are generally those which reimburse on a per-client basis in accordance with the usual fee of the provider. Occasionally, however, it has been this author's experience that some such agencies as cited above desire to contract on a flat-fee basis as determined by the anticipated number of clients who will require the audiologist's services, or the usual number of persons. That form of contract is generally more risky both on the part of the agency involved *and* the audiologist.

The forms of reimbursement discussed in this section are only viable today. What the future holds is not known. If changes in Medicare provisions occur relative to reimbursement for aural rehabilitation services, then appropriate modifications would be made.

CONCLUSION

With the future of reimbursement for audiology services showing signs of greater potential, with other health professionals realizing (with greater enthusiasm) that many elderly persons who are hearing impaired have the potential to benefit from the audiologist's services, that those persons deserve to regain their maximum potential as human beings, and, in light of the growing awareness of the federal government, that hearing impairment among the aging is a prime area of importance in health care, more of these persons will surely have the opportunity to receive the audiologist's services. These positive signs have not been observed before, and it is the audiologist's responsibility to assure that they do not dim, but become even brighter and more observable. Probably the most significant and positive sign is the ever-growing number of students in training who have as their goal the provision of audiology services on behalf of aging clients.

REFERENCES

Alpiner, J. G. Rehabilitation of the geriatric client, in J. G. Alpiner (Ed.), *Handbook of adult rehabilitative audiology*. Baltimore: Williams and Wilkins, 1978, p. 160.

Cutler, N. E., & Harootyan, R. A. Demography of the aged, in D. S. Woodruff & J. E. Birren (Eds.), *Aging—Scientific perspectives and social issues,* New York: D. Van Nostrand, 1975, pp. 31–69.

Hull, R. H. Aural rehabilitation for the aging hearing impaired person. *Journal of the Academy of Rehabilitative Audiology,* 1977, *10,* 46–50.

Hull, R. H. Aural rehabilitation of aging persons: Problems and strategies for their solution, in L. Bradford (Ed.), *Audiology—An audio journal for continuing education*. New York: Grune & Stratton, 1978.

Hull, R. H. Provisions and problems in medicare payments. *Journal of the Academy of Rehabilitative Audiology,* 1979, *12,* 32–37.

National Advisory Neurological Diseases and Stroke Council. *Human communication and its disorders: An overview*. National Institute of Neurological Diseases and Stroke. NINDS Monograph No. 10, 1970.

Pepper, C. Memorandum to Members of the U.S. House of Representatives Subcommittee on health and long-term care, in *Medical Appliances and the Elderly: Unmet Needs and Excessive Costs for Eyeglasses, Hearing Aids, Dentures and Other Devices*. Report of the Sub-Committee on Health and Long-Term Care of the Select Committee on Aging, House of Representatives, Ninety-fourth Congress, Washington, D.C.: U.S. Government Printing Office, September, 1976, p. v.

U.S. Bureau of Census. Demographic projections for the United States. *Current Population Reports*. Series P-25, No. 476. Washington, D.C.: U.S. Government Printing Office, 1974.

U.S. House of Representatives Special Committee on Aging. *Medical appliances for the elderly: Needs and costs. Hearing before the Sub-Committee on Health and Long-Term Care*. Washington, D.C.: U.S. Government Printing Office, 1976.

U.S. House of Representatives Special Committee on Aging. *Medical appliances and the elderly: Unmet needs and excessive costs for eye glasses, hearing aids, dentures and other devices. U.S. House of Representatives Report, Second Session, 94th Congress*. Washington, D.C.: U.S. Government Printing Office, 1976.

U.S. Office of Human Development Services. *The elderly population: estimates by county—1976*. National Clearing House on Aging, Administration on Aging, Pub. No. OHDS—78-20248. Washington, D.C.: Department of Health, Education and Welfare, 1978.

REFERENCE NOTES

1. Adams, J. K., & Hull, R. H. *National survey of audiology college training programs on preparation of students to work with the hearing impaired elderly*. Hyattsville, Maryland: Allied Health Training Branch, Department of Health and Human Services, 1977.
2. Gerhardt, S. L. V. *One solution*. Paper presented at the South Dakota Conference on Communication Problems of the Elderly, Sioux Falls, South Dakota, October 29–30, 1976.
3. Bracknell, L. *Congress and the elderly*. Paper presented at the Aspen Symposium on Aging, Aspen, Colorado, July 2–4, 1980.

APPENDIXES

Materials and Scales for Assessment of Communicative Abilities among Hearing Impaired Adults and Elderly Clients

Appendix A: CID Everyday Sentences*

List A

1. Walking's my favorite exercise.
2. Here's a nice quiet place to rest.
3. Our janitor sweeps the floors every night.
4. It would be much easier if everyone would help.
5. Good morning.
6. Open your window before you go to bed!
7. Do you think that she should stay out so late?
8. How do you feel about changing the time when we begin work?
9. Here we go.
10. Move out of the way!

List B

1. The water's too cold for swimming.
2. Why should I get up so early in the morning?
3. Here are your shoes.
4. It's raining.
5. Where are you going?
6. Come here when I call you!
7. Don't try to get out of it this time!
8. Should we let little children go to the movies by themselves?
9. There isn't enough paint to finish the room.
10. Do you want an egg for breakfast?

List C

1. Everybody should brush his teeth after meals.
2. Everything's all right.
3. Don't use up all the paper when you write your letter.
4. That's right.
5. People ought to see a doctor once a year.
6. Those windows are so dirty I can't see anything outside.
7. Pass the bread and butter please.
8. Don't forget to pay your bill before the first of the month.
9. Don't let the dog out of the house.
10. There's a good ball game this afternoon.

---

*Reproduced with permission by Davis, H. & Silverman, S. R. *Hearing and Deafness*. Philadelphia: Holt, Rinehart and Winston, 1965.

List D

1. It's time to go.
2. If you don't want these old magazines, throw them out.
3. Do you want to wash up?
4. It's a real dark night so watch your driving.
5. I'll carry the package for you.
6. Did you forget to shut off the water?
7. Fishing in a mountain stream is my idea of a good time.
8. Fathers spend more time with their children than they used to.
9. Be careful not to break your glasses.
10. I'm sorry.

List E

1. You can catch the bus across the street.
2. Call her on the phone and tell her the news.
3. I'll catch up with you later.
4. I'll think it over.
5. I don't want to go to the movies tonight.
6. If your tooth hurts that much you ought to see a dentist.
7. Put that cookie back in the box!
8. Stop fooling around!
9. Time's up.
10. How do you spell your name?

List F

1. Music always cheers me up.
2. My brother's in town for a short while on business.
3. We live a few miles from the main road.
4. This suit needs to go to the cleaners.
5. They ate enough green apples to make them sick for a week.
6. Where have you been all this time?
7. Have you been working hard lately?
8. There's not enough room in the kitchen for a new table.
9. Where is he?
10. Look out!

List G

1. I'll see you right after lunch.
2. See you later.
3. White shoes are awful to keep clean.
4. Stand there and don't move until I tell you.
5. There's a big piece of cake left over from dinner.
6. Wait for me at the corner in front of the drugstore.
7. It's no trouble at all.
8. Hurry up!
9. The morning paper didn't say anything about rain this afternoon or tonight.
10. The phone call's for you.

List H

1. Believe me!
2. Let's get a cup of coffee.
3. Let's get out of here before it's too late.
4. I hate driving at night.
5. There was water in the cellar after that heavy rain yesterday.
6. She'll only be gone a few minutes.
7. How do you know?
8. Children like candy.
9. If we don't get rain soon, we'll have no grass.
10. They're not listed in the new phone book.

List I

1. Where can I find a place to park?
2. I like those big red apples we always get in the fall.
3. You'll get fat eating candy.
4. The show's over.
5. Why don't they paint their walls some other color?
6. What's new?
7. What are you hiding under your coat?
8. How come I should always be the one to go first?
9. I'll take sugar and cream in my coffee.
10. Wait just a minute!

List J

1. Breakfast is ready.
2. I don't know what's wrong with the car, but it won't start.
3. It sure takes a sharp knife to cut this meat.
4. I haven't read a newspaper since we bought a television set.
5. Weeds are spoiling the yard.
6. Call me a little later!
7. Do you have change for a $5 bill?
8. How are you?
9. I'd like some ice cream with my pie.
10. I don't think I'll have any dessert.

Appendix B: The Denver Scale Quick Test*

Rehabilitative Audiology (Adults)

1. Good morning.
2. How old are you?
3. I live in (state of residence).
4. I only have one dollar.
5. There is somebody at the door.
6. Is that all?
7. Where are you going?
8. Let's have a coffee break.
9. Park your car in the lot.
10. What is your address?
11. May I help you?
12. I feel fine.
13. It is time for dinner.
14. Turn right at the corner.
15. Are you ready to order?
16. Is this charge or cash?
17. What time is it?
18. I have a headache.
19. How about going out tonight?
20. Please lend me 50 cents.

*Reproduced with permission by Alpiner, J. G. Evaluation of communication function, in J. G. Alpiner (Ed.), *Handbook of adult rehabilitative audiology*. Baltimore: Williams and Wilkins, 1978, p. 36.

Appendix C: The UNC Sentence Test of Speechreading Ability*

List 1

1. It was such a great day for hiking.
2. Have you read the sports page this morning?
3. The cost of living will make you poor.
4. He serves excellent food in all his restaurants.
5. What kind of a car do you drive?
6. The weather for the game was almost perfect.
7. Why was the picnic called off this time?
8. I like white houses with large covered porches.
9. Did the white-and-black cat have kittens?
10. Slow music always makes me feel like sleeping.
11. Why did you go there for your vacation?
12. How much snow did we have last night?

List 2

1. Will you come with me to see him?
2. Snow always looks pretty on the mountain sides.
3. Is your whole family getting together for Thanksgiving?
4. Do you have an umbrella with you today?
5. Fathers should spend more time with their children.
6. Are you going grocery shopping while in town?
7. The wind is blowing from the northeast again.
8. It is time to go back home now.
9. Did you forget to shut off the water?
10. (Name) has been considered this state's favorite sport.
11. Where do you usually work during the winter?
12. It is a good day for playing golf.

---

*Hull, R. H. Unpublished materials. University of Northern Colorado, 1976.

List 3

1. What time was it when you arrived?
2. Have you any brothers or sisters at home?
3. It has rained for the past 3 days.
4. Do you have a dog or a cat?
5. What does the judge say about him now?
6. A soft rain makes grass grow in spring.
7. Did you buy a new car this year?
8. You should brush your teeth three times daily.
9. Children go to school at around age 6.
10. He let the dog out of the house.
11. Hockey is often a rough and tumble sport.
12. Would you like to go to the show?

Appendix D: Hearing-Handicap Scale*

Form A

1. If you are 6 to 12 feet from the loudspeaker of a radio do you understand speech well?
2. Can you carry on a telephone conversation without difficulty?
3. If you are 6 to 12 feet away from a television set, do you understand most of what is said?
4. Can you carry on a conversation with one other person when you are on a noisy street corner?
5. Do you hear all right when you are in a street car, airplane, bus, or train?
6. If there are noises from other voices, typewriters, traffic, music, etc, can you understand when someone speaks to you?
7. Can you understand a person when you are seated beside him and cannot see his face?
8. Can you understand if someone speaks to you while you are chewing crisp foods, such as potato chips or celery?
9. Can you carry on a conversation with one other person when you are in a noisy place, such as a restaurant or at a party?
10. Can you understand if someone speaks to you in a whisper and you can't see his face?
11. When you talk with a bus driver, waiter, ticket salesman, etc, can you understand all right?
12. Can you carry on a conversation if you are seated across the room from someone who speaks in a normal tone of voice?
13. Can you understand women when they talk?
14. Can you carry on a conversation with one other person when you are out of doors and it is reasonably quiet?

---

*Reproduced with permission by High, W. S., Fairbanks, G., & Glorig, A. Scale for self-assessment of hearing handicap. *Journal of Speech and Hearing Disorders,* 1964, 29, 215–230.

15. When you are in a meeting or at a large dinner table, would you know the speaker was talking if you could not see his lips moving?
16. Can you follow the conversation when you are at a large dinner table or in a meeting with a small group?
17. If you are seated under the balcony of a theater or auditorium, can you hear well enough to follow what is going on?
18. When you are in a large formal gathering (a church, lodge, lecture hall, etc) can you hear what is said when the speaker *does not* use a microphone?
19. Can you hear the telephone ring when you are in the room where it is located?
20. Can you hear warning signals, such as automobile horns, railway crossing bells, or emergency vehicle sirens?

Form B

1. When you are listening to the radio or watching television, can you hear adequately when the volume is comfortable for most other people?
2. Can you carry on a conversation with one other person when you are riding in an automobile with the windows *closed*?
3. Can you carry on a conversation with one other person when you are riding in an automobile with the window *open*?
4. Can you carry on a conversation with one other person if there is a radio or television in the same room playing at normal loudness?
5. Can you hear when someone calls to you from another room?
6. Can you understand when someone speaks to you from another room?
7. When you buy something in a store, do you easily understand the clerk?
8. Can you carry on a conversation with someone who does not speak as loudly as most people?
9. Can you tell if a person is talking when you are seated beside him and cannot see his face?
10. When you ask someone for directions, do you understand what he says?
11. If you are within 3 or 4 feet of a person who speaks in a normal tone of voice (assume you are facing one another), can you hear everything he says?
12. Do you recognize the voices of speakers when you don't see them?
13. When you are introduced to someone, can you understand the name the first time it is spoken?
14. Can you hear adequately when you are conversing with more than one person?
15. If you are in an audience, such as in a church or theatre and you are seated near the *front,* can you understand most of what is said?
16. Can you carry on everyday conversations with members of your family without difficulty?
17. If you are in an audience, such as in a church or theatre and you are seated near the *rear,* can you understand most of what is said?
18. When you are in a large formal gethering (a church, lodge, lecture hall, etc) can you hear what is said when the speaker *does* use a microphone?
19. Can you hear the telephone ring when you are in the next room?
20. Can you hear night sounds, such as distant trains, bells, dogs barking, trucks passing, and so forth?

Appendix E: The Denver Scale of Communication Function*

Preservice ____________________ Postservice ____________________
Date ____________________ Case No. ____________________
Name ____________________ Age ________ Sex __________
Address ____

____
(City) (State) (Zip)

Lives Alone __________ In Apartment __________ Retired __________
(if no, specify)

Occupation ____

Audiogram (Examination Date ______________ Agency ________________)

Pure Tone:

	250	500	1000	2000	4000	8000	Hz
RE	______	______	______	______	______	______	dB (re:ANSI)
LE	______	______	______	______	______	______	

Speech:

SRT	*Discrimination Score* (%)
	Quiet Noise (S/N = ____)
RE __________dB	RE __________
LE __________dB	LE __________

Hearing Aid Information

Aided ________ For How Long ______________ Aid Type ________

Satisfaction ____

EXAMINER ____________________

The following questionnaire was designed to evaluate your communication ability as you view it. You are asked to judge or scale each statement in the following manner.

---

*Reproduced with permission by Alpiner, J. G., Chevrette, W., Glascoe, G., Metz, M., & Olsen, B. Unpublished materials. University of Denver, 1971.

If you judge the statement to be *very closely related* to either extreme, please place your check mark as follows:

Agree _X_ ____ ____ ____ ____ ____ ____ Disagree

or

Agree ____ ____ ____ ____ ____ ____ _X_ Disagree

If you judge the statement to be *closely related* to either end of the scale, please mark as follows:

Agree ____ _X_ ____ ____ ____ ____ ____ Disagree

or

Agree ____ ____ ____ ____ ____ _X_ ____ Disagree

If you judge the statement to be only slightly related to either end of the scale, please mark as follows:

Agree ____ ____ _X_ ____ ____ ____ ____ Disagree

or

Agree ____ ____ ____ ____ _X_ ____ ____ Disagree

If you consider the statement to be irrelevant or unassociated to your communication situation, please mark as follows:

Agree ____ ____ ____ _X_ ____ ____ ____ Disagree

PLEASE NOTE: Check a scale for every statement.
Put only one checkmark on each scale.
Make a separate judgment for each statement.

ALSO: You may comment on each statement in the space provided.

1. The members of my family are annoyed with my loss of hearing.
   Agree ____ ____ ____ ____ ____ ____ ____ Disagree
   Comments: ____________________
2. The members of my family sometimes leave me out of conversations or discussions.
   Agree ____ ____ ____ ____ ____ ____ ____ Disagree
   Comments: ____________________
3. Sometimes my family makes decisions for me because I have a hard time following discussions.
   Agree ____ ____ ____ ____ ____ ____ ____ Disagree
   Comments: ____________________
4. My family becomes annoyed when I ask them to repeat what was said because I did not hear them.
   Agree ____ ____ ____ ____ ____ ____ ____ Disagree
   Comments: ____________________
5. I am not an ''outgoing'' person because I have a hearing loss.
   Agree ____ ____ ____ ____ ____ ____ ____ Disagree
   Comments: ____________________
6. I now take less of an interest in many things as compared to when I did not have a hearing problem.

Agree _____ _____ _____ _____ _____ _____ _____ Disagree
Comments: ____

7. Other people do not realize how frustrated I get when I cannot hear or understand.
Agree _____ _____ _____ _____ _____ _____ _____ Disagree
Comments: ____

8. People sometimes avoid me because of my hearing loss.
Agree _____ _____ _____ _____ _____ _____ _____ Disagree
Comments: ____

9. I am not a calm person because of my hearing loss.
Agree _____ _____ _____ _____ _____ _____ _____ Disagree
Comments: ____

10. I tend to be negative about life in general because of my hearing loss.
Agree _____ _____ _____ _____ _____ _____ _____ Disagree
Comments: ____

11. I do not socialize as much as I did before I began to lose my hearing.
Agree _____ _____ _____ _____ _____ _____ _____ Disagree
Comments: ____

12. Since I have trouble hearing, I do not like to go places with friends.
Agree _____ _____ _____ _____ _____ _____ _____ Disagree
Comments: ____

13. Since I have trouble hearing, I hesitate to meet new people.
Agree _____ _____ _____ _____ _____ _____ _____ Disagree
Comments: ____

14. I do not enjoy my job as much as I did before I began to lose my hearing.
Agree _____ _____ _____ _____ _____ _____ _____ Disagree
Comments: ____

15. Other people do not understand what it is like to have a hearing loss.
Agree _____ _____ _____ _____ _____ _____ _____ Disagree
Comments: ____

16. Because I have difficulty understanding what is said to me, I sometimes answer questions wrong.
Agree _____ _____ _____ _____ _____ _____ _____ Disagree
Comments: ____

17. I do not feel relaxed in a communicative situation.
Agree _____ _____ _____ _____ _____ _____ _____ Disagree
Comments: ____

18. I do not feel comfortable in most communication situations.
Agree _____ _____ _____ _____ _____ _____ _____ Disagree
Comments: ____

19. Conversations in a noisy room prevent me from attempting to communicate with others.
Agree _____ _____ _____ _____ _____ _____ _____ Disagree
Comments: ____

20. I am not comfortable having to speak in a group situation.
    Agree ____ ____ ____ ____ ____ ____ ____ Disagree
    Comments: ____________________________________

21. In general, I do not find listening relaxing.
    Agree ____ ____ ____ ____ ____ ____ ____ Disagree
    Comments: ____________________________________

22. I feel threatened by many communication situations due to difficulty hearing.
    Agree ____ ____ ____ ____ ____ ____ ____ Disagree
    Comments: ____________________________________

23. I seldom watch other people's facial expressions when talking to them.
    Agree ____ ____ ____ ____ ____ ____ ____ Disagree
    Comments: ____________________________________

24. I hesitate to ask people to repeat if I do not understand them the first time they speak.
    Agree ____ ____ ____ ____ ____ ____ ____ Disagree
    Comments: ____________________________________

25. Because I have difficulty understanding what is said to me, I sometimes make comments that do not fit into the conversation.
    Agree ____ ____ ____ ____ ____ ____ ____ Disagree
    Comments: ____________________________________

Appendix F: Test of Actual Performance*

How well does he or she:

	Poor	Adequate	Good	Excellent
1. Pay attention in the group? (daydreams, restlessness, changes the subject)	______	______	______	______
2. Communicate ideas verbally?	______	______	______	______
3. Use speech intelligibly?	______	______	______	______
4. Respond to others? (shares similar experiences, agrees, disagrees)	______	______	______	______
5. Hear speech when noise was going on around him/her? (like at parties)	______	______	______	______
6. Understand speech when not able to see the speaker?	______	______	______	______
7. Monitor the loudness of his or her own speech?	______	______	______	______

*Reproduced with permission by Konditsiotis, C. Y. The use of hearing test to provide information about the extent to which an individual's hearing loss handicaps him. *Maico Audiological Library Series,* 1971, 9, 10.

Appendix G: The Hearing Measurement Scale*

Section 1—Speech Hearing

1. Do you ever have difficulty hearing in the conversation when you're with one other person at home?
2. Do you ever have difficulty hearing in the conversation when you're with one other person outside?
3. Do you ever have difficulty in group conversation at home?
4. Do you ever have difficulty in group conversation outside?
5. Do you ever have difficulty hearing conversation at work?

5a. Is this due to your hearing, due to the noise, or a bit of both?

6. Do you ever have difficulty hearing the speaker at a public gathering?
7. Can you always hear what's being said in a TV program?
8. Can you always hear what's being said in TV news?
9. Can you always hear what's being said in a radio program?
10. Can you always hear what's being said in radio news?
11. Do you ever have difficulty hearing what's said in a film at the cinema?

Section 2—Acuity for Nonspeech Sound

1. Do you have any pets at home? (Type ________) Can you hear it when it barks, mews, etc?
2. Can you hear it when someone rings the doorbell or knocks on the door?
3. Can you hear a motor horn in the street when you're outside?
4. Can you hear the sound of footsteps outside when you're inside?
5. Can you hear the sound of the door opening when you're inside that room?
6. Can you hear the clock ticking in the room?
7. Can you hear the tap running when you turn it on?
8. Can you hear water boiling in a pan when you're in the kitchen?

---

*Revised with permission. Noble, W. G. & Atherley, G. R. C. The hearing measurement scale: A questionnaire for assessment of auditory disability. *Journal of Audiological Research,* 1970, *10,* 229–250.

This scale cannot be used without reference to the manual of instructions. Copies of the Scale and the manual of instruction can be obtained from Dr. William Noble, Department of Psychology, University of New England, Armidale, N.S.W., 2351, Australia.

Section 3—Localization

1. When you hear the sound of people talking and they're in another room would you be able to tell from where this sound was coming?
2. If you're with a group of people and someone you can't see starts to speak would you be able to tell where that person was sitting?
3. If you hear a motor horn or a bell can you always tell in which direction it's sounding?
4. Do you ever turn your head the wrong way when someone calls to you?
5. Can you usually tell, from the sound, how far away a person is when he calls to you?
6. Have you ever noticed outside that a car you thought, by its sound, was far away turned out to be much closer in fact?
7. Outside, do you always move out of the way of something coming up from behind, for instance a car, a trolley, or someone walking faster?

Section 4—Reaction to Handicap

1. Do you think that you are more irritable than other people or less so?
2. Do you ever give the wrong answer to someone because you've misheard them?
3. When you do this, do you treat it lightly or do you get upset?
4. How does the other person react? Does he get irritated or make little of it?
5. Do you think people are tolerant in this way or do they make fun of you?
6. Do you ever get bothered or upset if you are unable to follow a conversation?
7. Do you ever get the feeling of being cut off from things because of difficulty in hearing?

7a. Does this feeling upset you at all?

Section 5—Speech Distortion

1. Do you find that people fail to speak clearly?
2. What about speakers on TV or radio? Do they fail to speak clearly?
3. Do you ever have difficulty, in everyday conversation, understanding what someone is saying even though you can hear what's being said?

Section 6—Tinnitus

1. Do you ever get a noise in your ears or in your head?

2a. to 2e. A series of items on nature and incidence of tinnitus.

3. Does it ever stop you from sleeping?
4. Does it upset you?

Section 7—Personal Opinion of Hearing Loss

1. Do you think your hearing is normal?
2. Do you think any difficulty with your hearing is particularly serious?
3. Does any difficulty with your hearing restrict your social or personal life?

4a. to 4f. A series of items on Temporary Threshold Shift, specifically for those with chronic acoustic trauma, on the relative importance of eyesight over hearing and on other difficult hearing situations not mentioned in the interview.

Appendix H: Profile Questionnaire for Rating Communicative Performance in a Home and Social Environment*

Home Environment

1. (a) In my living room, when I can see the speaker's face, I have

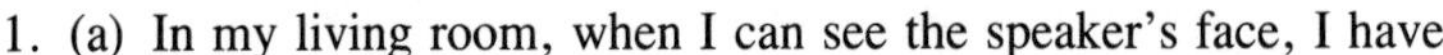

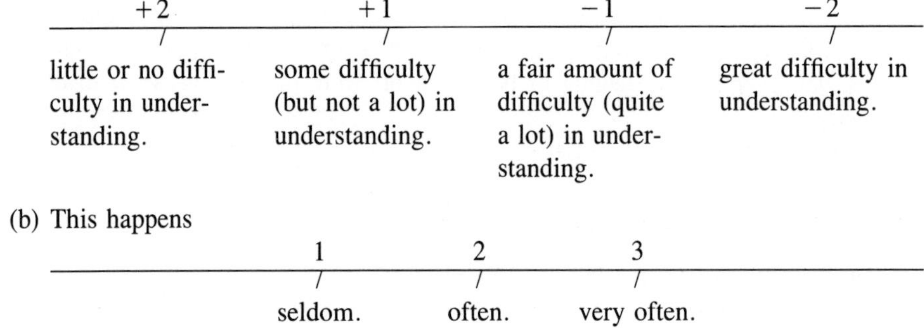

+2	+1	−1	−2
little or no difficulty in understanding.	some difficulty (but not a lot) in understanding.	a fair amount of difficulty (quite a lot) in understanding.	great difficulty in understanding.

(b) This happens

1	2	3
seldom.	often.	very often.

2. (a) If I am talking with a person in my living room or family room while the television, radio, or record player is on, I have

+2	+1	−1	−2
little or no difficulty in understanding.	some difficulty (but not a lot) in understanding.	A fair amount of difficulty (quite a lot) in understanding.	great difficulty in understanding.

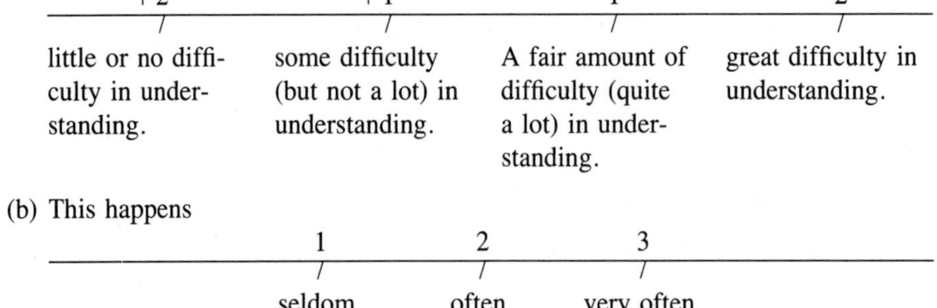

(b) This happens

1	2	3
seldom.	often.	very often.

---

*Reproduced with permission by Sanders, D. A. Hearing aid orientation and counseling, in M. C. Pollack (Ed.), *Amplification for the hearing impaired*. New York: Grune and Stratton, 1975, pp. 363–372.

3. (a) In a quiet room in my house, if I cannot see the speaker's face I have

+2	+1	−1	−2
little or no difficulty in understanding.	some difficulty (but not a lot) in understanding.	a fair amount of difficulty (quite a lot) in understanding.	great difficulty in understanding.

(b) This happens

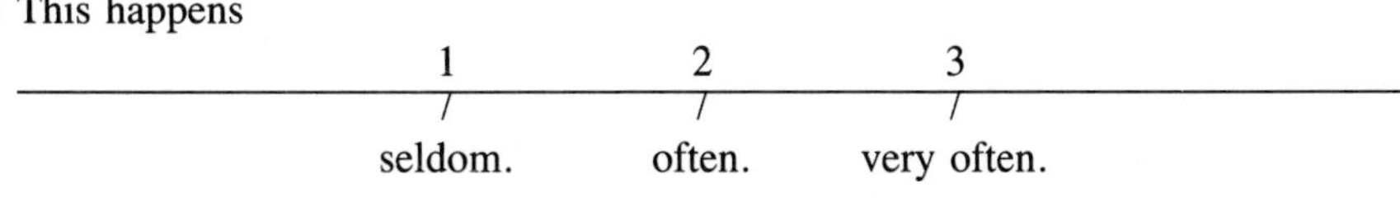

1	2	3
seldom.	often.	very often.

4. (a) If someone in my home speaks to me from another room on the same floor, I experience

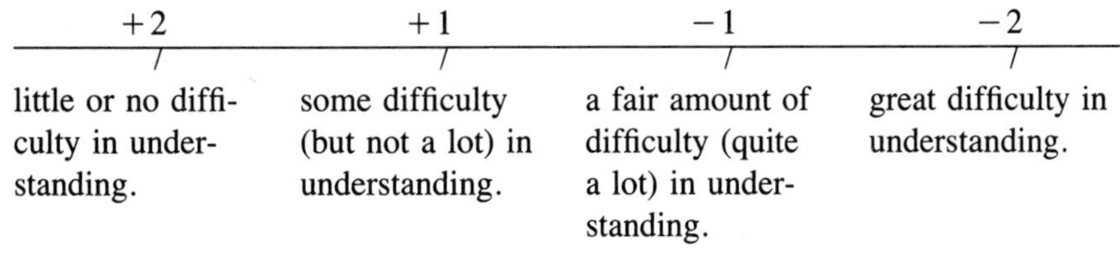

+2	+1	−1	−2
little or no difficulty in understanding.	some difficulty (but not a lot) in understanding.	a fair amount of difficulty (quite a lot) in understanding.	great difficulty in understanding.

(b) This happens

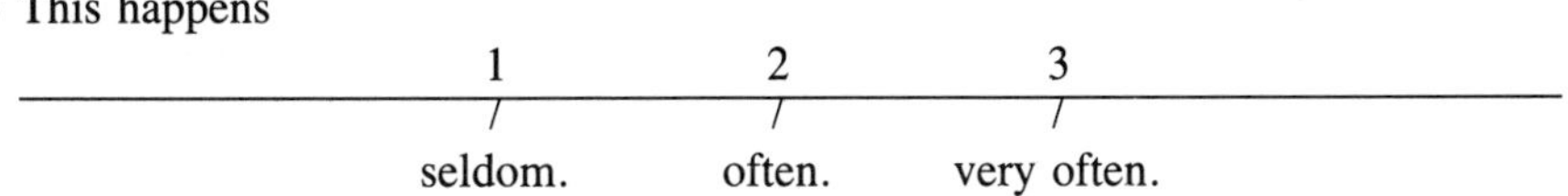

1	2	3
seldom.	often.	very often.

5. (a) If someone calls me from upstairs when I am downstairs, or from the window when I am in the garden, I will experience

+2	+1	−1	−2
little or no difficulty in understanding.	some difficulty (but not a lot) in understanding.	a fair amount of difficulty (quite a lot) in understanding.	great difficulty in understanding.

(b) This happens

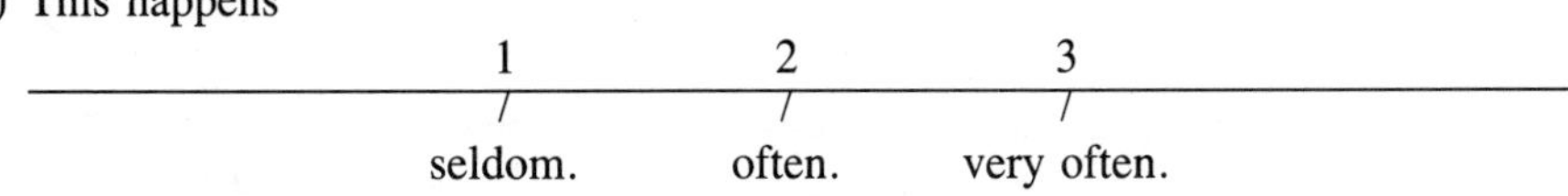

1	2	3
seldom.	often.	very often.

6. (a) Understanding people at the dinner table gives me

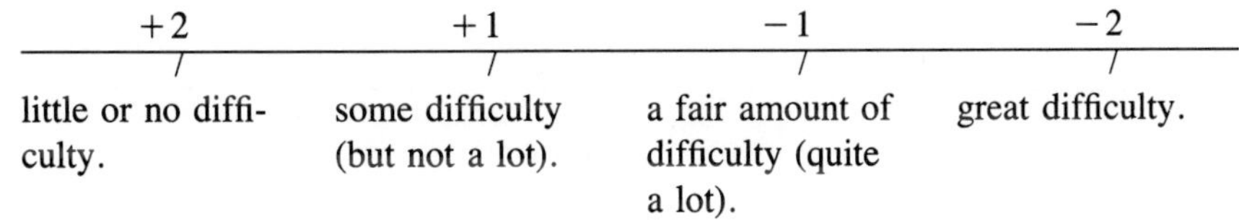

+2	+1	−1	−2
little or no difficulty.	some difficulty (but not a lot).	a fair amount of difficulty (quite a lot).	great difficulty.

(b) This happens

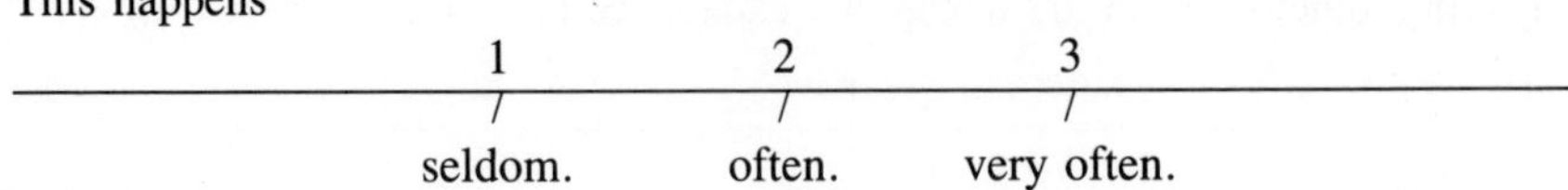

7. (a) When I sit talking with friends in a quiet room I have

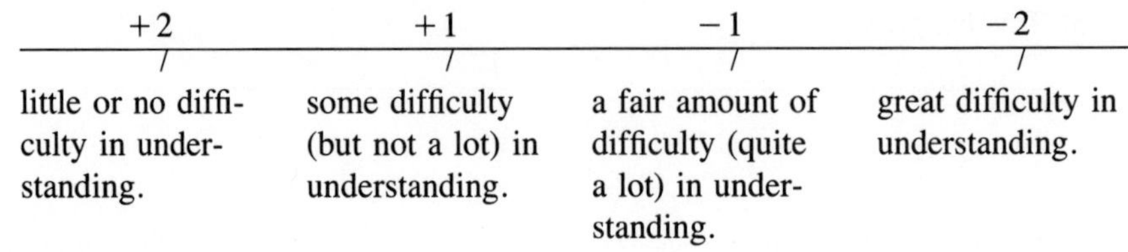

(b) This happens

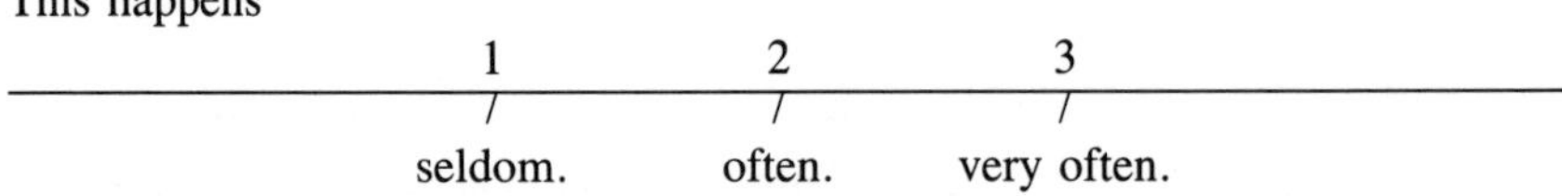

8. (a) Listening to the radio, record player, or watching TV gives me

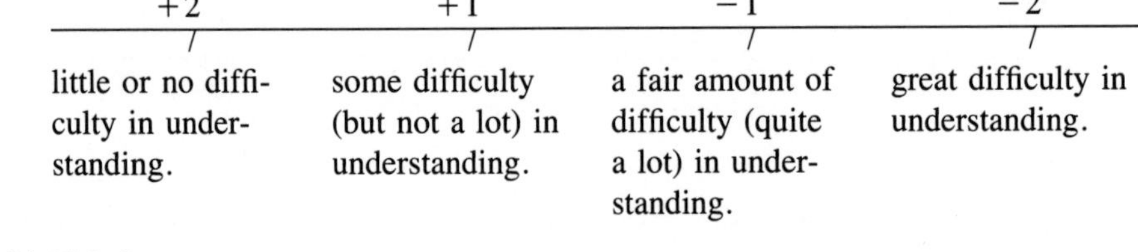

(b) This happens

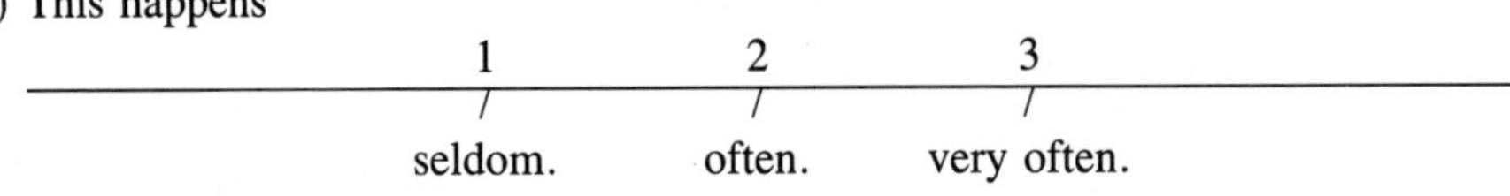

9. (a) When I use the phone at home, I have

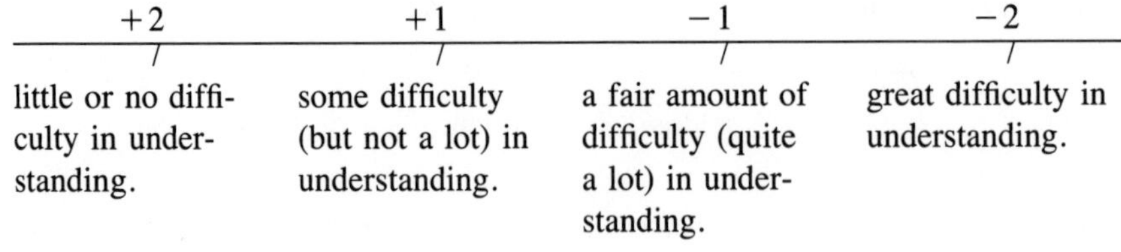

(b) This happens

1 — seldom. 2 — often. 3 — very often.

Social Environment

1. (a) If we are entertaining a group of friends, understanding someone against the background of others talking gives me

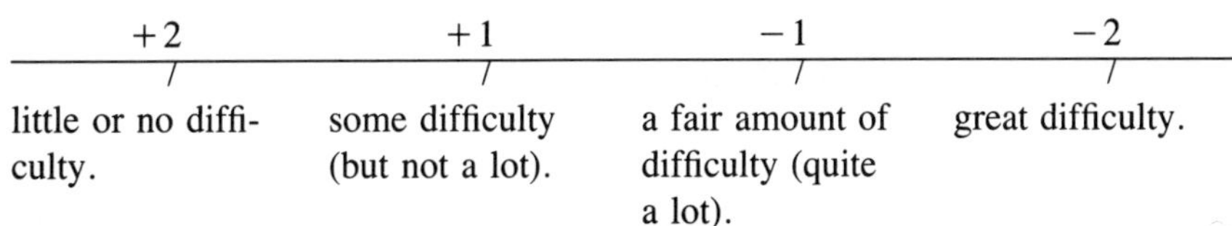

(b) This happens

1	2	3
seldom.	often.	very often.

2. (a) If we are playing cards, understanding my partner gives me

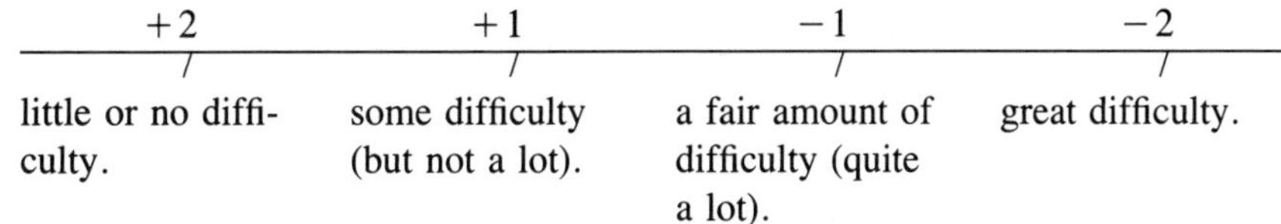

(b) This happens

1	2	3
seldom.	often.	very often.

3. (a) When I am at the theater or the movies, I have

+2	+1	−1	−2
little or no difficulty in understanding.	some difficulty (but not a lot) in understanding.	a fair amount of difficulty (quite a lot) in understanding.	great difficulty in understanding.

(b) This happens

1	2	3
seldom.	often.	very often.

4. (a) In church, when the minister gives the sermon, I have

+2	+1	−1	−2
little or no difficulty in understanding.	some difficulty (but not a lot) in understanding.	a fair amount of difficulty (quite a lot) in understanding.	great difficulty in understanding.

(b) This happens

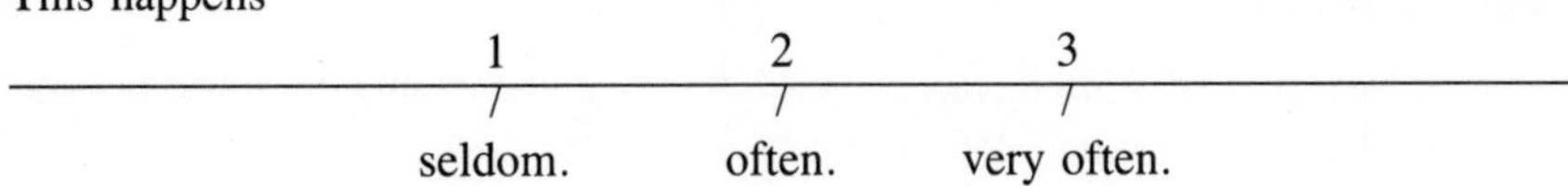

5. (a) When we eat out, following the conversation I have

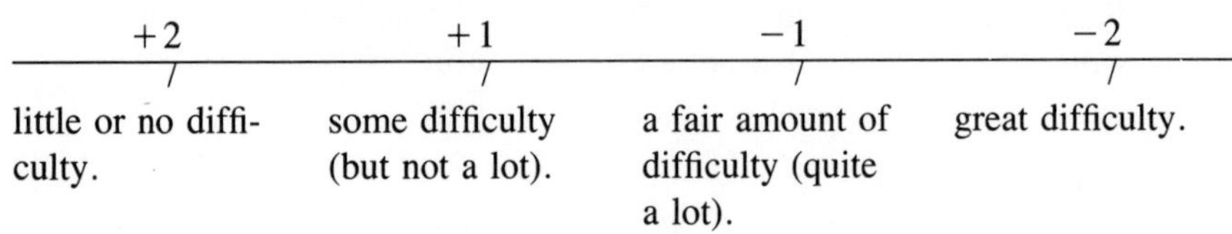

(b) This happens

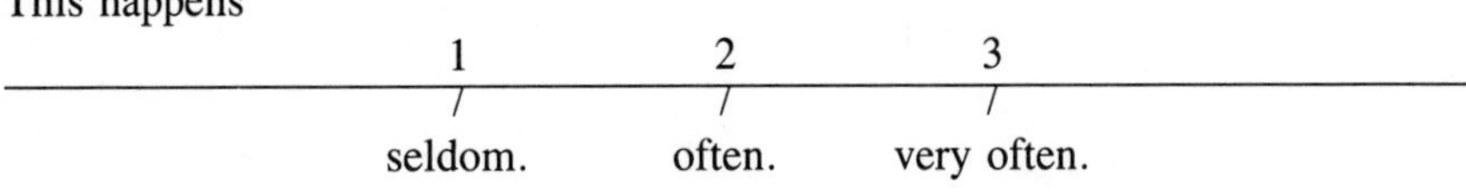

6. (a) In the car, I find that understanding what people are saying gives me

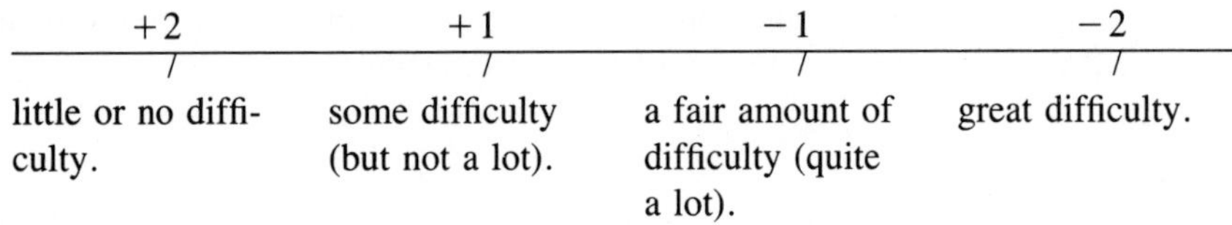

(b) This happens

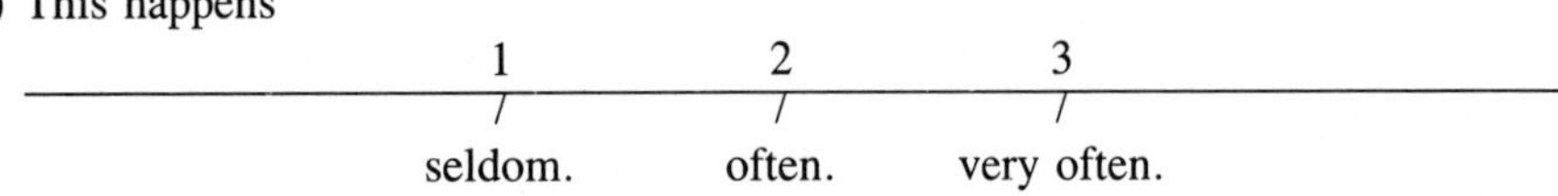

7. (a) When I am outside talking with someone I have

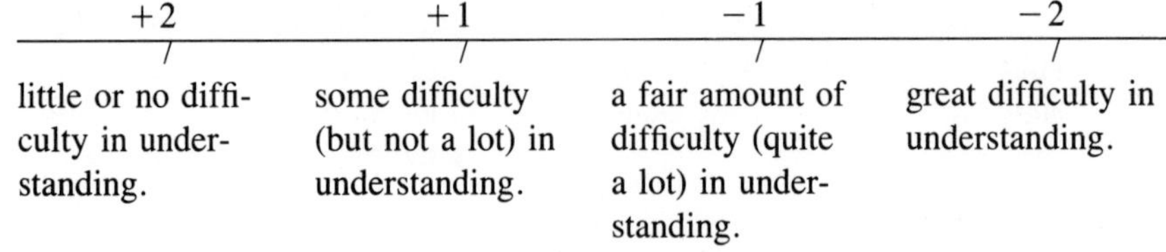

(b) This happens

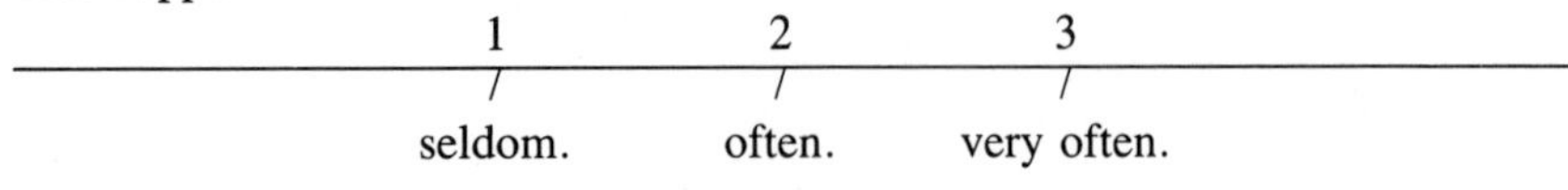

Appendix I: The Denver Scale of Communication Function for Senior Citizens Living in Retirement Centers*

Name ____________________ Date of Pretest ____________________
Address ____________________ Date of Post-test ____________________
Age ____________________ Examiner ____________________
Sex ____________________

1. Do you have trouble communicating with your family because of your hearing problem? Yes________ No________

   Probe Effect I

   a. Does your family make decisions for you because of your hearing problem? Yes________ No________
   b. Does your family leave you our of discussions because of your hearing problem? Yes________ No________
   c. Does your family get angry or annoyed with you because of your hearing problem? Yes________ No________

   Exploration Effect

   a. Do you have a family? Yes________ No________
   b. How often does your family visit you? ____________________
   c. How far away does your family live? In a city ________ Other ____________
   d. How often do you visit your family? ____________________

2. Do you get upset when you cannot hear or understand what is being said? Yes________ No________

---

*Reproduced with permission by Zarnoch, J. M. & Alpiner, J. G. The Denver scale of communication function for senior citizens living in retirement centers, in J. G. Alpiner (Ed.), *Handbook of adult rehabilitative audiology*. Baltimore: Williams and Wilkins, 1978, pp. 166–168.

Probe Effect I (to be used only if person responds yes)

a. Do your friends know you get upset? Yes________ No________
b. Does your family know you get upset? Yes________ No________
c. Does the staff know you get upset? Yes________ No________

Probe Effect II (to be used only if person responds no)

a. Do your friends realize you are not upset? Yes________ No________
b. Does your family realize you are not upset? Yes________ No________
c. Does the staff realize you are not upset? Yes________ No________

Exploration Effect (to be used only if person responds yes)

a. How does your behavior change when you become upset? ____________________

3. Do you think your family, your friends, and the staff understand what it is like to have a hearing problem? Yes________ No________

Probe effect

a. Do they avoid you because of your hearing problem? Yes________ No________
b. Do they leave you out of discussions? Yes________ No________
c. Do they hesitate to ask you to socialize with them? Yes________ No________

Exploration Effect

a. Family Yes________ No________
b. Friends Yes________ No________
c. Staff Yes________ No________

4. Do you avoid communicating with other people because of your hearing problem? Yes________ No________

Probe Effect

a. Do you communicate with people during meal times? Yes________ No________
b. Do you communicate with your roommate(s)? Yes________ No________
c. Do you communicate during the social activities in the home? Yes________ No________
d. Do you communicate with visiting family or friends? Yes________ No________
e. Do you communicate with the staff? Yes________ No________

Exploration Effect

a. Is your roommate capable of communication? Yes________ No________
b. What are the social activities of the home? ____________________
c. Which ones do you attend? ____________________

5. Do you feel that you are a relaxed person? Yes________ No________

Probe Effect

a. Do you think you are an irritable person because of your hearing problem? Yes________ No________
b. Do you think you are an irritable person because of your age? Yes________ No________

c. Do you think you are an irritable person because you live in this home? Yes________ No________

Exploration Effect

a. Do you have to live in this home? Yes________ No________

6. Do you feel relaxed in group communication situations? Yes________ No________

Probe Effect

a. Do you get nervous when you have to ask people to repeat what they have said if you have not understood them? Yes________ No________
b. Do you feel nervous if you have to tell a person that you have a hearing problem? Yes________ No________

Exploration Effect

a. Do you watch facial expressions? Yes________ No________
b. Do you watch gestures? Yes________ No________
c. Do you think you are a good listener? Yes________ No________ Why ________
d. Do you have a hearing aid? Yes________ No________
e. Do you wear your aid? Yes________ No________

7. Do you think you need help in overcoming your hearing problem? Yes________ No________

Probe Effect

a. If lipreading training was available, would you attend? Yes________ No________
b. Do you think this home provides adequate activities to make you want to communicate? Yes________ No________

Exploration Effect I

a. Can a person improve communication ability by using lipreading (or speechreading), which means watching the speaker's lips, facial expressions, and gestures when he or she is speaking? Yes________ No________
b. Do you agree with the above as a definition of lipreading? Yes________ No________

Exploration Effect II

a. Is your vision adequate Yes________ No________
b. Are you able to get around unassisted? Yes________ No________

Appendix J: University of Northern Colorado Communication Appraisal and Priorities*

Date ____________

Name ________________________ Age __________ Sex ____________
Address __________________________ Phone __________________________

Please indicate below those situations in which you are able to communicate best, those that are difficult for you in some instances, and those that are a definite problem. Under "explain," please tell us more if you desire, such as certain instances when you experience more difficulty than others, certain types of speakers, certain places, and so on.

	No problems	Only in specific instances	Definite problem	Priority
1. At parties or other social events	________	________	________	________
	Explain ________________________			
2. At the dinner table	________	________	________	________
	Explain ________________________			
3. On the telephone	________	________	________	________
	Explain ________________________			
4. At home	________	________	________	________
	Explain ________________________			

*Hull, R. H. Unpublished scale. Greeley: University of Northern Colorado, 1975.

5. With males ____ ____ ____ ____
Explain ____________________
____

6. With females ____ ____ ____ ____
Explain ____________________
____

7. With children ____ ____ ____ ____
Explain ____________________
____

8. In groups ____ ____ ____ ____
Explain ____________________
____

9. With certain important individuals ____ ____ ____ ____
Explain ____________________
____

10. At church ____ ____ ____ ____
Explain ____________________
____

11. At meetings ____ ____ ____ ____
Explain ____________________
____

12. Watching T.V. ____ ____ ____ ____
Explain ____________________
____

13. At the theatre ____ ____ ____ ____
Explain ____________________
____

14. At work ____ ____ ____ ____
Explain ____________________
____

15. Other (please specify) ____ ____ ____ ____
Explain ____________________
____

Do you have specific preferences in regard to things you would like to improve as they relate to your ability to communicate with others? ____________________
____

Index